Oxford Specialty Training: Training in Ophthalmology

Second Edition

Edited by

Venki Sundaram

Consultant Ophthalmic Surgeon
Luton and Dunstable University Hospital
UCL Partners, UK

Allon Barsam

Consultant Ophthalmic Surgeon
Luton and Dunstable University Hospital
UCL Partners, UK

Lucy Barker

Consultant Ophthalmic Surgeon
Rwanda International Institute of Ophthalmology
Dr Agarwal's Eye Hospital, Rwanda

Sir Peng Tee Khaw

Professor of Glaucoma and Ocular Healing, and Consultant Ophthalmic Surgeon
NIHR Biomedical Research Centre at Moorfields Eye Hospital and UCL Institute of Ophthalmology
London, UK

Series Editor

Matthew D. Gardiner

Specialty Trainee in Plastic Surgery, Imperial College London
Honorary Clinical Lecturer in Plastic Surgery, Kennedy Institute of Rheumatology, University of Oxford

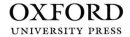

OXFORD
UNIVERSITY PRESS

OXFORD
UNIVERSITY PRESS

Great Clarendon Street, Oxford, OX2 6DP,
United Kingdom

Oxford University Press is a department of the University of Oxford.
It furthers the University's objective of excellence in research, scholarship,
and education by publishing worldwide. Oxford is a registered trade mark of
Oxford University Press in the UK and in certain other countries

© Oxford University Press 2016

The moral rights of the authors have been asserted

First Edition published in 2009
Second Edition published in 2016

Impression: 1

Published in the United States of America by Oxford University Press
198 Madison Avenue, New York, NY 10016, United States of America

British Library Cataloguing in Publication Data
Data available

Library of Congress Control Number: 2015946402

ISBN 978–0–19–967251–6

Printed in Great Britain by
Ashford Colour Press Ltd, Gosport, Hampshire

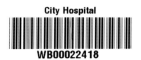
Oxford Specialist Training

Training in Ophthalmology

Second Edition

To my wife Champa, our boys Jay and Krish
and our families.
Venki Sundaram

To Sarah, Aron, Ezekiel, Raphael, and Joseph and
our families.
Allon Barsam

To my boys, Will and Rufus.
Lucy Barker

To Peggy, Ruth and Rachel.
Peng Khaw

Foreword

Training in Ophthalmology sets out a beautifully practical way to learn clinical ophthalmology. The experience of the authors translates into a welcome, much needed addition to the general ophthalmology text books genre and it deserves its place as an 'essential read'—not simply a new library book.

Each chapter covers the essentials—starting with basic sciences which are necessary to understand the subsequent clinical content in a meaningful way. Relevant clinical conditions and diagnoses are then drawn together in a combination of bullet points, clear descriptive text, tables, and illustrations. This extensive factual information is then supplemented by methods of clinical assessment which need to be mastered in order to elicit the appropriate clinical signs: and finally there are sections on practical and surgical skills which are a goldmine of tips and tricks to ensure that there is little room for error. The comprehensive content includes illustrations which are a mixture of high-quality clinical photographs, demonstrating relevant signs succinctly, and figures annotating critical detail—working well to complement the text.

Advances and newer treatments do not always feature in a teaching text, but these are reflected in the various chapters, such as refractive surgery, and it does not fail to omit the 'softer' professional skills, such as communication, governance, and understanding research, which are so important for everyone involved in patient care. The way that ophthalmology is delivered and taught is changing and this book demonstrates how this can be done effectively.

Although aimed at those in training—particularly, but not exclusively, ophthalmologists—the strength of this book is that it has something for everyone with an interest in this fascinating specialty and its layout and content make it eminently readable and pertinent. The authors are to be congratulated for this work which will help to shape the ophthalmic team of tomorrow.

Carrie MacEwen

Foreword: A Trainee's Perspective

Having thoroughly dissected the first edition of this book as a junior trainee and whilst preparing for my College exams, I am delighted to welcome this latest iteration.

Following on from its initial success as a bespoke training manual for UK trainees, this latest edition brings a fresh perspective that keeps up to date with the current curriculum and adds concise practical guidance in a number of key clinical and surgical skills. These summaries and protocols will be invaluable to the developing trainee learning new techniques and will also aid in the completion of work-based assessments.

Ophthalmic investigations and therapeutics have rapidly advanced in recent years and this new edition keeps up to date with these trends, summarising the latest evidence that not only emphasizes current clinical practice but also provides an important template for examination learning.

The last chapter covers important professional and practical skills that are typically not covered in other textbooks but form a growing part of our curriculum whilst new chapters in refractive surgery and microsurgical skills offer a unique perspective not commonly addressed in this format.

This book is wonderfully presented and easy to read with beautiful illustrations. It is a comprehensive yet compact text that mirrors the UK curriculum and will play a key role both as a daily reference and in preparing for College examinations. Being conveniently concise and portable, it is a book that belongs in the satchel of all budding ophthalmologists, as well as interested allied specialists and GPs

Oliver Bowes
Chairman, Ophthalmologists in Training Group (OTG),
Royal College of Ophthalmologists

Preface

We are pleased to introduce the second edition of *Training in Ophthalmology*. We introduced the first edition of this textbook to address the needs of ophthalmic trainees and relevant allied specialities, with particular emphasis on changes in ophthalmology training that occurred following the introduction of Modernising Medical Careers and the new Ophthalmic Specialist Training (OST) curriculum from the Royal College of Ophthalmologists.

With the relative lack of ophthalmology teaching at medical school and the often inconsistent formal teaching of fundamental examination and clinical techniques during initial posts, ophthalmology trainees often feel they are being 'thrown in at the deep end' early on in their career. In addition, trainees are now expected to clearly demonstrate evidence of having acquired the expected knowledge, clinical, technical, and surgical skills at each stage of their training in order to progress.

This book aims to help address these issues by mapping the stages of the OST curriculum and providing trainees with the core knowledge and clinical skills they will require to succeed. In this updated edition, we have included two new chapters, Refractive surgery (Chapter 4) and Microsurgical skills (Chapter 12), as well as expanding the strabismus section to create a dedicated paediatric ophthalmology and strabismus chapter (Chapter 9); and included additional practical and surgical skills that are required to be demonstrated in the final years of training.

As before, each chapter covers relevant basic science, history and examination techniques, and pertinent clinical conditions for each sub-speciality. Practical skills are highlighted with particular emphasis on the core competencies of the OST curriculum and we have provided an overview of the non-clinical yet increasingly important elements of 'being a doctor' in the professional skills chapter (Chapter 13).

Although this book is primarily aimed at trainees at all stages of their training, it will also be appealing for medical students, general practitioners, more senior ophthalmologists, optometrists, orthoptists, and other healthcare professionals with an interest in ophthalmology.

We hope that you enjoy and benefit from reading this book and we welcome any feedback on how it may be improved for the future.

VS
AB
LB
PTK

Acknowledgements

We would like to thank Fiona Richardson and Rachel Goldsworthy at OUP for their help and guidance throughout producing this book.

Thank you to all the chapter authors for their hard work and cooperation.

Contents

Contributors

James W. Bainbridge
Professor of Ophthalmology
UCL Institute of Ophthalmology and Moorfields
Eye Hospital
London, UK
Chapter 5

Lucy Barker
Consultant Ophthalmic Surgeon
Rwanda International Institute of Ophthalmology
Dr Agarwal's Eye Hospital, Rwanda
Chapters 9, 10, 13

Allon Barsam
Consultant Ophthalmic Surgeon
Luton and Dunstable University Hospital
UCL Partners, UK
Chapters 2–4

John Bladen
Trainee and Medical Student Mentoring Scheme
Faculty of Medical Leadership and Management
London, UK
Section 13.9

Fred K. Chen
Consultant Ophthalmologist
Perth, Australia
Chapter 5

Georgia Cleary
Specialty Registrar
London Deanery, UK
Chapters 2–4

Indran Davagnanam
Consultant Neuroradiologist
The National Hospital for Neurology and
Neurosurgery and Moorfields Eye Hospital
London, UK
Section 10.7

Eric Donnenfeld
Professor of Ophthalmology
New York University
New York, NY, USA and
Ophthalmic Consultants of Long Island
New York, NY, USA
Chapter 4

Daniel Ezra
Consultant Ophthalmic Surgeon
Moorfields Eye Hospital
London, UK
Chapters 1 and 11

Tarang Gupta
Locum Consultant Ophthalmic Surgeon,
Moorfields Eye Hospital
London, UK
Chapters 1 and 11

Joanne Hancox
Consultant Ophthalmic Surgeon
Moorfields Eye Hospital
London, UK
Chapter 9

Melanie Hingorani
Consultant Ophthalmologist
Moorfields Eye Hospital
London, UK
Chapter 13

Edward Hughes
Consultant Ophthalmologist
Sussex Eye Hospital
Brighton, UK
Chapter 7

Ronald Kam
Specialty Registrar
Moorfields Eye Hospital
London, UK
Chapter 12

Sir Peng Tee Khaw
Professor of Glaucoma and Ocular Healing, and
Consultant Ophthalmic Surgeon
NIHR Biomedical Research Centre at
Moorfields Eye Hospital and UCL Institute of Ophthalmology
London, UK
Chapter 8

Wanda Kozlowska
Consultant in Paediatric Respiratory Medicine
King's College Hospital
London, UK
Section 9.22

Sidath E. Liyanage
Vitreoretinal Department
Moorfields Eye Hospital
London, UK
Chapter 5

Kelly MacKenzie
Senior Orthoptist
Moorfields Eye Hospital
London, UK
Chapter 9

Michel Michaelides
Professor of Ophthalmology and Consultant Ophthalmic
Surgeon
UCL Institute of Ophthalmology and Moorfields Eye Hospital
London, UK
Chapter 6

Dania Qatarneh
Consultant Ophthalmologist
Alfred Hospital
Melbourne, Australia
Chapter 7

Gordon T. Plant
Consultant Neurologist, The National Hospital for Neurology and
Neurosurgery and Moorfields Eye Hospital
London, UK
Chapter 10

Ameenat Lola Solebo
NIHR Academic Clinical Lecturer,
UCL Institute of Child Health and UCL Institute
of Ophthalmology
London, UK
Chapter 13

Miles Stanford
Professor of Ophthalmology
St Thomas Hospital
London, UK
Chapter 7

Paul Sullivan
Consultant Ophthalmologist
Moorfields Eye Hospital
London, UK
Chapter 12

Venki Sundaram
Consultant Ophthalmic Surgeon
Luton and Dunstable University Hospital
UCL Partners, UK
Chapter 6

Andrew Tatham
Consultant Eye Surgeon
Princess Alexandra Eye Pavilion
Edinburgh, UK
Chapter 8, Section 9.26

Stephen Tuft
Consultant Ophthalmologist
Moorfields Eye Hospital
London, UK
Chapter 2

Contributors to the First Edition

Amar Alwitry
Consultant Ophthalmologist
Derby Hospitals NHS Foundation Trust
Derby

Simon D.M. Chen
Retina Specialist
Vision Eye Institute
Sydney
New South Wales
Australia

Claire Daniel
Adnexal Fellow
Moorfields Eye Hospital
London

John Elston
Consultant Ophthalmologist (paediatrics and neuro-
ophthalmology)
Oxford Eye Hospital
John Radcliffe Hospital, Oxford

Rebecca Ford
Specialist Registrar in Ophthalmology
Moorfields Eye Hospital
London

Matthew Gardiner
Clinical Research Fellow in Plastic and Reconstructive Surgery
Kennedy Institute of Rheumatology
Imperial College London
London

Saurabh Goyal
Glaucoma Clinical Fellow
Moorfields Eye Hospital
London

Julie Huntbach
Specialist Registrar in Ophthalmology
Queens Medical Centre
Nottingham

Moneesh Patel
Specialist Registrar in Ophthalmology
Derby Hospitals NHS Trust
Derby

Bheema Patil
Advanced Specialist Trainee in Ophthalmology
Nottingham University Hospital
Nottingham

Pankaj Puri
Consultant Ophthalmologist
Derbyshire Royal Infirmary
Derby

David Spalton
Consultant Ophthalmic Surgeon
St Thomas' Hospital
London

Jimmy Uddin
Consultant Ophthalmologist
Moorfields Eye Hospital
London

Abbreviations

AC/A ratio	accommodative convergence/accommodation ratio
ACE	angiotensin-converting enzyme
ACHM	achromatopsia
AIDS	acquired immunodeficiency syndrome
AION	anterior ischaemic optic neuropathy
AKC	atopic keratoconjunctivitis
ALPI	argon laser peripheral iridoplasty
ALT	argon laser trabeculoplasty
AMD	age-related macular degeneration
ANA	anti-nuclear antibody
ANCA	anti-neutrophil cytoplasmic antibody
AR	autosomal recessive
AREDS	Age-Related Eye Disease Study
AVM	arteriovenous malformations
BCC	basal cell carcinoma
BIO	binocular indirect ophthalmoscopy
BRAO	branch retinal artery occlusion
BRVO	branch retinal vein occlusion
BSS	balanced salt solution
CCC	continuous curvilinear capsulorrhexis
CCF	carotid–cavernous fistula
CCT	central corneal thickness
CDB	corneal dystrophy of Bowman's layer
CDR	cup/disc ratio
CHED	congenital hereditary endothelial dystrophy
CHRPE	congenital hypertrophy of retinal pigment epithelium
CIN	conjunctival intraepithelial neoplasia
CMV	cytomegalovirus
CNS	central nervous system
CNV	choroidal neovascularization
CPEO	chronic progressive external ophthalmoplegia
CRAO	central retinal artery occlusion
CRION	chronic relapsing inflammatory optic neuropathy
CRP	C-reactive protein
CRVO	central retinal vein occlusion
CSCR	central serous chorioretinopathy
CSF	cerebrospinal spinal fluid
CSMO	clinically significant diabetic macular oedema
CT	computed tomography
CXR	chest X-ray
DEXA	dual-energy X-ray absorptiometry
DR	diabetic retinopathy
DSAEK	Descemet's stripping automated endothelial keratoplasty
DSEK	Descemets stripping endothelial keratoplasty
DVD	dissociated vertical deviation

EBV	Epstein–Barr virus
ECCE	extracapsular cataract extraction
EOG	electro-oculogram
Epi-LASIK	epithelial laser-assisted in situ keratomileusis
EPR	electronic patient records
ERG	electroretinography
ESR	erythrocyte sedimentation rate
ETDRS	Early Treatment Diabetic Retinopathy Study
ETROP	Early Treatment for Retinopathy of Prematurity
FAF	fundus autofluorescence
FBC	full blood count
FFA	fundus fluorescein angiography
FOV	field of view
GA	geographic atrophy
GAT	Goldmann applanation tonometry
GCC	ganglion cell complex
GDD	glaucoma drainage devices
GI	gastrointestinal
GCA	giant cell arteritis
GMC	General Medical Council
GPS	glaucoma probability score
GVHD	graft-versus-host disease
HAART	highly active antiretroviral therapy
HIV	human immunodeficiency virus
HLA	human leucocyte antigen
HRT	Heidelberg retinal tomograph
HSCA	Health and Social Care Act
HSK	herpes simplex keratitis
HSV	herpes simplex virus
HZO	herpes zoster ophthalmicus
HZV	herpes zoster virus
ICG	indocyanine green
IFIS	intraoperative floppy iris syndrome
IL-1	interleukin 1
IL-2	interleukin 2
IOL	intraocular lens
IOP	intraocular pressure
IPD	interpupillary diameter
IR	inferior rectus
IRMA	intraretinal microvascular abnormalities
ITC	iridotrabecular contact
JIA	juvenile idiopathic arthritis
LASEK	laser-assisted subepithelial keratomileusis
LASIK	laser-assisted stromal in situ keratomileusis
LCD	limbal chamber depth
LE	left eye
LogMAR	logarithm of the mean angle of resolution

LPS	levator palpebrae superioris
LR	lateral rectus
LSM	laser spot magnification
MHC	major histocompatibility complex
MLF	medial longitudinal fasciculus
MMP	mucous membrane pemphigoid
MR	medial rectus
MRA	Moorfields regression analysis
MRI	magnetic resonance imaging
NHS	National Health Service
NICE	National Institute of Clinical Excellence
NMO	neuromyelitis optica
NPDR	non-proliferative diabetic retinopathy
NSAID	non-steroidal anti-inflammatory drug
NSR	neurosensory retina
NVD	neovascularization of the optic disc
NVE	new vessels elsewhere
OCA	oculocutaneous albinism
OCT	optical coherence tomography
OHT	ocular hypertension
OKN	optokinetic nystagmus
ONTT	Optic Neuritis Treatment Trial
OPP	ocular perfusion pressure
OTG	Ophthalmic Trainees' Group
PAC	perennial allergic conjunctivitis
PACG	primary angle closure glaucoma
PACS	primary angle closure suspect
PAS	peripheral anterior synechiae
PCO	posterior capsule opacification
PCR	polymerase chain reaction
PCT	prism cover test
PDR	proliferative diabetic retinopathy
PDS	pigment dispersion syndrome
PDT	photodynamic therapy
PED	pigment epithelial detachment
PHPV	persistent hyperplastic primary vitreous
PI	peripheral iridotomy
PM	pathological myopia
POAG	primary open-angle glaucoma
PORN	progressive outer retinal necrosis
PP	posterior pole
PPRF	paramedian pontine reticular formation
PR	peripheral retina
PRK	photorefractive keratectomy
PRP	pan-retinal photocoagulation

PUK	peripheral ulcerative keratitis
PVD	posterior vitreous detachment
PVR	proliferative vitreoretinopathy
PXF	pseudoexfoliation syndrome
RAPD	relative afferent pupillary defect
RD	retinal detachment
RE	right eye
RGC	retinal ganglion cell
RNFL	retinal nerve fibre layer
ROP	retinopathy of prematurity
RP	retinitis pigmentosa
RPE	retinal pigment epithelium
RRD	rhegmatogenous retinal detachment
SAC	seasonal allergic conjunctivitis
SAP	standard automated perimetry
SD-OCT	spectral domain optical coherence tomography
SITA	Swedish Interactive Thresholding Algorithm
SLT	selective laser trabeculoplasty
SO	superior oblique
SP	small pupil
SR	superior rectus
SS-OCT	swept source optical coherence tomography
STGD	Stargardt disease
SWAP	short-wavelength automated perimetry
TD-OCT	time domain optical coherence tomography
TGF	transforming growth factor
TIGR	trabecular-meshwork-inducible glucocorticoid response
TM	trabecular meshwork
TNF	tumour necrosis factor
tPA	tissue plasminogen activator
TPMT	thiopurine methyltransferase
TSH	thyroid-stimulating hormone
UBM	ultrasound biomicroscopy
UKPDS	UK Prospective Diabetes Study
VDRL	Venereal Disease Research Laboratory
VEGF	vascular endothelial growth factor
VEP	visual evoked potential
VFI	visual field index
VKC	vernal keratoconjunctivitis
VN	vestibular nucleus
VZV	varicella-zoster virus
WD	working distance

Chapter 1

Oculoplastics

Tarang Gupta and Daniel Ezra

1

Eyelid anatomy

The primary function of the eyelids is to protect the globe from injury, and the retina from excessive light. They also assist in the distribution of tears across the ocular surface during blinking. Additionally, the eyelids provide mechanical support for the globe, the lacrimal canaliculi, and the punctae that form part of the tear drainage system.

The upper and lower eyelids extend from the lateral to the medial canthi. The distance between the upper and lower lids is called the palpebral aperture and exhibits considerable racial variation. The eyelid consists of many layers, the most anterior being skin, which is followed by subcutaneous tissue and the orbicularis oculi muscle fibres, which together form the anterior lamella. The posterior lamella is formed by the tarsal plate and conjunctiva. The division of the eyelid into anterior and posterior lamellae is useful clinically as these structures are easily divided by a convenient surgical cleavage plane.

Skin

The eyelid skin is the thinnest in the body (<1 mm). Loose subcutaneous areolar tissue separates the skin from the underlying orbicularis. A plane can potentially form beneath the skin during local anaesthetic infiltration. Subcutaneous fat is sparse, and it is absent beneath the pretarsal skin.

Orbicularis oculi

The orbicularis oculi is one of the muscles of facial expression and may be divided into orbital, preseptal, and pretarsal portions (see Figure 1.1). These anatomical divisions also reflect functional and physiological differences. The pretarsal part is responsible for fast blink (90% of the muscle consists of Type 1 fast-twitch fibres). In contrast, the peripheral orbital part is responsible for forced sphincter closure. Orbital orbicularis oculi fibres interdigitate with those of the frontalis, the procerus, and the corrugator supercilii muscles superiorly and the lip elevators inferiorly.

Sweeping fibres of the orbicularis oculi run in a circular fashion from the medial canthal tendon inferiorly and superiorly, to join at the lateral palpebral ligament. Specialized fibres of the medial pretarsal orbicularis invest the canaliculi and insert into the lacrimal sac fascia. These fibres are known as Horners muscle, which is thought to mediate the lacrimal pump. The nerve supply of the orbicularis muscle is from the facial nerve (temporal and zygomatic branches).

Orbital septum

The orbital septum is a connective tissue extension of the thickened periosteum at the orbital rim (the arcus marginalis). It is a multi-laminated barrier between the eyelid and the orbit. The septum fuses with the levator aponeurosis near the eyelid margin (see Figure 1.2).

Tarsal plate

The tarsal plate forms the fibrous skeleton of the lids. The upper tarsal plate measures 10–12 mm centrally, and the lower tarsal plate measures about 5 mm. Both tarsal plates are attached to the orbital rim by medial and lateral palpebral ligaments. Each tarsus is 1 mm thick and contains approximately 30 meibomian glands. These glands produce a holocrine sebaceous secretion that constitutes the outer lipid layer of the precorneal tear film. The openings are located posterior to the grey line and just anterior to the mucocutaneous junction. The eyelash roots lie against the anterior surface of the tarsus and exit the skin at the anterior lid margin. The glands of Moll are modified sweat glands that open onto the lid margin between the lashes or into a lash follicle. The glands of Zeiss are sebaceous glands that open into each lash follicle.

Medial palpebral ligament

The medial palpebral ligament is formed by condensations of the pretarsal and preseptal orbicularis muscles. A superficial head inserts onto the frontal process of the maxilla whilst a deep head inserts into the lacrimal sac and posterior lacrimal crest.

Lateral palpebral ligament

The lateral palpebral ligament is a broad dense fibrous tissue that passes laterally, deep to the orbital septum, to insert into Whitnalls tubercle, 1.5 mm posterior to the orbital rim.

Upper lid elevators

Levator palpebrae superioris

The levator palpebrae superioris (LPS), a striated muscle, originates from the lesser wing of the sphenoid at the orbital apex. It shares a developmental origin and fibrous attachments with the superior rectus, which it passes above (see Figure 1.2). It then fans out, ending in an aponeurosis 10 mm behind the orbital septum. The muscle fibres change orientation from horizontal to vertical at Whitnalls ligament, which runs from the lacrimal gland fascia to the trochlea. The levator aponeurosis expands laterally and medially into horns which attach to Whitnalls tubercle and the posterior lacrimal crest, respectively. The levator aponeurosis inserts centrally into the upper third of the anterior surface of the tarsal plate. The LPS is supplied by the superior division of the oculomotor nerve.

Müllers muscle

This smooth muscle augments the action of the levator. It arises from the inferior aspect of the levator aponeurosis and inserts into the superior border of the tarsal plate. The peripheral vascular arcade is adherent to the lower border of Müllers muscle. It is innervated by sympathetic fibres from the superior cervical ganglion.

Lower lid retractors

There is no inferior equivalent to the levator. The lower lid retractors are connective tissue condensations that originate from the fascial sheath of the inferior rectus tendon. This sheath is continuous with Lockwoods suspensory ligament and extends anteriorly to envelop the inferior oblique muscle, ending at the inferior border of the inferior tarsus (see Figure 1.3).

Blood supply and lymphatic drainage

Arterial blood supply to the eyelids is provided by a marginal and peripheral arcade formed from the medial and lateral palpebral arteries. **Venous drainage** occurs medially into the ophthalmic and angular veins and laterally into the superior temporal vein. **Lymphatic drainage** from the lateral two-thirds of the upper and lower lids is to the superficial parotid (preauricular) lymph nodes, and lymphatic draining from the medial third is to the submandibular nodes.

Nasolacrimal system anatomy

The aqueous component of the tear film is produced by the lacrimal gland in the supero-lateral orbit. This gland comprises a large orbital lobe and a much smaller palpebral lobe. Tiny accessory lacrimal glands are also located in the conjunctival fornix. The nasolacrimal drainage system is a conduit for the flow of tears from the external surface of the eye to the nasal cavity (see Figure 1.4).

Lacrimal puncta

These are small openings that lie on the medial aspects of the upper and lower lids. Each punctum sits on an elevated pale mound called the papilla lacrimalis. The punctae are normally directed so as to be in contact with the tear meniscus.

Lacrimal canaliculi

The canaliculi begin at the punctum and pass vertically for 2 mm before turning through 90° to pass horizontally and medially for 8 mm before meeting at the common canaliculus. The common canaliculus continues medially to enter the lacrimal sac obliquely through the valve of Rosenmuller at the lateral wall of the lacrimal sac.

Lacrimal sac

The lacrimal sac is located in the lacrimal fossa in the anterior part of the medial orbital wall, between the anterior and posterior lacrimal crests formed by the frontal process of the maxilla and lacrimal bones, respectively. The sac measures 12 mm in length and is enclosed in fascia.

Nasolacrimal duct

The nasolacrimal duct connects the lower portion of the lacrimal sac with the nasal cavity. The duct passes inferiorly, posteriorly and laterally. The maxilla, lacrimal bone, uncinate process, and inferior turbinate form the canal. The duct opens into the inferior meatus of the nose. A flap of mucous membrane, called the valve of Hasner, prevents retrograde reflux of nasal contents and is commonly imperforate at birth, leading to epiphora.

Physiology

The main and accessory lacrimal glands secrete the tears, 10%–20% of which are lost through evaporation. The remainder pass across the ocular surface and across the tear strips on the upper and lower lid margins by capillarity. The contribution made by each canaliculus to total tear draining capacity is not known, but estimates vary from 50% to 80% for lower canalicular drainage. When the eyelids close during blinking, the Horners muscle fibres of the orbicularis muscle contract, causing expansion of the lacrimal sac. Negative pressure sucks tears into the canaliculi and sac. When the eyelids open, positive pressure within the sac then forces the tears down the nasolacrimal duct. This cycle is known as the lacrimal pump and becomes ineffective with increasing eyelid laxity.

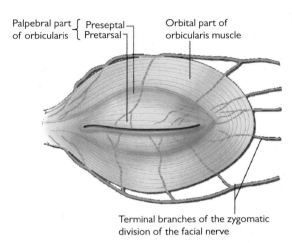

Fig 1.1 The orbicularis oculi muscle and the terminal branches of the facial nerve

Reproduced from *Colour Atlas of Ophthalmic Plastic Surgery*, 2008; A.G.Tyers and J.R.O. Collin p8 Butterworth Heinemann, copyright Elsevier

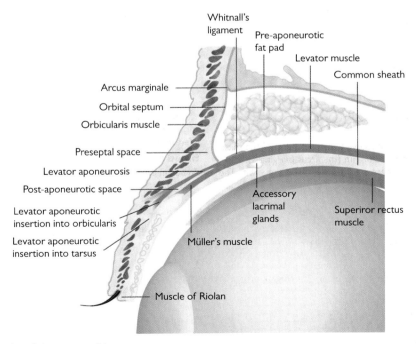

Fig 1.2 Vertical section of the upper eyelid

Reproduced from *Colour Atlas of Ophthalmic Plastic Surgery*, 2008; A.G.Tyers and J.R.O. Collin p18 Butterworth Heinemann, copyright Elsevier

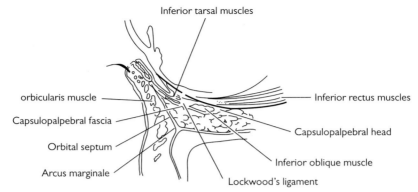

Inferior tarsal muscles

orbicularis muscle

Inferior rectus muscles

Capsulopalpebral fascia

Capsulopalpebral head

Orbital septum

Inferior oblique muscle

Arcus marginale

Lockwood's ligament

Fig 1.3 Cross section of lower eyelid

Reproduced from Gold D. and Lewis R., *Clinical Eye Atlas*, second edition, 2010, Fig. 1.5, p. 4, by permission of Oxford University Press, USA

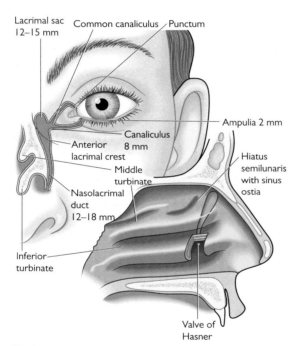

Lacrimal sac
12–15 mm

Common canaliculus

Punctum

Ampulia 2 mm

Canaliculus
8 mm

Anterior
lacrimal crest

Hiatus
semilunaris
with sinus
ostia

Middle
turbinate

Nasolacrimal
duct
12–18 mm

Inferior
turbinate

Valve of
Hasner

Fig 1.4 Normal anatomy of the lacrimal excretory system

Measurements are for adults

1.2 Lash abnormality

Trichiasis

Trichiasis is an acquired misdirection of **normally** sited eyelashes towards the globe. The most common underlying pathological process is posterior lamellae scarring but in children, particularly in those of Asian origin, epiblepharon is a common cause of trichiasis. Trichiasis is not to be confused with metaplastic lashes, which are aberrantly located lashes resulting from chronic eyelid margin inflammation.

Aetiology

* **Inflammatory:** chronic blepharitis, vernal and atopic keratoconjunctivitis, mucous membrane pemphigoid, Stevens–Johnson syndrome
* **Infective:** herpes zoster ophthalmicus, trachoma (can result in upper lid entropion; see Figure 1.5)
* **Traumatic:** post eyelid surgery (particularly transconjunctival approach), chemical (alkali burns, long-term eye drop use) or thermal injuries

Morbidity

The misdirected eyelashes cause repeated corneal trauma resulting in punctate epithelial erosions, microbial keratitis, and corneal scarring in chronic cases.

Management

As well as including the treatment of any underlying conditions, management is dictated by the pattern (segmental or diffuse) of the trichiasis, and the quality of the posterior lamella. Lubricants may reduce the irritation caused by lash contact but are often unsatisfactory if used in isolation.

In cases of focal trichiasis, lash follicle destruction is preferable, whereas diffuse trichiasis is best treated with lash repositioning.

Mechanical epilation

The initial treatment for a few misdirected lashes is removal with fine forceps at the slit lamp. Lash regrowth normally recurs in 3–4 weeks and the short, stiff lash cilia can be more irritating to the cornea than mature longer lashes.

Electrolysis

Modern electrolysis is delivered via a radio frequency probe to ablate the lash follicle. The probe should be inserted perpendicular to the eyelid margin, with sufficient depth to reach the follicle root (2.4 mm in the upper lid, 1.4 mm in the lower lid). The lash should fall away easily if sufficiently ablated. A direct cut-down and visualization of the follicle root prior to the application of electrolysis may be more effective with less collateral damage than electrolysis alone.

Repeated treatments can lead to scarring of the conjunctival surface, particularly in the presence of inflammatory conditions. To be most effective, treatment needs to be delivered at a time in the lash growth cycle when the lashes are actively growing.

Cryotherapy

This approach can be useful in segmental trichiasis. A grey line split is made in the area to be treated. A solid nitrous oxide cryoprobe is then applied in a double-freeze-thaw technique. The anterior lamella can be reattached with a double-armed 6–0 Vicryl suture through partial thickness tarsus and then out through the orbicularis and the skin and tied. Possible side effects include skin depigmentation, notching of the lid margin, and meibomian gland damage.

Surgery

Full-thickness wedge resection may be useful for segmental trichiasis. Generalized trichiasis may require anterior lamellar repositioning with or without a grey line split. This method does not disturb the conjunctival surface and may be preferable in mucous membrane pemphigoid.

Distichiasis

This relatively uncommon condition consists of an abnormal row of lashes originating from the meibomian gland orifices, posterior to the grey line (Figure 1.6). The lashes are often shorter and finer than normal lashes and tend to be directed towards the globe. Treatment options are similar to those for trichiasis. Congenital distichiasis is a rare autosomal dominant condition. It may be isolated or associated with ptosis, strabismus, chronic lymphoedema, spinal arachnoid cysts, and congenital heart defects.

Metaplastic lashes

Sometimes referred to as acquired distichiasis, this condition consists of aberrant, posteriorly directed lashes which result from chronic inflammation to the eyelid margin. The most common cause of metaplastic lashes is blepharoconjunctivitis, but other forms of cicatrizing conjunctivitis such as Stevens–Johnson syndrome and mucous membrane pemphigoid can also result in metaplastic lashes.

Madarosis

Madarosis is a complete loss or decrease in the number of lashes (see Figure 1.7). Causes include:
* **Ocular:** chronic blepharitis, infiltrating eyelid tumours
* **Traumatic:** chemical injuries, thermal injuries, trichotillomania (psychiatric disorder of habitual hair removal)
* **Iatrogenic:** following treatment of trichiasis or distichiasis; radiotherapy or cryotherapy of eyelid and surrounding facial tumours
* **Systemic:** psoriasis, generalized alopecia, hypothyroidism, lepromatous leprosy, syphilis, systemic or discoid lupus erythematosus

Eyelash ptosis

Eyelash ptosis is a downward misdirection of normally sited upper lid lashes, caused by anterior lamellar dissociation and slippage (see Figure 1.8). This condition is normally age related but can be associated with dermatochalasis, floppy eyelid syndrome, or facial nerve palsy. Treatment is with anterior lamellar repositioning surgery, which may be combined with eyelid ptosis correction where indicated.

Hypertrichosis

Hypertrichosis is a condition in which lashes are abnormally long and thick (trichomegaly) or there are an excessive number of lashes (polytrichosis). Causes may be congenital or pharmacological (prostaglandin analogues, ciclosporin, and phenytoin).

Poliosis

Poliosis is the premature whitening of hair and can involve the eyelashes as well as the eyebrows. Causes include:
* **Ocular:** sympathetic ophthalmitis, chronic anterior blepharitis
* **Systemic:** Vogt–Koyanagi–Harada syndrome, Waardenburg syndrome

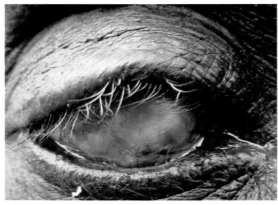

Fig 1.5 Trichiasis secondary to trachoma
Note the associated corneal opacification
Courtesy of Matthew Burton

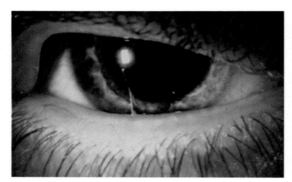

Fig 1.6 Distichiasis of the lower lid
Courtesy of Geoff Rose

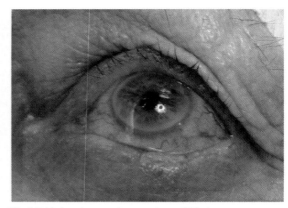

Fig 1.7 Madarosis secondary to a lower lid lesion

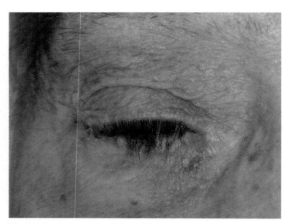

Fig 1.8 Eyelash ptosis of the right eye

1.3 Entropion

Entropion is an abnormal, inward rotation of the eyelid margin towards the globe. It commonly affects the lower lid but can also occur in the upper eyelid. Eyelash-corneal contact can lead to significant discomfort and, in severe cases, ulceration and scarring. Patients with significant punctate staining and poor corneal sensation or those who develop microbial keratitis should be referred urgently for correction of the entropion.

Aetiology

- Congenital
- Acute spastic
- Involutional
- Cicatricial

Congenital entropion

Congenital entropion is rare and should be distinguished from epiblepharon (see Section 1.13). It may be due to dysgenesis of the inferior retractors resulting in eyelid instability.

Treatment

Treatment involves excision of a strip of skin and orbicularis and then fixation of the skin to the tarsus (Hotz procedure).

Acute spastic entropion

Ocular irritation causes sustained eyelid orbicularis contraction and resultant inward rotation of the eyelid margin. The in-turned eyelashes cause a cycle of further irritation and orbicularis contraction. This condition commonly occurs in conjunction with involutional changes. Treatment options are similar to those for involutional entropion.

Involutional entropion

Several factors are thought to play a role in involutional entropion (see Figure 1.9):

1. **Horizontal eyelid laxity:** this condition can be assessed by using the 'snap-back' test, as follows. The eyelid is pulled away (distracted) from the globe. In patients without significant laxity the eyelid will 'snap' back to its original position. If horizontal laxity is present, the eyelid remains distracted until the patient blinks.
2. **Attenuation or disinsertion of eyelid retractors:** this condition can be identified when the lower lid has reduced downward excursion on down-gaze.
3. **Preseptal orbicularis overriding pretarsal orbicularis:** this condition may be evident when the patient squeezes the eyelids closed and can be elicited on instillation of topical anaesthetic.

Treatment

- Eyelid taping may be used as a temporary measure whilst awaiting definitive surgical repair.
- Botulinum toxin injection to the preseptal orbicularis muscle can temporarily relieve both spastic and involutional entropion. A low dose is injected just below the skin overlying the preseptal orbicularis muscle by using an insulin syringe. Avoid injecting below the punctum to prevent punctal ectropion. In cases where an alternative to surgery is required, repeated injections are usually sufficient to relieve symptoms.
- Everting suture techniques are quick and useful temporary measures that can be performed at the bedside if needed (e.g. in intensive therapy unit patients). However, when used alone, they are associated with a high recurrence rate. Infiltrate the lower lid with local anaesthetic. Three double-armed 4–0 or 5–0 Vicryl sutures are passed through the conjunctiva low in the fornix, exiting the skin 2 mm below the lashes (thus catching the inferior retractors). These sutures can be left to dissolve. The medial suture should be placed lateral to the punctum to avoid punctal ectropion.
- Horizontal eyelid tightening improves success rates and can normally be effectively achieved with a range of lid shortening procedures such as the lateral tarsal strip procedure, which involves shortening and fixation of the lateral tarsus.
- Retractors can be strengthened and directed anteriorly with retractor plication methods such as the Jones procedure. A subciliary incision is made 3 mm below the lid margin. The orbicularis is divided by blunt dissection, and the septum is opened to reveal the inferior retractors, which lie just anterior to the conjunctiva. Interrupted Vicryl sutures are then used to reattach the retractors to the lower border of the inferior tarsus. The skin is then closed, creating a scar that forms a barrier to prevent the preseptal orbicularis overriding the pretarsal orbicularis.

Cicatricial entropion

This condition is caused by conjunctival scarring and vertical tarsoconjunctival contracture. Causes include:

- **Traumatic:** chemical or thermal burns
- **Inflammatory:** Stevens–Johnson syndrome
- **Autoimmune:** mucous membrane pemphigoid
- **Infectious:** trachoma, herpes zoster
- **Iatrogenic:** post-enucleation, post-lid surgery (particularly transconjunctival approaches)

Treatment

Depending on the underlying cause, cicatricial entropion normally requires surgery; however, lubricating ointments and bandage contact lenses can be useful adjuncts. Mild-to-moderate cases may be treated with anterior lamellar rotation with retractor plication and a grey line split. Mucous membrane grafts or other spacers may be used in cases of significant forniceal shallowing due to symblepharon formation and scarring. Typically the graft is harvested from buccal mucosa, but nasal septum mucosa and amniotic membrane are also used. The graft is sutured to the posterior lamella once the symblepharons are divided. Care must be taken when operating on the conjunctiva in patients with mucous membrane pemphigoid, as it may trigger inflammation. Systemic immunosuppression may be advisable if there is significant risk of reactivation.

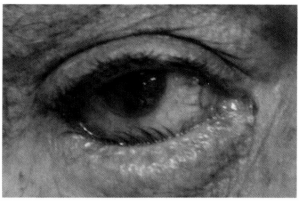

Fig 1.9 Right lower lid involutional entropion

1.4 Ectropion

Ectropion is an outward turning of the eyelid margin away from the globe. Corneal exposure and dryness can result in punctate epithelial erosions. Exposure of the palpebral conjunctiva results in keratinization.

Aetiology

- Congenital
- Paralytic
- Involutional
- Cicatricial
- Mechanical

Congenital ectropion

Congenital ectropion is rare and is usually associated with blepharophimosis syndrome or with ichthyosis. Often the cause is an underdeveloped anterior lamella. Treatment is therefore as for cicatricial ectropion.

Paralytic ectropion

Paralytic ectropion usually follows facial nerve palsy (see Figure 1.10). Paralysis of the orbicularis muscle may also result in lagophthalmos leading to corneal exposure (see Figure 1.10C).

Treatment

Regular lubrication and forced blinking can be used for mild or temporary cases. Taping of the lid (where the taping is applied horizontally) may also be useful for nocturnal lagophthalmos, as is a moisture chamber (created by applying lubricating ointment and then covering the eye with Clingfilm taped to the cheek and forehead). Cases with significant corneal exposure or permanent paralysis will need surgical treatment aimed at improving lid closure. Tarsorrhaphy can be temporary or permanent. It is vital to assess where the area of exposure is most profound when planning surgery. Poor orbicularis function may be addressed with levator recession or the insertion of a gold weight to aid downward lid excursion on blinking and forced eyelid closure. Lower lid ectropion and midface droop may require medial/lateral canthoplasty or fascial slings.

Tarsorrhaphy

Tarsorrhaphy is a procedure to oppose the upper and lower eyelids. It may be lateral, central, or complete (see Section 1.15)

Involutional ectropion

Involutional ectropion results from tissue relaxation, usually a combination of horizontal lid laxity and medial and lateral canthal tendon laxity (see Figure 1.11). Inferior retractor dehiscence may also play a part. Clinical examination can distinguish these entities as follows.

- Horizontal laxity can be assessed by the 'snap-back' test (see Section 1.3).
- Medial canthal tendon laxity can be assessed by the degree the punctum can be distracted laterally. In severe cases, the punctum may be pulled past the pupil.
- Lateral canthal tendon laxity is present when the lower lid can be pulled medially without significant resistance.
- Inferior retractor dehiscence can be identified when the lower lid has reduced downward excursion on down-gaze.

Treatment

Horizontal lid laxity can be managed with a lateral canthal strip procedure or a full-thickness wedge resection (see Section 1.15). The tarsal strip procedure will simultaneously address any lateral canthal tendon laxity. In cases of significant punctal ectropion, a lid shortening procedure can be combined with a medial spindle. The medial spindle procedure requires the excision of a horizontal diamond of conjunctiva below the punctum. The defect is then closed with a buried suture that catches the inferior retractors.

Cicatricial ectropion

Cicatricial ectropion is due to shortening of the anterior lamella (see Figure 1.12). It may occur secondary to a variety of causes, including sun damage, rosacea, atopic dermatitis, thermal/chemical burns, and trauma (including iatrogenic surgical trauma such as lower lid blepharoplasty).

Treatment

Treatment involves addressing the underlying cause. In cases of rosacea and dermatitis, liberal massage of the skin with an emollient can have a striking effect on reducing the ectropion. In localized cases due to scar formation, a relaxing procedure such as Z plasty can be used. More generalized cases require anterior lamellar lengthening using a skin graft, typically from the pre- or post-auricular areas. A midface lift can also be used to recruit more skin to the lower eyelid and has the advantage of not requiring any grafted tissue.

Mechanical ectropion

Mechanical ectropion may be caused by bulky tumours on or at the lid margin, or by poorly fitted spectacles.

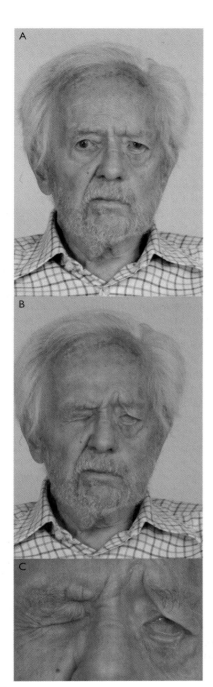

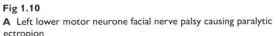

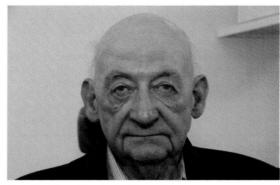

Fig 1.11 Bilateral involutional lower lid ectropion

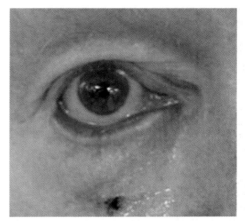

Fig 1.12 Right cicatricial ectropion secondary to a cheek basal cell carcinoma

Fig 1.10

A Left lower motor neurone facial nerve palsy causing paralytic ectropion

B Forced lid closure. Note that there is significant lagophthalmos but a good Bells phenomenon

C On close inspection, it can be seen that a small amount of cornea is exposed on forced closure. It is important to assess if there are signs of corneal exposure

Ptosis refers to drooping of any anatomical structure. Strictly speaking, the term blepharoptosis should be reserved specifically for an abnormally low position of the upper lid with respect to the globe. In adults, the upper lid normally sits 1–2 mm below the superior limbus. Ptosis is due to dysfunction of one or both of the eyelid elevators (the LPS and Müllers muscle).

History

Always ask about the nature of onset. Any sudden-onset ptosis may indicate a neurological cause. Pain must **always** be identified, as ptosis due to oculomotor nerve compressions (by a posterior communicating artery aneurysm) typically cause pain. A history of diplopia should also direct the clinician to consider any underlying neurological cause.

Ptosis examination

Introduction
Introduce yourself to the patient and explain the examination.

Observation
Look for:
* Scars (trauma, surgery)
* General facial asymmetry
* Anisocoria (third nerve palsy, Horner syndrome)
* Heterochromia (congenital Horner syndrome)
* Strabismus (myasthenia gravis, third nerve palsy)
* Frontalis overaction
* Chin lift (severe bilateral ptosis with superior visual field defects)
* Abnormal facial features (blepharophimosis syndrome, myotonic dystrophy)

If examining a child, ask them to chew and protrude their jaw to look for Marcus Gunn jaw-winking syndrome.

Measure
Measure the following (see Figure 1.13):
* The palpebral aperture in the primary position; measuring this aperture may require covering the other eye if the patient has a heterotropia as detected on cover test.
* The upper and lower marginal reflex distance (the distance between the centre of a light shone on the pupil and the upper and lower lid margin, respectively). Palpebral aperture measurements alone can be misleading e.g. in the context of lower lid ectropion or hypoglobus.
* The skin crease height (the distance between the lid crease and the upper lid margin in down-gaze). The lid crease is often high in aponeurotic dehiscence (see Figure 1.14).
* The upper lid show (the distance from the lid margin to the upper lid skin fold). This value may be zero in patients with significant dermatochalasis.
* Levator function (upper lid excursion as the patient is asked to look from extreme down-gaze to extreme up-gaze). It is important to prevent frontalis action during this measurement by placing a thumb firmly across the brow.

Bells phenomenon
Bells phenomenon is identified by asking the patient to close their eyes whilst the examiner holds the eyelid open. The phenomenon is positive if the eye rolls up under the upper lid. It is extremely useful in assessing the risk of post-operative corneal exposure. Patients with a poor or absent Bells phenomenon should have conservative lid raising to avoid corneal exposure.

Lid lift
Lift the ptotic eyelid to look for a contralateral ptosis being unmasked. This is an important test which can predict whether the fellow eyelid will become ptotic if the ptosis is corrected.

Fatigability
This test is performed by asking the patient to maintain up-gaze for 30 seconds and then observing if the ptosis is worse (which would suggest myasthenia gravis). After fatiguing the upper lid, ask the patient to make a quick downwards saccade, then back to primary position. An upward overshoot of the upper lid before taking up fixation occurs in myasthenia gravis (Cogans lid twitch sign). The ice pack test can also be used to aid diagnosis of myasthenia gravis. An ice pack is placed over the ptotic lid for 3 minutes. A rise in the lid position suggests myasthenia gravis.

Additional examination
* Exophthalmometry, to exclude enophthalmos
* Cover test to exclude hypotropia
* Ocular motility to exclude third nerve palsy, myasthenia gravis
* Pupillary reactions to exclude Horner syndrome, third nerve palsy
* Corneal sensation is important when deciding how high to surgically lift the eyelid.
* Evert the upper lid to exclude mechanical causes of ptosis, such as giant papillae or masses.
* Jaw-winking.

Consider pseudoptosis
Pseudoptosis is an apparent eyelid drooping that should be differentiated from true ptosis via:
* Ipsilateral hypotropia
* Contralateral hypertropia
* Contralateral upper lid retraction
* Volume deficiencies such as enophthalmos, microphthalmos, and phthisis bulbi
* Brow ptosis
* Dermatochalasis (when excess upper eyelid skin overhangs the eyelid margin and gives the appearance of a ptosis). Treatment is with blepharoplasty.

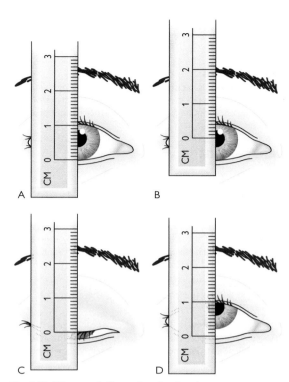

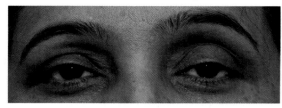

Fig 1.14 Left involutional ptosis
The preaponeurotic fat pad is pulled upwards into the orbit with the dehisced aponeurosis, resulting in a deep sulcus. Note also the raised skin crease and resulting increased upper lid show on the left caused by the dehisced aponeurosis. The left brow is raised in an attempt to clear the visual axis

Fig 1.13 Diagramatic illustration showing the necessary measurements for ptosis examination

A Interpalpebral fissure height
B Upper lid margin–corneal reflex distance
C, D Levator function

1.6 Ptosis II

Aetiology

Ptosis can be congenital or acquired. Congenital ptosis is discussed in Section 1.13. Acquired causes can be classified as aponeurotic, myogenic, or neurogenic.

Aponeurotic ptosis

Aponeurotic ptosis is the most common form of ptosis. It is caused by a defect in the transmission of power from a functioning levator muscle to the tarsal plate. This condition is most commonly due to involutional changes and dehiscence or disinsertion of the aponeurosis. Chronic inflammation, long-term contact lens use, and intraocular surgery necessitating the use of a speculum are all causes of stretching of the aponeurosis that can lead to dehiscence or disinsertion. The levator function is usually normal or near normal despite ptosis which may be severe. The skin crease is often high or indistinct in aponeurotic ptosis.

Myogenic ptosis

Myogenic ptosis may result from localized or systemic muscular disease. Levator function is often poor (<10 mm). Causes include:

- Myasthenia gravis
- Myotonic dystrophy
- Chronic progressive external ophthalmoplegia
- Ocular pharyngeal dystrophy

Neurogenic ptosis

Third nerve palsy

Third nerve palsy may be congenital or acquired. Causes of acquired third nerve palsies include trauma, intracranial artery aneurysm, vascular disease, demyelination, tumours, infection, and vasculitis. Third nerve palsies can be partial or complete and thus are associated with varying degrees of ptosis, mydriasis, and an inability to elevate and adduct the globe. Third nerve palsies can rarely be associated with aberrant regeneration where unusual eyelid movements accompany movements of the eye, for example, eyelid elevation on adduction or downgaze. Patients with pupil involvement or pain should be referred urgently to the neurologists for imaging to exclude an intracranial aneurysm (typically involving the posterior communicating artery).

Horner syndrome

Horner syndrome may be congenital or acquired. It arises due to an interruption of the sympathetic nerve supply to the head (see Chapter 10, Section 10.18). There are many causes, depending on the level of the interruption. The ptosis tends to be mild (1–2 mm) as a result of weakened Müllers muscle action. There is an associated miosis and pseudo-enophthalmos (due to upper lid ptosis and inverse ptosis of the lower lid) and hypohydrosis (see Figure 1.15). A posterior approach to surgery is often preferred in these cases.

Marcus Gunn jaw-winking syndrome

Marcus Gunn jaw-winking syndrome occurs in some cases of congenital ptosis. It is thought to result from a branch of the mandibular division of the fifth cranial nerve being misdirected to the levator muscle. The clinical manifestation is an elevation of the ptotic eyelid due to opening the mouth, chewing, and/or moving the jaw.

Mechanical ptosis

Mechanical ptosis is caused by masses or swellings weighing down the upper eyelid or restricting elevation. Causes of mechanical ptosis include chalazion, dermatochalasis, eyelid tumours, and oedema.

Management

Conservative

There is always an option of no treatment in cases where there is no functional visual loss or risk of amblyopia. Small doses of botulinum toxin to the pretarsal orbicularis can also be effective. Non-surgical options such as ptosis props (crutches attached to glasses) or shelved scleral contact lenses are rarely used today but still have role in the management of these conditions.

Surgical

The appropriate procedure depends on the type and degree of ptosis as well as the levator function. There are three main approaches.

Anterior (transcutaneous)

This approach is particularly useful for aponeurotic ptosis where levator function is near normal and the skin crease is high. It is the most commonly used approach. Dermatochalasis can be addressed simultaneously with blepharoplasty, and the skin crease can be reset at a lower, more desirable position. The tarsal plate is exposed and then the levator is identified. As the orbital septum is opened, the pre-aponeurotic fat pad is the defining landmark as the levator is found deep to it. The aponeurosis/levator is reattached to the tarsus with two or three sutures, and then the lid height is checked. In patients with poor levator function (5–12 mm), the levator often needs to be resected. The skin crease is then reformed using skin sutures that also pass through the aponeurosis.

Posterior (transconjunctival)

This approach is often useful for small degrees of ptosis (<2 mm), for example, in Horner syndrome. A good response to 2.5% phenylephrine in the clinic can indicate that this surgical approach may be effective. Müllers muscle resection is preferable to the Fasanella–Servat procedure, in which a small part of the upper tarsal border is excised together with the lower border of Müllers muscle and the conjunctiva, as the latter procedure makes further ptosis surgery difficult and may reduce upper lid stability.

Frontalis suspension

This approach is useful for severe ptosis with poor levator function (<4 mm). The eyelid is suspended by a sling running through the frontalis muscle. The eyelid then lifts when the brow is raised. Synthetic materials such as Supramid sutures may be used or autologous tissue such as fascia lata (although this tissue is not sufficiently developed until the age of 5 or 6). Patients should be warned of eyelid hang up on down-gaze and nocturnal lagophthalmos.

Complications of ptosis surgery

- Infection and scar (potential complications of all lid surgery)
- Lagophthalmos and resultant corneal exposure (especially with larger levator resections)

- Over/under correction, and lid asymmetry
- Lid contour defects
- Unmasking of contralateral ptosis (due to Herrings law of equal innervation)
- Lash ptosis/lash eversion
- Orbital haemorrhage (very rare)

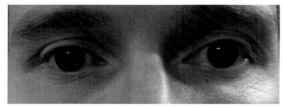

Fig 1.15 Right Horner syndrome. Note the subtle right ptosis and pupil miosis

Chalazion

Chalazion is a focal inflammatory cyst of the tarsus resulting from the obstruction of a meibomian gland orifice (see Figure 1.16). It is associated with posterior blepharitis and rosacea. Histologically it is a chronic lipogranulomatous inflammation.

Clinical evaluation

Chalazion may present with acute or chronic eyelid lumps, diffuse lid swelling, pain, and/or erythema. Look for signs of associated blepharitis and rosacea. A large chalazion may cause ptosis and obstruct the visual axis or induce astigmatism to affect vision. Identification of this condition is important in young children at risk of amblyopia.

Management

For acute inflammatory chalazion, warm compresses, gentle digital massage over the lump, and lid hygiene are appropriate in the first instance. The natural history of chalazion is for the lesion to resolve within weeks to months. If the lump persists or is causing significant symptoms, routine referral is indicated for surgical treatment. Referral guidelines will vary between regions. Surgery is performed with incision and curettage (see Figure 1.17).

Incision and curettage

- Mark the skin overlying the chalazion, as the lump may be difficult to localize following local anaesthetic infiltration.
- Instil topical proxymethocaine and tetracaine into the fornix.
- Inject premixed 2% xylocaine with 1 in 200 000 adrenaline subcutaneously. Allow sufficient time for the anaesthetic to work.
- The chalazion clamp is placed firmly over the chalazion, and the lid is everted.
- A vertical linear incision is made over the chalazion.
- A curette is used to remove the contents of the cyst.
- A tarsal biopsy should be considered for recurrent chalazia or lesions that do not produce typical contents on curettage.
- Instil a drop of chloramphenicol before removing the clamp.
- Firmly double-pad the eye.

Hordeolum

A hordeolum is an acute infection that is normally caused by staphylococcal infection of the eyelid glands.

External hordeolum (stye)

An external hordeolum involves the glands of Zeis. The infection is often centred on an eyelash follicle. Treatment is with eyelash epilation as well as warm compresses and topical antibiotics.

Internal hordeolum

An internal hordeolum involves the meibomian glands and is treated with hot compresses and topical antibiotics. In very rare cases, hordeola may be associated with secondary preseptal cellulitis, and systemic antibiotics may be required.

Xanthelasma

Xanthelasma is a cutaneous lipid deposit which may be idiopathic or associated with hyperlipidaemia, hypothyroidism, or primary biliary cirrhosis (see Figure 1.18). Treatment is only

for cosmetic reasons and may be with excision, argon laser, or trichloracetic acid application.

Molluscum contagiosum

Molluscum contagiosum is caused by a poxvirus. It manifests as a pale, umbilicated nodule often on the eyelid margin but can occur anywhere on the skin and can often be multiple. It has a higher prevalence in children, sexually active adults, and those who are immunodeficient. Individual lesions generally last for 2–3 months. However, the virus may propagate as a result of autoinoculation, and infections can last up to 18 months. Treatment options include excision, curettage, cauterization, and cryotherapy.

Other eyelid cysts

Cyst of Moll (apocrine hidrocystoma)

Cyst of Moll is a common, smooth-walled cyst originating from the gland of Moll at the eyelid margin. These cysts are translucent and may transilluminate (see Figure 1.19).

Cysts of Zeis

Cysts of Zeis are smooth-walled cysts of sebaceous material on the eyelid margin.

Milia

Milia are derived from hair follicle-associated glands and are visible under the skin as small white superficial cysts.

Management

As these lesions are benign, surgery is only indicated for cosmetic or diagnostic reasons. Complete cyst excision or deroofing with thermal cautery to the empty sac reduces the risk of recurrence.

Benign epithelial hyperplasia

Seborrheic keratoses

These lesions are classically described as having a smooth, greasy 'stuck-on-mud' appearance (see Figure 1.20). They may be sessile or pedunculated and have varying degrees of pigmentation.

Squamous cell papilloma

These lesions have multiple tiny projections, which giving them a frond-like appearance (see Figure 1.21). They can be sessile or pedunculated.

Exuberant hyperkeratosis (cutaneous horn)

This hyperkeratotic lesion protrudes from the skin. It can occasionally be associated with squamous cell carcinoma at its base and therefore the lesion should be always be sent for histology.

Management

All of these lesions can be removed with shave excision at the dermal-epidermal junction. If there is any doubt about the diagnosis, the specimen should be sent for histology.

Benign melanocytic lesions

Naevi

There are three main types of naevus: junctional (arising from the dermis-epidermis junction), compound (a mixture of junctional and intradermal proliferation), and dermal (arising solely from the dermis). Naevi are almost always benign, but occasionally malignant transformation of junctional or compound naevi may occur.

Dermal melanocytosis (naevus of Ota)

Dermal melanocytosis is a congenital diffuse blue/brown naevus of the periocular skin. It is within the distribution of the ophthalmic and/or maxillary branches of the trigeminal nerve. When associated with slate-grey episcleral pigmentation, it is known as oculodermal melanocytosis, which carries a 1 in 400 risk of uveal malignant melanoma.

Benign vascular lesions

Pyogenic granuloma

Pyogenic granuloma is a rapidly growing, bright red sessile or pedunculated lesion consisting of vascularized proliferation of granulomatous tissue (see Figure 1.22). Causes include prior trauma, surgery, and infection. Treatment is by excision.

Port-wine stain

Port-wine stain is a congenital subcutaneous cavernous haemangioma. It is normally unilateral, beginning as a pink patch and with age progressing to a dark purple colour. These lesions are seen in Sturge–Weber syndrome. When the periocular region is involved, there is a strong association with glaucoma. Treatment is with erbium laser.

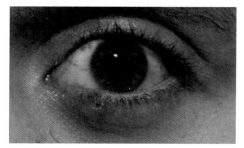

Fig 1.16 Left lower lid chalazion

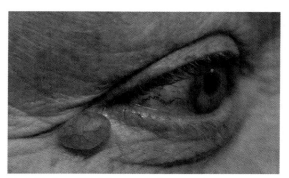

Fig 1.19 Cyst of Moll (apocrine hidrocystoma)

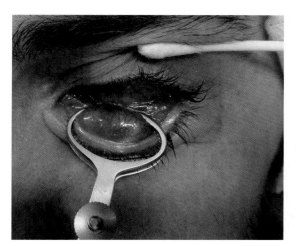

Fig 1.17 Incision and curettage of chalazion

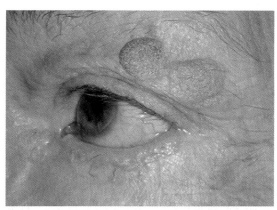

Fig 1.20 Seborrheic keratosis
Courtesy of Michele Beaconsfield

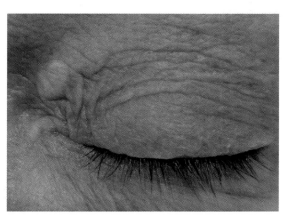

Fig 1.18 Xanthelasma of the left upper lid

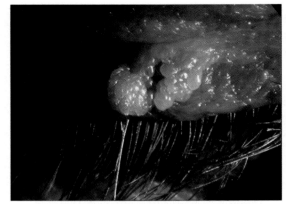

Fig 1.21 Squamous cell papilloma of the upper lid

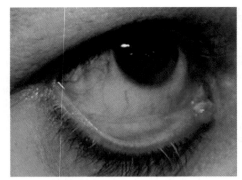

Fig 1.22 Pyogenic granuloma of the inferior canaliculus

1.8 Premalignant lesions

Actinic keratoses

Actinic keratoses are round, erythematous, scaly keratotic lesions with a rough surface (see Figure 1.23). These commonly affect elderly, fair-skinned individuals with a history of sun exposure. It is the most common precancerous skin lesion and is often described as a precursor to squamous carcinoma in situ. Although the majority of cutaneous squamous cell carcinomas arise from actinic keratosis, the risk of progression of actinic keratosis to squamous cell carcinoma is low. This risk is highest in those patients with multiple lesions (1 in 8 chance of transformation). Several options for treatment are available, including surgical excision, cryotherapy, and CO_2 laser. Topical treatments such as imiquimod and fluorouracil also have a role, but their use is limited by their potential to cause severe ocular surface inflammation.

Bowen disease

Bowen disease is squamous cell carcinoma in situ of the skin. It is a form of intraepidermal carcinoma which may ultimately progress to invasive squamous cell carcinoma (3%–5% progress). Patients often present with non-healing lesions and well-demarcated plaques of hyperkeratosis. Treatment is by complete surgical excision.

Keratoacanthoma

Keratoacanthoma is now considered a low-grade form of squamous cell carcinoma. The lesion typically begins as a pink papule that rapidly increases in size over a few days to become a firm, dome-shaped nodule (see Figure 1.24). During subsequent regression, a central keratin-filled crater may develop. UV radiation, trauma, human papilloma virus, and immunosuppression are all associated aetiological factors. Treatment is usually with complete excision.

Lentigo maligna

Lentigo maligna is a premalignant melanocytic lesion that is flat, irregularly shaped, unevenly pigmented, and slowly enlarging. It is often likened to a stain on the skin. It is a subtype of melanoma in situ. Up to 50% of these lesions pro-gress to lentigo maligna melanoma. It may be present for long periods before invasion occurs. Treatment is excision with adequate margins.

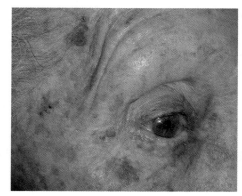

Fig 1.23 Actinic keratosis
Courtesy of Michele Beaconsfield

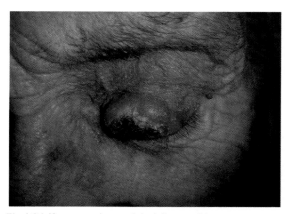

Fig 1.24 Keratoacanthoma of the left upper lid
Courtesy of Michele Beaconsfield

Basal cell carcinoma

Basal cell carcinoma (BCC) is the most common eyelid malignancy, accounting for 85%–90% of malignant eyelid tumours in Western populations. They typically appear on sun-exposed skin and so occur most frequently on the lower eyelid. They are epithelial tumours that invade the dermis but seldom metastasize. If neglected, tumours can grow to cause significant local tissue destruction. Patients at greatest risk are those with fair skin and a history of cumulative UV light exposure. There can be a latency of 25–50 years between sun exposure and the development of BCCs.

Aetiology

* Prolonged UV exposure causes DNA damage leading to the activation of oncogenes or the inactivation of tumour suppressor genes.
* Chronic immunosuppression (the risk of skin cancer is ten times higher in patients who have received organ transplantation compared to the rest of the population)
* **Xeroderma pigmentosum** is an autosomal recessive disorder that results in defective DNA repair and extreme hypersensitivity to UV radiation. Patients often have typical bird-like facies and develop multiple skin tumours at a young age as well as recurrent conjunctivitis with symblepharon formation.
* **Basal cell naevus syndrome (Gorlin syndrome)** is an autosomal dominant disorder involving the patched (*PTCH*) gene, which is a tumour suppressor. Patients develop multiple BCCs at a young age, as well as skeletal abnormalities.

Clinical evaluation

Patients typically present with a painless eyelid nodule or non-healing ulcer that bleeds after minimal trauma. The lesion may have been present for months or years. An essential sign of malignant eyelid lesions is disruption of normal anatomical structures. This is particularly diagnostic at the lid margin, where the complex and close arrangement of structures is often disrupted, even in the context of very small tumours. Lesions can cause eyelash loss, ulceration, telangiectasia, loss of meibomian orifices, and blunting of the grey line. In contrast, benign lesions do not destroy normal anatomical structures. Although patients will rarely present with pain, this is an important symptom suggestive of bony invasion as a result of late presentation. Several different histological subtypes of BCC are described which underlie differences in clinical presentation.

Nodular

Nodular BCC is the most common subtype, representing 60% of BCCs. These lesions present as raised nodules with well-demarcated, pearly telangiectatic borders (see Figure 1.25). As growth progresses, the centre becomes umbilicated and ulcerated. These lesions can often look similar to molluscum lesions on the eyelid margin.

Nodulo-ulcerative (rodent ulcer)

Nodulo-ulcerative BCC is characterized by central ulceration that can be extensive in advanced cases. If left untreated, the tumour can erode a large extent of the eyelid and beyond.

Morphoeic

Morphoeic BCCs are the next most common lesion. These can look innocuous and the borders are difficult to identify.

Morphoeic BCCs are often sore and crusted. For lesions close to the lid margin, the identification of anatomical destruction in the form of eyelash loss, lid margin blunting, and meibomian obliteration can be important signs signifying the extent of the lesion.

Other subtypes

Frequently, BCCs can present as pigmented lesions and BCC should be part of the differential diagnosis of periocular pigmented lesions. Occasionally, BCCs can present as a cystic lesions containing mucinous material that can be difficult to distinguish from other benign periocular cystic lesions without biopsy.

Prognosis

The prognosis is excellent, with a 95% cure rate at 5 years for BCCs under 10 mm in size.

Squamous cell carcinoma

Squamous cell carcinoma is a relatively uncommon malignant tumour of epithelial cells that typically affects fair-skinned elderly individuals. The main risk factor is cumulative UV radiation exposure. Lesions may appear many decades after the sun exposure. It can arise de novo or from premalignant sun-induced lesions such as actinic keratoses. It can also occur in patients who have undergone radiotherapy, those with genetic predispositions (e.g. xeroderma pigmentosum) or have been chronically immunosuppressed (transplant patients). The main differential diagnoses are actinic keratosis and keratoacanthoma.

Unlike BCCs, squamous cell carcinoma has potential to spread to regional lymph nodes and to metastasize to distant sites. Squamous cell carcinoma also has a predilection for perineural spread, and the main cause of mortality from this tumour is perineural spread into the CNS. Squamous cell carcinoma may be associated with skip lesions, whereby one lesion may be completely excised with 'clear margins' but another premalignant lesion may be present a few millimetres away. Long-term surveillance is therefore mandatory.

Clinical evaluation

Squamous cell carcinoma may appear as non-healing ulcers, plaques, or nodules (see Figure 1.26). A well-described feature is hyperkeratosis, and lesions present with varying degrees of scaling and crusting or sometimes keratin horn formation. Pain, numbness, and tingling are important diagnostic features, as they may signify perineural spread. Clinical assessment must include a full cranial nerve examination as well as examining the neck for enlarged lymph nodes.

Sebaceous cell carcinoma

Whilst sebaceous cell carcinoma is uncommon in the west, it comprises up to one-third of eyelid malignancies in southern and eastern Asia. Although this tumour can be aggressive, it is usually localized to the eyelid, with low mortality. It is very rare outside of the eyelid and is thought to arise from the meibomian glands.

Clinical evaluation

These tumours can masquerade as benign conditions such as chalazia, chronic blepharitis, or conjunctivitis (see Figures 1.27 and 1.28). Lesions are often firm and painless. Typically, the tumour can also be associated with meibomian gland orifice effacement and ulceration, and sometimes madarosis. An important feature of this tumour is its tendency to spread in a pagetoid fashion through the conjunctival epithelium. This pathological feature underlies its tendency to present as either blepharitis or a chronic conjunctivitis. A high index of suspicion of sebaceous cell carcinoma should be raised with chronic or recurrent lesions which are associated with unilateral blepharitis or conjunctivitis. Lesions typically mimic recurrent chalazia with similar lipogranulomatous contents on curettage. Any recurrent chalazion should have a tarsoconjunctival biopsy during curettage to exclude sebaceous cell carcinoma. Mapping biopsies should also be taken to determine the extent of pagetoid spread.

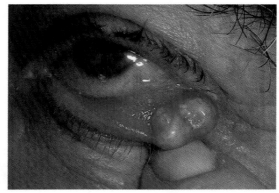

Fig 1.27 Discrete sebaceous cell carcinoma
Courtesy of Michele Beaconsfield

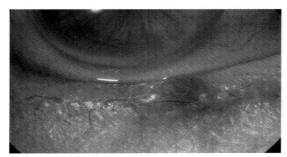

Fig 1.25 Nodular basal cell carcinoma
Note the telangiectatic vessels and loss of eyelashes

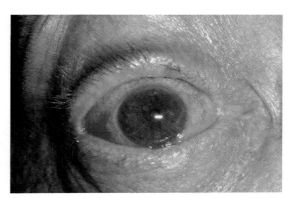

Fig 1.28 Intraepithelial sebaceous cell carcinoma mimicking unilateral conjunctivitis
Note the thickening of the medial bulbar conjunctiva
Courtesy of Michele Beaconsfield

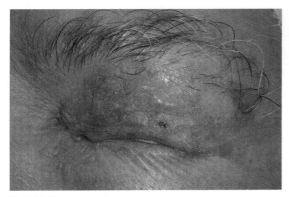

Fig 1.26 Squamous cell carcinoma
Note the areas of ulceration and madarosis

Management of malignant lid lesions

Patients with suspected eyelid malignancy should be seen by a specialist within 2 weeks.

The central objective of the evaluation of any eyelid lesion is to differentiate between benign and malignant lesions. Periocular skin tumours present unique difficulties in management owing to the proximity of the globe and orbital contents. The high-density innervation of the eyelids also makes perineural spread a significant problem for some tumour types. An accurate diagnosis is an essential initial step to the management of these lesions. Although only 15%–20% of eyelid lesions are malignant, an accurate clinical diagnosis and determination of malignant potential can be challenging. If there is any doubt, a biopsy should be taken as an initial step. Additional difficulties are presented with sebaceous cell carcinoma, where multiple conjunctival mapping biopsies are required to evaluate the presence or extent of any pagetoid tumour spread.

For larger or more aggressive tumours, imaging is essential to identify any orbital invasion. Any patients with suspected regional lymph node spread or distant metastases should be managed in the context of a multidisciplinary team.

Whilst there is significant variation in practice in the management of these tumours, the universal principle of treatment is to eradicate the tumour, with maximal preservation of function and physical appearance. After correct diagnosis, it is essential to ensure adequate clearance of the tumour.

Surgical excision

Surgical excision is usually the treatment of choice, allowing for complete removal of the tumour. Surgical excision has a lower rate of recurrence than other modalities. However, excision usually requires 2–3 mm of clear margin to ensure complete excision, and larger surgical defects will affect the cosmetic and functional outcome. To allow complete tumour removal whilst minimizing tissue loss, surgical excision is often performed with histology support services using a variety of techniques.

Frozen section

After the clinically apparent tumour has been excised with clear margins, the edges of the specimen are sectioned and examined by a histopathologist at the time of surgery for confirmation of tumour-free margins. The specimens are usually sent fresh or wrapped in a swab soaked in normal saline.

Paraffin section

Excision is as for frozen section but the specimen is sent in formalin and prepared in paraffin. It is then evaluated over 24 to 48 hours. Closure of the defect is delayed for 48 hours until the histology results are available. Paraffin sections allow for more accurate assessment than frozen sections. However, if standard 'bread-loaf' tissue sectioning is used, peripheral involvement may be missed, as only a small percentage of the margins is examined. Finger-like projections of tumour cells may be present in the unexamined intervals.

Mohs micrographic surgery

Mohs micrographic surgery has the lowest rate of recurrence of all modalities but is expensive and requires a trained team with expensive equipment. The clinically apparent tumour together with a thin rim of adjacent tissue is excised in horizontal layers and marked to provide three-dimensional mapping of the tumour. If any areas of tumour are seen at the margins, further tissue is removed from that area only. This technique is particularly useful for large tumours, those with ill-defined borders (such as infiltrative or morphoeic BCC) or to control occult tumour invasion which is a feature in the medial canthal area.

Surgical reconstruction

Defects are reconstructed using combinations of direct closure techniques, flaps, and free grafts.

Small defects

Defects of less than one-third the length of the eyelid can normally be closed directly. A lateral cantholysis can be performed to mobilize the tissue if necessary.

Moderate defects

Defects of less than half the eyelid length may be closed with a semicircular flap such as the Tenzel flap.

Large defects

Defects involving more than half the eyelid length for the lower lid can be repaired by transposition of a tarsoconjunctival flap from the upper eyelid into the posterior lamellar defect of the lower eyelid. The anterior lamella can then be created with either an advancement skin flap or a skin graft. For upper lid defects, a free tarsoconjunctival graft may be taken from the contralateral upper eyelid and covered with a skin-muscle flap.

Orbital invasion

Orbital invasion is a devastating complication of eyelid tumours and, where this is identified, the patient will need to undergo orbital exenteration (see Chapter 11, Section 11.10) to achieve surgical clearance, a circumstance which again highlights the importance of early recognition. Whilst exenteration improves survival outcomes for most tumours, there is evidence that it has no impact on survival in melanoma.

Radiotherapy

The recurrence rate with radiotherapy is higher than with surgical treatment, and new lesions may be more difficult to distinguish after the radiotherapy. Complications of this treatment include dry eyes, chronic keratitis, keratinization of the conjunctiva, and dermatitis.

Cryotherapy

The recurrence rate with cryotherapy is also high and, as for radiotherapy, it is thus reserved as treatment for patients who are otherwise unable to tolerate surgery. It is the treatment of choice for multiple BCCs such as Gorlin syndrome.

Uncommon malignant lesions

Malignant melanoma

Primary cutaneous malignant melanoma of the eyelids is rare (<1% of all eyelid tumours). Risk factors for melanoma are similar to those of other malignant tumours and include sun exposure, a family history, fair skin, and older age. Previous radiotherapy is also an important risk factor, particularly for patients previously treated for retinoblastoma, as they may have required high-dose external radiotherapy. Melanoma behaves aggressively and early identification is important.

Clinical evaluation

Lesions typically have irregular borders and variable pigmentation with dark and light regions within the lesion. A careful history is necessary in patients with suspicious pigmented lesions. If ulcerated, bleeding indicates a vertical (deep invasion into the dermis) component, which carries a worse prognosis. Breslow thickness is a strong predictor of survival outcome. There are several forms of cutaneous melanoma.

- **Lentigo maligna melanoma**: whilst these lesions often occur de novo, up to 50% of eyelid melanomas arise from a predisposing skin lesion such as lentigo maligna, congenital naevus, and rarely a naevus of Ota.
- **Superficial spreading melanoma**: this lesion normally manifests as an irregular plaque with variable pigmentation but with no vertical component.
- **Nodular melanoma**: this lesion can be amelanotic but is normally characterized by a pigmented nodule surrounded by normal skin.

Management
Any lesion that exhibits growth or change in colour suggests malignancy and should be biopsied. In histologically confirmed cases, wide surgical excision is required. The role of sentinel node biopsy is controversial.

Merkel cell carcinoma
Merkel cell carcinoma is a rare, aggressive primary skin tumour. Lesions are typically solitary red or purple dome-shaped nodules or firm plaques. Treatment is with wide local excision but, owing to its high malignancy, adjunct treatment may be required.

Kaposi sarcoma
Kaposi sarcoma is a tumour of probable endothelial cell origin that typically affects patients with AIDS. The lesions are purple or red and highly vascular with surrounding telangiectatic vessels (see Figure 1.29). They may be macular, plaque-like, or nodular. Treatment is with radiotherapy, as these lesions are exquisitely radiosensitive, or by excision.

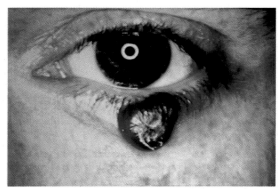

Fig 1.29 Kaposi sarcoma of the left lower lid
Courtesy of Geoff Rose

The term 'epiphora' refers to the symptom of a watery eye. It is caused by an imbalance between tear production and tear drainage. Tears are produced in the lacrimal gland and accessory lacrimal glands. Lacrimal gland secretions form the aqueous part of the tear film that wets the ocular surface. Capillarity draws the tears towards the puncta medially. Preseptal orbicularis fibres are attached to the lacrimal fascia surrounding the lacrimal sac so that, with each blink, orbicularis contraction causes negative pressure within the sac, drawing tears in from the tear meniscus ('the lacrimal pump'). Gravity and positive pressure within the sac upon orbicularis relaxation draw the tears into the nasolacrimal duct. Eyelid malpositions cause epiphora when the punctum is distracted from the tear lake. Eyelid laxity can also lead to epiphora owing to lacrimal pump failure even in the absence of frank eyelid or punctal malpositions.

Hypersecretion

Hypersecretion may be due to an excess of tear production due to abnormal stimulation of the lacrimal gland. Reflex tearing due to trigeminal nerve stimulation is a common cause of epiphora. Causes include trichiasis, ocular inflammation, tear-film instability, blepharitis, and corneal foreign bodies. Reflex tearing is often associated with burning, stinging, or itching. These conditions are discussed in Chapter 2.

Outflow obstruction

Outflow obstruction may be functional or anatomical. Anatomical obstruction refers to a demonstrable obstruction in outflow drainage; this obstruction can occur anywhere along the lacrimal drainage pathway, from the punctum to the nasolacrimal duct (see Section 1.1) and may be congenital (see Section 1.13) or acquired (Section 1.12). Functional nasolacrimal duct obstruction is diagnosed when patients have symptoms and signs suggestive of an anatomical obstruction but have a patent system on lacrimal syringing. In these patients, the nasolacrimal system may collapse during normal physiological conditions but is opened during the forced positive pressure created during syringing.

Evaluation of the patient with acquired epiphora

History
Table 1.1 details the important features in a history of epiphora, and their clinical relevance.

Examination
For cause of reflex tearing
Causes include trichiasis, blepharitis, tear-film instability (rapid tear-film break-up time), and punctate corneal erosions.

Marginal tear strip
- This structure can be elevated in outflow obstruction.
- The **fluorescein dye retention test** is useful in evaluating tear drainage in the physiological state (see Figure 1.30). A small drop of 2% fluorescein is instilled into the inferior fornix. A thin line of fluorescein should normally remain after 5 minutes (as viewed with the cobalt-blue filter on the slit lamp). Prolonged retention indicates lacrimal outflow failure.
- Examine the tear film for mucous debris, which may be a sign of nasolacrimal duct obstruction.

Puncta and lids
- Look for evidence of a small, stenosed, inflamed, or occluded punctum.
- Look for subtle punctal ectropion, where the punctum sits away from the tear lake.
- Look for an ectropion or an entropion.

Lacrimal sac
- Examine for evidence of a visibly distended lacrimal sac due to a mucocele or to acute dacryocystitis (see Section 1.12).
- Apply gentle pressure over the lacrimal sac and look for mucus reflux through either the upper or the lower punctum.

Jones dye test
Both the Jones 1 (primary) and Jones 2 (secondary) tests are described in Table 1.2. Despite sound principles, they give a variable diagnostic yield in clinical practice and so are rarely performed.

Syringing and probing
Syringing and probing procedures are detailed in Section 1.11 and Table 1.3.

Table 1.1 Symptoms and their likely underlying aetiology	
Symptom	Likely underlying cause of epiphora
Watering worse outdoors	Usually due to outflow obstruction. Outflow fails to match increased flow induced by tear hypersecretion.
Watering indoors and outdoors	Often due to outflow obstruction
Mucous discharge, particularly in the morning	Often due to nasolacrimal duct obstruction
Medial epiphora	Often due to outflow obstruction
Lateral epiphora	Often due to eyelid laxity
Intermittent symptoms	Often due to reflex tearing
Constant symptoms	Often due to outflow obstruction

Table 1.2 Jones dye tests		
Method	Result	Interpretation
Jones 1: 2% fluorescein instilled into fornix. At 5 minutes, a cotton-tipped applicator soaked in tetracaine inserted into the nose.	**Positive:** fluorescein recovered from the nose	Physiologically patent nasolacrimal system
	Negative: no fluorescein recovered	Anatomical or functional nasolacrimal duct obstruction or lacrimal pump failure
Jones 2: residual fluorescein is flushed by irrigation.	**Positive:** fluorescein recovered from the nose	Partial or functional nasolacrimal duct obstruction
	Negative: only saline recovered from the nose	Punctal/canalicular stenosis
	Negative: with reflux of fluorescein from the punctum	Complete nasolacrimal duct obstruction

Investigations

Dacryocystography

Dacryocystography is not commonly performed but can be useful if the diagnosis is inconclusive from history and examination alone. It allows visualization of the nasolacrimal system in great detail (see Figure 1.31). The technique involves irrigating the system with a contrast medium before obtaining radiographs at various intervals. It provides little information regarding function, as the contrast is injected directly into the system at forces that are not physiological.

Scintigraphy

Scintigraphy is a radionuclide test that can be useful in functional obstruction to determine if punctal pickup, lacrimal pump failure, or functional duct obstruction are the primary cause of epiphora. In pump failure, tears are not seen to drain into the lacrimal sac. In functional nasolacrimal duct obstruction, hold-up will be observed at the level of the lacrimal sac (see Figure 1.32).

Syringing and probing

- Explain the procedure to the patient and warn them they may taste salty water in the back of the throat.
- Ensure adequate anaesthesia with topical drops.
- Instil a single drop of 2% fluorescein and wait for a few minutes.
- Use a blunt-tipped lacrimal cannula on a 2.5 ml syringe filled with saline.
- Insert the cannula into the inferior punctum, at a 90° angle to the lid margin for the first 2 mm.
- If the punctum is too small to pass the cannula, a Nettleship dilator can be used to enlarge the punctum. As a general rule, if the lacrimal cannula passes without dilation, punctoplasty to enlarge the punctal is unnecessary.
- Pull the lower lid laterally with your other hand and angle the cannula tip parallel to the lid margin to advance into the inferior canaliculus.
- If there is resistance, pull back slightly and ensure the lid is taut; if lax, the canaliculus can become concertinaed, and the resistance you feel will be the canalicular wall rather than a 'soft stop' due to canalicular obstruction.
- Advance the tip gently until you feel a 'hard stop'. This is the medial wall of the lacrimal sac abutting the frontal process of the maxilla and lacrimal bones.
- Pull back slightly and gently irrigate. Table 1.3 details the outcomes that may be observed on irrigating the inferior punctum.

Table 1.3 Possible outcomes of syringe and probing

Outcome	Likely diagnosis
Free passage to the nose, no reflux	Patent nasolacrimal system
Passage into the nose but resistance felt or some reflux from the upper punctum	Partial nasolacrimal duct obstruction or stenosis
Fluorescein or mucous reflux from the upper punctum	Nasolacrimal duct obstruction with a dilated lacrimal sac
Clear reflux from the upper punctum	Common canalicular obstruction
Clear reflux from the lower punctum	Canalicular obstruction

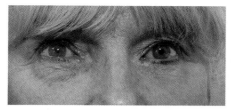

Fig 1.30 Prolonged fluorescein dye retention on the right

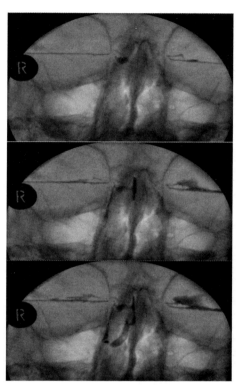

Fig 1.31 Dacryocystogram showing left common canalicular obstruction

On the left, the contrast medium is visibly refluxing around the eye. On the right, the patient has had dacryocystorhinostomy surgery. Contrast is seen to flow directly into the nasal cavity via a patent ostium. However, some contrast is still seen to flow into the nasolacrimal duct; this observation indicates that the lacrimal sac has not been fully opened during surgery

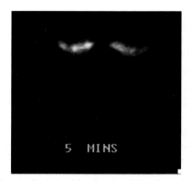

Fig 1.32 Lacrimal scintigraphy showing delayed transit from the lacrimal sac into the nasolacrimal duct

The patient's lacrimal sac is patent on syringing; this observation indicates functional nasolacrimal duct obstruction

Punctal stenosis

A common cause of epiphora is punctal stenosis. The punctum is visibly small on examination and may be covered with conjunctiva. If punctal dilation is possible, a Nettleship dilator may be used to enlarge the punctum size, and the patient may report a transient improvement in symptoms for a few days, but definitive treatment requires punctoplasty.

Treatment

The mainstay of treatment is a punctoplasty, which is usually performed as a 'three-snip' procedure in which the posterior wall of the canaliculus is opened (see Figure 1.33):

* Using Vannas scissors, insert one blade into the punctum, aiming vertically downwards for the first snip along the course of the vertical part of the canaliculus.
* The blade is then passed into the horizontal canaliculus for 2–3 mm, and a second snip is made to open it.
* The triangle of tissue is then removed with a third snip running from the punctum to the most medial part of the opened canaliculus. The lumen of the canaliculus should be visible.

Punctal eversion/medial ectropion

Punctal eversion may be subtle and only detectable on asking the patient to look up and down. The correct relationship between the punctum and tear film is essential if adequate tear drainage is to be achieved.

Treatment

In cases of punctal eversion, the restoration of the anatomical position of the punctum to lie in contact with the tear film may be achieved by removing a diamond-shaped piece of conjunctiva and tarsus inferior to the lower punctum. The wound edges are then approximated and tied either with a buried suture or by passing the sutures through the skin and tying them onto a bolster. The lower lid retractor is often incorporated into the suture before tying. This procedure is often combined with lid tightening procedures where appropriate (Section 1.15).

Canalicular obstruction

Causes of canalicular obstruction include ectodermal dysplasia, trauma, herpes virus infections, systemic cytotoxic drugs (e.g. fluorouracil), and cicatricial conjunctivitis (e.g. mucous membrane pemphigoid, lichen planus).

Nasolacrimal duct obstruction

Primary

This is the most common form of obstruction and is usually idiopathic with narrowing or obliteration of the nasolacrimal duct lumen as a common feature.

Secondary

* **Infection**: viral, bacterial (e.g. *Actinomyces*), fungal
* **Inflammation:** sarcoidosis, Wegeners granulomatosis
* **Neoplastic:** invasive squamous cell carcinoma of the eyelid, nasopharyngeal tumours
* **Other:** trauma, previous irradiation

Canaliculitis

Canaliculitis is normally a chronic condition. Patients present with a history of epiphora and copious discharge (typically string-like) and stickiness. Most commonly, it is due to infection with the anaerobic, Gram-negative rod *Actinomyces israelii*. There may be a history of punctal plug insertion or dry eye. On examination, the patient will have swelling of the medial eyelid margin, which may or may not be tender. The punctum is seen to be pouting, and a stringy discharge can be expressed from the punctum on gentle pressure over the canaliculus (see Figure 1.34).

Treatment

Definitive treatment requires a wide canaliculotomy, and expression of concretions, which can often be extensive (see Figure 1.35).

Dacryocystitis

Dacryocystitis is infection and distension of the lacrimal sac commonly associated with mucocele, which is a common sequelae of nasolacrimal duct obstruction. The accumulation of static mucous in the lacrimal sac predisposes to infection. Gram-positive bacteria are the most common pathogens.

Acute dacryocystitis

Patients present with epiphora and a raised, red, painful swelling in the medial canthal region (see Figure 1.36). There may be purulent discharge at the punctum, and an associated cellulitis. Extension of swelling above the medial canthal tendon is unusual and other pathologies should be considered in this context. Refer to a specialist and consider imaging in these cases.

Treatment

Lacrimal irrigation and probing should be avoided. Broad spectrum oral antibiotics such as co-amoxiclav are necessary for adequate treatment. Intravenous antibiotics may be indicated if there is significant associated cellulitis. When the acute infection has subsided, the definitive treatment requires a dacryocystorhinostomy procedure. Alternatively, where available, endoscopic endonasal dacryocystorhinostomy surgery can be an effective treatment for acute dacryocystitis.

Chronic dacryocystitis

In chronic cases, the patient may present with epiphora, mucous discharge, and a painless swelling in the region of the lacrimal sac. Gentle pressure over the mucocele normally results in reflux of mucous through the puncta, or directly on to the skin if a fistula has developed. If mucous is not expressed or if the swelling extends above the medial canthal tendon, consider other more sinister pathology and refer to a specialist for further evaluation.

Dacryocystorhinostomy

Principle

To create a channel for the flow of tears directly from the lacrimal sac to the nasal cavity, bypassing the nasolacrimal duct.

Indications

* Dacryocystitis
* Symptomatic partial or complete nasolacrimal duct obstruction, as demonstrated by lacrimal syringing

- Suspected functional nasolacrimal duct obstruction. Dacryo-cystorhinostomy has a lower success rate in relieving symptoms in these patients than in patients with demonstrable obstruction on syringing.

External dacryocystorhinostomy technique

1. A skin incision is made along the flat of the nose, medial to the medial canthus.
2. The superficial part of the medial canthal tendon is disinserted.
3. A bony window is created from the floor of the lacrimal fossa to the nasal mucosa (rhinostomy).
4. The lacrimal sac and nasal mucosa are incised to create anterior and posterior flaps. The corresponding posterior flaps are sutured together.
5. Silicone tubes are passed through the upper and lower canaliculi, tied, and then passed into the nasal cavity. This process prevents excessive scarring that might otherwise occlude the internal opening of the canaliculi into the nasal mucosa and which is a common cause of post-dacryocystorhinostomy failure.
6. The corresponding anterior flaps are sutured together and the skin is sutured (see Figure 1.37).

Post-operative epistaxis

- Post-operative epistaxis can be reduced by recovering upright, avoiding hot drinks and food for 48 hours after surgery, and avoiding active nose blowing for 2 weeks.
- If post-operative bleeding occurs, advising the patient to sit forwards, applying ice packs to the nasal bridge, and controlling pain and blood pressure will usually suffice.
- Packing should be considered if these measures fail to control bleeding.
- Patients should be carefully monitored for blood pressure and heart rate. Any sign of cardiovascular compromise should prompt referral to ENT surgeons for admission.

External versus endoscopic approach

Endoscopic dacryocystorhinostomy surgery has become increasingly popular for a number of reasons:

- No cutaneous scar
- Avoids disruption of the medial canthal tendon and orbicularis muscle. Thus the lacrimal pump remains intact.
- Rhinostomy can be performed using a drill, which can be more efficient when dealing with thick bone.
- Intraoperative time may be reduced, as flaps are not sutured.
- Nasal pathology (e.g. a deviated septum) may be corrected simultaneously.

However, the technique requires expensive equipment and surgeon expertise.

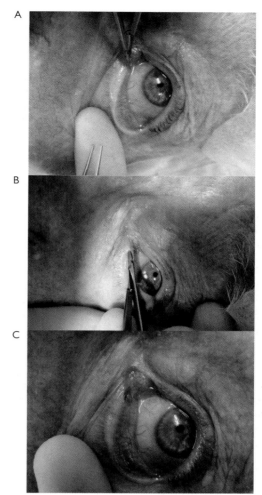

Fig 1.33 Three-snip procedure
A Vertical three-snip
B Horizontal three-snip
C Visible lumen of canaliculus at the end of the procedure

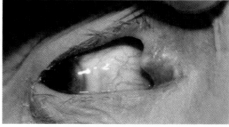

Fig 1.34 Canaliculitis involving the upper canaliculus
Note the pouting punctum and pus visible at the opening

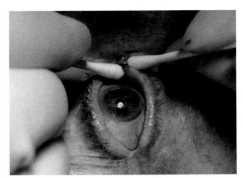

Fig 1.35 Milking of stones from the canaliculus using cotton-tipped applicators

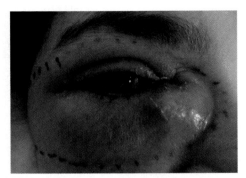

Fig 1.36 Acute dacryocystitis with abscess formation
Typically the swelling should not extend above the medial canthal tendon. Further extension warrants further investigation

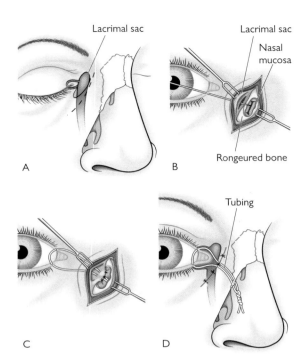

Fig 1.37 External dacryocystorhinostomy
A An incision is marked 10 mm from the medial canthus, starting just above the medial canthal tendon and extending inferiorly
B Bone from the lacrimal fossa and anterior lacrimal crest has been resected. Flaps have been fashioned in the nasal mucosa. A lacrimal probe extends through an incision in the lacrimal sac
C The anterior lacrimal sac flap is sutured to the anterior nasal mucosal flap after a silicone tube is placed
D Final position of the silicone tube following closure of the skin incision

Congenital ptosis

Congenital ptosis is most commonly due to idiopathic dysgenesis of the LPS, where the muscle fibres are replaced with fibroadipose tissue that has poor contractile ability. Levator function is reduced and, as the muscle fails to both contract and relax, the eyelid sometimes lags above the globe on down-gaze (see Figure 1.38). There may be associated superior rectus weakness. Associations of congenital ptosis include:

* Blepharophimosis syndrome
* Marcus Gunn jaw-winking syndrome. Misdirection of the nerve to the pterygoid muscle (a branch of the mandibular division of the trigeminal nerve) to the levator muscle causes elevation of the ptotic eyelid during mouth opening or chewing. Treatment is with levator disinsertion and brow suspension.
* Neurological causes, such as congenital oculomotor nerve palsy or Horner syndrome. Associated ocular motility abnormalities, anisocoria, and heterochromia are useful signs.

Clinical evaluation

Age-appropriate visual acuity, cycloplegic refraction, and dilated fundus examination are mandatory. The main issue governing the management of these conditions is the potential for sensory deprivation amblyopia.

Treatment

Early surgery is warranted for ptosis that occludes the visual axis or in cases where vision is persistently asymmetric. Patching is often necessary to promote visual development in the affected eye. Where levator function is reasonable (>4 mm), levator surgery (either advancement or excision) is performed. In cases of poor levator function (<4 mm), frontalis suspension is the procedure of choice. There is significant variation in the choice of suspension material for these cases, but generally synthetic material such as Supramid is used in children under 5 years of age, and autologous fascia lata is used for older children or adults.

Blepharophimosis Syndrome

Blepharophimosis syndrome is a rare autosomal dominant congenital disorder. It has characteristic features (see Figure 1.39) which include:

* Severe bilateral ptosis (often with poor levator function)
* Telecanthus (widening of the intercanthal distance owing to long medial canthal tendons)
* Epicanthus inversus (a fold of skin extending from the lower to upper eyelid in the medial canthal region)
* Other features including strabismus, lateral lower lid ectropion, a poorly developed nasal bridge, and hyperplasia of the superior orbital rims. Female patients with blepharophimosis are infertile.

Treatment

* Treating any amblyopia takes priority over any cosmetic correction.
* Staged surgical correction involves correction of the telecanthus with orbital wiring, Y-V plasty for the epicanthus inversus, and then bilateral frontal suspension for the ptosis.

Epiblepharon

Epiblepharon arises when the lower eyelid pretarsal muscle and skin override the lower eyelid margin to form a horizontal tissue fold, directing the lower lashes vertically upwards towards the globe (see Figure 1.40). It is common in children of Asian origin.

Treatment

The treatment for epiblepharon is normally conservative, as the condition tends to resolve as the child grows older. If there is lash-corneal touch, then lubricants can be useful. In more advanced cases, surgical correction is necessary (e.g. Hotz procedure, in which a strip of skin and orbicularis are removed).

Eyelid coloboma

An eyelid coloboma is a partial or full-thickness embryological eyelid defect. The most common site is at the junction of the medial and middle thirds of the eyelid. Upper eyelid defects that occur medially are normally an isolated anomaly. Lateral lower lid defects are often associated with systemic conditions such as Treacher Collins syndrome or Goldenhar syndrome. There may be associated congenital facial abnormalities such as cleft lip or palate. Patients may present with signs of corneal exposure.

Treatment

Small defects may be treated with primary closure. Larger defects may require lateral canthal semicircular flaps.

Capillary haemangioma

Aetiology

* A congenital hamartoma of vascular endothelial cells
* The most common benign orbital tumour in children
* Can be superficial (also known as 'strawberry naevus'; confined to the dermis) or deep (usually posterior to the orbital septum)
* Undergoes episodic periods of rapid growth in infants but mostly begin to slowly involute after children are age 2
* Fifty per cent of capillary haemangiomas will involute by the time the children are age 5, and 75% by the time the children are age 7.

Clinical evaluation

* Superficial lesions often present from birth or a few weeks later as a red mark on the eyelid that often blanches with pressure. Rapid growth usually occurs during the first year and there may be similar haemangiomas elsewhere on the body.
* Deep lesions may cause proptosis or globe displacement and increase in size during Valsalva manoeuvres or crying.
* May lead to anisometropia and amblyopia.

Investigations

* Ultrasound to exclude rhabdomyosarcoma (by showing vascularity). Regular ultrasound can also determine progression.
* Regular refraction and visual acuity to ensure amblyopia is not developing
* MRI shows a well-defined intra- or extraconal lesion in deep lesions.

Treatment

- Conservative, unless amblyopia is developing
- Intralesional steroid injections can lead to involution in up to 75% of cases, usually within 2 to 4 weeks. Repeated injections may be required. Side effects include lid and fat necrosis. Skin depigmentation as well as reports of central retinal artery occlusion.
- Systemic propranolol has been shown to be effective but requires monitoring by a paediatrician.

Congenital obstruction of the nasolacrimal system

Nasolacrimal duct obstruction

Nasolacrimal duct obstruction normally occurs because of delayed nasolacrimal duct canalization due to a membranous obstruction at the valve of Hasner.

Clinical evaluation

Presentation is with epiphora and matting of the eyelashes. Mucopurulent discharge may be present upon pressure over the lacrimal sac. Acute dacryocystitis is an uncommon sequela. It is important to rule out other causes of epiphora in infants, especially congenital glaucoma.

Treatment

Conservative measures include regular massaging of the lacrimal sac to try and encourage patency through the membranous obstruction. Topical antibiotics are indicated only if there is a concurrent conjunctivitis.

In approximately 90%–95% cases, the nasolacrimal duct canalizes by the age of 1 year. Therapeutic probing is therefore usually delayed until the child is 1 year old. Probing of the nasolacrimal duct results in perforation of the obstructing membrane and is successful in the vast majority of cases but may need repeating.

Dacryocystocele

A dacryocystocele is a collection of mucus (mucocele) or amniotic fluid (amniotocele) in the lacrimal sac and is due to an imperforate valve of Hasner.

Clinical evaluation

Patients present in the perinatal period with a dilated swelling below the medial canthal tendon.

Treatment

A dacryocystocele should be conservative initially, with local massage and topical antibiotics. If there is no response within 2 weeks or if infection develops, therapeutic probing is indicated.

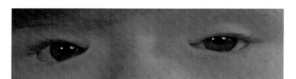

Fig 1.39 Blepharophimosis syndrome
Note the telecanthus, epicanthic folds, and bilateral ptosis

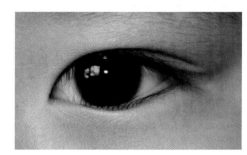

Fig 1.40 Epiblepharon
The lower lid fold misdirects the lashes to rub against the cornea

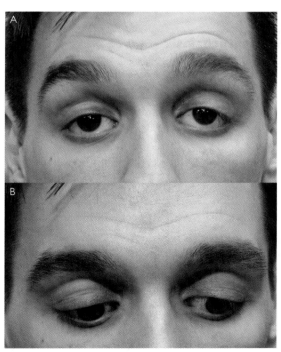

Fig 1.38 Bilateral congenital ptosis
A Note the significant frontalis overaction and markedly reduced levator function
B Both eyelids are high on down-gaze. Poor levator relaxation is a feature of congenital ptosis

1.14 Miscellaneous

Facial dystonias

Essential blepharospasm

Essential blepharospasm is a chronic condition that generally affects people over the age of 50, with a strong female preponderance. Patients report an increased blink frequency in response to everyday stimuli such as wind, light, and noise. This increase may be accompanied by photophobia or ocular discomfort. It has a well-described genetic association and is believed to be due to a maladaptive reflex response to chronic irritation in susceptible individuals. This response results in involuntary blinking and eyelid spasms that are bilateral and involve the orbicularis oculi, corrugator, and procerus muscles. Blepharospasm also commonly forms part of a segmental midface and orofacial dystonia which is sometimes referred to as **Meige** or **Breughel syndrome**.

Treatment

* Reduce ocular surface irritation that may trigger episodes (e.g. via artificial tears, blepharitis treatment, tinted glasses).
* Botulinum toxin injections.
* Orbicularis myectomy can be useful in resistant cases to further weaken the orbicularis muscle.
* Pharmacotherapy (e.g. GABA agonists, dopamine antagonists) is often unsatisfactory as a first-line treatment and is often reserved for those cases unresponsive to botulinum toxin.
* Patients who are unresponsive to botulinum toxin may have a component of apraxia of eyelid opening. In these patients, frontalis suspension may be considered.

Botulinum toxin

Botulinum toxin injection is highly effective at alleviating symptoms. The toxin blocks vesicular acetylcholine release at presynaptic nerve terminals, causing paralysis of the effector muscle. This treatment usually takes 5–7 days for maximal effect and often will give relief of symptoms for approximately 3 months. It can take a few cycles of treatment to establish the effective dosing protocol for that particular patient. A number of different botulinum toxin preparations are available.

Complications include subconjunctival haemorrhage, ptosis, lagophthalmos with associated corneal exposure, and rarely double vision.

Hemifacial spasm

Hemifacial spasm is an involuntary spasm of muscles supplied by the facial nerve. It affects patients in middle age and is almost always unilateral. The spasms can affect any muscle innervated by the facial nerve, including the platysma. Hemifacial spasm often presents to an ophthalmologist, as the first symptoms are noticed round the eye.

Hemifacial spasm is due to irritation of the facial nerve; the irritation may be caused by compressive lesions (e.g. tumours, vascular loops, or arteriovenous malformations) or non-compressive lesions (e.g. stroke, or multiple sclerosis plaques). The most common sites are at the exit of the nerve from the brainstem, where inferior cerebellar artery vascular loops can compress the nerve. Cerebellopontine angle lesions are also a common cause. It is essential that all patients have a full cranial nerve examination including a corneal sensation assessment, and all patients should have an MRI scan of the facial nerve pathway.

Treatment

Botulinum toxin injection is the treatment of choice. However, neurosurgical decompression of vascular anomalies can also be successful in alleviating symptoms.

Floppy eyelid syndrome

Floppy eyelid syndrome is characterized by lax upper eyelids, chronic papillary conjunctivitis, and symptoms of discomfort. The tarsal plate has a loss of rigidity, and the eyelid can be easily everted with minimal lateral traction (see Figure 1.41). Irritation occurs owing to spontaneous eversion during sleep, with the tarsal conjunctiva rubbing against the pillow. It is most commonly seen in obese men and there is an association with obstructive sleep apnoea. The condition is also associated with keratoconus; thus, chronic eye rubbing and mechanical trauma may be aetiological factors.

Treatment

Conservative treatment options, including eyelid patching, taping of the eyelids at night, lubricants, and blepharitis treatment, are usually ineffective. Surgical management is often needed to tighten the upper eyelids. Horizontal lid shortening procedures, such as an upper eyelid lateral canthal sling, are effective in up to 70% of cases.

Dermatochalasis

Dermatochalasis is a common condition normally occurring in elderly patients. It is characterized by excess eyelid skin, which may be associated with orbital fat prolapse. It can cause a mechanical ptosis or pseudoptosis. The upper lid show is reduced, and the overhanging skin may occlude the visual axis (see Figure 1.42). Blepharoplasty, in which the redundant skin is excised, may be performed for cosmesis or if the excess skin is causing a superior field defect. It is important to assess the brow position, as brow ptosis may worsen the dermatochalasis and it may be more appropriate to perform a brow lift in these patients.

Allergic lid swelling

Atopic dermatitis (eczema)

Atopic dermatitis is often associated with generalized eczema, asthma, and hay fever. Patients complain of itchy/dry/swollen eyelid skin. More severe cases result in thickening and fissuring of the eyelid skin. There may be associated vernal or atopic keratoconjunctivitis. Treatment for mild cases is with allergen avoidance advice together with emollients. More severe cases will require topical steroids.

Contact dermatitis

Contact dermatitis manifests in the eyelids as a Type 4 hypersensitivity reaction to allergens such as preservatives in topical medication. Patients present with swelling, erythema, and crusting of the eyelids. Symptoms normally resolve on withdrawal of the inciting cause.

Acute allergic oedema

Acute allergic oedema is characterized by acute, normally bilateral, painless lid oedema. This condition is usually due to contact allergy or an insect bite. Other causes include angioedema and drug reactions. Treatment is with systemic antihistamines.

Blepharochalasis

Blepharochalasis is a rare variant of angioneurotic oedema that occurs in young patients. It is characterized by idiopathic episodes of acute eyelid oedema. With time, the eyelid skin becomes chronically thinned and can take on the appearance of dermatochalasis.

Infectious lid swelling

Herpes simplex

Herpes simplex infection in the eyelid presents with crops of vesicles, which after a few days will rupture, crust, and heal. It can be associated with a variety of ocular surface conditions (see Chapter 2). Treatment is with topical and sometimes systemic acyclovir.

Herpes zoster ophthalmicus

Herpes zoster ophthalmicus (HZO) normally affects elderly or immunocompromised individuals. Presentation is with tingling followed by pain in the distribution of the ophthalmic division of the trigeminal nerve (V_1). The first sign is normally a raised erythematous rash in the distribution of the V_1 dermatome. The rash, but not necessarily the oedema, respects the midline. After a few days, vesicles form, which eventually crust over. Treatment is with acyclovir 800 mg orally five times a day for 1 week. A common sequela of HZO is postherpetic neuralgia, which can persist permanently.

Bacterial causes of lid swelling

There are a number of bacterial infections that can cause eyelid infections, including:

* Impetigo (*Staphylococcus aureus, Streptococcus pyogenes*)
* Erysipelas (*Strep.pyogenes*)
* Necrotizing fasciitis (*Strep. pyogenes, Staph. aureus*)

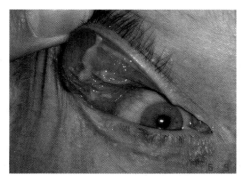

Fig 1.41 Floppy eyelid syndrome
The upper lid is easily everted on lateral traction. Note the tarsal conjunctival changes associated with chronic irritation

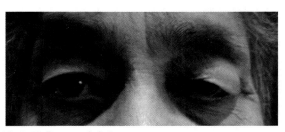

Fig 1.42 Dermatochalasis
Note the absent upper lid show on both sides and the frontalis overaction on the right. This reaction keeps the excess skin from affecting the visual field; however, this effect may be reduced as the patient tires towards the end of the day

1.15 Practical skills in oculoplastics

Using diathermy safely

Surgical diathermy or cautery uses a high-frequency alternating electric current to induce localized tissue burning. Depending on the current characteristics, it can be used to cut or coagulate tissue. The patient's body may form part of the electrical circuit.

- **Monopolar:** an electrical plate is placed under the patient and acts as an indifferent electrode. A current passes between the instrument and this electrode but, as the instrument tip is a great deal smaller than the electrode plate, heat is generated at the tip.
- **Bipolar:** two electrodes are combined in the instrument (e.g. forceps). The current passes between the tips and not through the patient. The tips must be held apart for the current to pass between them.

The handheld cautery devices use a direct current to heat a nichrome wire.

Diathermy can interfere with pacemaker function. In patients with metal implants, the electrode plate must be placed above the metal implant.

Removing sutures

For removing interrupted sutures, hold the suture with fine non-toothed forceps, cut it on one side of the knot as close to the skin as possible, and then remove it with a swift movement. If a continuous suture has been used, cut the suture at intervals to reduce discomfort of pulling the suture through a long distance.

Preparing a biopsy sample

When preparing a tissue biopsy, it is important to distinguish between an incisional and an excisional biopsy. For an incisional biopsy, no orientation is necessary, as the sample will be used to determine the diagnosis only. For excisional biopsies, try to limit manipulation of the tissue edges, as these will be examined to see if the pathological process extends to these margins. The surgeon should avoid grasping and re-grasping the tissue specimen. Avoid excessive local anaesthetic infiltration and inject from outside the area to be excised. The tissue should be orientated with sutures (see Figure 1.43)—preferably a non-braided suture made of Prolene or nylon. A long suture usually designates the lateral margin, and a short suture indicates the superior edge. A diagram should also be provided on the histology request form, to give as much information to the pathologist as possible. The specimen should be placed in the pot and the lid sealed to prevent leakage of formalin and subsequent desiccation of the tissue. Some specimens will be sent as 'fresh' (without formalin) for immunofluorescence studies or specialist solutions such as Michels medium for mucous membrane pemphigoid.

Surgical repair of lid trauma

Always check the patient's tetanus status and prescribe oral antibiotics (such as co-amoxiclav 375 mg three times per day or cephalexin 250 mg four times a day for 1 week). Careful exploration is essential to establish the extent of the wound (see Figure 1.44). This is best done with local anaesthetic and a cotton bud. **Always** evert the eyelids and ensure there is no underlying globe trauma.

Lacerations involving only anterior lamella (skin and/or orbicularis) can be closed with non-absorbable sutures. There should be no tension when closing the skin to avoid distortion of the lid, particularly in the lower lid, as there is a risk of cicatricial ectropion. In cases where there is tissue loss, undermining the skin, advancement flaps, or skin grafts may be required. Where possible, try to close the lower eyelid vertically rather than horizontally to minimize lid retraction and ectropion.

Full-thickness lid lacerations involving the eyelid margin require careful apposition of the lid margin edges to prevent notch formation, which can cause watering or ocular surface exposure (see Figure 1.45). A grey line suture is essential to align the eyelid for accurate placement of the tarsal plate sutures (see Figures 1.46). The grey line suture should ideally be long (e.g. a mattress suture) to prevent cheesewiring, and a non-absorbable suture should be used. A second 'lash line' suture can also be placed in the same manner. When tied, the wound edges should be slightly everted to reduce the risk of notching. The ends of the suture can be left long and then tied down with the skin sutures; 6–0 Vicryl can be used to appose the tarsal plate. Finally, the skin can be closed with 6–0 non-absorbable sutures that are removed after a week.

If the canaliculus is involved, repair should take place under general anaesthetic, as local anaesthetic will cause swelling and distortion of the cut ends of the canaliculus. First, try to identify the proximal cut end by direct visualization; often the operating microscope is essential in these cases. Additionally, topical adrenaline or phenylephrine can be used to differentiate the pale canaliculus from surrounding tissue. Monocanalicular stents such as the Mini Monoka stent can be used to oppose the cut ends and are secured in place with 6–0 Vicryl to the pericanalicular tissue and the orbicularis. Alternatively, a Barnard stent can be used to approximate the canaliculus, with the stents passed to the inferior meatus and tied off.

Protection of the ocular surface

A number of conditions can lead to corneal exposure, including thyroid eye disease, facial nerve palsy (see Figure 1.10), and cicatricial ectropion. Treatment options depend on many factors, such as severity of exposure, degree of Bells phenomenon, and the likelihood of spontaneous recovery.

Botulinum toxin injection

Botulinum toxin blocks synaptic vesicular acetylcholine release from nerve terminals, thus causing temporary paralysis of the treated muscles. Injection into the levator muscle can induce a ptosis to protect the cornea from further exposure. This treatment is only appropriate in patients who have good vision in their other eye as the effect can last for 3 months or longer.

The injection should be given through a posterior eyelid approach, with the eyelid everted to reduce the risk of superior rectus paralysis and globe perforation.

The procedure is as follows:

- Instil topical anaesthesia.
- The upper eyelid is everted and then the toxin injected via a tuberculin syringe above the upper border of the tarsus into the subaponeurotic space lateral to the midline. A dose of 40 units of Dysport or 5 units of Botox or Xeomin is typically used.
- The ptosis can take 3–5 days to develop.

The main complication of this procedure is superior rectus paralysis resulting in vertical diplopia. The underaction can persist after complete resolution of the ptosis.

Lateral tarsorraphy

Lateral tarsorraphy may be either temporary or permanent. It is cosmetically undesirable but can be very effective in reducing corneal exposure. However, it also reduces the visual field and can limit examination of the eye.

1. The length of the tarsorraphy is marked.
2. Local anaesthesia is infiltrated into the upper and lower eyelids.
3. A grey line split of the desired length is made in the upper and lower eyelids by using a feather blade.
4. The posterior lamella of the lid margin is shaved along the desired length to expose the tarsal plate.
5. A double-ended 5–0 non-absorbable suture made from materials such as Prolene or nylon is passed from 4 mm below the lower lid lash line through the exposed tarsal plate (partial thickness to avoid corneal irritation) to exit the grey line.
6. The suture is then passed through a corresponding point in the exposed tarsal plate of the upper eyelid to exit through the upper eyelid skin, 4 mm above the lash line.
7. The other end of the suture is passed through a piece of tarsorrhaphy tubing and then returned through the same tissue path to exit through the lower eyelid skin.
8. The two ends of the suture are then tied over another piece of tarsorrhaphy tubing.
9. The sutures are removed at 2 weeks.

The tarsorraphy can be opened at any time but can leave an irregular lid margin. For permanent tarsorraphy, the anterior lamella is excised from the lower lid, and the posterior lamella is excised from the upper eyelid. The upper and lower lids are then sutured with double-ended 6–0 Vicryl sutures.

Emergency lateral canthotomy/cantholysis

The orbit is a closed compartment; therefore, an increase in orbital volume can rapidly lead to a rise in orbital pressure as a result of a compartment syndrome. This increase in pressure can result in optic nerve ischaemia, causing irreversible blindness within 1–2 hours unless prompt treatment is given. Retrobulbar haemorrhage is the most common cause, occurring secondary to trauma, orbital surgery, and retrobulbar injections, as well as occurring spontaneously owing to vascular anomalies. Intense orbital infection and inflammation may also lead to an acute rise in orbital pressure.

Clinical presentation

Patients present with a tense orbit, severe pain, ophthalmoplegia, proptosis, chemosis, high intraocular pressure (IOP), and signs of optic nerve compromise.

Management

If an orbital compartment syndrome is suspected on clinical grounds, a canthotomy should be performed immediately, even before any imaging. The aim is to release the inferior limb of the lateral canthal tendon and associated septal components from the orbital rim to allow for expansion of the orbital contents and outflow of haemorrhage.

1. Consent should be obtained from the patient.
2. Infiltrate 2% xylocaine with 1:200,000 adrenaline into the lateral lower eyelid and lateral canthus.
3. Prep and drape the area.
4. Sit at the side of the patient.
5. Apply a straight artery clip to the lateral angle towards the lateral orbital rim for 20 seconds (see Figure 1.47).
6. Hold the lower lid with large forceps such as Addson forceps and, using sharp scissors, make a cut that extends 1 cm from the lateral canthal angle towards the orbital rim (see Figure 1.48).
7. The lower lid is then reflected to reveal the lateral canthal tendon, which is then cut with the scissors. Diathermy may be applied before successive cuts to minimize bleeding. The cantholysis is deemed sufficient if the lower lid can be freely detracted from the globe (see Figure 1.49).
8. IOP and optic nerve function should be reassessed. Further reduction in orbital pressure can be achieved by cutting the superior limb of the lateral canthal tendon.
9. Haemostasis can be achieved with either diathermy or prolonged pressure on the eyelid (but not the globe).
10. A dressing should be applied and the patient placed on prophylactic oral antibiotics (such as co-amoxiclav 375 mg three times a day).
11. The tendon can be reattached in the future once the acute event has subsided.

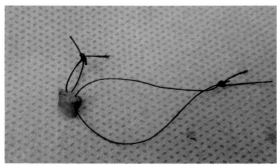

Fig 1.43 Orientation sutures for a biopsy specimenA long suture indicates the lateral edge, and a short suture, the superior edge

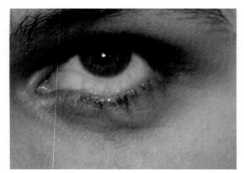

Fig 1.45 Ineffective approximation of the tarsal plate can lead to notch formation. The two ends of the tarsal plate are clearly visible. This condition can be avoided with careful positioning of tarsal plate sutures

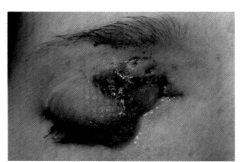

Fig 1.44 Eyelid lacerations may be extensive and involve the canaliculus. All patients must have a complete ophthalmic examination to rule out globe rupture

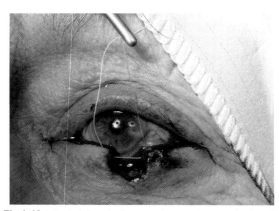

Fig 1.46 It is vital that the first tarsal suture is correctly aligned to avoid a notch

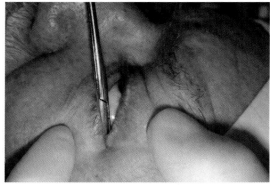

Fig 1.47 An artery clip is placed across the lateral canthal angle

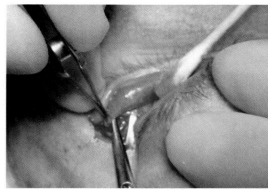

Fig 1.49 Cantholysis using Westcott scissors or sharp straight scissors

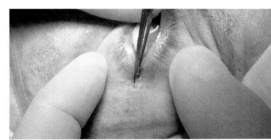

Fig 1.48 Canthotomy with sharp scissors

Chapter 2

Cornea and conjunctiva

Georgia Cleary, Allon Barsam, and Stephen Tuft

2.1 Corneal and conjunctival basic science

Corneal anatomy and physiology

Gross anatomy

The cornea is the transparent anterior portion of the eyeball. It has two main functions:

1. To protect the intraocular contents by providing a mechanical and chemical barrier
2. To provide two-thirds of the overall refractive power of the eye

In order to fulfil these functions, the cornea must maintain its shape, its strength, and its optical transparency. The cornea makes up approximately one-sixth of the external eye, with the sclera making up the other five-sixths. The junction of the cornea and the sclera is known as the limbus. The anatomical limbus lies slightly posterior to the surgical limbus.

The cornea is transversely oval, with an average horizontal diameter of 12.6 mm and an average vertical diameter of 11.7 mm in an adult. It is aspheric, with the greatest convex curvature in the central 3.0 mm zone. The cornea is thinnest in the centre (around 540 μm) and becomes progressively thicker towards the periphery (around 700 μm). The cornea provides 40–44 dioptres (D) of the refractive power of the eye (anterior surface, about +49 D; posterior surface, −6.0 D).

Corneal nutrition

The cornea is avascular. To maintain transparency, it derives its nutrition mainly from the tear film and the aqueous humour. The limbus is supplied by both internal (anterior ciliary branch of ophthalmic artery) and external (facial branch) carotid arteries.

Corneal innervation

The cornea has a rich sensory innervation (300–400 times that of skin). Sensory innervation is derived from the long ciliary nerves, a branch of the ophthalmic division of the trigeminal (the fifth cranial nerve). These nerves reach the cornea via the limbus. They pass radially forwards within the stroma before branching anteriorly to finish as free nerve endings within the corneal epithelium. Loss of corneal innervation reduces the stimulus for blinking, tear production, and epithelial proliferation.

Precorneal tear film

The surface of the corneal epithelium is irregular, with multiple finger-like projections (microvilli). In order to function as an optical surface, the covering precorneal tear film is required (see Figure 2.1). The air–tear interface is the major refractive interface of the eye. The tear film is 7 μm thick. The tear film is considered to have two distinct layers, plus a mucous gradient dispersed throughout the layers:

1. The outermost lipid layer (secreted by the meibomian glands) functions to reduce evaporation of the aqueous layer and acts as a surfactant for tear spreading and to contain the tear film on the lid margin
2. The middle aqueous layer (secreted by the main and accessory lacrimal glands) functions to supply oxygen and metabolites to the avascular corneal epithelium, carry antibacterial tear proteins (lactoferrin), and wash away debris and bacteria

Corneal histology

The cornea is a multilayered structure (see Figure 2.2) consisting from anterior to posterior of:

1. Epithelium
2. Bowman's layer
3. Stroma
4. Descemet's membrane
5. Endothelium

Epithelium

The epithelium (50 μm thick) comprises 5–6 cell layers of non-keratinized stratified squamous epithelium, which can be further subdivided into:

1. Two or three layers of superficial cells. Tight junctions between these cells prevent the flow of water into the stroma and consequent stromal oedema.
2. Two or three layers of wing cells
3. A monolayer of columnar basal cells which divide to replace continuous desquamation from the surface of the corneal epithelium. Basal cells adhere to the underlying basement membrane, which they also secrete. Central migration and then replication of basal cells act to repair epithelial defects. Limbal stem cells (see 'Limbal stem cells') are the source of new epithelial cells in wound healing.

Bowman's layer

Bowman's layer (10 μm thick) is an acellular layer of collagen fibres lying between the epithelial basement membrane and the stroma. Bowman's layer does not regenerate after injury, and breaks in this layer heal with cellular scar tissue.

Stroma

Stroma (450 μm thick) consists of extracellular matrix (mainly Type 1 collagen and proteoglycans: 65% keratin sulphate and 30% chondroitin/dermatin sulphate), keratocytes (modified fibroblasts), and nerve fibres. Corneal transparency is maintained as a result of the uniform size of and distance between the stromal collagen fibres (both the size and distance are less than half the wavelength of visible light). If the stroma becomes overhydrated, or distorted by injury/scarring, this regular architecture and transparency is lost and the stroma becomes opaque.

Stromal wound healing involves the laying down of Type 3 collagen by keratocytes. Collagen remodelling occurs and the tensile strength of the corneal stroma increases after injury for up to 6 months. In response to injury/inflammation/infection, activated keratocytes and other inflammatory cells (from the limbal vessels and tear film) may cause collagenolysis and stromal melting.

Descemet's membrane

Descemet's membrane is the basement membrane secreted by the endothelium. It consists of an anterior banded zone secreted during fetal life (2–4 μm), and a posterior non-banded zone that increases in thickness throughout life (12 μm in the elderly). Composed of mainly Type 4 collagen and laminin, it is a barrier to the penetration of cells but not water or small molecules from the aqueous layer to the stroma.

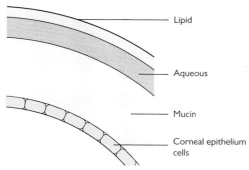

Fig 2.1 Precorneal tear film

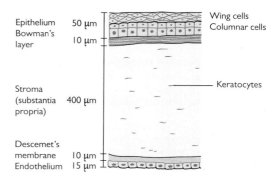

Fig 2.2 Corneal histology

Endothelium

The endothelium is a single layer of polygonal (mainly hexagonal) cells arranged in a mosaic. Cell density decreases with age (around 6000 cells/mm² at birth, and 2600 cells/mm² in adults). Endothelial cells do not proliferate but cell loss is compensated for by an increase in size when the cells become more irregular in shape (polymegethism). A minimum density of approximately 600 cells/mm² is required to maintain correct corneal hydration. Endothelial cells have sodium/potassium pumps and bicarbonate pumps that remove water from the stroma and maintain the optimum level of stromal hydration for transparency (78% water). Persistently high intraocular pressure damages the endothelium so that water can enter the stroma and cause the cornea to swell and become hazy.

Limbal stem cells

At the limbus, epithelial cells are thrown into folds by stromal ridges known as the palisades of Vogt. The corneal epithelial stem cells are thought to lie between these ridges. The function of the limbal stem cells is to provide a source of cells for epithelial regeneration. They also function as a junctional barrier that prevents the conjunctiva from growing onto the cornea (conjunctivalization).

Conjunctival anatomy and physiology

Gross anatomy

The conjunctiva is a thin mucous membrane that lines the eyelids (see Chapter 1, Section 1.1) and is reflected at the superior and inferior fornices onto the surface of the globe. Medially, the conjunctiva is folded to form the plica semilunaris. Medial to the plica semilunaris lies the caruncle, a fleshy tissue mass containing

fine hairs and sebaceous glands (see Figure 2.3). The conjunctiva can be further subdivided as follows:

- **Palpebral conjunctiva:** this structure starts at the lid margin and is firmly attached to the tarsal plates.
- **Forniceal conjunctiva:** this structure is loosely attached to the underlying fascial expansions of the levator and rectus muscle sheaths.
- **Bulbar conjunctiva:** this translucent layer lies over the anterior globe. It is loosely attached to Tenon's capsule except at the limbus, where Tenon's capsule and the conjunctiva fuse and are firmly attached to the sclera and the cornea.

Conjunctival histology

The conjunctiva has an epithelial surface of non-keratinizing stratified columnar cells (bulbar conjunctiva) or stratified squamous cells (palpebral and limbal conjunctiva) that rest on a lamina propria of loose connective tissue. The conjunctiva contains goblet cells that contribute to the mucin layer of the tear film. The accessory lacrimal glands of Krause and Wolfring are located within the substantia propria (see Figure 2.4).

Follicles

Follicles are subepithelial aggregations of hyperplastic conjunctival associated lymphoid tissue. They are encircled by blood vessels and are most clearly seen in the superior and inferotemporal fornix.

Papillae

Papillae result from epithelial hyperplasia and oedema and contain a vascular core.

Blood supply and lymphatic drainage

The blood supply and lymphatic drainage for conjunctiva is as for the eyelids (see Chapter 1, Section 1.1).

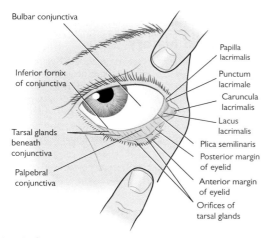

Fig 2.3 Conjunctival anatomy

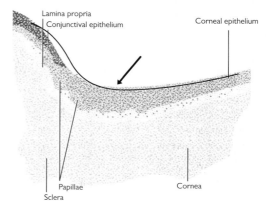

Fig 2.4 Conjunctival histology

2.2 History taking for anterior segment disease

A clinical history should be targeted to identify risk factors for disease, determine underlying aetiology, and gauge the severity of symptoms. A thorough history is instrumental in making the correct diagnosis and will guide individualized patient management.

When constructing a differential diagnosis, the usual surgical sieve should be considered: infectious, iatrogenic (drugs/surgery), autoimmune, traumatic, vascular, metabolic, neoplastic, and congenital.

Presenting complaint

Red eye
* **Infectious disease:** bacterial or viral conjunctivitis; microbial keratitis, especially from contact lens wear, secondary to lid/orbital infections (blepharoconjunctivitis, canaliculitis, preseptal/orbital cellulitis); blebitis; endophthalmitis
* **Iatrogenic:** drop allergy, drop/preservative toxicity, following any form of eye surgery
* **Autoimmune/hypersensitivity:** allergic conjunctivitis, staphylococcal hypersensitivity (marginal keratitis, rosacea keratitis), episcleritis, scleritis, anterior uveitis, ocular mucous membrane pemphigoid, Stevens–Johnson syndrome
* **Traumatic:** conjunctival/corneal abrasion, corneal/subtarsal foreign body, contact lens associated giant papillary conjunctivitis, corneal laceration, chemical injury, phototoxic keratopathy
* **Vascular:** subconjunctival haemorrhage, carotid–cavernous fistula, cluster headache
* **Other:** dry eye, hypoxic contact lens keratopathy, eyelash–ocular surface contact (trichiasis, entropion), inflamed pterygium/pingueculum, acute glaucoma, epithelial defect from corneal decompensation

Burning/sore eye
* Blepharitis, conjunctivitis, drop allergy, dry eye, non-infective contact lens related keratopathy, marginal keratitis, episcleritis, inflamed pterygium/pingueculum

Foreign body sensation
* As for burning/sore eye. Any disturbance of the corneal or conjunctival epithelial integrity will give a foreign body sensation.

Itchy eyes
* Allergic conjunctivitis, blepharitis, eyelid dermatitis, contact lens associated giant papillary conjunctivitis

Ocular pain/photophobia
Any corneal epithelial defect can give these symptoms. Causes include microbial keratitis, keratoconjunctivitis, corneal abrasion, and corneal foreign body. Other causes are anterior uveitis, scleritis, endophthalmitis, and acute glaucoma.

Blurred vision
Abnormalities of the tear film may cause blurred vision that improves or resolves with blinking. Corneal pathology (opacity or abnormal curvature) affecting the central part of the cornea will also produce blurred vision. Other causes include uncorrected refractive error, cataract, posterior capsular opacification after cataract surgery, severe iritis, acute glaucoma, and posterior segment/neurological disorders.

Watery eyes
Broadly, watery eyes may be due to outflow obstruction (see Chapter 1, Section 1.11) or excess lacrimation. Common anterior segment diseases causing excess lacrimation include blepharitis, conjunctivitis, corneal abrasion, chemical injury, corneal/subtarsal foreign body, and ectropion.

Discharge
* Blepharitis, conjunctivitis, mucous fishing syndrome, blepharoconjunctivitis, nasolacrimal outflow obstruction with mucocele

History of presenting complaint

Onset/duration
* Sudden (subconjunctival haemorrhage), acute (trauma, infection, angle-closure glaucoma), subacute (allergic conjunctivitis), herpes simplex keratitis (HSK), chronic (cataract), acute on chronic (rosacea keratitis), recurrent (epithelial erosion, HSK, anterior uveitis)

Associated features
* Severity, precipitating/relieving factors, response to previous treatment if recurrent, mechanism of injury for trauma

Past ocular history

Refraction
* Glasses, history of contact lens wear (type, duration of wear, overnight wear, cleaning regime, showering or swimming with lenses)

Trauma
* Physical (recurrent corneal erosion syndrome), chemical (limbal stem cell failure, corneal scarring), radiation (ocular surface disease, neoplasia, welding)

Surgery
* Intraocular surgery (endothelial dysfunction), corneal refractive surgery (post-LASIK dry eye/flap dehiscence)

Viral infection
* Previous HSK; herpes zoster ophthalmicus (HZO; interstitial keratitis)

Past medical history

General medical conditions that are associated with anterior segment pathology are discussed in more detail in State Chapter 7 for completeness and I think this has changed now to the medical ophthalmology /uveitis chapter – Venki/Lucy to advis-Sections 4.18, 4.19, and 4.22. Diseases that should be specifically elicited from the clinical history include:
* **Atopy:** asthma/eczema/hay fever associated with allergic conjunctivitis
* **Rheumatological disease:** dry eye, corneal melt, scleritis
* **Neurological disease:** facial nerve palsy, exposure keratopathy
* **Sexually transmitted disease:** chlamydial conjunctivitis, gonococcal conjunctivitis

- **Skin disease:** acne vulgaris or rosacea, eczema
- **Metabolic disease:** hypercalcaemia, band keratopathy

Drug history

Topical medications

- Toxicity caused by eye drops, particularly preservatives
- Topical steroid use may predispose to viral keratitis, fungal keratitis, glaucoma, and cataract.
- Corneal deposits (ciprofloxacin)

Systemic medications

- Systemic steroid (as for topical)
- Amiodarone (vortex keratopathy)

Previous allergies to systemic and topical medications (including preservatives) must be documented.

Family history

- Glaucoma, inherited corneal dystrophies, contact with infectious conjunctivitis

Social history

- Country of previous residence (sun exposure and pterygium/pingueculum/neoplasia, poor sanitation, trachoma)
- Occupation and hobbies; appreciation of these is needed to understand the patient's visual requirements (e.g. sports, driving, reading)
- Social and individual circumstances for compliance with treatment and follow-up
- Patients' expectations are an important consideration for any surgery.

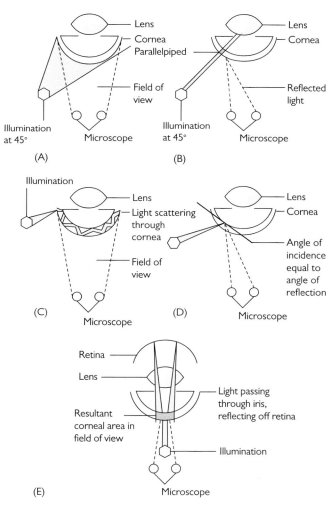

Fig 2.5 Diagrammatic representation of various slit lamp illumination techniques for corneal examination (see section 2.3): (A)diffuse illumination (B) direct focal illumination (C) sclerotic scatter, (D) specular reflection, (E) retroillumination

How to examine the anterior segment

The slit lamp has two main components: the biomicroscope (the viewing system) and the slit illuminator. Systematic examination of the anterior segment includes examination of the ocular adnexa, the conjunctiva, the episclera, the sclera, the tear film, the cornea, the anterior chamber, the iris, the lens, and the anterior vitreous.

Introduction
Introduce yourself to the patient.

Observation
General observation of the patient as a whole, aimed at identifying features of intercurrent or associated disease:
* **Skin:** atopic dermatitis (allergic conjunctivitis, keratoconus, cataract), acne vulgaris, seborrheic dermatitis, rosacea (blepharitis, rosacea keratitis)
* **Hands:** deformities in rheumatoid arthritis (dry eyes, corneal melt, scleritis) and nails (Stevens–Johnson syndrome)
* **Musculoskeletal:** kyphosis in ankylosing spondylitis (anterior uveitis)

Set up slit lamp
* Ensure examiner and patient comfort/position by adjusting the chair height, slit lamp height, and chin rest position.
* Ensure eyepieces are set for examiner's interpupillary distance and refraction so that binocularity is achieved.

Adnexa
* Set the slit lamp on low magnification with a neutral density filter (low illumination) and diffuse illumination.
* Eyelids: closure, position, blepharitis, tumour
* Eyelashes: trichiasis, madarosis, poliosis.
(See Chapter 1 for more details and definitions).

Conjunctiva
* **Palpebral conjunctiva:** evert upper lids (subtarsal foreign bodies, papillae, follicles, scarring)
* **Fornices:** chemosis/discharge/pseudomembrane (conjunctivitis), forniceal shortening/symblepharon/fibrosis (ocular cicatricial pemphigoid)
* **Bulbar conjunctiva:** hyperaemia, haemorrhage, pingueculum or pterygium, conjunctival stain with fluorescein (abrasion, drying, ulceration)
  Note: remember to lift the upper lid to look for a trabeculectomy bleb.
* **Limbal conjunctiva:** ciliary flush (anterior uveitis), Horner–Trantas dots (vernal conjunctivitis), Herberts pits (old trachoma)
  Note: Perform conjunctival swabs before instilling fluorescein if using immunofluorescent detection methods. If PCR is used, fluorescein will not affect the test result.

Episclera/sclera
* Examine for evidence of inflammation.

Tear film
* Examine tear meniscus for height and debris.
* Examine tear break-up time using fluorescein and a cobalt-blue filter.
* Schirmer test
See Section 2.6 for more details.

Cornea
See Figure 2.5 for a description of slit lamp techniques for corneal examination. Note: if patients are in significant discomfort from ocular surface disease, topical anaesthesia may be required to facilitate examination. It is important to test and document corneal sensation (herpetic/neurotrophic keratitis) prior to the instillation of anaesthetic.

Epithelium
* Defects are best seen with special staining (see 'Special dyes').
* Look for punctate epithelial erosions (non-specific signs of epithelial damage), microcysts (corneal oedema, epithelial erosion syndrome), mucous filaments (dry eye), and dendritic ulceration of herpes infection.
* **Iron lines:** Hudson–Stähli line, Fleischer ring (keratoconus); best seen with red-free (green) light

Bowman's layer
* Subepithelial corneal vascularization and fibrosis, termed pannus if at superior cornea border
* Look for band-shaped keratopathy (chronic anterior uveitis, hypercalcaemia).
* Look for anterior scars and raised areas of Salzmann nodular degeneration.

Stroma
* Infiltrates (sterile, infected), opacities (dystrophies and degenerations)
* Stromal oedema (corneal decompensation after endothelial damage), herpes simplex disciform keratitis
* Stromal vascularization (interstitial keratitis, contact lens overwear, infection, inflammation)
* Stromal scarring
* Ectasia
* With the exception of oedema, all of these processes can be associated with stromal thinning.

Descemet's membrane
* Folds (hypotony, stromal oedema)
* Breaks: trauma, advanced keratoconus, congenital glaucoma (Haab's striae)
* Thickening associated with guttata (Fuchs endothelial dystrophy)

Endothelium
* Pigment deposits: Krukenberg spindle (pigment dispersion syndrome)
* Keratic precipitates (anterior uveitis)
* Endotheliitis (HSK)

Anterior chamber
* Set slit lamp on high magnification and high intensity, with a 1 mm wide, 3 mm long slit.
* Look for flare, cells, hypopyon, and hyphaema.
* Check anterior chamber depth.

Iris
* Distorted pupil (anterior segment dysgenesis, iridocorneal endothelial syndrome)
* Aniridia

- Deposits at pupil margin (pseudoexfoliation syndrome)
- Vessels (rubeosis iridis, vascular tufts)
- Peripheral iridotomy (superior for trabeculectomy or acute glaucoma, inferior after the use of silicone oil to treat retinal detachment in an aphakic eye)
- Nodules (Koeppe and Busacca nodules in anterior uveitis)
- Transillumination (pigment dispersion, trauma)
- Adhesions: Anterior or posterior synechiae

Lens and anterior vitreous

- Look for lens capsule abnormalities, pseudoexfoliation, lens opacities, an intraocular lens, and cells in the anterior vitreous.

Slit lamp techniques for anterior segment examination

Diffuse illumination

Indication

- This initial examination is performed with white light to scan the ocular surface tissues, providing an overview.
- Use a cobalt-blue filter for examination with fluorescein.

Technique

- Place a full-height, broad, low-brightness beam onto the ocular surface, with illumination angled at 45° From the nasal or temporal side.

Direct focal/slit illumination

Indication

- Examining the depth of lesions
- Qualitative assessment of corneal thickness/thinning
- Also used for episcleral/scleral examination, anterior segment examination, crystalline lens examination, and anterior vitreous examination

Technique

Direct a full-height, medium-width, bright beam obliquely into the cornea so that a block of light illuminates the cornea. The beam can be thinned further and placed on high magnification to provide a thin optical section giving a high-clarity view of a cross section of the cornea.

Specular reflection

Indication

- For examination of the corneal endothelium for guttata
- Can also be used for examining the anterior surface of the cornea or lens

Technique

Direct a narrow beam (thicker than the optical section) from the temporal side. The angle of illumination must be 50°–60° From the viewing system, which should be offset nasally. High magnification with a 16× eyepiece is preferable. Look at the image of the reflected light. Specular reflection is a monocular technique.

Normally the illumination is directed at the point of focus of the viewing arm (parfocal). For the following techniques, dissociating the two can be achieved by adjusting the centring screw of the slit lamp.

Indirect illumination

Indication

- Translucent lesions such as subtle stromal opacities

Technique

The light is directed adjacent to the lesion to be examined.

Sclerotic scatter

Indication

- Detecting subtle corneal opacities and translucent cysts

Technique

The illumination is directed at the limbus whilst the central corneal area is observed. When sclerotic scatter is achieved (by total internal reflection of light), the opposite limbus glows.

Retroillumination

Indication

- Detection of microcystic epithelial oedema
- Detection of abnormalities of posterior surface of the cornea, such as guttata
- Detection of posterior capsular opacification

Technique

A medium-width beam of light is projected onto structures posterior to the area to be examined. Reflected light is then used to backlight the area to be examined. To examine the cornea in this way, the iris or fundus can be used as the reflective surface. When using the fundus, it is preferable to have the pupil dilated.

Transillumination

Indication

- Detecting iris defects, the position of peripheral iridotomy, and iris atrophy

Technique

The technique used is as for retroillumination, using the fundus as the reflective surface.

Special dyes

Fluorescein

Fluorescein is available as a 0.25% solution ready-mixed with proxymetacaine. It is also available in impregnated strips and as 1% and 2% single-use eye drops. Fluorescein does not stain healthy corneal or conjunctival epithelium. It readily stains epithelial defects and may penetrate the intercellular spaces when epithelial cells loosen or desquamate or when the epithelial mucous layer is absent.

Indication

- To detect a corneal/conjunctival epithelial defect (punctate epithelial erosions, corneal abrasion, corneal ulcer)
- To assess tear-film break-up time
- Seidel's test: 2% fluorescein is applied directly to the area in question; if a defect (e.g. bleb leak, surgical wound, corneal perforation) is present, aqueous humour will dilute the stain.
- To assess rigid contact lens fit
- Goldman applanation tonometry

Rose bengal

The availability of this dye is limited. It stains devitalized epithelium and de-epithelialized areas (which also can be stained with fluorescein). It also stains mucus. It can be used to assess dry eye disease but it may cause discomfort and its use should be preceded by topical anaesthetic drops.

Lissamine green

The staining characteristics of lissamine green are similar to those of rose bengal but lissamine green causes less irritation than rose bengal does.

2.4 Blepharitis

Blepharitis (inflammation of the lid margins) is common. The term blepharitis is generally used to describe chronic lid inflammation but can also be used for acute lid infections. This chapter will focus on chronic blepharitis and associated conditions.

Blepharitis can be divided anatomically into anterior or posterior blepharitis. Anterior blepharitis refers to inflammation around the base of the eyelashes. Posterior blepharitis involves the meibomian gland orifices. There is considerable overlap between the divisions and subdivisions, with many patients manifesting both 'types' of blepharitis.

Blepharitis can be associated with systemic diseases (rosacea, seborrhoeic dermatitis, acne vulgaris) and can cause secondary ocular disease (dry eye syndrome, chalazion, trichiasis, conjunctivitis, keratitis).

Anterior blepharitis

Pathophysiology

Anterior blepharitis involves bacterial colonization of the lash follicles. *Staphylococcus aureus* is the most common pathogen found in this condition (see Figure 2.6), although *Staph. epidermidis*, *Propionibacterium*, *Corynebacterium*, and the parasite *Demodex follicularum* are also potential pathogens. The immune-mediated inflammation is caused by the presence of bacterial toxins. In addition, bacterially modified lipids can result in an unstable tear film.

Seborrhoeic blepharitis (see Figure 2.7) is seen in association with seborrhoeic dermatitis (generally older people) as compared to staphylococcal disease (which is seen in younger adults and occasionally children).

Clinical evaluation

History

Clinical features are normally fairly symmetrical and are characterized by chronic, low-grade symptoms with exacerbations. Symptoms are normally worse first thing in the morning. They include:

- A burning, itching, foreign body sensation
- Mild photophobia, crusting, redness of the lid margins

Examination

- Erythema and thickening of the anterior lid margin
- Hard and brittle scales (collarettes) surrounding the base of the lashes in staphylococcal disease. When these are removed in severe cases, there may be small ulcers beneath, on the lid margin.
- Soft and greasy scales (scurf) that cause matting together of the lashes in seborrheic disease
- A 'sleeve' of homogenous smooth material surrounding the eyelash base may indicate demodex infestation.
- An external hordeolum (stye) may develop if the lash follicles or glands of Zeis/Moll become infected (see Section 1.7).
- Decreased tear break-up time, and evaporative dry eye
- In chronic and severe cases: scarring and irregularity of the lid margin, madarosis (loss of eye lashes), poliosis (whitening of lashes), and trichiasis (misdirected eyelashes)
  - Corneal changes can occur secondary to dryness and trichiasis but are often immune-mediated (see Section 2.5)

- Skin changes: seborrhoeic dermatitis is characterized by oily skin and flaking from the scalp, nasolabial folds, brows, and behind the ears.

Differential diagnosis

- Dry eye disease
- Basal cell carcinoma, squamous cell carcinoma, sebaceous cell carcinoma

Note: sebaceous gland carcinoma can occasionally mimic chronic blepharitis in the absence of a significant mass. 'Blepharitis' in such cases is resistant to treatment and may be associated with localized madarosis (see Section 1.9).

Management

For all types of blepharitis, the severity of symptoms correlates poorly with the clinical signs; consequently, management can be frustrating. Treatment of blepharitis is aimed at control rather than cure. Acute exacerbations require aggressive management, whilst chronic disease requires maintenance therapy.

Lid hygiene is the mainstay of treatment. Cleaning with a flannel, cotton bud, or commercially available wipe can remove the scales and reduce the bacterial load. A selenium-containing shampoo is only indicated in cases of seborrhoeic blepharitis.

Topical antibiotics, for example chloramphenicol or azithromycin, (applied on the lid margin after lid hygiene) are useful for acute exacerbations.

Tear-film supplements treat symptoms of dry eye.

Topical corticosteroids are useful acutely, especially if there are signs of staphylococcal hypersensitivity.

Posterior blepharitis

Pathophysiology

Posterior blepharitis is characterized by meibomian gland dysfunction (see Figure 2.8). Obstruction of the meibomian glands is caused by hyperkeratinization of the duct orifice and alters the tear-film physiology, resulting in tear-film instability. The stagnant material can also become a growth medium for bacteria. Posterior blepharitis can be associated with acne rosacea.

Clinical evaluation

History

- As for anterior blepharitis
- Recurrent chalazia

Examination

- Capping of meibomian gland orifices by oil globules, oily tear film, foam on the lid margin
- Rounding, thickening, and telangiectasia of the lid margin. On lid pressure, turbid, thick, or paste-like fluid oozes out.
- Decreased tear break-up time, corneal punctate epithelial erosions, corneal vascularization and infiltrates
- Conjunctival papillae, concretions, chalazia
- Skin changes: rosacea is characterized by facial erythema, rhinophyma, telangiectasia, and pustules.

Differential diagnosis

- As for anterior blepharitis

Management

- **Lid massage after heat:** this is the mainstay of treatment for posterior blepharitis. A warm compress is applied to the lids for several minutes to melt the thick lipid secretions. Then, meibomian secretions are expressed by pressing a fingertip/cotton bud along the marginal tarsal plate.

- **Topical antibiotics/steroids:** short courses of these are particularly useful in cases of staphylococcal hypersensitivity (see Section 2.5).
- **Tear-film supplements:** indicated in the presence of an unstable tear film
- **Systemic tetracyclines:** useful in persistent or severe cases. A 3–6 month course of oral doxycycline 100 mg once a day can bring symptoms under control. Side effects include photosensitivity and stomach upset. Tetracyclines are contraindicated in children under 12 years, and during pregnancy and breast feeding, because of the risk of tooth enamel abnormalities.

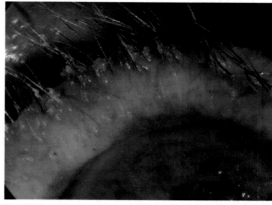

Fig 2.7 Seborrhoeic anterior blepharitis
Note the greasy scales and matting of the lashes

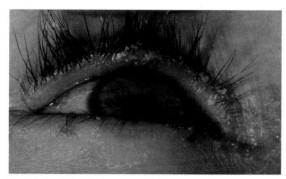

Fig 2.6 Staphylococcal anterior blepharitis
Note the collarettes surrounding the base of the lashes and the surrounding erythema

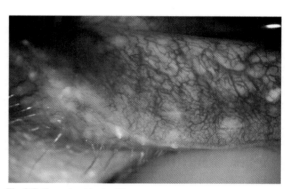

Fig 2.8 Posterior blepharitis
Note the telangiectasia of the posterior lid margin and the thickened meibomian gland secretions being expressed

2.5 Staphylococcal hypersensitivity disorders

There are a variety of disorders characterized by ocular surface inflammation and which occur in patients with coexisting blepharitis. The exact pathophysiology of these conditions has not been fully elucidated but a Type 4 hypersensitivity reaction to staphylococcal antigens is believed to be responsible for them. The exact antigenic stimulus for rosacea keratitis is not known but it is included in this section as it represents an ocular surface inflammation that can occur with blepharitis. Many of these conditions can coexist.

Staphylococcal hypersensitivity syndrome

Staphylococcal hypersensitivity syndrome is characterized by conjunctival injection and a punctate epithelial keratopathy that predominantly affects the inferior cornea, where it is in close physical contact with the eyelids. Occasionally, a diffuse punctate keratopathy and peripheral vascularization can occur. The condition can be bilateral, asymmetrical, or unilateral. The extent of corneal involvement can be significant despite only mild eyelid disease. Symptoms range from mild irritation to foreign body sensation, watering, and photophobia.

Treatment

Depending on the degree of inflammation, treatment may involve a short course of topical steroids, together with treating the blepharitis.

Marginal keratitis

Marginal keratitis classically presents as a grey-white anterior stromal sterile corneal infiltrate (see Figure 2.9). It commonly occurs on the peripheral cornea, leaving a 1 mm clear area between the infiltrate and the limbus. Symptoms are mild irritation, watering, redness, and photophobia. Initially, the epithelium is intact but it can break down to produce a defect. After prolonged inflammation, the ulcer may spread circumferentially with small blood vessels growing towards the infiltrate.

Treatment

Resolution often occurs spontaneously after several days. However, a short course of topical steroid with antibiotic cover can speed recovery. Treat associated staphylococcal blepharitis.

Phlyctenulosis

Phlyctenulosis occurs in children and young adults as a result of Type 4 hypersensitivity to microbial antigens (most commonly *Staph. aureus* but also *Mycobacterium tuberculosis* in endemic areas). Phlyctenules are single/multiple grey-yellow elevated inflammatory lesions at the limbus or conjunctiva and which are surrounded by an intense injection of blood vessels (see Figure 2.10). They present with watering, redness, and photophobia. The lesion ulcerates and then heals with vascularization in the involved area over 2–3 weeks. Recurrences can occur at the edge of an area of vascularization associated with a previous scar and can progress centrally on the cornea.

Treatment

Treatment is as for marginal keratitis (consider investigations for tuberculosis in endemic areas).

Rosacea keratitis

Rosacea is a chronic idiopathic condition that affects the facial skin and eyes in adults (normally, adults aged 30–60 years old). Cutaneous features include midfacial erythema, telangiectasia, papules, nodules, and rhinophyma (thickened skin and connective tissue of the nose). It is thought to be due to dysfunction of the meibomian glands of the skin and eyelids, with secondary inflammation. The ophthalmic manifestations can occur in the presence of minimum skin changes and include posterior blepharitis and telangiectasia of the lid margin; recurrent chalazia; tear-film dysfunction; marginal keratitis; superficial, wedge-shaped, peripheral vascularization with its base at the limbus; thinning; scarring; and even perforation (see Figure 2.11).

Treatment

* Treatment is with topical corticosteroids and may be intensive in cases with advancing corneal inflammation. The steroids should be quickly tapered as symptoms permit.
* A course of systemic tetracycline
* Tear supplements and lubricants

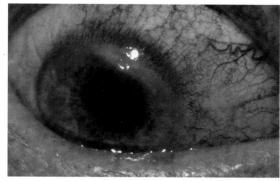

Fig 2.9 Marginal keratitis

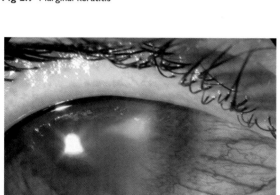

Fig 2.10 Phlyctenulosis
Corneal phlyctenule

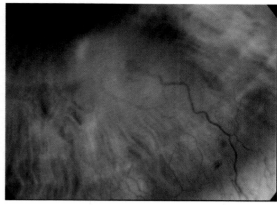

Fig 2.11 Rosacea keratitis

2.6 Dry eye disease

Dry eye disease (also called keratoconjunctivitis sicca) is a common, multifactorial disease. It is a disorder of the tear film that occurs because of:

1. Deficient production of aqueous tears *or*
2. Excessive evaporation of tears due to poor tear composition *or*
3. A combination of the two
   Inflammation and damage of the ocular surface may be either a cause or consequence of the dry eye state.

Pathophysiology

Aqueous tear deficiency
The main lacrimal glands produce the majority of the aqueous component of tears. There is also significant production of aqueous tears by the accessory conjunctival lacrimal glands. There is both a basal and a reflex component to aqueous tear production. The reflex component occurs in response to any irritation of the ocular surface.

Sjögren dry eye syndromes
Sjögren syndrome is an autoimmune exocrinopathy characterized by immune-mediated inflammation of the lacrimal and salivary glands. It produces dry eyes and a dry mouth. Women are mostly affected. It can be classified further into primary and secondary forms.

- **Primary Sjögren syndrome:** occurs in the absence of other autoimmune or connective tissue disease
- **Secondary Sjögren syndrome:** its clinical features are identical to those of primary Sjögren syndrome, but it occurs in the presence of another autoimmune disease. Rheumatoid arthritis is the most common autoimmune disease that it occurs with; others include systemic lupus erythematosus and anti-neutrophil cytoplasmic antibody (ANCA)-positive vasculitides.

Non-Sjögren dry eye syndromes
- **Lacrimal gland disease:** congenital, infiltrative (lymphoma, sarcoidosis), infective (HIV, EBV), inflammatory (thyroid eye disease)
- **Lacrimal duct obstruction:** cicatricial diseases (trachoma, ocular cicatricial pemphigoid, Stevens–Johnson syndrome and graft-versus-host disease (GVHD), postirradiation fibrosis) and goblet cell destruction (vitamin A deficiency; also known as xerophthalmia)
- **Drug related:** anticholinergics, antihistamines, diuretics, oral contraceptives
- **Loss of reflex tearing, due to decreased surface innervation:** herpetic disease, diabetic neuropathy, topical anaesthesia, fifth cranial nerve disease, post-excimer laser refractive surgery

Evaporative tear dysfunction
- Meibomian gland dysfunction
- Contact lens wear
- Disorders of eyelid closure: exposure, ectropion, lagophthalmos, proptosis
- Reduced blink rate (Parkinsons disease)

Clinical evaluation
The spectrum of clinical manifestations of dry eye disease ranges from minimal ocular surface disease to sight-threatening corneal complications.

History
- Burning, foreign body sensation, photophobia, red eye, blurred vision (usually intermittent), occasionally pain (filamentary keratitis)
- Excessive watering (paradoxical reflex watering)
- Symptoms worse with prolonged reading, using a VDU (decreased blink rate), in cold, windy weather, with central heating, with air conditioning, or in an airplane cabin (increased tear evaporation, decreased humidity)
- Symptoms from aqueous tear deficiency tend to be worse at the end of the day. Those from meibomian gland dysfunction (evaporative dry eye) tend to be worse at the beginning of the day.
- Dry mouth, difficulty in swallowing dry food (Sjögren syndrome)
- Contact lens intolerance

Examination
- Hyperaemia of the bulbar conjunctiva, redundant folds of bulbar conjunctiva (conjunctival chalasis)
- Decreased tear meniscus
- Decreased tear break-up time: assessed by instilling fluorescein into the conjunctival fornix. After several blinks, measure the time taken from the last blink to the first dry patch appearing on the cornea. A tear break-up time of less than 10 seconds may be considered abnormal.
- Schirmer test: this is performed by having the patient retain a folded strip of filter paper (No. 41 Whatman) behind the lower lid margin in the tear film with eyes closed for 5 minutes. The amount of wetting is then assessed. It is abnormal if <5 mm (suggestive of aqueous tear deficiency). If anaesthetic is instilled first, then basal secretion alone is tested. Without anaesthetic, basal and reflex secretions together are tested (Schirmer 1 test). Stimulation of the nasal mucosa tests reflex secretion (Schirmer 2 test).

Keratopathies
- Punctate epithelial erosions
- **Filamentary keratopathy:** Corneal filaments are grey threads attached to the epithelium and move with blinking (see Figure 2.12). They are composed of mucous debris and devitalized epithelium and are thus most readily seen with rose bengal if available (see Figure 2.13). Fluorescein also stains filaments.
- Mucus plaques: semi-transparent elevated lesions that occur on the surface of the cornea often associated with filamentary keratopathy
- Severe cases can result in an epithelial defect or a sterile corneal infiltrate or ulcer. Secondary infectious keratitis can also develop. Both sterile and infectious corneal perforations can occur.

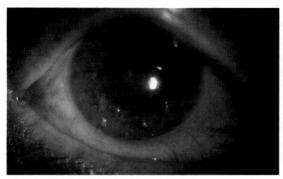

Fig 2.12 Filamentary keratopathy

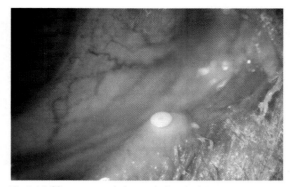

Fig 2.14 Silicone punctal plug occluding the lower punctum

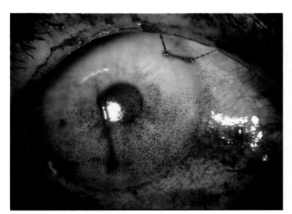

Fig 2.13 Rose Bengal staining of a dry eye
Note the punctate epithelial erosions on the inferior corneal surface and the inferior bulbar conjunctiva

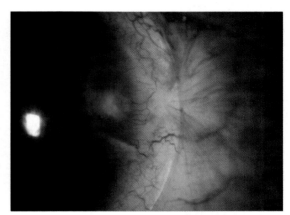

Fig 2.15 Dellen managed with soft contact lens

Investigations

Dry eye disease is predominantly a clinical diagnosis. If there are symptoms of Sjögren syndrome (dry eye and dry mouth), then consider investigations to establish primary or secondary causes:

- **Primary Sjögren syndrome:** positive anti-Ro and/or anti-La antibodies
- **Secondary Sjögren syndrome:** measure rheumatoid factor, inflammatory markers, autoantibodies (including anti-nuclear antibodies), and anti-neutrophil cytoplasmic antibodies

Management

Management needs to be directed depending on severity and aetiology. Underlying disease such as blepharitis must be adequately treated.

Mild disease

- Standard artificial tears such as carbomer gel or hypromellose 0.3%, four times daily
- Lubricating ointment, such as paraffin-based ointment, at night

Moderate disease

- Preservative-free artificial tears (e.g. carmellose 0.5%) as required, up to every hour; lubricating ointment at night
- If large filaments or mucous strands are present, they can be gently removed with a cotton bud. Mucolytics such as acetylcysteine 5% four times daily are also useful.

- Punctal occlusion: temporary punctal plugs should be used in the first instance to ensure there is no epiphora (see Figure 2.14). If effective then punctal cautery can be performed.
- Topical steroids or ciclosporin can be useful to modulate the inflammatory component of the condition.
- Dietary omega-3 fatty acids

Severe disease

- All of the treatments for moderate disease
- Moist chamber goggles, humidifier
- Autologous serum eye drops
- Lateral tarsorrhaphy (see Chapter 1, Section 1.15).

Dellen

Dellen is caused by localized tear-film instability, which results in a focal area of stromal dehydration and consequent thinning (see Figure 2.15). It usually occurs adjacent to a raised lesion present on the conjunctiva, limbus, or cornea (e.g. a filtering bleb, pterygium, or pingueculum). Symptoms are normally of mild irritation. On examination, there is no epithelial defect but a focal corneal depression with poor surface wetting.

Treatment

The aim is to restore the continuity of the overlying tear film with tear supplements or in some cases soft contact lenses. The causative elevated lesion may need to be removed surgically if symptoms persist.

51

Conjunctivitis classification

Conjunctivitis is a non-specific term for inflammation of the conjunctiva. The general clinical features include:

1. Vascular dilatation (conjunctival hyperaemia)
2. Oedema (chemosis)
3. Exudation (discharge)

Conjunctivitis may be classified in various ways:

Age

* Neonatal (ophthalmia neonatorum), childhood, and adult conjunctivitis

Duration

* Acute (<4 weeks duration) or chronic (>4 weeks)

Aetiology

* Infective (viral, bacterial, chlamydial, parasitic)
* Allergic (seasonal, perennial, vernal, giant papillary)
* Autoimmune (ocular cicatricial pemphigoid, Stevens–Johnson syndrome)
* Toxic (drop toxicity, chemical injury, postirradiation)
* Mechanical (eye rubbing, mucous fishing syndrome, foreign body, entropion)
* Neoplastic (sebaceous gland carcinoma, conjunctival malignancies)

Morphology

* **Papillary:** this is a non-specific feature of many causes of conjunctivitis. Giant papillae (papillae >1 mm) occur in chronic cases when individual papillae become confluent; they are a characteristic feature of giant papillary conjunctivitis and vernal conjunctivitis.
* **Follicular** (viral, chlamydial, drop allergy)
* **Pseudomembranous:** pseudomembranes are not true membranes but rather coagulated exudates which adhere to the conjunctival epithelium. They can be peeled off without causing trauma to the underlying epithelium. Causes include adenoviral conjunctivitis, gonococcal conjunctivitis, and the acute stage of Stevens–Johnson syndrome.
* **Membranous:** true membranes are continuous with the conjunctival epithelium and cannot be removed without traumatizing the conjunctiva. Causes include *Streptococcus pyogenes* and diphtheria.
* **Cicatricial** (trachoma, ocular cicatricial pemphigoid, Stevens–Johnson syndrome)
* **Haemorrhagic** (enterovirus, adenovirus, haemophilus, gonococcus)
* **Granulomatous** (sarcoidosis, tuberculosis)

Discharge

Classifying conjunctivitis according to the type of discharge is not specific but can be helpful where a more complete examination is not possible, for example in very young children.

* Purulent (acute bacterial infections)
* Mucopurulent (bacterial, chlamydial)
* Mucoid (allergic, viral)
* Watery (viral)

Adenoviral conjunctivitis

Pathophysiology

Adenoviruses are the most common cause of viral conjunctivitis. They are double-stranded DNA viruses, with over 50 serotypes. The incubation period for adenoviruses is about 8–9 days. The virus is shed for up to 2 weeks following the onset of conjunctivitis. Adenovirus is transmitted by close contact with ocular/respiratory secretions or fomites. The virus is extremely contagious, and care must be taken in the eye clinic to minimize spread of the virus to staff and to other patients.

Clinical evaluation

Adenoviral conjunctivitis presents clinically as one of three possible syndromes:

* **Simple follicular conjunctivitis:** no systemic involvement. Corneal involvement is mild if present.
* **Pharyngoconjunctival fever:** fever, pharyngitis, and follicular conjunctivitis. Corneal involvement is mild if present.
* **Epidemic keratoconjunctivitis:** may be preceded by an upper respiratory tract infection. The hallmark with this syndrome is significant corneal involvement.

In reality, these syndromes are difficult to distinguish clinically, especially in the early stages of disease. General features of adenoviral conjunctivitis and keratitis are considered below.

History

* Watery discharge and mild-to-moderate burning, which usually begins in one eye; often becomes bilateral owing to autoinoculation of the fellow eye
* Red eye, lid oedema, photophobia
* Pain and blurred vision if the cornea is involved

Examination

* Palpable, tender preauricular and submandibular lymph nodes
* Conjunctiva: follicles (see Figure 2.16), papillae (see Figure 2.17), chemosis, injection, and subconjunctival petechial haemorrhages. Conjunctivitis normally resolves within 2 weeks.
* In severe cases, there may be pseudomembranes (see Figure 2.18).

Keratitis may present in two forms:

1. Punctate epithelial erosions occur 7–10 days after the onset of symptoms and normally resolve after 2 weeks.
2. Round subepithelial infiltrates: these are thought to represent an immunological response to the virus and persist for several weeks (occasionally years) before complete resolution (see Figure 2.19). Rarely, large persistent lesions can leave a residual scar and blurred vision.

Investigations

Diagnosis is usually clinical but may be confirmed by PCR performed on a conjunctival swab. Point-of-care tests are available for immediate diagnosis of adenoviral infection.

Management

* Cool compresses and artificial tears for symptomatic relief
* Topical antibiotics are often given, as there is some overlap with the clinical manifestations of bacterial conjunctivitis.

- Topical steroids can be used to treat pseudomembranes and severe/persistent keratitis associated with decreased vision. The use of steroids accelerates resolution but does not otherwise affect the natural course of the disease.
- All equipment and surfaces should be carefully cleaned to prevent cross-infection between patients.
- Patients should be educated about hygiene measures to prevent transmission of the virus.

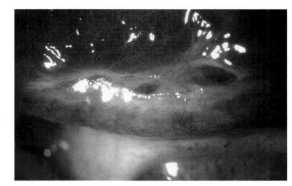

Fig 2.18 Conjunctival scarring following severe adenovirus infection

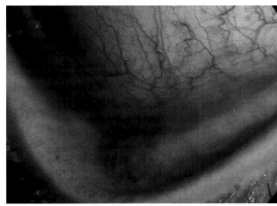

Fig 2.16 Follicles on the inferior palpebral conjunctiva in a case of adenoviral conjunctivitis

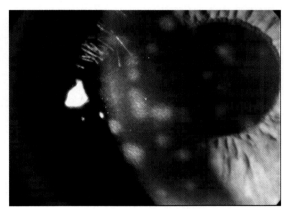

Fig 2.19 Subepithelial scars in adenoviral keratitis

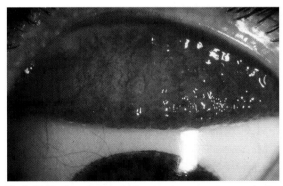

Fig 2.17 Papillary conjunctivitis secondary to ocular prosthesis

2.8 Conjunctivitis II: Other infectious causes

Herpes simplex conjunctivitis

Herpes simplex blepharoconjunctivitis occurs either as a primary infection or, more commonly, as a result of viral reactivation. Clinical features include:

- Unilateral follicular conjunctivitis
- Preauricular lymphadenopathy
- Lid/eyelid margin vesicles
- Dendritic epithelial keratitis (see Section 2.18)

The condition is normally self-limiting, with the conjunctivitis resolving within 1 week. Treatment to shorten the duration of symptoms is with topical acyclovir ointment five times daily for 1 week.

Molluscum contagiosum conjunctivitis

Molluscum contagiosum is a poxvirus, transmitted by direct contact or autoinoculation. Clinical features include pearly umbilicated nodules at/near the lid margin, and ipsilateral follicular conjunctivitis. In long-standing cases, punctate epithelial erosions and corneal pannus may occur. Spontaneous resolution takes months to years. Removal of lid lesions by shave excision, incision, or curettage is curative. Multiple mollusca in the chin-strap region can be a feature of AIDS.

Chlamydial conjunctivitis

Chlamydia trachomatis is an obligate intracellular bacterium. It causes three conjunctivitis syndromes:

1. Trachoma: Serotypes A–C
2. Adult inclusion conjunctivitis: Serotypes D–K
3. Chlamydial ophthalmia neonatorum: Serotypes D–K

Trachoma

Trachoma is the most common cause of preventable blindness in the world, with 150 million people estimated to be affected. In endemic areas, it occurs in communities with poor access to facilities for hygiene and sanitation. It is transmitted by direct contact, flies, or fomites.

Clinical evaluation

Primary infection usually occurs during childhood.

- Recurrent severe follicular conjunctivitis with follicles predominantly on the superior tarsal conjunctiva and limbus. Follicles can be obscured by diffuse papillary hypertrophy.
- With time, linear or stellate scarring over the tarsal plate occurs (see Figure 2.20). Broad confluent scars are known as Arlt lines.
- Involution and necrosis of limbal follicles result in depressions known as Herberts pits (see Figure 2.21).
- Progressive scarring of the conjunctiva results in trichiasis, entropion, and dry eye, which in turn lead to corneal disease.
- Corneal findings include punctate epithelial erosions, scarring, and vascularization.

Management

- Public health preventative measures such as increased hygiene (face washing) and access to clean water.
- Treatment for acute infection is azithromycin 1 g orally as a single dose.
- Treatment for dry eye is often necessary, and entropion or trichiasis may require surgical intervention.

Adult inclusion conjunctivitis

Adult inclusion conjunctivitis is a sexually transmitted disease which typically affects young adults. It often occurs in conjunction with urethritis or cervicitis.

Clinical evaluation

The onset is subacute. If untreated, symptoms can persist for up to 18 months. Clinical features include:

- Follicular conjunctivitis and preauricular lymphadenopathy
- Potential corneal involvement, which includes fine or coarse epithelial and/or subepithelial infiltrates

Investigations

The investigation of choice is PCR, but a variety of laboratory tests are available. These include culture, ELISA, and direct fluorescent antibody microscopy (note: topical fluorescein can interfere with immunofluorescent tests).

Management

- Patients with laboratory-confirmed infection should be investigated for coinfection with other sexually transmitted diseases before systemic antibiotic treatment is initiated and should be managed at a specialist genitourinary clinic. Sexual partners need to be traced and treated to prevent reinfection.
- Azithromycin ointment may be used in the first instance until review in the genitourinary clinic.
- Systemic treatment is azithromycin 1 g orally as a single dose.

Chlamydial ophthalmia neonatorum

Chlamydial ophthalmia neonatorum is the most common cause of neonatal conjunctivitis and, like the other causes of infectious ophthalmia neonatorum, is acquired during passage of the baby through the birth canal.

Clinical evaluation

- The time from birth until the onset of signs is variable but is typically subacute, starting at 5 days postnatal.
- There is no follicular response in neonates.
- There is a significant mucopurulent discharge.
- If the condition is associated with systemic chlamydial infection, there is a risk of chlamydial pneumonitis.

Management

- Treatment is with systemic erythromycin (50 mg/kg/day orally or intravenously four times a day for 14 days) under the supervision of a paediatrician.
- Both the mother and her partner(s) need to be examined and treated by a physician for genital infections.

Bacterial conjunctivitis

Simple bacterial conjunctivitis

Simple bacterial conjunctivitis is a common condition (particularly in children). It can be caused by a wide range of bacteria, including both Gram-positive and Gram-negative bacteria. Common causative organisms include *Staph. aureus*, *Strep. pneumoniae*, and *Haemophilus influenzae*. Spread occurs by direct contact.

Clinical evaluation

- Onset is acute/subacute, coming on over hours to days.
- There is usually bilateral (or sequential) involvement.
- The discharge may initially be watery but soon becomes classically mucopurulent, with matting of the eyelashes.

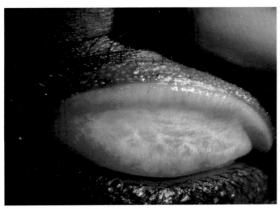

Fig 2.20 Trachomatous scarring
Courtesy of Matthew Burton

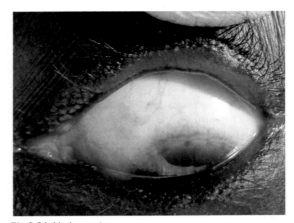

Fig 2.21 Herberts pits
Courtesy of Matthew Burton

- There is papillary conjunctival reaction, and chemosis with variable lid oedema.
- There is usually no preauricular lymphadenopathy.
- There may be mild punctate epithelial erosions on the cornea.
- *Staph. aureus* conjunctivitis is commonly associated with blepharitis (blepharoconjunctivitis), and these cases may develop recurrent infections if the blepharitis is left untreated.

Management
Simple bacterial conjunctivitis is usually a self-limiting condition, resolving within 2 weeks. The following treatment can reduce the duration of symptoms:
- Cleaning of lids and removal of discharge
- Application of a broad spectrum, topical antibiotic ointment or drops (e.g. chloramphenicol, four to six times daily)

Note: Ointments blur vision, and therefore drops may be preferable for adults during the day. However, if there is considerable watering, then ointment is more useful. *H. influenzae* conjunctivitis should be treated with oral amoxicillin because of the potential for extraocular infection.

Hygiene measures are important to prevent spread to contacts.

Adult gonococcal conjunctivitis

Adult gonococcal conjunctivitis (see Figure 2.22) is a sexually transmitted disease resulting from genital to eye contact. It is caused by the Gram-negative diplococcus *Neisseria gonorrhoeae*, which can invade the healthy cornea. It is an ophthalmic emergency, as infection can lead rapidly to perforation of the cornea.

Clinical evaluation
Onset is hyperacute (<24 hours), with severe mucopurulent conjunctivitis. Features include marked lid swelling, preauricular lymphadenopathy, copious purulent discharge, and pseudomembranes.

Corneal involvement starts as a peripheral ulcer that progresses to become a ring ulcer. Corneal perforation and endophthalmitis can occur. There may be associated genital infection.

Management
- Investigations include conjunctival swabs for urgent Gram stain, for culture, and for sensitivities.
- If there is no corneal involvement, treatment is with intramuscular ceftriaxone 250 mg daily for 3 days, or oral cefotaxime 400 mg as a single dose.

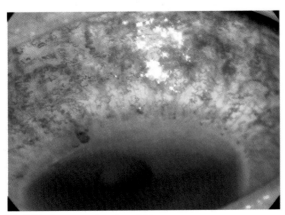

Fig 2.22 Gonococcal conjunctivitis
Note the intense vascular dilatation and conjunctival haemorrhages

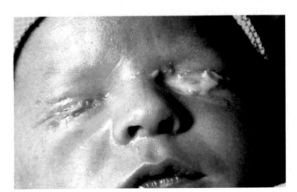

Fig 2.23 Gonococcoal ophthalmia neonatorum
Courtesy of Volker Klauss

- If there is corneal involvement, admission is necessary, and treatment is with ceftriaxone 1 g intravenously twice a day for 3 days.
- Frequent irrigation of the conjunctival sac with saline may be necessary to remove discharge.
- Topical treatment is with cefuroxime 5% drops.
- Patients and their sexual partners must be investigated by the genitourinary clinic and treated for other sexually acquired infections.

Gonococcal ophthalmia neonatorum

Clinical evaluation

- Typically presents within 1–3 days of birth, with a bilateral, initially serosanguinous conjunctival discharge which becomes purulent (see Figure 2.23).

- As with adult disease, there is also significant risk of corneal involvement.
- Disseminated gonococcus rarely occurs, with potentially life-threatening meningitis, pneumonia, and sepsis.

Management

- Investigations include conjunctival swabs for urgent Gram stain, for culture, and for sensitivities.
- Urgent treatment with intramuscular (or intravenous) ceftriaxone (25–50 mg/kg daily for 3 days)
- Admission and intravenous ceftriaxone is required if corneal involvement is present.
- Regular irrigation of the conjunctival sac is necessary.
- Topical treatment is as for adult gonococcal conjunctivitis.

  Note: ophthalmia neonatorum is no longer a notifiable disease but should be managed in conjunction with a paediatrician.

2.9 Conjunctivitis III: Allergic and miscellaneous

Allergic conjunctivitis represents a spectrum of disease that can be classified into:

1. Seasonal allergic conjunctivitis (SAC)
2. Perennial allergic conjunctivitis (PAC)
3. Vernal keratoconjunctivitis (VKC)
4. Atopic keratoconjunctivitis (AKC)

SAC and PAC have overlapping clinical features and will be considered together.

SAC and PAC

These conditions are common forms of acute allergic conjunctivitis.

Pathophysiology

Both conditions are Type 1 IgE-mediated immediate hypersensitivity reactions that occur in response to airborne antigens. SAC causes symptoms during pollination in late spring and summer. PAC causes symptoms throughout the year, with exacerbation in the autumn in response to greater levels of dust and fungal antigens. Both conditions can be associated with other atopic conditions such as eczema, asthma, and hay fever.

Clinical evaluation

History

- The hallmark symptom is itch, which is often associated with increased lacrimation, slight red eye, and occasionally mucous discharge.
- It can also be associated with sneezing, nasal itch, and rhinorrhoea.

Examination

- Mild conjunctival injection and oedema, with papillary reaction of the tarsal conjunctiva
- Corneal disease is uncommon.

Management

Patients should be advised against rubbing their eyes.

Allergen avoidance

- Patients with SAC can be counselled to limit their outdoor activity on high pollen count days.
- Patients with PAC should be advised on measures to reduce dust mites (avoid carpets, feather bedwear, etc.).
- A cold compress can provide symptomatic relief.

Medical treatment

- Artificial tears are beneficial in diluting and flushing away allergens and other inflammatory mediators from the ocular surface.
- Topical vasoconstrictors can provide temporary symptomatic relief, but prolonged use can result in a compensatory rebound hyperaemia.
- The mainstay of treatment is a topical antihistamine, a topical mast cell stabilizer, or a drug that has both effects, such as olopatadine.
- It is important to start mast cell stabilizers prophylactically at least 2 weeks before the time when allergy normally occurs. These agents are less useful for acute exacerbations, as their onset of action is delayed.

- Topical steroids are reserved for severe exacerbations.
- Oral antihistamines are useful, especially for associated symptoms of rhinitis.

VKC

Pathophysiology

This condition is a bilateral chronic inflammation of the conjunctiva, often with secondary corneal involvement. Symptoms can occur year-round, with a marked seasonal component with exacerbations during the spring (vernal). It occurs more frequently in males than females (2 : 1), and those affected commonly have a personal or family history of atopy. VKC is caused by both Type 1 (IgE-mediated) and Type 4 (cell-mediated) hypersensitivity reactions.

Clinical evaluation

History

- Severe itch and copious mucoid discharge
- With corneal involvement, there may be photophobia and blurring of vision.

Examination

There are two forms of VKC, corresponding to the anatomical location where clinical signs are most prominent:

Limbal VKC

- This form occurs more commonly in black and Asian patients and is more prevalent in hot climates.
- In this form, there is a thickened, fleshy appearance to the limbus, with scattered papillae.
- In active disease, papillae have white apices (Horner–Trantas dots), which are aggregates of eosinophils and necrotic epithelial cells (see Figure 2.24).

Palpebral VKC

- Conjunctival hyperaemia and chemosis associated with diffuse papillary hypertrophy; more prominent on the upper tarsus
- In more severe cases, the papillae can coalesce, giving rise to giant 'cobblestone' papillae (see Figure 2.25).
- There may be a mechanical ptosis.

Both limbal VKC and palpebral VKC can occur in isolation or together.

Keratopathy

Keratopathy is more common with palpebral disease and includes:

- Punctate epithelial erosions, most common superiorly
- Pannus, and corneal vascularization
- Sterile epithelial breakdown with calcification of the exposed stroma (shield ulcer; see Figure 2.26). Stromal opacification, infection, and vascularization are potentially sight-threatening complications.
- Pseudogerontoxon is an arc-like opacification of the peripheral cornea adjacent to an area of limbus previously affected by inflammation.
- Severe allergic conjunctivitis is associated with both keratoconus and cataract.

Management

- For mild-to-moderate disease, the treatment is as for SAC/PAC.
- For more severe disease, and where there is significant corneal involvement, there are the following treatment options:
- Topical steroids should be administered initially at high frequency and then rapidly tapered.
- Topical ciclosporin 0.05%–2% may act as a steroid-sparing agent.
- Topical acetylcysteine 5% is useful for mucous plaque.
- Surgical debridement or superficial keratectomy may be necessary to remove a calcified plaque. A supratarsal steroid injection given at this time can help prevent recurrence.

AKC

Pathophysiology

This chronic condition typically presents in early adulthood and is strongly associated with severe atopic dermatitis. Atopic individuals have systemic depressed cell-mediated immunity, which makes them susceptible to herpes simplex viral keratitis, and colonization of the eyelids with *Staph. aureus*. The pathophysiology is otherwise similar to vernal keratoconjunctivitis. The differences between AKC and VKC are shown in Table 2.1.

Clinical evaluation

History

- History is as for VKC, with the exception being that disease tends to occur year-round, with minimal or no seasonal exacerbation.

Examination

- **The skin** of the eyelids is thickened, macerated, and fissured.
- **The eyelid margin** often has staphylococcal blepharitis.

Table 2.1 Differences between vernal keratoconjunctivitis and atopic keratoconjunctivitis

Feature	Vernal keratoconjunctivitis	Atopic keratoconjunctivitis
Age of onset	Before 10 years	25–50 years
Duration	Lasts 2–10 years (resolves by puberty)	Chronic
Sex	M>F	Equal
Exacerbations	Spring exacerbations	Minimal or no exacerbations
Conjunctival involvement	Upper tarsus, scarring rare	Upper and lower tarsus, scarring common

- **The conjunctiva** is often pale and featureless. During exacerbations, there is hyperaemia, chemosis, and a small-to-medium-sized papillary reaction on the upper and lower palpebral conjunctivas. In severe cases, conjunctival scarring can prevent the papillary response over the upper tarsus. Forniceal shortening and symblepharon formation can occur.
- **The cornea** may display punctate epithelial erosions in mild disease. More extensive disease may result in persistent epithelial defects, stromal scarring, and pannus formation. Corneal disease may be further complicated by microbial or HSK.

Management

- Management of AKC is as for VKC but there may be a poor response to treatment.
- Patients with AKC also require treatment for associated infections such as staphylococcal blepharitis.
- In a minority of patients with severe disease, systemic immune suppression may be necessary, especially prior to corneal surgery.

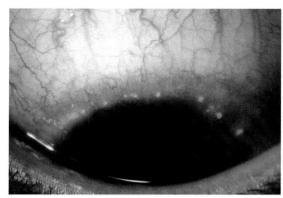

Fig 2.24 Horner–Trantas dots in limbal vernal keratoconjunctivitis

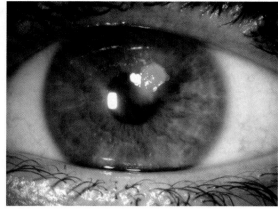

Fig 2.26 Shield ulcer in vernal keratoconjunctivitis

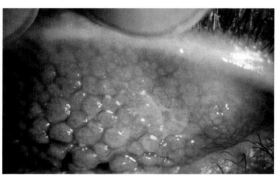

Fig 2.25 Giant cobblestone papillae in palpebral vernal keratoconjunctivitis

Superior limbic keratoconjunctivitis

Pathophysiology

Superior limbic keratoconjunctivitis (see Figure 2.27) is a chronic condition occurring mostly in young adult to middle-aged women. It is associated with hyperthyroidism and dry eye. It is thought to be due to mechanical trauma caused by friction between the superior palpebral conjunctiva and the bulbar conjunctiva. It is often bilateral but asymmetrical and tends to resolve spontaneously after relapsing and remitting over 1–10 years.

Clinical evaluation

History

- Redness, foreign body sensation, photophobia, and/or pain
- Blepharospasm may be present, especially if there is associated filamentary keratitis.

Examination

Signs are best seen with the patient looking down and with the upper lid elevated. Signs include:

- Papillary reaction and congestion on the superior tarsal conjunctiva
- Hyperaemia/thickening/loosening of the superior bulbar conjunctiva. Hyperaemia is maximal at the limbus.
- Punctate staining (fluorescein or rose bengal) of the superior limbal conjunctiva and cornea
- Filamentary keratopathy of the superior cornea
- There may also be signs of associated tear film dysfunction and/or thyroid eye disease.

Treatment

A variety of potential treatments exist. These include:

- Tear-film supplements/lubricants, mucolytics, topical steroid, and punctal occlusion
- Topical vitamin A, ciclosporin, pressure patching, large-diameter bandage contact lens, and/or thermal cauterization of the superior bulbar conjunctiva
- Superior conjunctival resection (3–4 mm strip) may be effective in patients who do not respond to these treatments.

Toxic keratoconjunctivitis

Pathophysiology

Toxic keratoconjunctivitis develops in response to a variety of topical or systemic medications. Toxic conjunctivitis is more commonly papillary but can also be follicular or cicatrizing in morphology.

Commonly implicated medications include:

- Aminoglycoside antibiotics (gentamycin, tobramycin)
- Fortified antibiotics and antifungals
- Antivirals
- Topical anaesthetics (see 'Topical anaesthetic abuse')
- Intraocular pressure (IOP) lowering agents (pilocarpine, apraclonidine, brimonidine, dorzolamide)
- Preservatives (especially benzalkonium chloride and thiomersol)

Clinical evaluation

- Toxic papillary keratoconjunctivitis normally takes 2 or more weeks to develop and causes punctate staining of the infero-nasal conjunctiva and the cornea (where medications gravitate with tear flow). There is redness, papillary reaction, and mucoid discharge.
- Toxic follicular conjunctivitis usually takes several weeks to develop in response to topical medications, eye make-up, or environmental pollutants. Follicles are most prominent in the inferior fornix and on the inferior palpebral conjunctiva. There is normally mild conjunctival hyperaemia and punctate staining.

Treatment

Treatment includes withdrawal of the medications, substitution with preservative-free formulations, and use of preservative-free artificial tears.

Patients can also become allergic to topical medications (e.g. chloramphenicol, neomycin) and mount a hypersensitivity response.

Topical anaesthetic abuse

Topical anaesthetic agents should not be prescribed as a form of analgesia for ocular surface disease or trauma, as their use can retard epithelial healing and mask deterioration of disease. Prolonged use of topical anaesthetic agents may lead to:

- Punctate keratitis
- Neurotrophic ulceration
- Corneal melting
- Increased risk of infection

Prophylactic topical antibiotics and occasionally oral analgesia are useful for breaking the pain cycle.

Mucous fishing syndrome

Mucous fishing syndrome results from a cycle of mechanical irritation from repeated attempts to remove mucus from the fornix in patients with chronic conjunctivitis (e.g. keratoconjunctivitis sicca, blepharitis, allergic conjunctivitis). Rubbing and 'fishing' causes mechanical damage to the conjunctival epithelium and exacerbates the underlying conjunctivitis.

Treatment

- Patients should be educated to stop rubbing and removing mucus.
- Treatment of underlying conjunctival disease
- Topical acetylcysteine and lubrication as required

Factitious keratoconjunctivitis

In factitious keratoconjunctivitis, conjunctival inflammation is caused by self-inflicted physical or chemical harm. It may occur in the context of psychiatric disease or in those seeking to avoid work or financial gain (malingering). Self-induced harm can be in the form of medication, chemical injury, or mechanical injury (e.g. corneal or conjunctival abrasions or lacerations).

Factitious keratoconjunctivitis can be difficult to diagnose and treat. It should be suspected if there is unexplained poor ocular surface healing or recurrent epithelial breakdown. It is usually present in the inferior or nasal quadrants. Twenty-four hour observations may be necessary to allow healing to occur. Psychiatric referral should be considered.

Parinauds oculoglandular syndrome

Pathophysiology

Parinauds oculoglandular syndrome is a rare unilateral nodular/ulcerative conjunctivitis with adjacent submandibular or preauricular lymphadenopathy. It is most frequently due to cat scratch disease (*Bartonella* spp.) and tularaemia. There are a variety of other infectious causes, such as sporotrichosis, tuberculosis, and syphilis.

Clinical evaluation

- The disease has a self-limiting course over weeks to months.
- Presentation is with unilateral conjunctivitis, mild fever, and/or a rash.
- Conjunctival granulomas (red/whitish yellow nodules, 3–4 mm in diameter) appear together with adjacent lymphadenopathy.

Treatment

- Treatment should be directed at the underlying cause.
- *Bartonella* species are sensitive to oral doxycycline, ciprofloxacin, and co-trimoxazole.

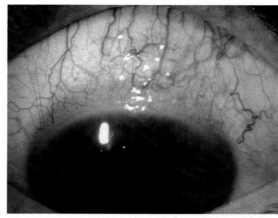

Fig 2.27 Superior limbic keratoconjunctivitis

Cicatrization literally means scarring. There are a variety of conditions that can cause conjunctival scarring.

- **Infection:** severe infection with trachoma, adenovirus, or streptococcal conjunctivitis
- **Trauma:** chemical or thermal injury
- **Iatrogenic:** radiotherapy or ocular surface surgery, chronic topical medications (pilocarpine, adrenaline), or GVHD
- **Blepharokeratoconjunctivitis:** severe chronic rosacea or AKC
- **Autoimmune:** ocular mucous membrane pemphigoid (MMP) or Stevens–Johnson syndrome
- **Neoplastic:** conjunctival neoplasia/carcinoma or sebaceous gland carcinoma

This section will focus on MMP, Stevens–Johnson syndrome, and GVHD. The other causes of cicatrizing conjunctivitis are covered in other sections.

Ocular MMP

Ocular MMP was previously known as ocular cicatricial pemphigoid (see Figure 2.28). MMP is a systemic autoimmune disease characterized by chronic blistering and scarring of the mucous membranes and less commonly the skin. It is a progressive, bilateral (although it can be asymmetric), and potentially blinding condition.

Pathophysiology

MMP affects women twice as often as men, and most patients are over the age of 60.

It is a Type 2 autoimmune disease in which autoantibodies target the mucosal basement membrane zone, resulting in subepithelial blistering, inflammation, and subsequent fibrosis. Conjunctival inflammation and scarring cause destruction of conjunctival goblet cells and obstruction of lacrimal ductules. This damage in turn causes mucous and aqueous tear deficiency and keratinization of the conjunctiva and corneal epithelium. The mouth, oropharynx, genitalia, and anus can also be involved.

Clinical evaluation

History

The course of disease can be chronic and unremitting. Diagnosis of this rare disease is typically delayed because of misdiagnosis, which also delays treatment.

- Onset is with redness, foreign body sensation, watering, and photophobia, consistent with chronic conjunctivitis.
- Cicatricial entropion may distort the lid contour, and patients may complain of ingrowing lashes.
- There may be symptoms of systemic disease (e.g. dysphagia).

Examination

The progression of disease can be categorized into four stages based on clinical signs (Foster staging):

- **Stage 1:** subconjunctival scarring and fibrosis. Loss of the plica and flattening of the caruncle is an early sign.
- **Stage 2:** cicatrization with shortening of the fornices
- **Stage 3:** symblepharon formation (adhesion between tarsal and bulbar conjunctiva; see Figure 2.29)
- **Stage 4:** ankyloblepharon, that is, dense adhesions to the lid margin, limiting eye movement (frozen globe)

Data from *Transactions of the American Ophthalmology Society*, 84, C S Foster, 'Cicatricial pemphigoid', 1986.

Severe keratopathy develops owing to eyelid/lash malposition, aberrant eyelash growth, cicatricial entropion, dry eye, exposure, and limbal stem cell deficiency. Persistent epithelial defects, corneal ulceration, and neovascularization can occur.

Investigations

Conjunctival and buccal mucous membrane biopsies must be performed to confirm the diagnosis. Direct immunofluorescence shows linear deposits of IgG, IgA, and/or complement component 3 at the epithelial basement membrane zone. Indirect immunofluorescence may also be performed on blood samples to detect circulating autoantibodies.

Treatment

Systemic immune suppression is essential for this progressive and potentially blinding disease. Topical treatment is inadequate.

- **Mild inflammation:** Dapsone is commonly used (contraindicated in glucose-6-phosphate dehydrogenase deficiency). Alternatives include sulphapyridine and methotrexate.
- **Moderate inflammation:** in cases of moderate inflammation or those not responding to the agents listed, treatment may be stepped up to include mycophenolate or azathioprine (check thiopurine methyltransferase or thiopurine S-methyltransferase levels before commencing treatment).
- **Severe/resistant inflammation (conjunctival necrosis, limbitis):** cyclophosphamide or a short course of oral steroids may be used.
- Intravenous immunoglobulin therapy for refractory cases

Adjuvant therapy

- Treatment for dry eye (tear-film supplements, lubricants, punctal occlusion if not already stenosed from conjunctival scarring)
- Treatment of coexisting blepharitis

Surgery

Surgery may be required in the following cases:

- Cicatricial ectropion and forniceal loss may require complex adnexal surgery including lamellar repositioning and fornix reconstruction (see Chapter 1, Sections 1.2, 1.3).
- Penetrating keratoplasty has an extremely guarded prognosis if there is severe surface disease. A keratoprosthesis (artificial cornea) may be the only option to restore vision in advanced cases.

Stevens–Johnson syndrome

Stevens–Johnson syndrome is a potentially fatal acute mucocutaneous disorder. The most severe manifestation of this disease is toxic epidermal necrolysis.

Pathophysiology

Stevens–Johnson syndrome is an immune complex mediated (Type 3) hypersensitivity reaction with immune complex deposition in the skin and mucous membranes.

The most common known aetiological factors include:

- Drug hypersensitivities (sulphonamides, penicillin, phenytoin)
- Viral infection (herpes simplex, AIDS, influenza)
- Malignancy

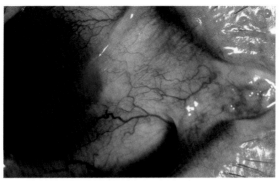

Fig 2.28 Ocular mucous membrane pemphigoid
Note the loss of normal conjunctival anatomy with effacement of the caruncle and loss of the plica. Also note the corneal vascularization and opacification

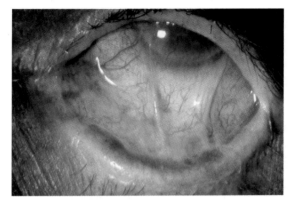

Fig 2.29 Symblepharon formation in a case of ocular mucous membrane pemphigoid

The precipitating cause is not identified in up to one-half of cases.

Clinical evaluation

* Initial presentation is with a 1–14 day prodrome of upper respiratory tract symptoms.
* Mucocutaneous lesions develop abruptly. Skin lesions are classically erythematous maculopapules described as 'target

lesions'. Severe cases of toxic epidermal necrolysis lead to desquamation of skin and mucous membranes.

* The ocular acute phase lasts 2–3 weeks and consists most commonly of a transient, self-limiting bilateral conjunctivitis.
* Occasionally, there may be more severe conjunctival involvement, with bullae, necrosis, and membrane formation. There may be secondary ocular surface infection.
* Long-term ocular surface scarring may occur depending on the severity of the disease. All of the features of ocular MMP may be present but these are **usually** non-progressive after the acute event.
* Ocular surface disease can lead to progressive corneal scarring and vascularization.

Management

* Diagnosis is clinical.
* The mainstay of acute treatment is systemic and supportive. Systemic immune suppression is usually managed by intensive care physicians and dermatologists.
* Ocular treatment involves intensive artificial tears and lubricants, prophylactic topical antibiotics, and topical steroids. Frequent review, at least daily in the acute stages, is required.
* Early amniotic membrane grafting should be considered for eyes with persistent epithelial defects.
* Any associated long-term dry eye, lash abnormality, and lid abnormality are managed as for ocular MMP.
* Systemic immunosuppression for ophthalmic disease is only indicated if there are signs of recurrent conjunctival inflammation. Chronic conjunctival inflammation is a known sequela of Stevens–Johnson syndrome.

GVHD

GVHD is a complication of allogeneic bone marrow transplantation. In this condition, the grafted cells attack the patient's (host) tissues; most commonly affected are the skin, the gastrointestinal system, and the eyes. Ocular complications tend to occur if GVHD becomes chronic. There are two main components:

* Conjunctival inflammation, possibly with cicatrization
* Severe dry eye from lacrimal gland failure

Ocular treatment is as for dry eye disease (artificial tears, punctal plugs, or cautery) plus topical steroids or ciclosporin to control the local inflammation. Occasionally, systemic immune suppression may be required; this therapy is usually managed by a haematologist.

All of the following conditions are common and are often asymptomatic findings.

Pingueculum

Pathophysiology

A pingueculum is a conjunctival degeneration in the exposed interpalpebral zone (see Figure 2.30). The conjunctival stromal collagen undergoes elastoid degeneration and even calcification in response to prolonged exposure to UV light. The overlying conjunctival epithelium can be normal.

Clinical evaluation

* Pinguecula are located adjacent to the limbus more often on the nasal side. There is no corneal involvement.
* The appearance is of a subepithelial, yellow-white nodule.
* Occasionally, they become inflamed (pingueculitis) and irritated because of surface drying.

Management

* Artificial tears/lubricants for ocular surface irritation
* Short course of weak topical steroids for pingueculitis
* Excision is very rarely necessary for cosmesis or chronic inflammation/irritation.

Pterygium

Pathophysiology

A pterygium is a triangular fibrovascular proliferation that grows from the conjunctiva onto the cornea (see Figure 2.31). It arises most often from the nasal conjunctiva. There is subepithelial elastoid degeneration. The cornea shows destruction of Bowman's layer by fibrovascular ingrowth. The major aetiological factor is chronic exposure to UV light.

Clinical evaluation

History

* Cosmetic concern
* Ocular irritation and redness if the pterygium has become inflamed
* Reduced vision is rare in developed countries but may occur due to encroachment of the pterygium onto the visual axis and consequently induced astigmatism.

Examination

* Usually nasal; less often temporal
* Localized decreased tear wetting, in some cases leading to a defect of the overlying epithelium, and/or dellen
* Localized conjunctival hyperaemia
* There may be iron deposition (Stockers line) in the corneal epithelium adjacent to the pterygium.

Differential diagnosis

* Pseudopterygia may occur following trauma, chronic conjunctival inflammation, rosacea, or chemical injury. They can occur in any location around the limbus. Pseudopterygia are fixed only at the apex to the cornea, whereas true pterygia are fixed to underlying structures throughout.
* Conjunctival intraepithelial neoplasia and carcinoma growing onto the cornea

Management

* Patients should be reassured that visual loss from pterygia is uncommon.
* **Advise** wearing UV-blocking sunglasses.
* **Topical treatment** is as for pinguecula.
* **Surgical excision** is the only definitive treatment option.

Pterygium excision with conjunctival autograft

Indications

* Cosmesis
* Chronic/recurrent redness and irritation
* Blurred vision from induced astigmatism
* Encroachment onto the visual axis

Pterygia have an unacceptably high recurrence rate following simple excision. This rate is reduced significantly by conjunctival autografting. This procedure usually involves harvesting a free conjunctival graft from the superior bulbar conjunctiva (note the superior conjunctiva should be avoided in patients with glaucoma). The graft is sized according to the conjunctival defect created by removal of the pterygium. The graft may be fixed by suturing with 10–0 Vicryl sutures or with biological fibrin glue. This procedure may also be augmented by application of mitomycin C intraoperatively if recurrence is considered likely.

Concretions

Concretions are epithelial inclusion cysts filled with lipid and keratin debris. They occur in the elderly or following chronic conjunctivitis/blepharitis. They manifest clinically as multiple discrete white/yellow deposits in the palpebral conjunctiva. They are normally asymptomatic. If they erode through the overlying conjunctival epithelium, they may cause a foreign body sensation. In symptomatic cases, they can be removed under topical anaesthesia at the slit lamp, with a 25-gauge needle.

Inclusion cyst

Inclusion cysts are discrete clear fluid filled cysts which, if symptomatic (ocular surface irritation), should be surgically excised.

Lymphangiectasia

Lymphangiectasias are local dilatations of thin-walled conjunctival lymphatic vessels. They appear as single or multiple lobular clear fluid filled cysts.

Conjunctivochalasis

In conjunctivochalasis, folds of redundant conjunctiva lie on the margin of the lid, typically inferiorly. This condition occurs with ageing and/or with chronic ocular surface inflammation. The mobile, redundant conjunctiva can result in a foreign body sensation and there may be fluorescein staining of the inferior cornea and conjunctiva.

Treatment of associated blepharitis and use of tear supplements may result in remission. If these do not alleviate symptoms, then the redundant conjunctiva may be excised surgically.

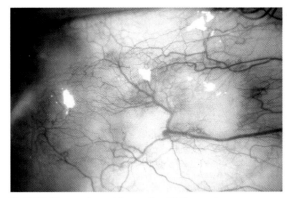

Fig 2.30 Pingueculum with associated inflammation

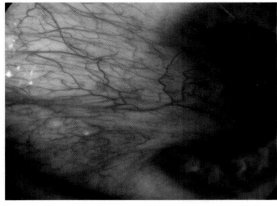

Fig 2.31 Large pterygium encroaching onto the centre of the cornea

Conjunctival neoplasia can be classified according to the cell type that the lesion arises from and then subclassified into benign, premalignant, or malignant.

Epithelial neoplasia

Conjunctival papilloma

Conjunctival papillomas are **benign** lesions. There are two forms of conjunctival papilloma, each caused by a different strain of the human papilloma virus (HPV):

1. Sessile: normally found at the limbus, these lesions are flat and shiny (see Figure 2.32A). Beneath the epithelium, there are numerous dilated fronds of abnormal capillaries. Dysplastic change (more common with sessile lesions than with pedunculated lesions) can occur and is suggested by symblepharon formation, inflammation, and invasion.
2. Pedunculated: these are normally found in the inferior fornix and are fleshy, multilobulated, exophytic growths emanating from a stalk with a fibrovascular core.

Treatment

These lesions can regress spontaneously and can be observed if asymptomatic. If necessary, complete surgical excision with adjunctive cryotherapy is the treatment of choice. Recurrences are treated by repeat excision, interferon alpha, topical mitomycin C, or oral cimetidine.

Conjunctival intraepithelial neoplasia

Conjunctival intraepithelial neoplasia (CIN), which is a **premalignant** process, occurs when dysplastic cells are present but do not invade the underlying epithelial basement membrane. The process is graded histologically as mild, moderate, or severe, depending on the extent of cellular atypia. When the full thickness of the epithelium is involved, CIN is known as carcinoma in situ. Risk factors implicated include light skin, chronic UV exposure, smoking, immunosuppression (including HIV infection), HPV infection, and xeroderma pigmentosum.

Clinical evaluation

There are three clinical variants, all of which are slow-growing:

1. En plaque: this is the most common type. The appearance is of a raised, gelatinous, or leukoplakic (white) lesion with a 'stuck-on' appearance and tufts of superficial vessels (see Figure 2.32B).
2. Papilliform: here the CIN arises from an existing dysplastic sessile papilloma.
3. Diffuse: this variant is the least common of the three. The appearance is of an indistinct, diffusely thickened conjunctiva.

All these lesions are commonly associated with a granular, translucent epithelial sheet with fimbriated edges that extends onto the cornea. There is no corneal neovascularization associated with these lesions

Treatment

* Surgical excision with a 1–2 mm margin of clinically uninvolved tissue. Rose bengal staining can be used to help delineate tumour margins.
* Adjunctive cryotherapy should be applied to the conjunctival margins in a double freeze-thaw technique at the time of surgery.
* If there is corneal involvement, then the affected corneal epithelium should be removed with absolute alcohol.

* Recurrence is common, especially with more advanced lesions.
* Topical: interferon alpha, mitomycin C, or fluorouracil can be used as adjuncts or alternatives to surgical treatment in select cases.

Squamous cell carcinoma

This **malignant** neoplasm arises from a CIN lesion that has either broken through the basement membrane to involve the subepithelial tissue or has metastasized. Morbidity is related primarily to local involvement of the conjunctiva and the cornea. Regional spread and distant metastasis are a rare possibility. The risk factors are as for CIN.

Clinical evaluation

* Many patients are asymptomatic and are diagnosed incidentally on routine optician/ophthalmic examination.
* Possible symptoms include ocular surface irritation, a mass, or blurred vision if the central cornea is involved.
* The appearance may be consistent with any of the forms of CIN described in 'Conjunctival intraepithelial neoplasia'.
* One feature particularly suggestive of malignancy is the presence of prominent conjunctival/episcleral feeder vessels.

Treatment

Treatment is as for CIN. If malignancy is suspected, wide (3 mm) surgical margins are advisable to prevent recurrence. An episclerectomy must be performed in these cases along with a superficial sclerectomy if there is tethering to underlying structures; Absolute alcohol can be applied to the scleral base. In rare cases of globe or orbital invasion, more radical surgery may be necessary.

Lymphoma

Conjunctiva-associated lymphoid tissue can act as a reservoir or source of lymphoproliferative neoplasia that ranges histologically from lymphoid hyperplasia (formerly known as reactive hyperplasia) through to lymphoma (see Figure 2.32C). Conjunctival lymphomas represent a monoclonal proliferation predominantly of B-cells. Most conjunctival lymphomas are non-Hodgkin. Lymphomas may be limited to the conjunctiva or may be associated with systemic involvement.

Clinical evaluation

* Benign (lymphoid hyperplasia) and malignant lesions cannot be distinguished clinically.
* Most tumours will be marginal zone B-cell lymphomas (MALToma), which are more common in young people.
* The classical presentation is a slow-growing, salmon-coloured, diffuse, mobile, subepithelial mass with moderate vascularization.
* The lesions may be localized to the conjunctiva or may extend into the orbit.

Treatment

* Patients must be referred to a haematologist for systemic investigation and staging.
* Incisional biopsy is necessary for histopathological diagnosis.
* Local radiotherapy is usually successful in treating lesions confined to the conjunctiva. Systemic chemotherapy may be required if there is systemic involvement.

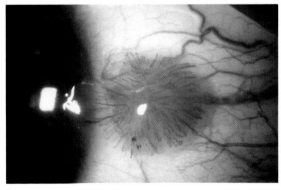

A

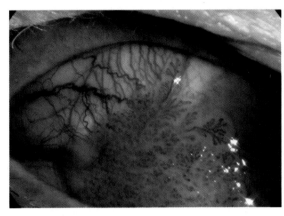

B

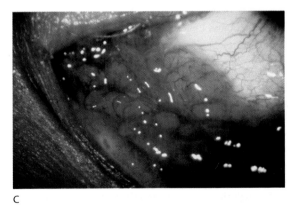

C

Fig 2.32
A Sessile conjunctival papilloma
B En plaque conjunctival intraepithelial neoplasia. Note the prominent episcleral feeder vessels.
C Conjunctival lymphoma

Melanocyte-associated neoplasia

Naevi

These **benign** lesions are composed of melanocytes, naevus cells, and epithelial cells (see Figure 2.33). They can be histologically classified into junctional, compound, or subepithelial. They arise during childhood and adolescence.

Clinical evaluation

They appear as solitary, variably pigmented, well-demarcated lesions. The most common location is at the limbus, where they tend to be flat. In other locations, they are elevated. Increased pigmentation may occur at puberty, together with rapid enlargement due to the development of epithelial down-growth cysts, which are common in conjunctival melanocytic naevi.

Treatment

Malignant transformation is rare. Lesions can often be photographed and observed. Indications for surgical excision include:
- Change in appearance, suspicious of malignancy (increase in size, change in pigmentation, vascularization)
- Lesions of the palpebral conjunctiva (as naevi are rare here)
- Cosmesis

Congenital epithelial melanosis

Also known as a conjunctival freckle, congenital epithelial melanosis is a **benign** lesion that appears within the first few years of life as a flat brown patch normally near the limbus.

Benign melanosis

Benign melanosis is a condition in which there is a bilateral, diffuse increase in the pigmentation of the conjunctiva; it tends to occur in darkly pigmented, middle-aged individuals. It is characterized by light-brown pigmentation of the perilimbal and the interpalpebral bulbar conjunctiva. Streaks of pigmentation can extend into the peripheral corneal epithelium (striate melanokeratosis).

Ocular melanocytosis

Ocular melanocytosis is a **benign** congenital pigmentation of the episclera and occurs most commonly in pigmented individuals. It is caused by a subepithelial proliferation of normal melanocytes (see Figure 2.34).

Clinical evaluation

Patches of episcleral pigmentation have a slate-grey appearance through the conjunctiva. The iris and choroid may also show increased pigmentation. Approximately 50% of affected patients also have ipsilateral dermal melanocytosis (oculodermal melanocytosis, also known as naevus of Ota; see Chapter 1, Section 1.7). Malignant transformation is rare but, when it occurs, usually takes place in the uveal tract. Very occasionally, primary orbital malignant melanoma arises in association with melanocytosis.

Primary acquired melanosis

Primary acquired melanosis is a **premalignant,** predominantly unilateral condition that normally occurs in middle-aged, fair-skinned individuals. It arises owing to a proliferation of abnormal melanocytes in the basal conjunctival epithelium. It is classified histologically depending on whether the cells exhibit atypia. If atypia is present, there is a significantly greater chance of malignant transformation (to melanoma; see 'Melanoma'; see Figure 2.35).

Clinical evaluation

- Multiple, flat, brown, noncystic patches of pigmentation; can occur on any area of the conjunctiva

- Malignant transformation should be suspected when there is enlargement, fixation of the conjunctiva to deeper structures, nodularity, increased vascularization, and/or haemorrhage.

Treatment

- Discrete areas can be surgically excised with a technique similar to that used for CIN.
- More diffuse lesions that are too extensive to permit surgical excision can be treated with cryotherapy or topical mitomycin C.

Melanoma

Melanoma is a rare, potentially fatal **malignant** neoplasm (see Figure 2.36) which can arise de novo (approximately 10% of cases), from a pre-existing naevus (approximately 20% of cases), or from primary acquired melanosis with atypia (60%–70% of cases). It typically occurs in fair-skinned individuals in their 50s.

Clinical evaluation

- Presentation is variable depending on the presence of pre-existing lesions and the extent, nature, and location of the tumour. Melanomas can occur in any part of the conjunctiva. The most common location is the bulbar conjunctiva, at the interpalpebral limbus.
- Typical presentation is a solitary, dark nodule which is fixed to the episclera and associated with dilated feeder vessels.
- Lesions can be amelanotic with a pink, fleshy appearance.

Treatment

- The primary treatment is surgical resection, as for squamous cell carcinoma of the conjunctiva.
- Extensive lesions that invade the globe or orbit may require exenteration, although this procedure does not improve survival.
- Topical mitomycin C may have a role as an adjunct to surgery.

Prognosis

- Mortality is approximately 15% at 10 years.
- Poor prognostic factors include tumours not involving the limbus, multifocal lesions that arise de novo, residual involvement at the surgical margins, and lymphatic or orbital spread.

Epibulbar choristomas

Epibulbar choristomas are **benign** congenital lesions that occur when normal tissue grows in an abnormal location during embryogenesis.

Epibulbar dermoid

Epibulbar dermoids result from displaced embryonic tissue that was otherwise destined to have become skin tissue. They are composed of fibrous tissue and can also contain hair follicles or sebaceous glands. They are embedded in the superficial sclera and/or the cornea.

Clinical evaluation

- Typical presentation is in infancy/early childhood, with a smooth, well-demarcated, white-to-yellow coloured lesion that is fixed to underlying structures.
- They normally occur beneath the conjunctiva at the inferotemporal limbus. They can also be found on the cornea or in the orbit.

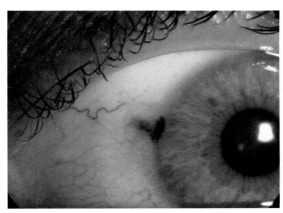

Fig 2.33 Conjunctival naevus

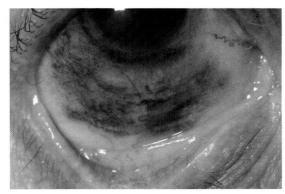

Fig 2.35 Primary acquired melanosis

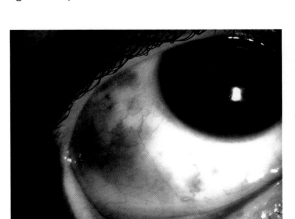

Fig 2.34 Ocular melanocytosis

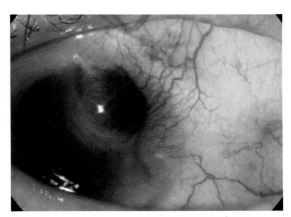

Fig 2.36 Invasive melanoma occurring in an area of primary acquired melanosis

- They may interfere with normal lid function, obscure the visual axis, or induce astigmatism and subsequent amblyopia.
  Limbal dermoids may be associated with Goldenhar syndrome (oculoauriculovertebral dysplasia), which is a congenital disorder of the first branchial arch. Other features include upper lid colobomas, preauricular skin tags, and vertebral anomalies.

Treatment

- Treatment is indicated for obstruction of the visual axis, ocular surface irritation, astigmatism, or cosmesis.
- The elevated portion of a dermoid can be excised but there is often deep extension into underlying tissues, preventing complete removal. Lamellar keratoplasty may be necessary if there is significant corneal involvement.

Dermolipoma (lipodermoid)

Dermolipomas predominantly contain adipose tissue, in addition to other skin elements. They are normally found at the outer canthus, where they have a gelatinous appearance. There is classically an indistinct posterior border, with the lesion extending into the orbit. There is a well-demarcated anterior border several millimetres behind the limbus. These lesions tend to be more extensive than simple epibulbar dermoids are. It is important to distinguish these lesions from prolapsed orbital fat, which has a very similar clinical appearance but, unlike dermolipomas, can be moved freely over the sclera beneath. Treatment for dermolipomas is as for epibulbar dermoid.

Vascular lesions

Kaposi sarcoma

Kaposi sarcoma is also described in Chapter 1, Section 1.10. It **is a malignant** neoplasm of vascular endothelium which affects the skin and mucous membranes. It occurs following infection with the human herpes virus 8. In young patients, it often occurs with AIDS.

When present on the conjunctiva, the appearance is of a bright red, highly vascular subconjunctival lesion that may simulate a chronic subconjunctival haemorrhage. It most commonly presents in the inferior fornix. Options for treatment include surgical debulking, cryotherapy, and radiotherapy.

Pyogenic granuloma

Pyogenic granuloma is an inflammatory vascular proliferation. It is a misnomer because it is not suppurative nor does it contain giant cells. The lesion may occur over a chalazion or when minor trauma or surgery stimulates an excessive healing reaction. It is a rapidly growing lesion that is red, smooth, and pedunculated. Treatment is with topical steroids alone or surgical excision combined with topical steroids.

Metastatic tumours

Secondary metastatic deposits in the conjunctiva from primary tumours elsewhere such as the breast, lung, and kidney do occur very rarely. Treatment is palliative.

2.15 Corneal degeneration

Corneal degeneration presents as usually bilateral (often asymmetric) corneal changes. It commonly occurs with increasing age. It can be categorized as follows:

- **Primary age-related corneal degeneration:** arcus senilis, shagreen, white limbal girdle, and corneal farinata
- **Inflammatory corneal degeneration:** band keratopathy, lipid keratopathy, and Salzmann nodular degeneration
- **UV radiation-related corneal degeneration:** climatic keratopathy

Arcus senilis

Pathophysiology
Arcus senilis is an extremely common, age-related condition that is caused by the deposition of lipid in the peripheral corneal stroma (see Figure 2.37). It affects nearly everyone over the age of 80 years. It is not usually associated with any underlying systemic disorder. However, arcus in young patients is occasionally secondary to hyperlipoproteinaemia. Unilateral arcus is rare and is associated with ocular hypotony or carotid artery disease.

Clinical evaluation
- This condition is first seen at the superior and inferior corneal periphery and progresses to encircle the entire corneal circumference.
- The arcus has a hazy white appearance with a sharp peripheral border and an indistinct central border.
- There is a clear corneal zone between the arcus and the limbus, which may show mild thinning (a furrow).

Management
Arcus senilis has no effect on vision and no treatment is required. Young patients (<40 years old) with a family history of cardiovascular disease should have a serum lipid profile performed.

Corneal shagreen

Corneal shagreen is characterized by bilateral, polygonal, greyish-white stromal opacities separated by clear zones (see Figure 2.38). These opacities are usually centrally located and are asymptomatic. The lesions can be located in the anterior stroma (anterior form) or the posterior stroma (posterior form). No treatment is required.

White limbal girdle (of Vogt)

White limbal girdle (of Vogt) is a crescent-shaped, white, chalky band that occurs along the nasal or temporal limbus in the interpalpebral fissure (see Figure 2.39). No treatment is required.

Corneal farinata

Corneal farinata is characterized by bilateral, asymptomatic, tiny deposits located in the posterior stroma and which look like grains of flour. The lesions are more prominent centrally and are best seen using oblique diffuse illumination.

Band keratopathy

Pathophysiology
Band keratopathy is a common condition that occurs as a result of precipitation of calcium salts from the tear film into Bowman's layer (see Figure 2.40). It is often idiopathic, occurring commonly with increasing age. It has a number of known causes:

- Ocular: chronic anterior uveitis (especially in children), phthisis bulbi, intraocular silicone oil, alkali injury
- Systemic: hypercalcaemia, hyperphosphatemia, and hyperuricaemia (urate rather than calcium is deposited)
- Hereditary

Clinical evaluation
- The first appearance is of a peripheral, white, granular, superficial deposition nasally and/or temporally, with a clear zone separating the peripheral edge of the lesion from the limbus. There are often clear holes within the lesion.
- Eventually, the nasal and temporal deposits can coalesce to form a horizontal, band-shaped plaque across the entire cornea. If the optical zone of the cornea is affected, patients may complain of glare or reduced vision.
- When the band is long-standing, there may be flakes of calcium that break through the overlying epithelium and result in discomfort and foreign body sensation.

Investigations
Only investigate for systemic disease (serum calcium, phosphate, renal function) if there is no identifiable ocular cause.

Treatment
Any underlying systemic disease must be treated. Ocular treatment is only indicated if the patient is symptomatic. For mild symptoms of discomfort, use ocular lubricants. If lubricants are ineffective then the band can be removed surgically:

- **EDTA chelation of band keratopathy:** this procedure is performed under topical anaesthesia. Dilute a solution of 15% EDTA to create a 3% mixture. Debride the corneal epithelium with a scalpel. Rub a cellulose sponge saturated with EDTA over the band until the cornea clears (may require 20–30 minutes).
- **Phototherapeutic keratectomy** is quick and effective if the surface is regular. Ablating an irregular surface will tend to leave irregular astigmatism.

Lipid keratopathy

Lipid keratopathy is caused by lipid deposition in the stroma. It normally occurs in a pre-existing vascularized scar such as those seen following herpetic keratitis or other causes of interstitial keratitis. The blood vessels are incompetent and leak lipids. The clinical appearance is of a yellow/cream-coloured deposit within the corneal stroma.

Treatment should be aimed at any underlying inflammatory process to prevent further leakage of lipids. Feeder vessel occlusion by argon laser photocoagulation or cautery can sometimes induce regression or limit progression. Penetrating or lamellar keratoplasty can be considered for visually significant corneal opacities.

Climatic keratopathy

Climatic keratopathy is a bilateral condition caused by prolonged exposure to environmental UV light. Patients also often have pterygia. Climatic keratopathy is characterized by the presence of numerous yellow-golden spheres in the anterior interpalpebral stroma. It is usually asymptomatic but can cause discomfort because of surface irregularity or reduce vision (if it progresses to form a band across the pupil). Treatment options include lamellar keratoplasty, lubricants, or having the patient wear UV-blocking sunglasses (with good side protection).

Salzmann nodular degeneration

Salzmann nodular degeneration is caused by localized degeneration at the level of Bowmans layer in conjunction with the deposition of hyaline and fibrillar material. It can be idiopathic or occur as a late sequel of chronic keratitis (VKC, trachoma). The clinical appearance is classically that of discrete, elevated, grey-white, subepithelial nodules in the paracentral cornea or at the edge of a corneal scar (see Figure 2.41). Treatment for ocular surface discomfort is with lubricants. If vision is affected, then superficial keratectomy or lamellar keratoplasty may be required.

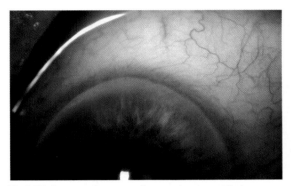

Fig 2.37 Arcus senilis seen at the superior corneal limbus

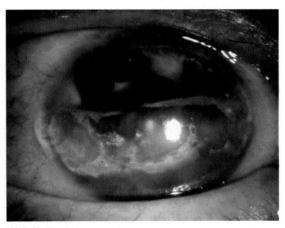

Fig 2.40 Band keratopathy

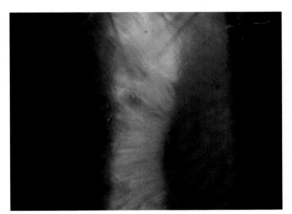

Fig 2.38 Corneal shagreen seen in the area of diffuse illumination

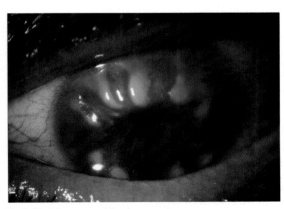

Fig 2.41 Salzmann nodular degeneration

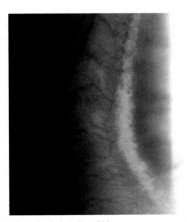

Fig 2.39 White limbal girdle of Vogt

2.16 Infectious keratitis I: Bacterial

The term 'infectious keratitis' is an umbrella term for all cases of keratitis caused by infection. The term 'microbial keratitis' applies to corneal infections caused by bacteria, fungi, or protozoa, but not viruses. There are a wide variety of potential pathogens and host responses involved in this sight-threatening disease. Although polymicrobial keratitis is common, the various causative organisms will be covered separately.

Bacterial keratitis

Bacterial keratitis is the most common form of infectious keratitis (see Figure 2.42). Onset and disease progression may be rapid. Corneal destruction may be complete in less than 24 hours, with the most virulent of bacteria.

Pathophysiology

Disruption of the corneal epithelium permits the entrance of bacteria into the corneal stroma, where they proliferate. Invading bacteria secrete proteases and attract neutrophils that migrate into the cornea from the limbal vasculature and tear film. Matrix metalloproteinases are released, breaking down the extracellular matrix and causing inflammatory necrosis. Progressive inflammation may result in corneal perforation and secondary endophthalmitis. When bacterial replication is controlled, wound healing processes begin, but this may be accompanied by corneal neovascularization and scarring.

Risk factors

* Contact lens wear (especially soft contact lenses and overnight wear; less common with daily disposable lenses)
* Trauma (including foreign bodies)
* Immunosuppression
* Corneal surgery
* Dry eye or other causes of ocular surface disease; e.g.:
  - HSK
  - Exposure
  - Neurotrophic keratitis
  - Bullous keratopathy

Bacterial keratitis is rare in the absence of these risk factors.

Common causative organisms

* *Pseudomonas aeruginosa* (most common organism in soft contact lens wearers)
* *Staph. aureus / Staph. epidermidis*
* *Strep.* spp.
* Enterobacteriaceae (*Proteus, Enterobacter,* and *Serratia*)

Clinical evaluation

History

* Typical presentation is with increasing foreign body sensation, pain, photophobia, and reduced vision.

Examination

* The typical presentation is with a sharply demarcated epithelial defect (termed 'ulcer' if there is associated stromal tissue loss) and an underlying, focal, dense, white stromal infiltrate consisting of neutrophils and bacteria (stromal abscess) with surrounding stromal oedema.
* Other signs that may be present include intense conjunctival injection, eyelid oedema, an endothelial inflammatory plaque, anterior chamber reaction, hypopyon (normally sterile in the absence of perforation), and corneal thinning.

* Patients who are immunocompromised (including those taking topical steroid medication) who present with a stromal melt should be suspected of having infectious keratitis until proven otherwise. These patients do not necessarily mount the inflammatory response necessary to produce the classical signs listed.

Differential diagnosis

* Other causes of infectious keratitis (fungal, viral, protozoal)
* Sterile keratitis (contact lens related, marginal keratitis)

Investigations

* Corneal cultures should be taken in all cases to provide material for microbiological diagnosis. Taking samples for culture may also help to remove necrotic tissue and enhance antibiotic penetration.
* Corneal scrapes for PCR, if PCR is available, should also be taken in atypical or unresponsive cases.
* Baseline indices of disease, such as size of epithelial defect, extent of thinning, and infiltrate size, should be recorded.
* The technique for corneal scraping is as follows:
  - Instil non-preserved topical anaesthetic.
  - Use 21-gauge (green) needles or no. 15 blades, using a new needle/blade for each medium.
  - Scrape at the edge and the base of the ulcer (avoid the base if there is significant thinning).
  - Spread material onto a glass slide for Gram staining.
  - For culture, spread material directly as several 'C' shapes onto the culture medium (avoiding breaking the surface).
* Use the following culture media:
  - Blood agar (most aerobic bacteria and fungi will grow on this medium)
  - Liquid broths (e.g. thioglycolate broth, cooked meat broth) will preserve anaerobes
  - The following types of media are only necessary if specific organisms are suspected or if initial cultures have been negative: chocolate agar (*Haemophilus* spp., *Neisseria* spp.), Löwenstein–Jensen medium (mycobacteria). Samples for *Acanthamoeba* or fungi will be discussed in Section 2.17.
* Send contact lens and case (if available) for culture

Treatment

The aims of treatment are (1) to sterilize the wound and (2) to promote healing:

Sterilization phase

* Commence intensive broad spectrum antibiotics. Treatment is usually monotherapy with a fluoroquinolone (e.g. levofloxacin or moxifloxacin eye drops, 0.5%) hourly day and night for 2 days then reducing as signs permit over the next 7 days. Alternatively, a fortified cephalosporin (e.g. cefuroxime 5%) and an aminoglycoside (e.g. gentamicin 1.5%) will cover most Gram-positive or Gram-negative pathogens.
* Topical cycloplegic drops for comfort
* Consider systemic antibiotics (e.g. ciprofloxacin 750 mg twice a day or moxifloxacin 400 mg once a day) if there is

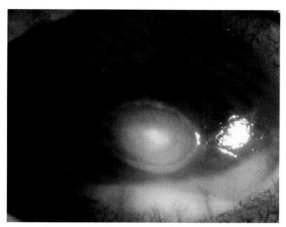

Fig 2.42 Bacterial keratitis
Note the associated hypopyon

an actual or threatened perforation, to reduce the risk of endophthalmitis.

- Consider admission for intensive treatment if there is concern with compliance or in complicated cases (e.g. only eye, unable to administer drops).
- Review in 48 hours to assess the clinical response and the initial culture results. Features suggestive of positive response to antibiotic treatment include reduced pain, sharper margins/decreased infiltrate intensity, and decreased inflammatory signs. Antibiotic treatment should be reassessed if there is clinical progression despite treatment or if culture results indicate resistance to the initial antibiotic therapy.
- Review as required (e.g.g. after one week) to confirm recovery is continued. In cases that do not improve, consider stopping all antibiotics for 24 hours and reculturing. If progression continues and cultures are negative, consider a corneal biopsy for culture and histology.

Healing phase
The aim of this phase is to promote healing and re-epithelialization of the ulcer by using the following measures:
- Reduction of inflammation: cautious addition of topical steroids (e.g.g. prednisolone 0.5% four times a day), once it is clear that the infection is responding to the antibiotics (steroids may potentiate herpetic or fungal infection)
- Prevention of drop toxicity: reduce the frequency of aminoglycoside treatment to four times a day, within 48 hours
- Treat associated ocular surface disease.

Complications
- **Threatened/actual perforation:** should be referred urgently to a corneal specialist. Corneal glue may seal a small corneal perforation (see 'Corneal glue'), allowing time for the infection to be controlled and potentially avoiding the need for surgery. Emergency keratoplasty may be necessary but, in the presence of active infection, the prognosis for graft survival is poor and this procedure should be avoided if possible.
- **Endophthalmitis:** bacteria, unlike fungi, do not penetrate an intact Descemet's membrane and do not cause endophthalmitis unless there is a concurrent perforation.

- **Irregular astigmatism:** from stromal loss during infection
- **Scar formation:** if the scar results in a significant effect on vision, then surgical options such as lamellar or penetrating keratoplasty may be required.

Infectious crystalline keratopathy

Infectious crystalline keratopathy is a specific and rare form of corneal stromal infection. It is typically caused by slow-growing beta haemolytic streptococci (viridans streptococci), but it may also be caused by mycobacterium or other organisms. It classically occurs in patients that have undergone corneal graft surgery and who have been on long-term topical steroid treatment, which suppresses the usual response to infection. It presents as densely packed, white, branching aggregates of organisms, with an almost complete absence of an inflammatory response (see Figure 2.43).

Corneal glue

Background/indication
- Applied to restore the integrity of the globe in corneal perforations up to 1 mm in diameter
- To avoid or delay more definitive surgery (e.g. tectonic keratoplasty) and to buy time whilst other treatments such as antibiotics and/or immunosuppression take effect
- Tissue adhesives (e.g. Dermabond, Histoacryl) are long-chain derivatives of cyanoacrylate. Commercial 'superglue' (methyl cyanoacrylate) is toxic and should not be used.

Technique
- Apply at a slit lamp or with the patient supine under the operating microscope.
- Instil topical anaesthetic. Debride the epithelium over the area to which the glue is to be applied. Dry the area with a cellulose sponge and apply the glue immediately.
- The application technique depends on the size of the perforation. For microperforations (<0.25 mm) the glue can be applied directly with the tip of a 30-gauge needle.
- For larger perforations, a patch technique is required. A small disc of polythene from the non-adhesive portion of a sterile surgical drape is cut out with a 3–4 mm skin biopsy trephine (the disc must be large enough to cover the perforation, with a 1 mm surround). The patch is placed on top of the wooden end of a cotton-tipped applicator that has been dipped in K-Y gel (to prevent the patch sticking to the applicator). A very thin layer of glue is applied to the exposed surface of the patch with a 30-gauge needle. The applicator is then used to firmly press the patch onto the cornea. Pressure is maintained until the glue can be seen to 'set'.
- Minimal iris adhesions at the site of perforation can usually be left, as they will break when the anterior chamber reforms. If the adhesions are extensive, they may need to be repositioned in theatre.
- Place a bandage contact lens on the cornea for comfort
The glue can normally be left in situ until it spontaneously detaches as the cornea heals (see Figure 2.44).

Further reading

1. Allan BD, Dart JK: Strategies for the management of microbial keratitis. *Br J Ophthalmol* 1995 Aug; **79**(8): 777–86.

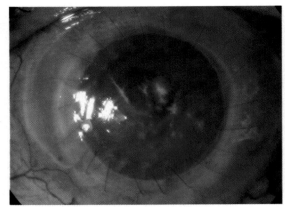

Fig 2.43 Infectious crystalline keratopathy

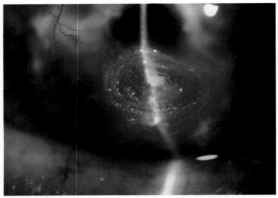

Fig 2.44 Patch of corneal glue in situ

Acanthamoeba keratitis

Pathophysiology

Acanthamoeba is a genus of free-living protozoa. These organisms are ubiquitous and can be found in tap water, fresh water, swimming pools, air, and soil. Acanthamoebas exist in two forms: (1) active trophozoites and (2) dormant cysts. Trophozoites produce enzymes that aid tissue penetration and destruction. They are thought to feed on keratocytes. Cysts are extremely resilient and are able to survive in unfavourable conditions such as extremes of temperature and chlorine. The major risk factor for developing *Acanthamoeba* keratitis is contact lens wear, which is implicated in 85% of cases in developed countries. The risk is increased by poor contact lens hygiene, including improper storage/disinfection, and swimming or showering in lenses. In developing countries, *Acanthamoeba* keratitis is associated with corneal trauma contaminated by soil or water.

Clinical evaluation

Acanthamoeba keratitis should be considered in all cases of progressive keratitis not responding to first-line antimicrobial therapy.

History

* Gradual increase in discomfort over a course of weeks. Patients are frequently misdiagnosed initially. HSK is a common misdiagnosis. Misdiagnosis delays appropriate treatment.
* Severe pain in some patients (disproportionate to clinical signs), redness, and photophobia

Examination

* In early cases, the disease is localized to the epithelium, with heaped epithelial irregularity, punctate epithelial erosions, or pseudodendrites (mimicking HSK). Corneal sensation may be reduced. Infiltrates along the corneal nerves (radial keratoneuritis; see Figure 2.45) are highly suggestive of *Acanthamoeba* infection.
* Stromal infection normally occurs centrally. Early cases present with grey-white diffuse stromal infiltrate with an overlying epithelial defect. This condition can progress to an abscess with stromal melting. In advanced cases, this area may become surrounded by a characteristic dense ring infiltrate (see Figure 2.46).
* Other clinical signs include limbitis, diffuse/nodular scleritis, anterior uveitis, and hypopyon.
   Note: patients with suspected HSK who have recently worn contact lenses should also always be investigated for *Acanthamoeba* infection.

Investigations

Definitive diagnosis of *Acanthamoeba* keratitis requires positive culture, histology, or PCR (where available).

In early cases, the epithelium should be debrided and sent for investigation. The stroma should be sampled in eyes with a corneal abscess, or biopsied in cases in which the initial culture was negative. Culture contact lenses and solutions if available.

1. Culture on non-nutrient agar with *Escherichia coli* overlay (plate directly onto non-nutrient agar or send a sample in saline for the laboratory to plate).
2. Histology (Gram/Giemsa/calcofluor white stains; send samples in formalin)

In vivo confocal microscopy can detect cysts and trophozoites and can be useful if available. However, a definitive diagnosis cannot be made on clinical findings and confocal microscopy alone.

Treatment

Early diagnosis and treatment is the most important prognostic indicator for a successful outcome. Cysts are relatively resistant, and prolonged treatment is required (6 months or more). Treatment is initially hourly and consists of the following two components:

* **Biguanide:** polyhexamethylene biguanide 0.02% *or* chlorhexidine 0.02%
* **Diamidine:** propamidine 1% (Brolene) *or* hexamidine 1%
   Ocular surface toxicity is common with these drops. Topical steroid should only be use if there is uncontrolled inflammation, stromal melting, or vascularization. Steroid use may contribute to the persistence of viable cysts.
   Oral NSAIDs may help control discomfort.
   Keratoplasty is indicated for impending perforation or for significant central corneal scarring once infection has been eradicated.

Fungal keratitis

Fungal keratitis (see Figure 2.47) is rare in temperate countries, chronic, and difficult to treat. Fungal keratitis is more common in the tropics and in agricultural workers. Fungi gain entry through an epithelial defect. The most common pathogens are filamentous fungi (*Fusarium* and *Aspergillus* spp.) or yeast (*Candida albicans*).

Risk factors include:

* Agricultural trauma
* Contact lens wear
* Topical steroid use
* Immunosuppression
* Diabetes
* Chronic keratitis or ocular surgery

Clinical evaluation

* There may be foreign body sensation, watering, pain, photophobia, and a visible corneal opacity. Inflammatory manifestations of fungal keratitis are milder in the initial period than those of bacterial keratitis but may progress to signs of intense inflammation.
* **Filamentous fungal keratitis** presents as a grey-white infiltrate with irregular feathery margins. The stroma may have a dry, rough texture before melting begins. Additional manifestations include multifocal/satellite lesions, deep stromal infiltrate in the presence of an intact epithelium, endothelial plaques, and/or hypopyon. As the keratitis progresses, it becomes clinically indistinguishable from bacterial keratitis. Fungi may penetrate Descemet's membrane and enter the anterior chamber to cause endophthalmitis.
* **Yeast keratitis** presents with white infiltrates similar in appearance to those associated with bacterial keratitis. Patients often have a history of chronic ocular surface disease treated with topical steroid.

Investigations

Samples are collected as for bacterial keratitis and should be sent for:

1. Stain: fungal cell walls stain with Gomori methenamine silver. Gram stain highlights *Candida* but not filamentary fungal species.
2. Culture: blood agar, Sabourauds agar, and brain–heart infusion media

   Consider corneal biopsy for histology and culture.

Treatment

* Superficial corneal debridement: removal of the epithelium aids penetration of antifungals and reduces the fungal load.
* Topical antifungal therapy is commenced hourly and tapered slowly over 6–8 weeks. Initial treatment is with natamycin eye drops, 1%, (active against *Candida* spp., *Aspergillus* spp.,and *Fusarium* spp.) or amphotericin 0.15% (active against *Candida* spp. and *Aspergillus* spp.). Voriconazole (as eye drops) is an alternative agent. Chlorhexidine eye drops, 0.2%, may be added in severe cases.
* If a topical steroid is already being used by the patient, its use should be stopped, if possible.
* Severe disease (deep peripheral corneal lesions, scleral or intraocular invasion) requires adjunctive systemic therapy with oral voriconazole or itraconazole.

Advice from a microbiologist should be sought once the isolate has been identified.

A penetrating keratoplasty to excise infected tissue may be required in cases that continue to progress despite maximal medical therapy. The prognosis is poor in these cases.

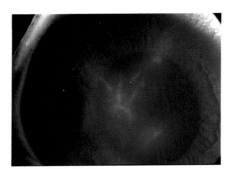

Fig 2.45 *Acanthamoeba* keratitis
Radial keratoneuritis

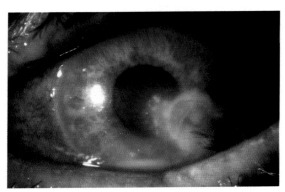

Fig 2.47 Fungal keratitis secondary to aspergillus
Note the satellite lesions

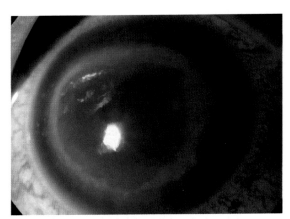

Fig 2.46 *Acanthamoeba* keratitis.
Ring infiltrate

Pathophysiology

The herpes simplex virus (HSV) is a double-stranded DNA virus. Ocular disease is caused by HSV-1, which causes orofacial (and rarely genital) disease. HSV-2 causes genital (rarely, orofacial and ocular) disease.

Primary infection with HSV-1 generally occurs in childhood through skin and mucous membrane contact with oral lesions and secretions. Primary infection is normally with a non-specific upper respiratory tract infection but can result in orofacial, ocular (blepharoconjunctivitis, rarely keratitis) or rarely systemic (encephalitis, meningitis, myelitis, hepatitis) manifestations. The virus then ascends via sensory nerve axons to establish latent infection in the corresponding ganglion (trigeminal ganglion for orofacial/ocular exposure). Viral reactivation can later occur whereby the virus travels along the nerve axon to the sensory nerve endings and then to the epithelium, where it replicates. Various factors including sunlight, trauma, surgery, heat, menstruation, infectious diseases, and emotional stress have all been implicated as potential triggers for reactivation.

HSK can be classified according to the layer of the cornea that is predominantly affected: epithelial, stromal, or endothelial. Epithelial HSK occurs through the reactivation and replication of virus (and rarely as a manifestation of primary infection). The pathophysiology of stromal and endothelial HSK remains poorly understood but is believed to be immune-mediated.

Epithelial keratitis

Clinical evaluation

History

Presentation is with foreign body sensation, watering, redness, blurred vision, and/or photophobia.

Examination

* Corneal sensation may be reduced or absent.
* The earliest visible manifestations are areas of punctate epithelial keratitis; these coalesce into one or more linear, branching, dendritic epithelial ulcers with terminal bulbs at the end of each branch.
* There is swollen, heaped-up epithelium around the edge of the ulcer, which stains with rose bengal. The base of the ulcer stains with fluorescein (see Figure 2.48).
* There may be an anterior stromal infiltrate under the ulcer; this infiltrate normally resolves when the epithelium has healed.
* Areas of dendritic keratitis can coalesce and enlarge to form a large geographic ulcer; this condition is more likely with topical steroid therapy.
* After resolution of the epithelial dendrite, subepithelial scarring may persist.
* A neurotrophic keratopathy may occur (see Section 2.23).

Differential diagnosis

There are a variety of conditions that may result in dendrite-like (dendritiform) lesions. These include:

* Varicella-zoster virus (VZV) infection
* A healing epithelial abrasion
* *Acanthamoeba* keratitis; this condition must be considered in all contact lens wearers or following agricultural trauma

* Neurotrophic keratopathy
* Rarely adenovirus or Epstein–Barr virus

Investigations

Diagnosis is clinical. In atypical cases, perform viral PCR.

Treatment

* Epithelial debridement should be performed by gently wiping the surface of the dendrite with a cellulose sponge.
* Topical antiviral: aciclovir 3% ointment five times a day, until epithelial healing has occurred. This treatment should normally be discontinued after 10–14 days, after which time it can result in toxic keratopathy. Topical alternatives include ganciclovir 0.15% gel five times a day or trifluorothymidine 1% drops six times a day.
* If there are signs of toxicity, an alternative to topical treatment is oral antiviral treatment with aciclovir 400 mg five times a day. The aciclovir is secreted in the tear film but at a lower concentration than with topical therapy.
* Consider long-term oral aciclovir prophylaxis (400 mg twice a day) for recurrent epithelial disease (this treatment reduces the risk of recurrence by 50%).
* Topical corticosteroids are contraindicated in the presence of an active dendrite. If the patient was already using topical steroids before the development of the dendrite, the steroids should not be stopped immediately, as the rebound inflammatory response may result in additional damage. Instead, the steroids should be weaned down gradually or a weaker preparation used.

Stromal keratitis

Stromal keratitis can be either non-necrotizing (interstitial keratitis; see Section 2.20) or, rarely, necrotizing.

Herpes simplex interstitial keratitis

Herpes simplex interstitial keratitis classically presents with pain and decreased vision (see Figure 2.49). On examination, there is unifocal or multifocal stromal haze in the absence of epithelial ulceration. There may be mild stromal oedema and an anterior chamber reaction. Long-standing/recurrent cases can result in corneal thinning, scarring, vascularization, and/or lipid keratopathy.

Treatment

* Start with a topical antiviral and then introduce a topical steroids such as dexamethasone eye drops, 0.1%, four times a day (depending on the degree of inflammation) comprise the mainstay of treatment. The steroids must be slowly tapered depending on the clinical response. A long-term low dose such as prednisolone eye drops, 0.1%, daily/alternate days may be required to prevent recurrence of inflammation.
* When topical steroids are used in a patient with a history of HSK, it is necessary for the patient to take a prophylactic oral dose of acyclovir 400 mg twice a day to prevent disease recurrence. This dose can also be used for prophylaxis in recurrent stromal disease and after corneal surgery.

Necrotizing stromal keratitis

Necrotizing stromal keratitis, which is a rare condition, is caused by active viral replication together with a host immune response that produces tissue necrosis. The clinical presentation is that of a dense stromal infiltration that may be clinically indistinguishable from bacterial or fungal keratitis, and secondary infection must be excluded. The overlying epithelium may be intact or ulcerated. Necrosis and ulceration may result in rapid thinning and perforation.

Treatment

• Treatment of necrotizing stromal keratitis is with oral aciclovir 400 mg five times a day (the potential for corneal drop toxicity makes topical antiviral therapy undesirable in the presence of ulceration and necrosis).

• A low dose of topical steroid such as dexamethasone eye drops, 0.1%, twice a day is usually sufficient to control inflammation.

Disciform endothelial keratitis

Disciform endothelial keratitis is a primary inflammation of the endothelium (see Figure 2.50). The exact aetiology is unknown. It may be due to viral infection of endothelial cells or may represent an immune response to a viral antigen. It presents with stromal and epithelial oedema in a round/oval distribution. There are keratic precipitates on the endothelium underlying the zone of oedema. There is often a mild associated anterior uveitis and, if the trabecular meshwork is also inflamed, there may be a raised intraocular pressure.

Treatment

Treatment of disciform endothelial keratitis is with a topical antiviral and a topical steroid, initially four to six times a day and then gradually tapered down, depending on the clinical response. Raised IOP should also be treated. Oral acyclovir should be used if iridocyclitis is present.

Note also:

1. If visually significant stromal scarring results from any of the subtypes of HSK, a penetrating or lamellar keratoplasty may be required.

2. Herpetic iridocyclitis can occur independently or together with epithelial, stromal, or endothelial inflammation.

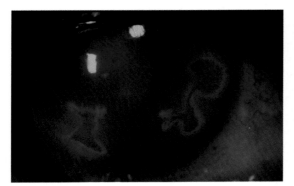

Fig 2.48 Geographic ulcer staining with fluorescein
Courtesy of John Dart

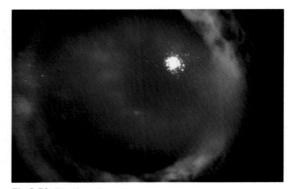

Fig 2.50 Disciform keratitis

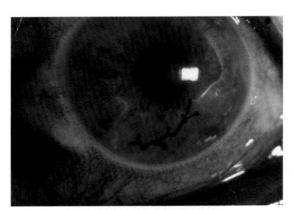

Fig 2.49 Herpes simplex epithelial keratitis
Dendrite staining with rose bengal

Pathophysiology

VZV is a double-stranded DNA virus from the herpes family. It causes chicken pox as the primary infection, which is usually acquired in childhood. With the exception of eyelid vesicles and follicular conjunctivitis, ocular involvement is uncommon during primary VZV infection. Following resolution of chicken pox, the virus then remains latent in the dorsal root ganglion; reactivation causes herpes zoster (shingles). Reactivation most commonly occurs in the thoracolumbar region. Cranial nerve involvement occurs in up to 20% of cases of shingles, with the ophthalmic division of the trigeminal nerve (V_1) being most commonly involved (HZO).

The skin manifestations of HZO (described more fully in Section 1.14) may occur with or without ocular involvement. The nasociliary branch of V_1 innervates the skin on the tip of nose as well as the intraocular structures. Therefore, skin vesicles on the tip of the nose (Hutchinson's sign) are associated with a high risk (50%–75%) of ocular involvement.

The ocular manifestations of HZO may follow the acute skin rash by weeks, months, or even years. Occasionally, they can precede the skin rash. Other extra-corneal manifestations of HZO include:

- **Conjunctiva:** papillary or follicular conjunctivitis, membranes, vesicles, haemorrhage, conjunctival scarring, and/or symblepharon
- **Episclera/sclera:** episcleritis, scleritis, or sclerokeratitis
- **Other:** uveitis, sectorial iris atrophy, trabeculitis (with ocular hypertension or glaucoma), retinitis, choroiditis, optic neuritis, cranial nerve palsies, encephalitis, and postherpetic neuralgia

Risk factors for HZO include increasing age and immunosuppression.

Epithelial keratitis

Epithelial keratitis develops within the first few days of the onset of the rash and resolves spontaneously a few days later. It is characterized by punctate epithelial erosions and pseudodendrites (it differs from HSV dendrites in being more superficial, with tapered ends that lack terminal bulbs).

Nummular keratitis

Nummular keratitis usually occurs around 10 days after the onset of the rash. It is characterized by multiple round granular subepithelial deposits surrounded by stromal haze (see Figure 2.51). They can resolve spontaneously or become chronically inflamed, with vascularization and lipid infiltration.

Disciform keratitis

Disciform keratitis occurs around 3 weeks after the onset of the rash and is usually preceded by nummular keratitis. It is indistinguishable clinically from herpes simplex disciform keratitis. If untreated, disciform keratitis becomes chronic.

Mucous plaque keratitis

Mucous plaque keratitis occurs between 3 and 6 months after the onset of the rash. It is characterized by elevated mucous plaques that stain brightly with rose bengal. The plaques can take on a linear, grey branching appearance.

Other corneal manifestations of HZO

Other corneal manifestations of HZO include profound corneal anaesthesia and neurotrophic keratitis, exposure keratopathy (due to cicatricial lid changes), or lipid keratopathy.

Treatment

- Systemic antiviral therapy with aciclovir 800 mg five times a day (alternatively, valaciclovir 1 g three times a day or famciclovir 500 mg three times a day) for 7 days is indicated as soon as the rash starts. This approach is particularly effective at reducing the duration of the disease as well as the potential sequelae if commenced within 72 hours of the onset of the rash.
- If the patient is systemically unwell, vomiting, and/or immunosuppressed, admission under the care of the general physicians for administration of intravenous acyclovir (15–20 mg/kg/day) may be necessary.

Epithelial disease

- Topical aciclovir 3% five times a day is only indicated in acute disease.
- Unpreserved lubricants

Stromal disease/ keratouveitis/ disciform keratitis/trabeculitis/ sclerokeratitis

- Topical steroids (dose tailored to the degree of inflammation). A low maintenance dose may be required to prevent recurrence.
- Topical antiviral not indicated
- Unlike the case for HSK, oral antiviral therapy is not useful in preventing recurrence with HZO and does not need to be given after surgery or along with topical steroid therapy.

Mucous plaques

- Mucous plaques are treated by gentle removal if possible, lubricants, mucolytics, and, if necessary, topical steroids.

Neurotrophic keratitis

- See Section 2.15.

Postherpetic neuralgia

- Topical capsaicin cream (0.025%–0.075% three times a day/ four times a day) and amitriptyline 10–25 mg four times a day
- Early referral for specialist pain management, as the neuralgia can become chronic
- Note: significant corneal scarring may require penetrating or lamellar keratoplasty.

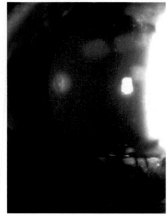

Fig 2.51 Nummular keratitis seen on retroillumination
Courtesy of John Dart

2.20 Interstitial keratitis

Pathophysiology

Interstitial keratitis is non-ulcerative inflammation of the corneal stroma without significant involvement of the epithelium or endothelium (see Figure 2.52). The inflammation causes focal or diffuse cellular infiltration with or without vascularization. It can be infectious, immune, or both. The distribution and depth of stromal involvement together with any associated systemic signs can be helpful in identifying the cause.

Aetiology

Infectious

- **Viral:** herpes simplex, herpes zoster, or Epstein–Barr virus
- **Bacterial:** syphilis, Lyme disease, or brucellosis
- **Mycobacterial:** tuberculosis, leprosy, or atypical mycobacteria
- **Parasitic:** onchocerciasis, microsporidia, or leishmania

Non-infectious

- Phlyctenular keratitis
- Cogan syndrome (see 'Cogan syndrome')
- Sarcoidosis
- Lymphoma
- Contact lens related

Many of these conditions are described in more detail in other sections. The remainder of this section will focus on syphilitic interstitial keratitis (the first infection to be linked with interstitial keratitis, and a classical example of the disease process) and Cogan syndrome.

Syphilitic interstitial keratitis

Most cases of syphilitic interstitial keratitis are due to congenital syphilis from mothers with primary, secondary, or early latent disease. It occurs rarely in acquired syphilis.

Congenital syphilis

Pathophysiology

Interstitial keratitis is a delayed immune-mediated response, not a manifestation of active infection. Onset is at around 5–20 years of age.

Clinical evaluation

- Interstitial keratitis is usually bilateral.
- Initial symptoms are pain, watering, photophobia, and redness.
- In early disease, the clinical manifestations include sectoral superior stromal inflammation and keratic precipitates.
- Later in the disease process, deep stromal vascularization develops. The surrounding inflammatory infiltrate and stromal oedema obscure the outline of the vessels, making the stroma appear pink ('salmon patch').
- Sequelae of stromal keratitis include corneal thinning, ghost vessels, stromal opacification, Descemet's membrane scrolls, endothelial cell loss, and reduced vision.
- Pigmentary chorioretinopathy may be present because of prior chorioretinitis.
- Other non-ocular features of congenital syphilis may be seen, such as deafness, dental abnormalities (e.g. notched incisors, mulberry molars), bone and cartilage abnormalities (e.g. saddle nose, palatal perforation, frontal bossing), and mental retardation (Hutchinson's triad refers to deafness, interstitial keratitis, and notched teeth).

Acquired syphilis

Interstitial keratitis is rare in acquired syphilis. Uveitis and retinitis are more common manifestations of this disease.

Investigations

The Venereal Disease Research Laboratory (VDRL) test and rapid plasma reagin test are positive in active disease, whilst the fluorescent treponema-specific antibody test remains positive even after treatment.

Treatment

- Intense topical steroids (e.g. dexamethasone 0.1%/prednisolone 1% six to eight times a day) can reduce the inflammation, limit the opacification, and improve vision. Tapering steroids may be needed for several months to keep the inflammation under control. Penetrating keratoplasty can be considered in patients with sequelae of interstitial keratitis.
- Systemic penicillin does not treat the interstitial keratitis but is used to treat systemic infection or prevent neurosyphilis.
- Physicians should be involved in investigations and management of suspected syphilis.

Cogan syndrome

Cogan syndrome is an uncommon idiopathic autoimmune disorder of young adults (mean 30 years old), characterized by interstitial keratitis, vertigo, tinnitus, and hearing loss.

Non-specific interstitial keratitis can be the presenting feature or follow the otological symptoms, as both usually develop within a few months of each other. The interstitial keratitis is bilateral and starts as peripheral and superficial nummular lesions (differential diagnosis: adenoviral keratitis) before developing deep multifocal stromal nodules and later vascularization. The diagnosis is one of exclusion and is based on positive ocular and otological features.

Treatment of the keratitis is with topical steroids. Prompt treatment of otological disease with systemic steroids is essential to prevent hearing loss. Steroid-sparing immunosuppression may be needed. Ten per cent of patients develop large vessel vasculitis (like polyarteritis nodosa) many weeks or years later.

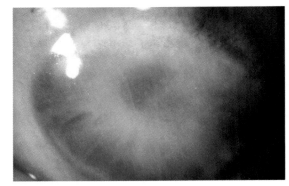

Fig 2.52 Interstitial keratitis

2.21 Peripheral ulcerative keratitis

Peripheral ulcerative keratitis is a potentially blinding disorder consisting of crescent-shaped destructive inflammation located in the peripheral corneal stroma and associated with an overlying epithelial defect (see Figure 2.53).

Pathophysiology

The peripheral cornea has structural characteristics that predispose it to immunological inflammation. The limbal vasculature is a source of immunocompetent cells. Any inflammatory stimulus in the peripheral cornea (e.g. infection, immune complex deposition in systemic immune diseases, trauma, malignancy, or dermatologic conditions) can result in neutrophil recruitment and complement activation. This inflammatory process results in the release of enzymes that cause destruction of the corneal stromal architecture, thinning, and eventually perforation.

Aetiology

There are a variety of conditions that can result in peripheral ulcerative keratitis (PUK):

- **Systemic:** rheumatoid arthritis, systemic vasculitides (e.g. relapsing polychondritis, Wegeners granulomatosis, polyarteritis nodosa), inflammatory bowel disease, neoplasia, infection (e.g. bacillary dysentery, hepatitis C, tuberculosis, syphilis)
- **Ocular:** Mooren's ulcer, rosacea keratitis, trauma, surgery, infection (herpetic/bacterial/fungal keratitis)

Connective tissue and vasculitic diseases are the major risk factors. Many of the other aetiological conditions are discussed elsewhere in the chapter. This section will focus on PUK with systemic autoimmune disease and Moorens ulcer. Other forms of keratitis due to rheumatoid arthritis will also be included in this section.

PUK with systemic immune-mediated disease

Pathophysiology

As described, inflammatory cells and mediators are recruited from the limbal vasculature. Biopsy specimens of the conjunctiva adjacent to the involved cornea typically show evidence of immune-mediated vaso-occlusive disease.

Clinical evaluation

History

- There is often a history of autoimmune, connective tissue, or vasculitic disease, which is usually active when PUK occurs.
- Ocular symptoms are variable and may be minimal. The most common symptoms are a subacute onset of watering, photophobia, reduced vision, and a foreign body sensation with or without eye pain.
- There may be associated scleritis, in which case eye pain may be more pronounced.

Examination

- The disease normally presents as a crescent-shaped epithelial defect with variable underlying stromal thinning and infiltrate, often limited to one quadrant of the juxtalimbal cornea. The disease may extend to involve the paralimbal sclera.
- There may be varying degrees of adjacent conjunctival injection.
- Limbal ischaemia due to vasculitic vaso-occlusion may also be present.

- There may be signs of systemic autoimmune disease.

Investigations

- Corneal scrape (to rule out primary or secondary infectious keratitis). Note that an infiltrate may not always be visible in a thinning cornea in the presence of infection.
- Investigations to detect underlying systemic disease should be performed in consultation with a rheumatologist. The investigations should include an urinalysis (renal vasculitis), a full blood count, the erythrocyte sedimentation rate, urea and electrolyte levels, a rheumatoid factor test, a test for anti-nuclear antibodies, an ANCA test, a VDRL test, hepatitis C serology, and a chest X-ray.

Treatment

There are three main aims for treating PUK:

1. **Ocular surface wetting:** Intensive tear-film supplements are important not only for the treatment of aqueous tear deficiency (which may coexist with rheumatoid arthritis) but also to dilute the effect of inflammatory cytokines in the tear film. Wetting may also help treat a dellen effect at the ulcer base.
2. **Re-epithelialization:** Lubricants or a bandage contact lens can be utilized for this purpose. Systemic collagenase inhibition with doxycycline may be of value. A topical broad spectrum antibiotic is used as prophylaxis against secondary infection.
3. **Systemic immune suppression:** This approach is the mainstay of treatment. It is necessary to treat the PUK as well as the underlying systemic disease. For rapidly progressing cases, high-dose oral or intravenous corticosteroid is required, and cyclophosphamide or monoclonal antibody treatment should be considered.

For severe disease with actual or impending perforation, there are a variety of surgical options performed in conjunction with immunosuppression:

- Cyanoacrylate glue (limits ulceration by protecting the ulcer bed from leukocytes and inflammatory mediators in the tear film)
- Peripheral lamellar keratoplasty
- Amniotic membrane grafting and/or limbal conjunctival excision or recession

Mooren's ulcer

Mooren's ulcer (see Figure 2.54) is a rare PUK of unknown aetiology. Mooren's ulcer is a diagnosis of exclusion and therefore can only be made after excluding other systemic/ocular causes of PUK.

Pathophysiology

The pathophysiology of Mooren's ulcer has not been fully elucidated. Autoimmune corneal destruction may occur in response to previous infection or trauma which alters the expression of corneal antigens.

Clinical evaluation

- Mooren's ulcer is a chronic progressive painful (often severe) ulceration of peripheral corneal epithelium and stroma.
- The ulceration begins in the corneal periphery before spreading circumferentially and then centrally. The peripheral base of the ulcer becomes vascularized.
- It can be distinguished from other causes of PUK by the absence of scleral involvement. Another distinguishing feature is that the leading central edge of the ulcer is undermined.

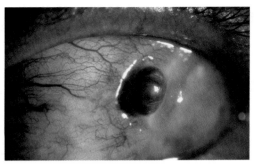

Fig 2.53 Peripheral ulcerative keratitis with systemic immune-mediated disease
Corneal perforation has occurred with iris prolapse

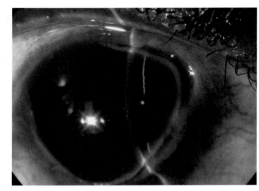

Fig 2.54 Mooren's ulcer
Courtesy of John Dart

* Two clinical types of Moorens ulcer have been described. The first is unilateral and typically occurs in elderly patients. The second is bilateral, rapidly progressive, and poorly responsive to therapy. This second type typically occurs in younger patients.

Treatment
Treatment for Mooren's ulcer is as for PUK associated with systemic, immune-mediated disease. In addition, topical steroids and/or topical ciclosporin can be used to treat Mooren's ulcer.

Other forms of keratitis in rheumatoid arthritis

Other forms of keratitis in rheumatoid arthritis include:
* **Limbal guttering:** characterized by peripheral stromal thinning without epithelial loss or infiltration. It can occur without conjunctival injection or other signs of inflammation. When involving the entire limbus, it resembles a contact lens on the cornea (see Figure 2.55). It may perforate in severe cases.
* **Sclerosing keratitis:** characterized by gradual opacification and neovascularization of peripheral cornea adjacent to an area of scleritis without thinning
* **Acute stromal keratitis:** initially presents with stromal infiltrates and oedema, with an intact epithelium associated with non-necrotizing scleritis. It can progress to PUK.
* **Acute corneal melting:** can occur with or without signs of inflammation, especially in the very dry eye. It is characterized by acute stromal thinning beneath an epithelial defect and it usually occurs centrally.

The treatment for all these forms is as for PUK with systemic disease.

Terrien marginal degeneration

Terrien marginal degeneration (see Figure 2.56) is a rare, non-inflammatory condition; it is included in this section as it forms an important part of the differential diagnosis for PUK.

It is a slowly progressive, idiopathic peripheral corneal thinning disorder occurring mostly in men in the second or third decade of life. It is normally bilateral, though often asymmetrical. It begins superiorly before spreading circumferentially. The earliest sign is peripheral anterior stromal yellow-white deposits that progress to peripheral guttering parallel to the limbus. The guttering has a steep central edge and a shallow sloping limbal edge. The gutter is 1–2 mm wide, with an intact epithelium. Fine vessels cover the area of thinning and there is often secondary lipid deposition. Unlike PUK, there is rarely pain or inflammation associated with this disease. Patients may complain of mild irritation and progressive blurred vision due to increasing against-the-rule astigmatism. Spontaneous corneal perforation is rare but can occur secondary to even minor trauma.

Treatment
Treatment for Terrien marginal degeneration is only required in the case of disabling astigmatism or perforation. A scleral lens can be used for visual correction. Crescent-shaped lamellar/full-thickness corneo-scleral patch grafts or annular lamellar keratoplasty may be needed, depending on the extent and depth of thinning.

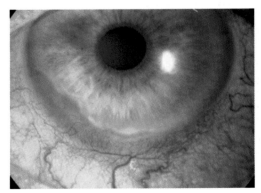

Fig 2.55 Limbal guttering in rheumatoid arthritis

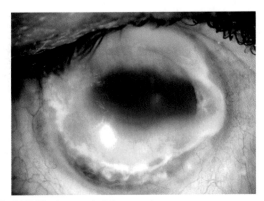

Fig 2.56 Terrien marginal degeneration

Vortex keratopathy (cornea verticillata)

In vortex keratopathy (see Figure 2.57) bilateral, whorl-like, grey-brown epithelial deposits accumulate in the lower half of the cornea, sparing the limbus. Histopathology shows deposition of complex lipids in the basal epithelial layer. Medications that induce this condition include:

* Amiodarone
* Chloroquine
* Chlorpromazine

This condition is asymptomatic and is not an indication to discontinue the drugs. If the patient does complain of reduced vision, other causes of ocular morbidity associated with these drugs (optic neuropathy with amiodarone, retinopathy with chloroquine) should be sought. If the drugs are discontinued, the deposits gradually disappear.

Vortex keratopathy also occurs in Fabrys disease, an X-linked recessive multisystem disorder (corneal changes occur in both the affected males and carrier females).

Ciprofloxacin deposits

Topical ciprofloxacin therapy can result in chalky white deposits within an epithelial defect. The deposit is composed of ciprofloxacin crystals and may be irreversible even after cessation of therapy.

Corneal chrysiasis

Corneal chrysiasis is the deposition of gold in the cornea; this condition occurs after prolonged administration of systemic gold in the treatment of rheumatoid arthritis. It is characterized by asymptomatic, glittering purple granules/dust-like opacities in the corneal stroma.

Adrenochrome deposition

Adrenochrome deposition results from long-standing administration of topical adrenaline compounds, which were used historically to treat glaucoma. It is characterized by dark-brown/black granules on Bowmans layer or in conjunctival cysts. It is an innocuous finding.

Wilson's disease (hepatolenticular degeneration)

Wilson's disease is an autosomal recessive disorder resulting in abnormal copper transport and in the deposition of copper in multiple tissues. Extraocular features include hepatic (cirrhosis, hepatitis, hepatosplenomegaly) and neurological disease (tremors, rigidity, chorea, psychosis).

Corneal involvement in the form of yellow-brown/green deposits (Kayser–Fleischer ring) in the peripheral cornea is the most consistent disease finding (occurs in 95% of cases). The deposits are located at the level of Descemet's membrane in the peripheral cornea. It can be detected earliest by gonioscopy as deposits at Schwalbes line. Later it can be seen at the slit lamp, and in advanced cases it may be visible to the naked eye. Patients may have associated green anterior capsular cataracts (sunflower cataract).

The combination of a sunflower cataract and a Kayser–Fleischer ring can also occur in association with an intraocular copper foreign body (chalcosis).

Immunoprotein deposition

Immunoprotein deposition is an uncommon manifestation of several systemic diseases, including paraproteinaemia, from amiodarone multiple myeloma and leukaemia. It is characterized by multiple, flake-like opacities in the peripheral corneal stroma. Treatment is directed at the underlying disease.

Cystinosis

Cystinosis is a rare autosomal recessive disorder characterized by widespread cysteine crystal deposition within tissues. Systemic features include growth retardation, renal failure (Fanconi syndrome), and hepatosplenomegaly. Ocular features include the deposition of myriads of minute crystals within the conjunctiva and the cornea, resulting in photophobia, epithelial erosions, and blurred vision. Crystals can also be deposited in the iris, lens capsule, and retina. Treatment is with topical cysteamine 0.2%.

Iron deposition

Epithelial iron deposition is common, occurring in areas where tears pool due to irregularities in the contour of the corneal surface. It is visible as a yellow-brown epithelial line.

This line can be seen in:

* The interpalpebral fissure in normal eyes (the Hudson–Stähli line)
* At the head of a pterygium (Stockers line)
* Around the cone in keratoconus (the Fleischer ring; see Figure 2.58)
* In front of a filtering bleb (Ferrys line)
* After refractive corneal surgery

Iron staining can also develop around a metallic corneal foreign body.

Siderosis

Siderosis occurs secondary to the presence of an intraocular iron-containing foreign body. Iron is deposited in intraocular epithelial structures (lens capsule, retina, and iris).

Mucopolysaccharidoses

Mucopolysaccharidoses are rare lysosomal storage diseases due to a deficiency or dysfunction of lysosomal enzymes which are essential for the breakdown of glycosaminoglycans. The deficiency/dysfunction leads to the deposition of glycosaminoglycans in various tissues. Excessive dermatan and keratin sulphate results in corneal stromal clouding.

There are seven distinct types and several subtypes of mucopolysaccharidoses. All have autosomal recessive inheritance except for Hunter syndrome (which is X-linked recessive). Corneal clouding occurs in all except Hunter syndrome and Sanfilippo syndrome. Corneal clouding is particularly severe (onset within first few years in life) in Hurler syndrome and Scheie syndrome. Other associated ocular features include pigmentary retinopathy, optic atrophy, and glaucoma. Systemic features include skeletal dysplasia, facial dysmorphism, mental retardation, hepatosplenomegaly, and cardiac disease.

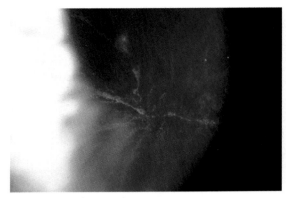

Fig 2.57 Vortex keratopathy

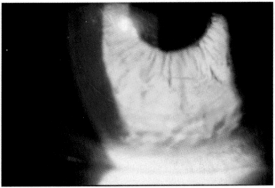

Fig 2.58 Iron line around the cone in keratoconus (Fleischer ring)

2.23 Miscellaneous

Thygeson superficial punctate keratitis

Thygeson superficial punctate keratitis is a condition of unknown aetiology, characterized by recurrent episodes of bilateral coarse punctate keratopathy without vascularization or conjunctival injection. Symptoms consist of watering, foreign body sensation, photophobia, and blurred vision. There may be several white-grey, superficial slightly elevated epithelial lesions (see Figure 2.59). Each lesion, if untreated, persists for 1–2 months. The overall course of the disease is usually 2–3 years. The lesions stain with fluorescein during the acute exacerbations. During remissions, they can completely disappear.

Treatment

The lesions resolve with mild topical steroid therapy, a finding which suggests an immune-mediated aetiology. Steroid treatment may prolong the course of the disease and should be used for a short course during acute exacerbations. Topical lubricants, a bandage contact lens, or topical ciclosporin are alternative treatments.

Exposure keratopathy

Pathophysiology

Inability to close the lids (lagophthalmos) leads to corneal drying, epithelial breakdown, secondary infectious keratitis, and even perforation (see Figure 2.60). Lagophthalmos with or without exposure keratopathy can be present at night in some healthy individuals (nocturnal lagophthalmos). Potential causes of exposure keratopathy include:

* Facial nerve palsy (e.g. Bell's palsy)
* Reduced facial nerve tone in comatose/intubated patients (e.g. in intensive care units)
* Lid abnormalities: ectropion, iatrogenic (post surgery), cicatricial lid/conjunctival disease, or proptosis

Clinical evaluation

* Presentation is with irritation, foreign body sensation, burning, and watering, especially upon waking.
* The degree of lagophthalmos should be assessed with normal blinking, gentle lid closure, and tight lid closure.
* Patients with poor Bell's phenomenon are particularly at risk (see Chapter 1, Section 1.5).
* The classical examination findings are interpalpebral, inferior punctate corneal and conjunctival epitheliopathy, with or without conjunctival injection. If severe, there can be corneal opacification, ulceration, and even perforation.

Treatment

* In mild cases, frequent artificial tears by day with a lubricating ointment at night may suffice. In more severe cases, the ointment can be applied hourly by day.
* Exposure may be reduced by temporary measures such as taping the eyelid shut at bedtime, a temporary tarsorrhaphy, or by inducing a ptosis with botulinum toxin injection into the upper lid.

* More permanent measures include lateral and/or medial tarsorraphy or gold weight insertion into the upper lid.
* Topical antibiotics should be given in severe cases if coexisting infectious keratitis is present.

Neurotrophic keratopathy

Pathophysiology

An intact corneal nerve supply is vital for the maintenance of epithelial integrity, reflex tear production, and blinking. Persistent corneal anaesthesia or hypoaesthesia results in degradation of the epithelial surface and the quality of the tear film. Such degradation can lead to epithelial breakdown, stromal lysis, thinning, and perforation (with or without secondary infection; see Figure 2.61).

Causes of reduced corneal sensation include:

* Herpes simplex and zoster keratitis
* Fifth cranial nerve pathology (e.g. iatrogenic trauma during acoustic neuroma surgery)
* Systemic disease (e.g. diabetes mellitus)
* Iatrogenic from ocular surgery (e.g. LASIK, corneal surgery, damage to ciliary nerves by retinal laser and surgery)
* Topical medications (e.g. anaesthetic abuse)
* Chemical burns and chronic epithelial injury or inflammation
* Congenital syndromes (e.g. familial dysautonomia)

Clinical evaluation

There is reduced corneal sensation (may be sectorial in HSK). Progressive signs include rose bengal staining of the inferior conjunctival surface, punctate corneal staining, acute epithelial loss, and chronic non-healing corneal ulceration with raised rolled edges. Rarely, stromal lysis, thinning, and perforation can occur. There can be a secondary microbial keratitis.

Treatment

* Treatment of mild cases is as for dry eye: tear supplements, lubricants, and, if necessary, punctal plugs.
* More advanced cases require further intervention to promote epithelial healing: botulinum induced ptosis, tarsorraphy, and/or autologous serum drops.
* If there is significant stromal lysis, amniotic membrane grafting, penetrating or lamellar corneal grafting, or, as a last resort, a conjunctival flap may be required (see 'Conjunctival flaps').

Non-healing epithelial defect

A non-healing (persistent) epithelial defect can be due to a variety of causes including intrinsic corneal disease (e.g. bullous keratopathy), mechanical causes (e.g. trichiasis, exposure, dry eye), chemical causes (e.g. stem cell failure post chemical injury, drop toxicity), or neurotrophic, inflammatory, infectious, or neoplastic factors. The cause should be established, and treatment should be aimed at correcting the underlying aetiology and promoting healing (as shown in 'Neurotrophic keratopathy' in this section).

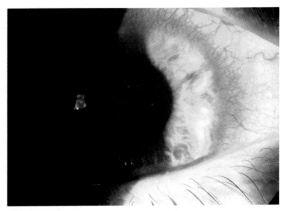

Fig 2.59 Thygeson superficial punctate keratitis

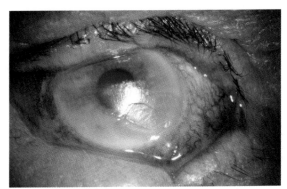

Fig 2.60 Exposure keratopathy following lower lid surgery

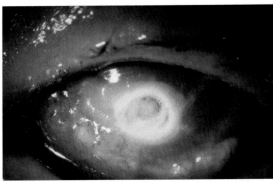

Fig 2.61 Neurotrophic keratopathy with a persistent epithelial defect.

Conjunctival flap

Advancement of the conjunctiva over the cornea can be performed to provide pain relief and/or aid healing in a variety of ocular surface disease where restoration of vision is not the priority. Such cases include corneal oedema, severe neurotrophic keratitis, non-healing epithelial defects, and/or indolent infective keratitis. The flaps can be partial (e.g. advancement flaps, uni-/bi-pedicle) or total. Partial advancement flaps can be helpful in peripheral corneal disease, for example peripheral melt. Total conjunctival flaps/conjunctival hooding (also referred to as Gundersen's flap) are fashioned by dissecting the superior conjunctiva from Tenon's capsule and advancing it to the inferior limbus after removing the corneal epithelium and superficial stroma.

Amniotic membrane transplantation

Amniotic membrane harvested from placenta is used for surface reconstruction in a variety of ocular conditions including fornix reconstruction in cicatrizing conjunctivitis, neurotrophic keratitis, and non-healing epithelial defects. It is also used as a base for the proliferation and transplantation of autologous limbal cells in ocular surface reconstruction. It reduces inflammation, neovascularization, and scarring and promotes wound healing and epithelialization. The amniotic membrane is gradually absorbed. Contraindications to its use include severe dry eye, exposure, and severe stromal necrosis.

Anterior chamber paracentesis

Background/indication

- Performed for diagnosis (obtaining an aqueous sample in endophthalmitis) or therapy (to reduce IOP in a central retinal artery occlusion)

Technique

- Can be done at the slit lamp or under the operating microscope
- Instil topical povidone iodine (5%) and topical anaesthetic.
- Enter at the temporal limbus with an insulin syringe (26–30-gauge needle) with its plunger drawn out.
- Aim towards the inferior iris, keeping the needle bevel up over the iris to reduce the risk of damage to the crystalline lens.
- IOP itself will force aqueous into the syringe. Withdraw after 0.1–0.2 ml of aqueous humour has been collected or when the anterior chamber begins to collapse.
- Instil stat topical antibiotic and prescribe topical antibiotics for 4–5 days.

Corneal dystrophies comprise a group of bilateral, normally symmetrical, inherited conditions that result in progressive corneal opacification commencing between the first and fifth decades of life. The dystrophies can be classified according to the anatomical layer of the cornea that is involved. Molecular genetics has led to a reassessment of the traditional clinical groupings.

Epithelial dystrophies

Epithelial basement membrane dystrophy

Epithelial basement membrane dystrophy/degeneration is the most common anterior dystrophy, occurring in over 2% of the general population (see Figure 2.62). It is also known as Cogan's microcystic or map-dot-fingerprint dystrophy.

Pathophysiology

Inheritance may be autosomal dominant (with incomplete penetrance) but most cases are sporadic. The genetic cause is unknown. Histology shows a thickened and reduplicated basement membrane, absent/abnormal hemidesmosomes on the basal epithelial cells, and fibrillar material between the basement membrane and Bowman's layer. The combination of these features results in weak anchoring of the epithelium to the underlying basement membrane.

Clinical evaluation

* The onset of disease is in the second decade of life.
* Patients may be asymptomatic or may present with symptoms of recurrent corneal erosions (see end of Section 2.25). Clinical manifestations of disease can be asymmetrical.
* Approximately 10% of patients with this dystrophy will develop recurrent corneal erosions, and 50% of patients with recurrent corneal erosions have evidence of this dystrophy.
  There are four types of corneal abnormality that may be observed:

1. **Epithelial microcysts**
2. **Dots:** collapsed microcysts
3. **Fingerprints:** these consist of thickened/multilaminar strips of epithelial basement membrane
4. **Geographic areas** of thickened and irregular basement membrane deposit

Treatment

No treatment is required in asymptomatic cases. Treatment in the presence of symptoms is as for recurrent corneal erosions.

Meesmann dystrophy

Meesmann dystrophy is a rare autosomal dominant dystrophy with onset during early childhood. The disease manifests as discrete clear epithelial microcysts (best seen with retroillumination). It is usually asymptomatic but can cause mild ocular irritation, photophobia, and reduction of vision. Treatment is usually not required.

Corneal dystrophy of Bowman's layer

Corneal dystrophy of Bowman's layer type 1 (Reis–Bücklers dystrophy)

Pathophysiology

Corneal dystrophy of Bowman's layer (CDB) type 1 (Reis–Bücklers dystrophy) is an autosomal dominant dystrophy linked to a mutation of the transforming growth factor beta induced (TGFBI) gene on Chromosome 5. Histologically, degenerative changes can be seen in the deep epithelium. Bowman's layer is disrupted or absent and replaced by irregular bands of collagen, which stains blue with Massons trichrome (see Figure 2.63).

Clinical evaluation

Onset is in early childhood. Recurrent epithelial erosions, surface irregularity, and anterior stromal scarring/oedema result in progressive, grey-white, superficial, honeycomb-shaped opacification by the first or second decade of life.

Treatment

Initial treatment is as for recurrent corneal erosions. More advanced cases require excimer laser phototherapeutic keratectomy or lamellar keratoplasty. Recurrence of disease in the graft is common.

CDB type 2 (Theil-Behnke dystrophy)

CDB type 2 (Theil-Behnke dystrophy) is usually clinically indistinguishable from CDB type 1, and the treatment is the same. Inheritance is also autosomal dominant.
The main difference between this condition and CDB type 1 are:

1. Different appearances under the electron microscope (rod-like granules in Bowman's layer in CDB type 1, and curly filaments in CDB type 2).

Stromal dystrophies

Granular dystrophy and Avellino dystrophy

Pathophysiology

Granular dystrophy (see Figure 2.64) and Avellino dystrophy show autosomal dominant inheritance and are, like CDB type 1, linked to the TGFBI gene on Chromosome 5. The different clinical manifestations shown by the different dystrophies are due to distinct changes in adjacent mutation hotspots on the same gene.

Histology shows the granular material within the stroma to be amorphous hyaline deposits that stain bright red with Massons trichrome

Clinical evaluation

* Onset is in early life, with white, well-demarcated, crumb-like, central anterior stromal deposits. The intervening stroma is clear.
* With age, the lesions increase in number and depth and spread towards the corneal periphery but do not reach the limbus
* Anterior lesions can break through Bowmans layer and result in recurrent corneal erosions.
* Lesions gradually coalesce, resulting in decreased vision.
* **Avellino dystrophy:** this is histologically and clinically the same as granular dystrophy, with the addition of amyloid deposits typical of lattice dystrophy (see 'Lattice dystrophy'). It is thus also referred to as granular–lattice dystrophy.

Treatment

Superficial disease can be treated as for recurrent corneal erosions. Visually significant opacification is treated with deep anterior lamellar keratoplasty or penetrating keratoplasty.

Lattice dystrophy

Pathophysiology

Inheritance is autosomal dominant with variable expression. Light microscopy reveals amyloid deposits primarily located in

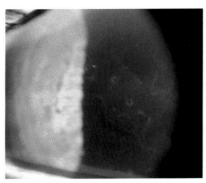

Fig 2.62 Epithelial basement membrane dystrophy

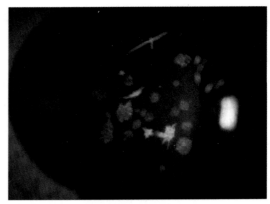

Fig 2.64 Granular dystrophy

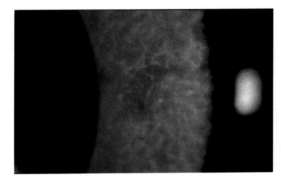

Fig 2.63 Reis–Bücklers dystrophy

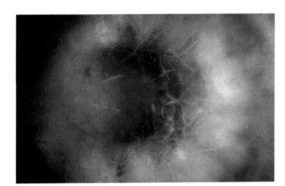

Fig 2.65 Lattice dystrophy

the anterior stroma (see Figure 2.65). Amyloid may also accumulate beneath the epithelium, affecting epithelial adhesion. Amyloid stains orange-red with Congo red dye and it exhibits apple-green birefringence with polarized light.

Clinical evaluation

The classical clinical appearance is of central anterior stromal fine-branching refractile lattice lines best seen with retroillumination. There is also a variable diffuse anterior stromal haze that does not affect the peripheral cornea.

There are two main causes of lattice corneal lines

* **Lattice corneal dystrophy Type 1 (Biber–Haab–Dimmer):** this is the most common form of lattice, and inheritance is autosomal dominant. Onset is within the first decade of life, with recurrent corneal erosions that precede the development of corneal opacities and reduced vision.
* **Meretoja syndrome:** this is a rare autosomal dominant disease due to mutations in the gelsolin gene. There is coexisting systemic amyloidosis. Onset of disease is in the third decade of life. In this form, the lattice lines are more peripherally located. Extraocular features include cranial nerve palsies, pendulous ears, dry/lax skin, and a mask-like facial expression.

Treatment

Treatment is as for granular dystrophy.

Macular dystrophy

Macular dystrophy (see Figure 2.66) is less common than the other classic stromal dystrophies described.

Pathophysiology

Inheritance is autosomal recessive change in the CHST6 gene. The deposits are glycosaminoglycans which stain with Alcian blue and colloidal iron.

Clinical evaluation

Onset is in the first decade of life, initially with focal grey-white anterior stromal opacities. These progress to involve the entire stromal thickness, also extending peripherally up to the limbus. The stroma between the opacities is hazy. The cornea is diffusely thinned.

Treatment

Treatment is as for granular dystrophy.

Schnyder crystalline dystrophy

Schnyder crystalline dystrophy is a rare autosomal dominant disease due to mutations of the UBIAD1 gene. It is thought to result from a local disorder of corneal lipid metabolism. There is a strong association with systemic hypercholesterolaemia. Clinical presentation is in the second decade, with central corneal opacification, fine polychromatic cholesterol crystals in the anterior stroma, and a dense corneal arcus. Treatment is with phototherapeutic keratectomy or lamellar keratoplasty.

Gelatinous droplike dystrophy

Gelatinous droplike dystrophy is an autosomal recessive subepithelial amyloidosis due to mutations of the TACSTD2 gene. It is uncommon outside of Japan. Presentation is in the first decade, initially with a band keratopathy-like picture, which is followed by the development of protruding, mulberry-like subepithelial deposits. Management is difficult due to recurrence. Keratoprosthesis may be required.

2.25 Corneal dystrophies II

Endothelial dystrophies

Fuchs' endothelial dystrophy

This common dystrophy occurs more frequently in females than in males.

Pathophysiology

Fuchs' usually occurs sporadically but can be inherited in an autosomal dominant fashion. It is characterized by reduced endothelial cell density and pump function and increased endothelial permeability. Descemet's membrane is thickened, and posterior excrescences are visible clinically as guttata. Corneal oedema occurs as a result of endothelial dysfunction (see Figure 2.67).

Clinical evaluation

Fuchs' dystrophy manifests clinically after the age of 50, progressing through three stages:

* **Stage 1:** asymptomatic increase in central guttata and spread towards the corneal periphery. Confluence of guttata produces a 'beaten-metal' appearance on indirect or retroillumination. Pigment may adhere to the abnormal endothelium.
* **Stage 2:** endothelial decompensation and corneal oedema resulting in blurred vision. Vision is initially worse on waking and clears as the day progresses. The oedema is initially confined to the stroma, with accompanying Descemet's folds. Epithelial microcystic oedema can cause acute discomfort.
* **Stage 3:** Persistent epithelial oedema results in bullous keratopathy (see 'Bullous keratopathy').

Investigations

* Endothelial cell density can be measured by specular microscopy.
* Corneal thickness can be measured by ultrasound pachymetry. Along with clinical features, these parameters can be used to monitor progression of the disease.

Treatment

* Topical sodium chloride 5% drops or ointment is useful for increasing the tonicity of the tear film and dehydrating the cornea. The same effect can also be achieved with warm dry air from a hairdryer held at arm's length from the cornea for a few minutes in the morning.
* Bandage contact lenses provide temporary relief from discomfort by protecting exposed corneal nerve endings.
* Corneal graft surgery is the definitive treatment. Penetrating keratoplasty was once the mainstay of treatment; however, this procedure has been superseded by lamellar grafting techniques (Descemet's stripping (automated) endothelial keratoplasty, Descemet's membrane endothelial keratoplasty; see Section 2.28).
* An amniotic membrane graft or a conjunctival flap can be used to control pain in eyes with poor visual potential.

Posterior polymorphous dystrophy

Posterior polymorphous dystrophy is an autosomal dominant inherited condition. Histologically, the multilayered endothelial cells have some features normally seen in epithelial cells (e.g. microvillae). On specular microscopy, there are isolated grouped vesicles, or broad bands with grey scalloped edges. This condition is normally asymptomatic and treatment is not then needed. Astigmatism and corneal decompensation can develop rarely.

Congenital hereditary endothelial dystrophy

Congenital hereditary endothelial dystrophy (CHED) is a bilateral congenital primary dysfunction of corneal endothelial cells that results in corneal opacification.

* **CHED** is an autosomal recessive condition due to a mutation in SLC4A11 gene. presents from birth or within the first few weeks of life. Expression is with marked oedema, significantly increased corneal thickness, and severely decreased vision that can lead to amblyopia and nystagmus. Deafness can be a feature.

The differential diagnosis of bilateral early-onset corneal opacification includes congenital glaucoma, forceps injury, congenital infections, early-onset posterior polymorphous dystrophy, and metabolic diseases.

Treatment of CHED was historically with penetrating keratoplasty; however, there is increasing use of lamellar grafting techniques in these paediatric cases.

Clinical syndromes associated with corneal dystrophies

Recurrent corneal erosion syndrome

Pathophysiology

Recurrent corneal erosion syndrome, which is a common condition, occurs in eyes with a pre-existing corneal dystrophy (especially epithelial basement membrane dystrophy), eyes that have suffered a previous traumatic corneal abrasion (especially via a fingernail injury), or eyes that have a combination of these two conditions. Poor adhesion of the epithelium is thought to result from abnormalities of the underlying basement membrane and its associated network of attachment complexes (hemidesmosomes, basal lamina, laminin).

Clinical evaluation

* Clinical manifestations may occur soon or many years after the initial injury and there may be numerous recurrences.
* Presentation is with the sudden onset of pain, lacrimation, photophobia, redness, and foreign body sensation, at night or upon first waking. Symptoms may resolve over a few hours, with apparent healing of the epithelium, or may be severe and last for several days.
* Upon examination, the epithelium may have already healed or there may be an area of epithelial microcysts and other signs of epithelial basement membrane dystrophy (note: it is important to examine the fellow eye carefully). More severe attacks are characterized by heaped-up loose epithelium with or without an epithelial defect.

Treatment

* **Acute stage:** regular prophylactic lubricating antibiotic ointment and topical cycloplegia if there is significant photophobia and pain

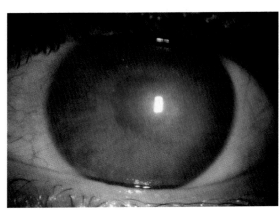

Fig 2.66 Macular dystrophy
See Section 2.24

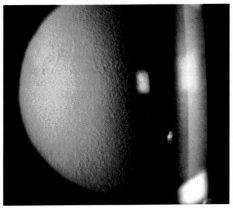

Fig 2.67 Fuchs' endothelial dystrophy

- **Prophylaxis:** tear-film supplements during the day, and lubricating ointment at night for 6–12 months to prevent recurrences and allow normal epithelial basement membrane adhesion
- Hypertonic saline ointment at night is an alternative to lubricating ointment.
- Systemic doxycycline is of theoretical benefit to help reduce inflammation, especially if there is coexisting blepharitis (acts by inhibiting matrix metalloproteinase activity).
- Bandage contact lenses are helpful for symptoms as well as promoting epithelial adhesion. They should be used continuously for 2 months for this purpose.

Interventional options
These options are indicated for severe/recurrent cases that are resistant to other forms of treatment:

- Epithelial debridement in the acute phase, if sheets of loose epithelium are present
- Phototherapeutic keratectomy: the epithelium is removed and about 5–10 μm of Bowman's layer is ablated with an excimer laser to help adhesion of new epithelium.
- Anterior stromal micropuncture can be useful, but only if there is a localized area of abnormal epithelium away from the visual axis. It is performed with the bent tip of a

25-gauge needle. Non-continuous punctures are made in the abnormal area and extending 1–2 mm into the surrounding, apparently unaffected cornea.

Bullous keratopathy
Pathophysiology
Bullous keratopathy (see Figure 2.68) results from endothelial dysfunction. Corneal oedema begins in the stroma and then progresses to the epithelium. Epithelial oedema is initially microcystic and then advances to macrocystic (bullous) oedema. Fuchs' endothelial dystrophy is the most common cause. Other causes include:

- Intraocular surgery: aphakic and pseudophakic bullous keratopathy occur particularly following complicated cataract surgery with vitreous loss and/or placement of an anterior chamber intraocular lens (IOL)
- Endotheliitis: herpetic (simplex/zoster)
- Corneal graft failure/rejection
- Chronic anterior uveitis
- Trauma

Clinical evaluation
Symptoms are worse in the morning and include blurred vision, lacrimation, photophobia, and pain (particularly due to rupture of macrobullae).

On examination, there is stromal oedema (Descemet's folds/striate keratopathy) in the initial stages followed by epithelial oedema. In long-standing cases, there may be subepithelial scarring with superficial corneal neovascularization.

Treatment
Replacement of the dysfunctional corneal endothelium is with lamellar grafting, as for Fuchs' dystrophy. Other underlying conditions (e.g. herpetic endotheliitis, poor-fitting anterior chamber IOL) should be treated.

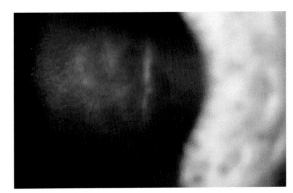

Fig 2.68 Bullous keratopathy

2.26 Contact lenses

Contact lenses can be used for various optical and therapeutic purposes. There are a variety of complications associated with contact lens wear. Soft contact lenses are the most common type of lens worn. Rigid gas permeable lenses have a smaller diameter (9–10 mm) and have a variety of indications that are outlined in this section.

Optical uses

The majority of contact lenses are used to correct simple refractive error, as an alternative to glasses. Contact lenses can also be used to improve visual acuity that cannot otherwise be improved by spectacles in the following circumstances:

* **High or irregular astigmatism:** e.g. keratoconus, corneal scar, following penetrating keratoplasty. Rigid gas permeable lenses are most suitable for this purpose.
* **Anisometropia:** this condition occurs when there is a significant difference in the refractive error between eyes, e.g. if one eye is aphakic. Correction with glasses results in aneisokonia (a disparity in the image size between each eye). This effect is greatly reduced with contact lenses.
* **Superficial corneal irregularities** such as that occurring with superficial corneal scarring can be neutralized with a rigid gas permeable lens to provide a more optically regular refractive interface.

Non-optical therapeutic uses

Bandage contact lenses are plano (i.e. no refractive power) lenses. Silicone hydrogel soft lenses are the most frequently used but rigid lenses are occasionally indicated. Bandage contact lenses can be used for a variety of therapeutic purposes:

* **Pain relief:** e.g. in bullous keratopathy, where the contact lens protects exposed free nerve endings from lid movement
* **Protect the ocular surface:** e.g. after cyanoacrylate corneal glue application, and after corneal or conjunctival surgery
* **Promote epithelial healing:** e.g. with persistent epithelial defects, recurrent corneal erosions, and post surgery (e.g. refractive surgery). In these circumstances, the lens acts to protect the healing epithelium from the constant rubbing action of the eyelids.
* **Maintain corneal integrity:** e.g. with a descemetocele (corneal thinning down to the level of Descemet's membrane), small corneal perforation, or post-operative wound leak

Additional considerations

* Bandage contact lenses are available in various sizes and materials. The design used is determined by the location and nature of the disease process (e.g. large 14 mm lenses for a leaking filtering bleb). Silicone hydrogel lenses have a high oxygen permeability, are suitable for extended wear, and are an appropriate first choice for most indications. The lens should centre on the cornea, and a good fit is confirmed by judging the degree of movement upon blinking (should be

0 5 mm). In general, a lens with a flat base curve will move more than one with a steep base curve.
* Use preservative-free medications where possible (as soft contact lenses retain preservatives and can cause corneal toxicity) and avoid ointments as they will be retained by the lens and blur vision.
* Use topical antibiotics prophylaxis if there is an epithelial defect.
* Warn the patient regarding the risk of infection and replace extended wear soft lenses every 1–2 months.

Complications of contact lens wear

Microbial keratitis

Microbial keratitis is the most serious complication associated with contact lens wear (see Sections 2.16–17). The risk is least with rigid gas permeable lenses and greatest with extended wear soft lenses. The risk is increased by sleeping with the lenses in as well as with poor lens hygiene. It is important to rule out infection in any patient with an acute painful eye associated with contact lens wear. As most infections associated with contact lenses are caused by Gram-negative bacteria, do not treat an abrasion or suspected infection in a contact lens wearer with chloramphenicol (ineffective).

Epithelial defects

* Mechanical trauma, especially whilst removing/inserting lenses can cause micro/macro abrasions.
* Cleaning/disinfectant solutions (hydrogen peroxide, surfactants, enzymes) if inadvertently instilled into the eye can cause diffuse punctate staining (toxic epitheliopathy).
* Tightly fitting lenses or lens overwear can cause corneal hypoxia. There may discomfort, bulbar conjunctival injection, multiple peripheral corneal and conjunctival punctate epithelial erosions and microcysts, and even central epithelial necrosis.
* Treatment involves avoiding lens wear until the condition has resolved (may take days to weeks), topical lubricants, prophylactic antibiotics, and ensuring that the lens fit is correct and that the lenses are not being overworn.

Sterile keratitis

Sterile keratitis may occur as a hypersensitivity reaction to bacterial exotoxins. Symptoms consist of an acutely red eye and a foreign body sensation. Clinical signs are characterized by peripheral, often multiple, epithelial, subepithelial, or anterior stromal, well-demarcated, white-grey infiltrates (see Figure 2.69). There is minimal or no overlying epithelial defect. Treatment is as for epithelial defects (above), leaving the lens out, with the additional options of a mild topical steroid when infection has been excluded and of improving lens hygiene.

Note: infectious infiltrates are typically more central than sterile infiltrates, larger with a definite epithelial defect, and have an anterior chamber reaction. If unsure whether an infiltrate is sterile, treat as infective.

Corneal neovascularization

Corneal neovascularization is caused by chronic corneal hypoxia. It is most common with soft contact lenses and most pronounced superiorly (see Figure 2.70). It is generally

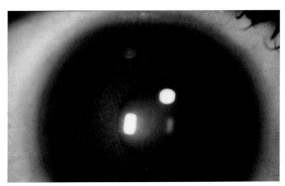

Fig 2.69 Sterile contact lens related keratitis

Courtesy of John Dart

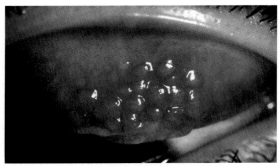

Fig 2.71 Giant papillary conjunctivitis

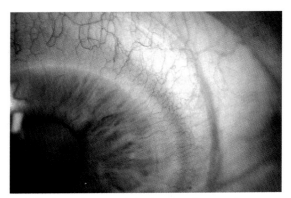

Fig 2.70 Corneal neovascularization secondary to soft contact lens

asymptomatic. If deep new vessels grow more than 2 mm inwards from the limbus, the contact lenses fit must be modified or lens wear discontinued.

Allergic conjunctivitis

Allergic conjunctivitis is caused by an allergy to thiomersal (a preservative that has now generally been removed from contact lens solutions). This condition can occur within days or many months after first exposure to thiomersal. Symptoms of redness, itching, and burning occur soon after lens insertion. On examination, there is evidence of papillary conjunctivitis.

Giant papillary conjunctivitis

Pathophysiology

Giant papillary conjunctivitis is thought to be caused by mechanical trauma between the lens and the upper tarsal conjunctiva, along with a hypersensitivity response to allergens on the lens surface (see Figure 2.71). It is usually seen with soft contact lenses but can also be seen with hard contact lenses, ocular prostheses, or from protruding corneal sutures.

Clinical evaluation

* Presentation may be months or years after commencing lens wear.
* Symptoms include contact lens intolerance, itching, and mucous discharge. Blurred vision may occur because of lens deposits.
* Signs include papillary conjunctivitis (giant papillae of greater than 0.3 mm may be present), conjunctival injection, and, in severe cases, a mechanical ptosis.

Treatment

Treatment is with a break in contact lens wear or a switch to a different type of contact lens. If there is a non-contact lens related cause, it must be addressed (i.e. polish and clean the prosthesis, remove a protruding suture). Topical mast cell stabilizers are useful in mild disease. Topical steroid can be used if there is a prosthesis but should otherwise be reserved for acute severe attacks only.

Other complications of contact lens wear

* Ptosis: especially with rigid gas permeable lenses
* Lost lens: can become decentred, fall out, or migrate into the superior fornix. The problem of a lost lens may be compounded if repeated attempts by the patient to remove the lens cause abrasion to the ocular surface
* Chronic contact lens use can result in irregular astigmatism due to mechanical moulding of the cornea (warpage). The effect usually regresses after the lens is removed but may take weeks to months to resolve

The term 'corneal ectasia' refers to progressive thinning, weakness, and protrusion of the cornea. There are a variety of corneal ectatic disorders.

Keratoconus

Keratoconus (see Figure 2.72) is the most common corneal ectatic disorder; it is characterized by the conical protrusion of the central cornea and is associated with apical thinning and progressive myopia with irregular astigmatism. The cone is usually displaced inferiorly.

Pathophysiology

Keratoconus is bilateral but usually asymmetric. Onset is in the teens or twenties, with a variable rate of progression. There is no gender predisposition, and prevalence is estimated to be 1 : 1000, but it is more common in South Asians. The aetiology is unknown but there are both genetic and environmental influences. Eye rubbing (e.g. from allergic eye disease, Leber amaurosis, Down syndrome) may be a contributory factor. Offspring are affected in about 8% of cases. The inheritance may be autosomal dominant with incomplete penetrance.

Associations

See Box 2.1 for associations of keratoconus.

Clinical evaluation

History

- Blurred vision that cannot be fully corrected by glasses
- Progressive astigmatism measured by the optometrist
- Glare and monocular diplopia
- A sudden decrease in vision with pain and photophobia may occur in acute corneal hydrops (see 'acute corneal hydrops').

Examination

- In early disease (forme fruste keratoconus), clinical signs are absent and the diagnosis is topographic.
- Refraction shows high myopic astigmatism which is often irregular (i.e. the two axes are not 90° apart) and progressive.
- Retinoscopy reveals a scissoring reflex.
- Direct ophthalmoscopy: an 'oil droplet' reflex is visible

Box 2.1 **Associations of keratoconus**
Ocular
Vernal keratoconjunctivitis
Atopic keratoconjunctivitis
Retinitis pigmentosa
Leber amaurosis
Retinopathy of prematurity
Floppy eyelids
Systemic
Atopy: Eczema, hay fever, asthma
Down syndrome (15% have signs)
Connective tissue diseases: • Ehlers–Danlos syndrome • Osteogenesis imperfecta • Marfan syndrome

- Munson's sign: this is a protrusion of the lower lid by the cone upon down-gaze (a sign of advanced keratoconus; see Figure 2.73)
- Slit lamp examination: central or inferior corneal thinning is the hallmark of the disease and may be visible in more advanced disease using a thin optical section

Other slit lamp manifestations of keratoconus that may be present in moderate or severe disease include:

- Vogt's striae: fine vertical lines in the posterior stroma that disappear if the globe is gently pressed
- Apical scars (due to previous hydrops)
- Fleischer ring (epithelial iron deposition at the base of the cone, best seen with cobalt-blue light)

Acute corneal hydrops

Acute corneal hydrops is a complication of advanced and progressive keratoconus (see Figure 2.74). It develops when the Descemet's membrane and endothelium of the ectatic cornea splits, allowing aqueous humour to enter the corneal stroma and resulting in stromal oedema and bullous epithelial oedema.

Acute corneal hydrops normally resolves spontaneously over several months. Treatment (e.g. hypertonic saline) does not improve outcome, although topical steroid is indicated if there is vascularization. Corneal graft surgery may eventually be indicated but it should be delayed until the optical effect of any corneal scarring can be assessed.

Investigations

- Refractive astigmatism: more than 1 D change is suggestive of progression
- Best-corrected visual acuity: more than one line lost is suggestive of progression
- Scheimpflug tomography/keratometry is the most widely used method for detecting early disease (forme fruste keratoconus) and monitoring progression. Measurements ideally obtained after contact lenses have been removed for 1 week (soft lenses) or 2 weeks (rigid gas permeable lenses). Relevant parameters include:
  - **Keratometry:** reveals irregular high astigmatism. A value of 47 D or greater is suggestive of keratoconus. An increase in the Pentacam anterior K2 or Kmax of more than 1.5 D is suggestive of progression. An increase in the posterior K2 of more than 0.5 D is suggestive of progression.
- **Pachymetry:** corneal thickness is reduced, especially in the inferior half of the cornea. Thinning of the central or minimum corneal thickness by more than 13 μm is suggestive of progression.

Glasses

Glasses improve vision in mild cases only.

Contact lenses

Rigid gas permeable lenses are the mainstay of treatment, although they are not tolerated by all patients. Soft lenses are less useful as they drape over the contour of the cone, reducing their refractive effect. Other options include 'piggyback' contact lenses (rigid lens worn on top of a soft lens) and scleral lenses.

Corneal collagen cross-linking

Cross-linking treats corneal ectasia by stiffening the cornea, thus increasing its biomechanical stability. Riboflavin (vitamin B_2)

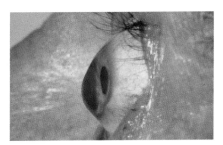

Fig 2.72 Keratoconus

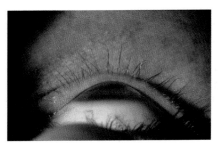

Fig 2.73 Munson's sign
Courtesy of John Dart

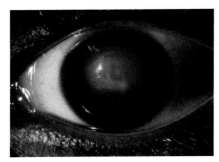

Fig 2.74 Acute corneal hydrops

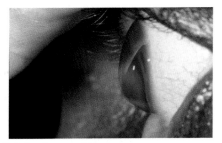

Fig 2.75 Pellucid marginal degeneration

visual acuity; rather, this treatment aims to improve quality of vision, contact lens fit, and tolerance of contact lenses.

Corneal grafting

Keratoconus is the most common indication for corneal graft surgery and has the best prognosis and lowest rate of graft rejection (89% graft survival at 10 years). Indications for keratoplasty in keratoconic eyes include:

* Contact lens intolerance
* Central corneal scarring, particularly after acute hydrops
* Non-resolving hydrops

Penetrating keratoplasty was once the procedure of choice for keratoconus. However, deep anterior lamellar keratoplasty is now preferred, as the risk of post-operative endothelial rejection is eliminated.

Phakic intraocular lens implantation

Phakic intraocular lens implantation is a useful option in eyes with stable keratoconus and good corrected visual acuity.

Pellucid marginal degeneration

Pellucid marginal degeneration is an uncommon bilateral inferior band of thinning of the cornea, whilst the central cornea appears normal (see Figure 2.75). It presents in the second to fifth decade of life, with reduced vision due to increasing astigmatism. Large-diameter rigid contact lenses or scleral lenses may be required to improve vision. Surgical options include large eccentric lamellar keratoplasty or lamellar excision of a wedge of stroma over the thinned area of cornea.

Keratoglobus

Keratoglobus is a bilateral, rare, ectatic disorder characterized by marked thinning of the entire cornea, which is thus made susceptible to rupture from minor trauma. Treatment is with protective eyewear, scleral contact lenses, and lamellar keratoplasty. The differential diagnosis includes:

* x-linked Megalocornea (diameter >13 mm, with normal IOP and reduced corneal thickness)
* Congenital glaucoma (diameter >12.5 mm, with raised IOP, Haab's striae, corneal thinning, and secondary corneal oedema)

Posterior keratoconus

Posterior keratoconus is a very rare, developmental, non-progressive, usually unilateral, localized anterior protrusion of the posterior corneal surface with a normal anterior surface. Acquired cases can occur following trauma. Other ocular associations include aniridia, ectropion uveae, anterior lenticonus, and anterior polar cataract. Patients have mild astigmatism or posterior scarring. Posterior keratoconus usually does not require treatment unless scarring is central, in which case a penetrating keratoplasty may be required.

reacts with UVA radiation and is thought to increase the interfibrillary or possibly interlamellar collagen bonds.

The aim of cross-linking is to stabilize keratoconus. Thus, it is only suitable for patients in whom progression has been documented. It is of no value for patients with stable disease. Cross-linking stabilizes keratoconus in 90% of treated eyes.

Various treatment protocols are in use; they vary in the duration of the riboflavin soak and the duration and intensity of the UVA exposure. The treatment comprises the following steps:

* The central 9 mm of the corneal epithelium is debrided.
* The cornea is soaked with isotonic riboflavin 0.1% solution (with or without dextran).
* UVA irradiation is applied over the central cornea.
* A bandage contact lens can be applied to reduce post-operative pain and promote epithelial healing.

Accelerated treatment protocols have been developed to reduce the procedure time. Epithelium-on cross-linking is also used in some centres, although the efficacy of this is uncertain.

The long-term effects of cross-linking are unknown.

Intracorneal ring segments

These C-shaped segments are inserted into the cornea to achieve a flattening effect at the centre of the cone. They do not predictably achieve a significant improvement in uncorrected

2.28 Keratoplasty

Keratoplasty (corneal transplantation or grafting) is an operation that replaces abnormal corneal host tissue with healthy cadaveric donor tissue. As the cornea is avascular, it is an immunologically privileged site and keratoplasty is thus one of the most successful types of human organ transplant operation. A corneal graft may be full thickness (penetrating) or partial thickness (lamellar).

Indications for keratoplasty

* **Optical:** to establish a clear visual axis or reduce distortion that cannot be corrected with other means. Disease indications for keratoplasty include keratoconus, bullous keratopathy, Fuchs endothelial dystrophy, other dystrophies, and scarring from trauma or infection.
* **Therapeutic:** removal of diseased tissue may be necessary for advanced microbial keratitis that is not responsive to antimicrobial therapy (e.g. fungal)
* **Tectonic:** to provide structural support with corneal thinning, or imminent or actual perforation

Preoperative considerations
It is important to evaluate and treat **factors associated with a poor prognosis** prior to surgery. These factors include:

* **Ocular surface abnormalities:** blepharitis, trichiasis, entropion, ectropion, lagophthalmos, dry eye and/or conjunctivitis, loss of corneal sensation
* **Corneal neovascularization:** the greater the extent (number of involved quadrants and stromal depth of vessels), the worse the prognosis
* **Previous surgery:** particularly a previous failed graft. Survival rates fall with each successive graft.
* **Glaucoma:** should be controlled before surgery
* **Uveitis:** should be well controlled before and after surgery
  Other factors to consider include:
* **Visual potential:** check for other conditions that may be responsible for poor vision in the presence of corneal disease (e.g. retinal dysfunction, macular dysfunction, optic nerve dysfunction)
* **Pre-existing cataract:** if this is present, consider a triple procedure (keratoplasty, cataract extraction, and intraocular lens insertion)

Penetrating keratoplasty

Historically, penetrating keratoplasty has been the most common type of corneal transplantation (see Figure 2.76).

Intraoperative management
* Surgery is usually performed under general anaesthesia (as there is less intraoperative orbital pressure under those conditions) but can be performed under local anaesthesia.
* Instil topical miotic (e.g. pilocarpine 2%) or mydriatics if combined cataract surgery is planned.
* Inspect the graft material for any obvious defects (storage media and graft should be clear).
* Consider stabilization of the eye with a scleral fixation ring (e.g. a Flieringa ring) if the eye is aphakic (to prevent scleral collapse).
* Select host bed and donor graft size. There is a greater risk of glaucoma, vascularization, and rejection with a larger

graft (>8.5 mm), and more astigmatism with smaller grafts (<6.5 mm). In keratoconus, the size and location of the cone must be taken into account. In general, a 7.5 mm recipient bed size is suitable for most cases, with the graft centred on the cornea. The graft size should be 0.25–0.5 mm larger than the recipient bed.

* Manual or automated trephines are available to prepare the host and donor buttons. Femtosecond lasers may also be utilized to cut the buttons, using a range of incision profiles.
* Suturing of the donor to the graft is carried out as follows: four cardinal sutures are placed at 12, 6, 3, and 9 o'clock, with 10–0 nylon. Additional sutures are placed with either interrupted alone (a total of 16–24 sutures), continuous running or a combination of interrupted sutures (8–16 sutures) and a continuous running suture. The depth of the suture should be to 90% of the corneal thickness. All knots should be buried in the host stroma.

Post-operative management
Medications
* Topical steroids are necessary to reduce the risk of graft rejection. The intensity of treatment should be tailored to the individual and the perceived risk of rejection. Drops are often instilled every 1–2 hours for the first few days after surgery and then reduced to four times a day for several weeks and slowly tapered down, stopping after 1 year or more if possible.
* Prophylactic topical antibiotic drops are necessary in the first few weeks after surgery.
* Oral acyclovir (400 mg two times a day) is used as prophylaxis in patients who have previously had HSK.
* Oral steroid and immunosuppression are used in high-risk cases.

Follow-up
Follow-up also needs to be tailored to the patient. Follow-up is usually at 1 day post-operatively, then 1 week, 2 weeks, 1 month, monthly for 2–3 months, and then every 3–6 months thereafter.

It is essential to educate patients about the symptoms of graft rejection and advise them to present promptly if these symptoms occur.

Suture removal
Loose or broken interrupted sutures must be removed immediately because of the risk of infection or graft rejection. A broken continuous suture should be spliced if it is too early to remove it. Sutures are normally left in situ for around 18 months, at which time, depending on the degree of astigmatism and the level of wound healing, they are removed selectively or completely.

Contact lenses
Rigid gas permeable lenses may be needed to correct high astigmatism once all sutures have been removed. Refractive procedures (see Chapter 4) may be used to reduce post-graft astigmatism.

Lamellar keratoplasty

The principle of lamellar keratoplasty is to replace only those corneal layer(s) affected by disease.

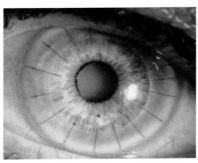

Fig 2.76 Clear corneal graft following penetrating keratoplasty

Advantages of lamellar keratoplasty

1. Shorter rehabilitation time
2. Reduced risk of immunological graft rejection
3. Strengthens the eye and increases its ability to resist trauma
4. Material with a low endothelial cell count and thus unsuitable for penetrating keratoplasty can be used for anterior lamellar surgery.
5. Less post-operative astigmatism with posterior lamellar grafts

Disadvantages of lamellar keratoplasty

1. Lamellar techniques are technically more demanding than other methods.
2. The risk of interface opacification and poor final acuity may not be as good as with penetrating keratoplasty.
3. Posterior lamellar discs can dislocate post-operatively and there is a higher risk of primary graft failure than after penetrating keratoplasty, owing to the increased amount of manipulation in lamellar keratoplasty.

There are a variety of techniques for lamellar graft surgery. Current techniques include:

Descemet's stripping endothelial keratoplasty

Descemet's stripping endothelial keratoplasty (DSEK) has overtaken penetrating keratoplasty as the most common keratoplasty procedure for Fuchs endothelial dystrophy and pseudophakic bullous keratopathy in some developed countries.

The host posterior corneal lamella (endothelium and Descemet's membrane) is stripped manually and is replaced by a donor lenticule of endothelium and Descemet's membrane which remains attached to a thin layer of posterior stroma (around 150 μm). The donor cornea is cut into anterior and posterior lamellae using a manual dissection method. The donor tissue is then trephined (usually to a diameter of 8.0–8.5 mm) and inserted into the anterior chamber with a dedicated insertion device. Air is injected into the anterior chamber to tamponade the graft against the host cornea. DSEK grafts may dislocate in the early post-operative period, requiring repositioning. Best visual outcomes are achieved with thinner grafts.

Descemet's stripping automated endothelial keratoplasty

Descemet's stripping automated endothelial keratoplasty is identical to DSEK except the donor lenticule is cut using an automated microkeratome.

Descemet's membrane endothelial keratoplasty

In Descemet's membrane endothelial keratoplasty, the donor lenticule consists only of Descemet's membrane and endothelium. This thin scroll of tissue is difficult to handle and the graft frequently dislocates in the early post-operative period, requiring reinjection of air ('rebubbling'). The steep learning curve and high complication rates associated with this procedure have limited its uptake; however, it is gaining in popularity.

Deep anterior lamellar keratoplasty

In deep anterior lamellar keratoplasty, the anterior corneal lamella (epithelium and ideally all of the stroma) is replaced, leaving the host Descemet's membrane and endothelium intact. Indications for this technique include keratoconus, anterior corneal dystrophies/degenerations, and superficial corneal scarring. Dissection of the host corneal stroma from Descemet's membrane is achieved either by manual dissection (Melles technique) or by injecting air into the stroma ('big bubble' technique).

Keratoprostheses

Keratoprostheses are artificial corneal implants which are used as a last resort in patients who are unsuitable for conventional keratoplasty.

* **Boston K-Pro (Type 1):** a specialized lens comprising a front plate and a stem is inserted through a full-thickness donor button, secured with a back plate, and sutured into the eye as for penetrating keratoplasty. Patients must have adequate tear production to support the donor button.
* **Boston K-Pro (Type 2):** the lens passes through the cornea and the upper lid, which is permanently closed with a tarsorraphy. This procedure is indicated for eyes with a very dry, compromised ocular surface (e.g. advanced cicatrizing conjunctivitis).
* **Osteo-odonto-keratoprosthesis:** this complex surgery is performed in several stages. Briefly, an optical cylinder is implanted into a rod fashioned from the patient's tooth root and alveolar bone. The cylinder is then implanted into the diseased cornea.

It is not possible to measure IOP in patients implanted with a keratoprosthesis, and glaucoma is a significant post-operative problem. Surgery may be combined with tube drainage surgery.

Removal of corneal sutures

Background/indication

Loose sutures can stimulate neovascularization and act as a focus for infection. Tight sutures induce corneal astigmatism, which is relieved by suture removal.

* **Phaco wound:** remove at the first post-operative visit.
* **Extracapsular cataract extraction wound:** remove selective sutures (guided by astigmatism) or all sutures after 2 months.
* **Keratoplasty:** see 'Penetrating keratoplasty'.

Technique

* Removal of sutures can be performed at the slit lamp or under the operating microscope.
* Instil topical anaesthetic and povidone iodine 5%.
* Use a 25-gauge needle advanced parallel to the corneal surface to lift and cut the suture.
* Pull the cut end in the direction of the suture (not perpendicularly) with fine forceps (e.g. Max Fine or tying forceps). If the suture breaks, leave the buried part but remove any exposed ends.
* Apply topical antibiotic stat. Prescribe topical antibiotic (chloramphenicol eye drops four times a day for 3 days).

In corneal graft patients, also give topical steroid (dexamethasone eye drops, 0.1%, four times a day for two weeks and then twice a day for two weeks). Warn the patient of the risk of infection or rejection.

Early post-operative complications

Wound leak/suture track leak

Wound leak/suture track leak presents with a low IOP, a shallow anterior chamber, and a positive Seidels test. Conservative treatment with a bandage contact lens may suffice but resuturing is indicated if the leak persists.

Persistent epithelial defects

Persistent epithelial defects are common if there is a pre-existing ocular surface disease, such as dry eye or exposure. If there is also stromal loss, it is important to exclude microbial keratitis. Treatment is with intensive tear-film supplements, bandage contact lenses, tarsorraphy, botulinum toxin ptosis, and addressing the underlying ocular surface disease.

IOP rise/glaucoma

IOP rise/glaucoma can occur in the immediate post-operative period and/or in the long term. Potential mechanisms include angle closure, retained viscoelastic in the anterior chamber, inflammation, or suprachoroidal haemorrhage. Treatment should be tailored to the underlying cause.

Suture infiltrates

Suture infiltrates can be either immune-mediated (multiple sutures affected, usually on host side, no epithelial defect) or infectious (solitary with epithelial defect).

Primary (early) graft failure

Primary (early) graft failure presents with irreversible corneal oedema in the immediate post-operative period (from Day 1–2). It is caused by inadequate endothelial function, which may be pre-existing in the donor graft or induced by surgical trauma. Treatment is with a regraft if the oedema persists.

Other early complications

Other early complications include inflammation, cystoid macular oedema, infection (including endophthalmitis), hyphaema, iris ischaemia with fixed dilated pupil (Urrets-Zavalia syndrome), and loose/broken sutures.

Late post-operative complications

Late graft failure

Late graft failure is usually due to graft rejection (see 'Graft rejection'). Other causes include late endothelial failure, recurrence of the primary disease (e.g. HSK, corneal dystrophy), infection, or persistent epithelial defect.

Other late complications

Other late complications include astigmatism, glaucoma, or retrocorneal membranes.

Graft rejection

Pathophysiology

Graft rejection is caused by a Type 4 immune hypersensitivity reaction. It rarely occurs within 2 weeks of surgery but it can occur at any time after corneal grafting. The vast majority of cases occur within 1 year of surgery, and the risk then reduces. It occurs in about 30% of all grafts and is the most common cause of graft failure. It can be epithelial, stromal, or endothelial.

Most episodes of graft rejection do not cause irreversible graft failure if recognized early and treated aggressively. Thus, it is imperative that graft patients have a clear understanding of the symptoms of graft rejection, and access to emergency care if these symptoms occur.

Risk factors

* Young age
* Previous graft surgery
* Preoperative deep stromal vascularization
* Glaucoma
* Post-operative loose/broken/vascularized sutures
* Large/eccentric grafts
* Previous/current active inflammation
* Non-compliance with topical steroid therapy post-operatively

Clinical evaluation

Symptoms include redness, photophobia, irritation, and/or decreased vision. Rejection episodes may rarely be asymptomatic.

Most episodes are directed against the endothelium; however, a combination of epithelial, stromal, and endothelial rejection may be present. For the sake of simplicity it is useful to consider the clinical features of each type of rejection individually.

Epithelial rejection

Epithelial rejection is relatively uncommon in isolation and is characterized by a linear epithelial ridge that advances centrally. It occurs within the first post-operative year. It rapidly responds to topical steroid treatment.

Stromal rejection

Stromal rejection normally accompanies epithelial rejection and rarely occurs in isolation. It is characterized by subepithelial circular opacities and there may also be anterior uveitis.

Endothelial rejection

Endothelial rejection is the most common form of graft rejection (see Figure 2.77). It is also the most serious form of rejection, as endothelial cells that are destroyed by the host response can only be replaced by a further graft procedure. It may be characterized by an endothelial rejection line (Khodadoust line) that often begins at a vascularized portion of the peripheral graft–host junction and progresses across the endothelial surface over several days (see Figure 2.78). The rejection line consists of white cells that damage endothelial cells as they move across the cornea. The donor cornea is clear ahead of the rejection line and is cloudy and oedematous behind it. A mild/moderate anterior chamber reaction is present.

Another variant of endothelial rejection is the diffuse formation of keratic precipitates on the donor endothelium, with an anterior chamber reaction. In this type of rejection, stromal oedema is generalized throughout the graft.

Treatment

The clinician should have a low threshold for initiating treatment against graft rejection in any graft patient with significant signs of inflammation.

* Intensive topical steroids (e.g. prednisolone, eye drops, 1%, or dexamethasone, eye drops, 0.1%, hourly) comprise the mainstay of treatment. These are tapered slowly depending on the initial response.
* Consider periocular/systemic steroids in severe cases or if there are doubts about compliance.

- Oral steroid or pulsed steroid are often used but probably do not improve the outcome compared to topical treatment alone.
- Treat inciting factors, such as loose vascularized sutures (see Figure 2.79).

Prognosis
Some 5%–10% of all cases of rejection result in graft failure. The earlier and more aggressively the rejection episode is treated, the better the prognosis is.

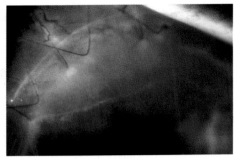

Fig 2.78 Endothelial graft rejection
Note the endothelial rejection line (Khodadoust line)

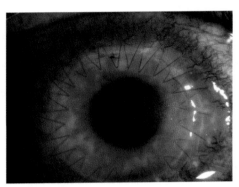

Fig 2.77 Endothelial graft rejection
Note the vascularization at the graft–host junction

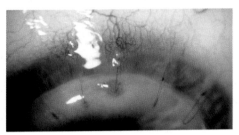

Fig 2.79 Vascularization associated with a suture

2.30 Anterior uveal tumours

Uveal melanomas are malignant neoplasms that arise from neuroectodermal melanocytes within the iris, ciliary body, and choroid (see Chapter 5, Section 5.15 for choroidal melanoma). Uveal melanomas are much more common in Caucasians (blue/grey iris) than in Africans. They are an important diagnosis as they have the potential to metastasize.

Iris melanoma

Iris melanomas are the least common (approximately 5%) of all uveal melanomas and typically present in patients who are in their 40s–50s (10–20 years earlier than ciliary body and choroidal melanomas). Histologically, most iris melanomas are composed of a mixture of spindle and epithelioid melanoma cells.

Risk factors for developing iris melanoma include exposure to UV light, ocular melanocytosis, and dysplastic naevus syndrome.

Clinical evaluation

History

- Usually asymptomatic or incidental finding on examination
- Enlargement/change in pre-existing spot on iris
- Visual disturbance due to secondary cataract
- Occasionally pain from raised IOP

Examination

- Pigmented (occasionally non-pigmented) iris lesion, usually well circumscribed, with a smooth or irregular surface
- Raised IOP may occur because of pigment clumping in the trabecular meshwork, direct invasion of the angle, or neovascular angle closure (see Chapter 8).
- Spontaneous hyphaema may occur from abnormal vessels within the tumour.
- Features associated with malignant potential include large size (>3 mm), thickness (>1 mm), irregularity, vascularity, fast growth, and effect on adjacent structures (e.g. localized cataract, pupil distortion, ectropion uveae). However, pupil distortion, ectropion uveae, and incomplete pupil dilation in the zone of the lesion can also occur with benign naevi.

Investigations

- **Anterior segment photography** (including gonioscopic views, if relevant) to document and monitor location, size, shape, colour, and vascularity
- **Ultrasound biomicroscopy (UBM)** to assess size, shape, extension, and internal characteristics; differentiates solid from cystic lesions
- **Anterior segment fluorescein angiography:** may be helpful for assessing the vascularity of the lesion and differentiating benign from malignant lesions
- **Tissue diagnosis:** options for obtaining tissue/cells for diagnosis include fine needle aspiration cytology, aqueous sampling, and incisional or excisional biopsy.

Differential diagnosis

- Iris naevus: small (<3 mm in diameter, <0.5 mm thick), pigmented, and well-defined stromal lesion (see Figure 2.80)
- Ciliary body melanoma with iris invasion (see 'Ciliary body melanoma').
- Lisch nodules: small, multiple, bilateral iris lesions in patients with neurofibromatosis type 1

- Freckles: smaller than naevi, frequently multiple and bilateral
- Cysts of theiris pigment epithelium: unilateral, solitary, dark-brown cysts that transilluminate
- Cyst of the iris stroma: presents in the first year of life as a solitary unilateral cyst with a translucent anterior wall and which contains fluid; can remain dormant for many years and later enlarge, causing glaucoma or corneal decompensation
- Metastatic carcinoma to iris: rare, pink/yellow, solitary deposit(s) which can grow rapidly; can cause hyphaema, pseudohypopyon, and raised IOP (see Figure 2.81)
- Leiomyoma of iris: rare benign tumour arising from smooth muscle
- Juvenile xanthogranuloma: a rare dermatological disorder with possible uveal nodules
- Inflammatory granulomas (e.g. sarcoidosis, tuberculosis)
- Adenoma/adenocarcinoma of the iris pigment or ciliary epithelium

Treatment

- Observation of suspicious lesions for growth
- Excision: iridectomy for small lesions with iris reconstruction (suturing or prosthesis); iridocyclectomy for those involving the angle
- Plaque radiotherapy or external radiation for surgically non-resectable tumours
- Enucleation is occasionally required for diffuse tumours, extensive seeding into the aqueous humour, ring angle invasion, trans-scleral extension, or blind, painful eyes due to tumour related complications.

Prognosis

- Most patients who undergo tumour excision do not develop metastatic disease.
- Mortality is 0%–3% in the absence of ciliary body involvement.
- Indicators of worse prognosis include large lesions, involvement of the ciliary body, ring angle invasion, and extrascleral extension.
- Monitoring is required to look for recurrence or satellite lesions (every 6 months for the first 3–5 years and then annually).

Ciliary body melanoma

Ciliary body melanomas account for approximately 10% of uveal tumours, presenting most commonly in the sixth decade. Histologically, they are more commonly composed of epithelioid melanoma cells than uveal melanomas at other sites are.

Ciliary body melanomas have the worst prognosis of all uveal melanomas. This characteristic may be due to a delay in diagnosis, as the tumour is hidden behind the iris. Further, the ciliary body is highly metabolically active, a feature which increases the likelihood of haematogenous spread.

Risks factors include uveal naevi, congenital ocular melanocytosis, dysplastic naevus syndrome, xeroderma pigmentosum, and a family history of uveal melanoma.

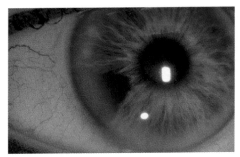

Fig 2.80 Benign iris naevus

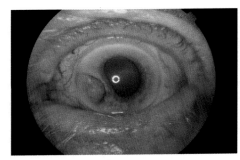

Fig 2.81 Amelanotic iris melanoma

Clinical evaluation

History

- Asymptomatic until the melanoma impinges on neighbouring ocular structures or the visual axis
- Blurred vision from lenticular astigmatism, cataract, or intraocular haemorrhage
- Gradual visual loss if posterior extension occurs
- Pain from acute secondary angle-closure glaucoma
- Red eye from dilated episcleral vessels ('sentinel vessels') overlying the tumour
- Systemic features of malignancy: weight loss and night sweats

Examination

- Gonioscopy and dilated fundus examination are required in all cases.
- Transillumination of any lesions should be attempted, to distinguish solid from cystic lesions.
- 'Sentinel vessels'
- A dark pigmented mass posterior to the pupil
- An epibulbar mass, due to extraocular extension of the tumour (may mimic conjunctival melanoma)

- Erosion through the iris root (can mimic iris melanoma)
- Pressure on the lens can cause subluxation and/or cataract.
- Raised IOP

Differential diagnosis

- Other ciliary body tumours: medulloepithelioma (from non-pigmented ciliary epithelium), melanocytoma (benign), adenoma, metastases
- Iridociliary cysts can be identified by their ultrasound appearance.
- Uveal effusion syndrome: rare, idiopathic condition with choroidal and exudative retinal detachments

Investigations

- **B-scan:** appears as a solid, acoustically dark mass. A B-scan can help estimate tumour size and extraocular extension.
- **UBM:** can help differentiate between ciliary body and choroidal melanomas
- Consider incisional or excisional biopsy.
- Chest X-ray, liver function tests, and liver ultrasound, if malignant spread is suspected (although 98% of patients have no detectable extraocular metastatic disease at time of diagnosis of ocular tumour)

Treatment

- There are many considerations when planning treatment: patient characteristics (age, health, systemic metastasis) and tumour characteristics (size, location, intra/extraocular extension, histological type).
- Observation, only if the tumour is less than 2 mm and suspicious features are absent
- Plaque brachytherapy for medium-sized tumours (10–15 mm)
- Sclerouvectomy: block excision leaving 2–3 mm clear margin in tumours involving less than 4 clock hours of circumference
- External beam irradiation by protons or gamma knife, but side effects may be severe. This procedure may be used for medium-sized tumours.
- Enucleation (it is uncertain whether this improves survival)
- Exenteration: if extensive extrascleral extension or recurrence after enucleation

Prognosis

- Mortality rate of 30%–50% at 10 years from the time of diagnosis
- Poor prognostic factors include large size, extrascleral extension, increased age, metastatic spread.
- Visual prognosis is guarded.
- Follow up initially every 3 months and then every 6 months, with liver function test monitoring for metastatic spread.

A variety of terms are used to describe the mechanisms and manifestations of ocular trauma. These are not necessarily mutually exclusive (e.g. a laceration can result in an open injury).

* **Closed injury:** the walls of the globe (cornea and sclera) are intact; usually due to blunt trauma.
* **Open injury:** a full-thickness defect in the corneo-scleral wall; can be due to blunt rupture or a sharp perforating/penetrating/lacerating injury
* **Penetrating injury:** a single full-thickness defect caused by an object which enters the globe without exiting; occurs with a retained foreign body (see Figures 2.82 and 2.83)
* **Perforating injury:** caused by an object entering and then exiting the globe through two separate sites; occurs with a gunshot/missile injury
* **Laceration:** a partial- or full-thickness defect in the corneo-scleral wall; caused by a sharp object at the site of impact
* **Rupture:** a full-thickness defect in the corneo-scleral wall; occurs secondary to blunt injury. The defect is at a weak point on the globe (previous surgical wounds, insertion of rectus muscles), not necessarily at the site of impact.

Open-globe injury

Clinical evaluation

Ocular trauma can occur in isolation or it can occur with head and/or systemic injury. The diagnosis and treatment of potentially life-threatening injuries takes precedence over the management of eye injuries.

History

Note the exact mechanism of injury. Risk factors for open-globe injury include metal striking metal (e.g. hammering, grinding), high-velocity projectile (e.g. squash ball, bullet), lack of eye protection, and/or previous intraocular surgery, as the old wound may rupture.

Examination

* Evaluate associated facial/orbital injuries.
* Visual acuity must be measured and documented. In eyes with poor vision, check that projection of light can be appreciated in all four quadrants.
* Check for an afferent pupillary reaction.
* Examine the eye for signs **suggestive** of an open-globe injury. These include full-thickness eyelid laceration, conjunctival or corneal laceration, shallow anterior chamber, hyphaema (see Figure 2.84), iridocorneal contact, hypotony, lens capsule defect, and/or lenticular opacity.
* Signs **diagnostic** of an open-globe injury include exposed uvea and/or vitreous, positive Seidel test and visualization of an intraocular foreign body.
* If an open-globe injury is suspected, pressure should not be applied to the eye during examination.

Investigations

A B-scan ultrasound scan may be useful if there is no fundal view to assess signs of posterior segment trauma (see Chapter 5, Section 5.17). It can also be of use for detecting intraocular foreign bodies.

Plain X-rays are useful for detecting metallic intraocular foreign bodies. At least two X-rays should be performed in at least two positions of gaze.

Computed tomography scanning of the orbit has largely superseded X-rays for detecting non-metallic intraocular foreign bodies; it is also useful for assessing the integrity of the surrounding orbital bones.

Treatment

Preoperative care

If surgery is indicated, it should be performed as soon as practical to reduce pain, devitalization of prolapsed uveal tissue, and inflammation, and to reduce the risk of suprachoroidal haemorrhage and endophthalmitis.

The following measures should be taken prior to surgery:

* Analgesia and anti-emetic as required
* Tetanus prophylaxis if needed
* Apply an eye shield (avoid padding which puts pressure on the globe)
* Admit and prepare for theatre: the patient should take nil by mouth. Inform theatres and inform the anaesthetist.
* Consent: discuss examination under anaesthesia, guarded prognosis for visual recovery, the need for evisceration/enucleation if the eye is beyond repair, and the need for further treatment/surgery
* Consider performing biometry (see Chapter 3, Section 3.9) on the fellow eye if there is a possibility that lens extraction along with IOL insertion may be considered at the time of primary repair.
* Start systemic antibiotics (e.g. moxifloxacin 400 mg once a day or ciprofloxacin 750 mg twice a day).

Non-surgical care

Small, self-sealing partial-thickness or full-thickness wounds can be observed without surgical intervention. A bandage contact lens, topical antibiotic therapy, topical cycloplegia, and close observation are necessary.

General principles of primary repair of corneo-scleral lacerations

* The primary goal for initial repair is to restore the integrity of the globe (i.e. to close the eye). A secondary goal is to restore vision by means of repairing damaged intraocular structures.
* All reasonable attempts must be made to perform a primary repair, even in cases of severe trauma, because the loss of an eye is a highly traumatic event psychologically.
* In cases of severe trauma, it may be impossible to perform a primary repair; rarely, primary evisceration or enucleation may be required (see Chapter 11, Section 11.10).
* Evisceration or enucleation after severe trauma reduces the risk of sympathetic ophthalmia.
* General anaesthesia is almost always required, as periocular anaesthesia will increase the pressure on the open globe.

Surgical principles of primary repair of corneo-scleral lacerations

* Place 5% povidone iodine in the conjunctival sac.
* Try to minimize pressure on the globe during draping and speculum insertion.

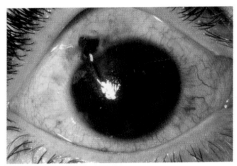

Fig 2.82 Penetrating globe injury
Note the full-thickness corneo-scleral laceration with iris prolapse

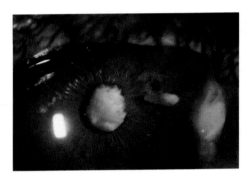

Fig 2.83 Sequelae of penetrating globe injury
Note the raised corneo-scleral scar, the full-thickness iris defect, and the traumatic cataract

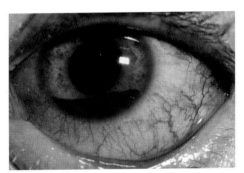

Fig 2.84 Hyphaema
Also see Chapter 8

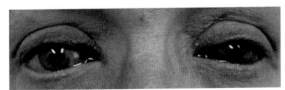

Fig 2.85 Bilateral subconjunctival haemorrhage

- Clean and remove any debris including foreign bodies from the periocular area.
- Make a paracentesis and re-form the anterior chamber with viscoelastic.
- An anterior chamber maintainer may be useful in some cases.

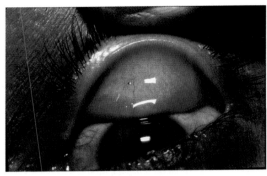

Fig 2.86 Subtarsal foreign body

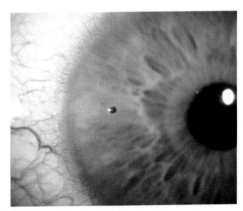

Fig 2.87 Corneal foreign body

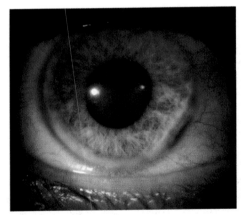

Fig 2.88 Iridodialysis

- Vitreous should be removed from the wound with a vitreous cutter in the anterior chamber. Triamcinolone may be used to aid visualization of the vitreous.
- If the uvea or retina has prolapsed from the eye, it should be gently repositted using the paracentesis. Only when the uveal tissue is necrotic should it be excised.
- Repair the limbus first (9–0 nylon) then the cornea (10–0 nylon interrupted). Bury the knots away from the visual axis.
- Scleral lacerations must be explored by performing a conjunctival peritomy, extending posteriorly until the entire laceration is exposed.

- The sclera is thin beneath the insertion of the rectus muscles; this area is a common site of globe rupture.
- Repair the sclera with 9–0 nylon or an absorbable suture. Begin anteriorly and progress posteriorly.
- If the laceration extends underneath a rectus muscle, the muscle must be placed on a suture and disinserted. Once the sclera is closed, the muscle can be reinserted.
- The conjunctiva should be closed with 8–0 Vicryl.
- Once the globe has been closed, the intraocular structures can be repaired during the primary procedure or later as a secondary procedure. Potential anterior segment procedures include removal of anterior intraocular foreign bodies, iris repair, lens extraction, anterior vitrectomy, and intraocular lens insertion.
- Administer subconjunctival steroid and antibiotic.
- Intravitreal antibiotic injection should be considered for contaminated wounds involving the vitreous.

Post-operative care

- Topical steroid, antibiotics, and cycloplegia; oral antibiotic for open injuries

Specific anterior segment injuries

Note: cyclodialysis, angle-recession glaucoma, and hyphaema are not covered here but instead are covered in Chapter 8. Traumatic uveitis is covered in Chapter 7.

Subconjunctival haemorrhage

Subconjunctival haemorrhages are common and usually innocuous (see Figure 2.85). Their appearance is often alarming to the patient; however, most resolve spontaneously over 10–14 days.
Causes include:

- Spontaneous/idiopathic
- Trauma (conjunctival (including eye rubbing), iatrogenic/post-surgical, orbital, cranial (base of skull fracture))
- Valsalva (vomiting, coughing)
- Infectious conjunctivitis (e.g. adenoviral, streptococcal)
- Systemic disease (bleeding diathesis, hypertension)

There is often no identifiable predisposing factor. If there is a history of trauma, it is important to rule out other ocular injuries (including globe rupture under an elevated subconjunctival haemorrhage).

No treatment is generally required except reassurance. Lubrication may be needed to prevent dellen in cases of elevated haemorrhage.

Conjunctival/corneal foreign body

It is essential to evert the upper eyelid in all patients in whom a foreign body is suspected. Vertical linear superior corneal abrasions are commonly seen when there is a superior subtarsal foreign body (see Figures 2.86 and 2.87). Double eversion of the upper lid with a Desmarres retractor may be necessary to visualize the foreign body if it is high on the tarsus or in the superior fornix. The technique for removal of the foreign body is explained in 'Removal of corneal foreign bodies'. After complete removal of the foreign body, the patient should be treated with chloramphenicol ointment four times a day for one week.

Corneal abrasion

Corneal abrasions cause acute pain, lacrimation, photophobia, and blepharospasm. Common causes include trauma by fingernails, paper or cardboard edges, and plants. They are also associated with contact lenses (e.g. tight lens, overwear, attempts at insertion/removal). Corneal abrasions can occasionally result in recurrent corneal erosions (see Section 2.25). They stain brightly with fluorescein and should be examined carefully on the slit lamp to exclude a deeper corneal laceration or a corneal ulcer secondary to infection/inflammation (infiltrate present).

Loss of the corneal epithelium may allow water from the tear film to enter the stroma, causing stromal oedema and Descemet's folds in some cases. Depending on the size (large abrasions take longer to heal than small ones) and location (peripheral abrasions heal more quickly than central ones), healing normally occurs within 7 days.

Treatment

- Topical antibiotics (e.g. chloramphenicol ointment three to four times a day) and cycloplegic (e.g. cyclopentolate, eye drops, 1%, twice a day)
- Pressure patching is of no benefit and prolongs the healing time.
- Abrasions related to contact lens wear should be monitored for infection (consider broad spectrum antibiotics, e.g. levofloxacin).
- Topical anaesthetics should not be used for pain relief (except to facilitate examination).

Iridodialysis

Iridodialysis refers to the separation of the iris root from the ciliary body and occurs as a result of trauma (including surgical; see Figure 2.88). It is usually associated with hyphaema. It may be asymptomatic or may cause glare and/or monocular diplopia. A small dialysis may be left untreated but a large dialysis causing symptoms may need surgical repair. It is important to exclude associated injuries such as retinal dialysis.

Iris sphincter damage

Iris sphincter damage is caused by blunt trauma and is characterized by small notches in the pupillary margin; these notches represent defects in the sphincter pupillae muscle. These defects can result in an increase in pupil size (mid-dilated) and/or distortion of the pupil. Usually no treatment is needed. If there is significant glare from increased pupil size, pilocarpine drops, a painted contact lens or surgical repair are therapeutic options.

Removal of corneal foreign bodies

- Instil topical anaesthetic.
- Ensure that the patient fixates with the fellow eye.
- Ideally, one hand should be used to hold open the eyelids and the needle, leaving the other hand free to control the slit lamp.
- Superficial and loose foreign bodies can be irrigated away with sterile saline or manually removed with a moist cotton bud.
- Impacted/deep foreign bodies can be removed with the tip of a 25-gauge needle. The needle can be mounted on a syringe to allow easier handling. The tip of the needle can be bent over to create a hook by pressing on the inside of the plastic needle sheath.
- The needle is advanced parallel to the surface of the cornea, with the bevel up and the foreign body removed.
- If there is an associated rust ring, it can be removed with a needle if it is very superficial or with a dental burr if the rust has penetrated the anterior stroma.

2.32 Chemical injury

Chemical injuries are potentially blinding events, usually occurring in the context of industrial or domestic accidents and assaults (see Figure 2.89). They are time-critical ophthalmic emergencies; prompt early management may improve the long-term prognosis.

Pathophysiology

The effect of chemicals on the eye depends on the pH (alkali injuries are worse than acid injuries), concentration, duration and area of contact, and associated injury (thermal and mechanical trauma).

Alkali injuries are the most serious. Alkalis cause saponification of cell membranes, resulting in cellular disruption. Once the surface epithelium is breached, alkalis continue to penetrate deep into the stroma, destroying the proteoglycan ground substance and collagen fibres of the stromal matrix. The limbal stem cells are also vulnerable. They can be damaged directly by the alkali or secondarily by ischaemia from destruction of the limbal vasculature. Alkalis may also penetrate through the cornea into the anterior chamber and cause intraocular inflammation and toxicity, trabecular meshwork injury, and cataract.

Acids cause immediate coagulation of tissue proteins upon contact with the eye, limiting further penetration. Strong acids like sulphuric acid and hydrochloric acid can however still cause severe injury.

Acidic agents
- **Sulphuric acid (H_2SO_4):** battery fluid and industrial use
- **Hydrochloric acid (HCl):** bleach, pool-cleaning fluid, and industrial use
- **Hydrofluoric acid (HF):** glass/metal manufacturing and semiconductors. It is a weak acid but one of the most destructive agents due to the highly reactive F^- anion. This anion is able to penetrate deeply through the cornea, conjunctiva, and skin, causing severe ocular and systemic injury.

Alkali agents in decreasing order of severity
- **Ammonia (NH_3):** fertilizer, refrigerant; used in the chemical industry
- **Sodium hydroxide (NaOH, caustic soda):** drain and oven cleaner; used in the paper industry; soap/detergent
- **Potassium hydroxide (KOH, caustic potash):** alkaline batteries, soaps/detergent
- **Calcium hydroxide ($CaOH_2$, lime):** plaster, cement

Initial management

Initial management should be commenced immediately at the site of the incident. Copious irrigation with normal saline is ideal; if saline is unavailable, water should be used. The eye should be held open and irrigated for at least half an hour during transfer to hospital. The pH should be determined as soon as possible on arrival (i.e. before further history and examination is elicited) and further irrigation continued (aided by a lid speculum if necessary) until the pH is normal (pH 7–7.5) and remains so.

Topical anaesthesia should be applied and particulate matter removed with forceps or a swab. Double evert the lid to remove debris (cement/lime/plaster) from the fornices.

Note: CS gas (similar to tear gas, used by police) should be treated by drying in front of a fan rather than irrigation.

Clinical evaluation
- Determine the mechanism/nature/duration of chemical injury.
- Corneal epithelial defects can range from scattered superficial punctate epithelial erosions to sloughing of the entire epithelium.
- The cornea is clear in mild injuries and hazy to opaque in more severe injuries (see Figure 2.90).
- There are focal or diffuse areas of conjunctival chemosis and injection in mild injuries. In moderate-to-severe injuries, there are areas of conjunctival blanching (see Figure 2.91) and limbal ischaemia (see Figure 2.92). Limbal ischaemia is classified according to the proportion of the limbus that is affected. (Note: the eye may appear white in severe chemical injuries because of complete blanching of the limbal and conjunctival vessels).
- There may be anterior chamber inflammation, raised IOP (due to alkali-mediated destruction of the trabecular meshwork), or hypotony (alkali destruction of ciliary body epithelium).
- Note: do not ignore associated facial skin burns and refer promptly for specialist management.

Grading of alkali injury
Chemical injuries can be graded according to the Roper-Hall classification system. In grade I injuries the cornea is clear, there is no limbal ischaemia and the prognosis is good. In grade II injuries the cornea is hazy, iris details are visible, there is less than a third limbal ischaemia and the prognosis is good. In grade III injuries the cornea is opaque, there is a third to half limbal ischaemia and the prognosis is guarded. In grade IV injuries the cornea is opaque, there is more than a half limbal ischaemia and the prognosis is poor. If in doubt treat as Grade II or worse.

Treatment
- In the initial stages, the aim is to relieve pain, promote epithelialization, control IOP, and limit secondary damage due to inflammatory mediators.
- Admit if severe injury or concern regarding compliance.
- Use preservative-free drops wherever possible.
- Intensive preservative-free artificial tears
- Prophylactic topical antibiotics (e.g. chloramphenicol four times a day)
- Topical mydriatic (e.g. cyclopentolate 1% three times a day) and oral analgesia
- IOP control: use aqueous suppressants (e.g. oral acetazolamide, topical timolol).

Grade 2 injury or worse
Use the following:
- Topical steroids (e.g. dexamethasone 0.1% four to eight times a day for a minimum of 10 days)
- Topical ascorbate (e.g. sodium ascorbate 10% every 1–2 hours) and oral ascorbic acid (1–2 g four times a day) until

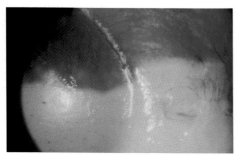

Fig 2.89 Corneal and conjunctival epithelial loss secondary to chemical injury, staining brightly with fluorescein

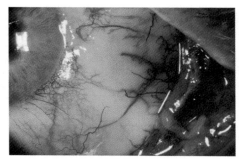

Fig 2.91 Conjunctival blanching

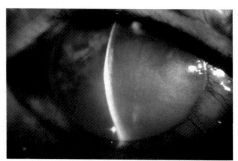

Fig 2.90 Corneal opacification in severe chemical injury

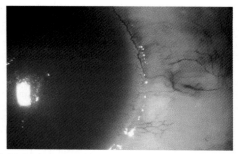

Fig 2.92 Limbal ischaemia in a severe chemical injury

epithelization is complete. Ascorbate promotes the synthesis of mature collagen by corneal fibroblasts.

- Topical sodium citrate 10% (given every 2 hours for 10 days) inhibits neutrophil activity and migration.
- Oral doxycycline may help prevent collagenolysis.

Additional management

- Amniotic membrane onlay (to help reduce inflammation and promote reepithelization)
- Glue, patch graft, or tectonic graft to treat melting and perforation

Long-term management

Limbal stem cell transplantation, keratoplasty (poor prognosis), keratoprosthesis, glaucoma control (augmented trabeculectomy, drainage devices).

Complications

Dry eye, symblepharon, corneal opacification, vascularization, corneal melt, exposure, perforation, glaucoma, and/or cataract

Further reading

1. Roper-Hall MJ: Thermal and chemical burns. *Trans Ophthalmol Soc UK* 1965; **85**: 631–653

Chapter 3

Cataract

Georgia Cleary and Allon Barsam

3.1 Lens anatomy and embryology

Cataract is the pathological opacification of the crystalline lens. The word cataract is derived from *cataracta*, which is Latin for waterfall. Cataract is an important cause of visual impairment and blindness worldwide, in both developed and developing countries. According to the latest WHO estimates, age-related cataract accounts for 47% of world blindness, affecting approximately 18 million people. Fortunately, acquired cataract is a reversible cause of visual impairment.

The majority of cataracts are age related. In developed countries, cataract surgery is the most commonly performed elective surgical procedure. Cataract surgery incurs considerable cost to health services, and this cost will rise as populations continue to age. However, cataract surgery is a highly cost-effective health intervention. In poor countries, many people remain cataract blind because of a lack of access to ophthalmic services.

Lens anatomy

The function of the crystalline lens is to focus images onto the retina. After the cornea, it is the second most powerful refractive structure in the human eye.

The crystalline lens undergoes considerable changes with age. At birth, the crystalline lens measures 6.5 mm in diameter, and is 3.5–4.0 mm thick. It is a highly elastic structure, and is capable of changes in shape and thus refractive power. The ability of the eye to change focus from distance to near is known as accommodation, and this process is achieved by an increase in the axial thickness of the lens, steepening of its anterior and posterior radii of curvature, and a net forwards shift.

The axial thickness of the lens increases throughout life. Its diameter stabilizes in early adulthood at 9–10 mm. With increasing age, there is progressive hardening of the crystalline lens. This process is accompanied by loss of accommodation and therefore loss of clear near vision. This usually begins in the fifth decade, and is called presbyopia.

Macroscopic anatomy

The crystalline lens lies posterior to the iris and anterior to the vitreous body (see Figures 3.1, 3.2, and 3.3). It is a transparent, biconvex disc. Fine glycoprotein fibres, the zonules, support the lens within the eye. They insert onto the lens equator circumferentially and are attached to the ciliary body via the ciliary processes.

The lens is surrounded by a capsule which varies in thickness, measuring approximately 15 μm at the anterior pole and 3 μm at the posterior pole. Beneath the capsule lies the lens cortex. The most central portion of the lens is the nucleus.

Microscopic anatomy

The entire crystalline lens is composed of cells of a single type. Lens fibres arise from the anterior lens epithelium, and are progressively laid down throughout life. As they mature, these cells lose their nuclei and become densely packed with lens proteins called crystallins. Each lens fibre is conserved throughout life, and it is the stability, resilience, and precise organization of the crystallins that allow the lens to remain transparent into adult life. The oldest, most differentiated cells lie deep within the lens nucleus, whilst the youngest cells are most superficial (see 'Lens embryology').

The basement membrane of the lens epithelial cells forms the lens capsule, which surrounds the lens completely, and provides a surface for insertion of the zonular fibres.

Lens embryology

The crystalline lens arises from surface ectoderm (see Figures 3.4 and 3.5).

Day 27

A small region of surface ectoderm overlying the optic vesicle thickens, to form the lens placode.

Day 29

The lens placode invaginates to form the lens vesicle and lens pit above the retinal disc.

Day 33

The lens pit closes, and the lens vesicle moves into the developing eye, forming the embryonic lens. The lens vesicle is surrounded by a basal lamina, the future lens capsule. All cells are orientated with their base adherent to the lens capsule, and their apices towards the lens cavity.

Days 33–47

Anterior and posterior cells of the lens vesicle display different behaviours.

Posterior cells

Posterior cells elongate and grow anteriorly, closing the lens cavity and forming the primary lens fibres. Nuclei of these elongated cells migrate anteriorly to form the lens bow.

Anterior cells

Anterior cells form the anterior lens epithelium, the source of secondary lens fibres. Secondary lens fibres originate from anterior lens epithelium at the lens equator. Each lens fibre grows anteriorly and posteriorly, meeting with other lens fibres at the anterior and posterior surfaces of the lens to form the Y-sutures.

Sequential lamellae of secondary lens fibres are laid down throughout embryonic development; this process continues throughout life.

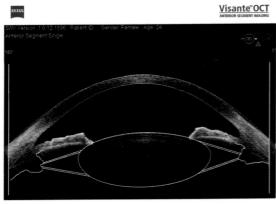

Fig 3.1 Anterior segment anatomy, superimposed on an anterior segment optical coherence tomography scan

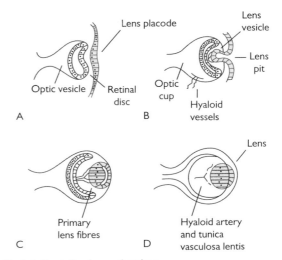

Fig 3.4 Crystalline lens embryology

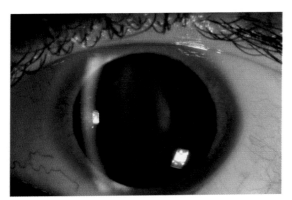

Fig 3.2 Clear crystalline lens

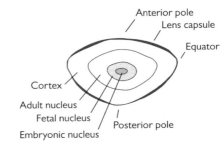

Fig 3.5 Anatomy of the crystalline lens

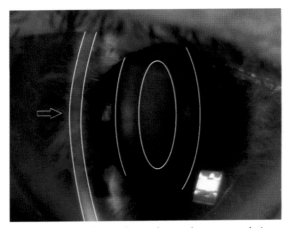

Fig 3.3 Crystalline lens, indicating lens nucleus, as seen during slit lamp examination (arrow indicates direction of light)

3.2 Acquired cataract

Broadly, cataract aetiology can be divided into congenital and acquired causes. The majority of cataracts encountered in clinical practice are acquired, and most acquired cataracts are age related.

Clinical classification

Acquired cataracts may be classified in terms of morphology, aetiology, and maturity.

Morphology

A morphological classification is used commonly in the clinic setting and provides useful information when planning for cataract surgery.

Nuclear cataract

Nuclear cataract (see Figures 3.6 and 3.7) is a common type of senile cataract and may be associated with increasing myopia as the refractive index of the lens nucleus increases. Also referred to as nuclear sclerosis, these cataracts may be very hard when advanced, requiring a large amount of ultrasound energy during phacoemulsification cataract surgery. They may progress to be brown in colour (brunescent).

Cortical cataract

The opacities in cortical cataracts (see Figures 3.8 and 3.9) are typically arranged radially, in the soft outer cortical zone of the lens.

Subcapsular cataract

Posterior subcapsular cataracts (see Figures 3.10 and 3.11) lie just anterior to the posterior capsule and often develop as a side effect of corticosteroid use. Small, central posterior subcapsular cataracts can be highly symptomatic, owing to their proximity to the nodal point of the eye. Anterior subcapsular cataracts are less common than posterior ones.

Polar cataract

Posterior polar cataracts are rare and involve the lens capsule as well as the underlying lens matter. The risk of posterior capsule rupture is very high in these cases and therefore they must be distinguished from posterior subcapsular cataracts.

Various formal classification systems have been developed to objectively grade cataracts; for example the Lens Opacities Classification System III. These classifications systems are utilized primarily as research tools.

Aetiology

- Age related (senile)
- Drugs
  - Corticosteroids (topical or systemic)
  - Chlorpromazine
  - Amiodarone
  - Aspirin
  - Topical glaucoma medications
  - Miotic agents (e.g. pilocarpine)
- Trauma
  - Iatrogenic (e.g. pars plana vitrectomy, trabeculectomy, intravitreal injection (see Figure 3.12))
  - Penetrating injury
  - Blunt injury (see Figure 3.13)
  - Chemical injury
  - Electrocution (see Figure 3.14)
  - Irradiation (e.g. X-rays)
- Secondary to systemic disease
  - Diabetes mellitus (see Figure 3.17)
  - Myotonic dystrophy
  - Wilsons disease (sunflower cataract)
  - Atopic dermatitis
  - Neurofibromatosis type 2
  - Fabry disease
- Secondary to ocular disease
  - Uveitis (see Figure 3.15)
  - Myopia
  - Acute angle-closure glaucoma
  - Retinal dystrophies (e.g. retinitis pigmentosa)

Maturity

Immature cataract

Most cataracts seen in UK practice are immature, characterized by incomplete opacification of the lens.

Mature cataract

A mature cataract is a dense, white cataract which obstructs the red reflex and the view of the fundus (see Figure 3.16).

Hypermature cataract

As a mature cataract continues to age, water leaks from the lens, the cataract is accompanied by shrinkage and wrinkling of the capsule.

Morgagnian cataract

With further progression from hypermaturity, the cortical lens matter liquefies, with inferior displacement of the nucleus in the capsular bag.

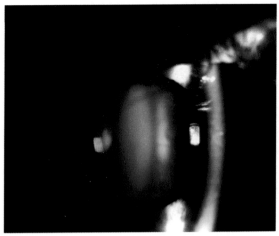

Fig 3.6 Nuclear cataract

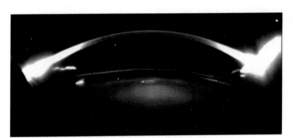

Fig 3.7 Nuclear cataract, imaged with a Scheimpflug camera
Courtesy of L. Pelosini

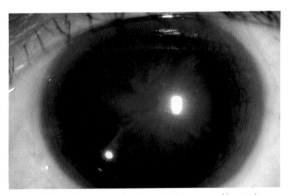

Fig 3.8 Cortical cataract, showing radial pattern of lenticular opacification

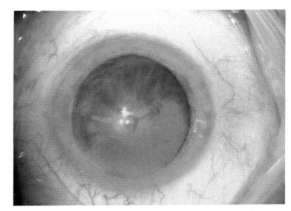

Fig 3.9 Cortical cataract viewed intraoperatively

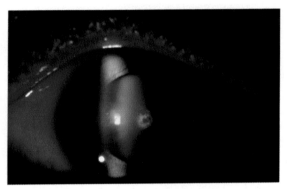

Fig 3.10 Small central posterior subcapsular cataract

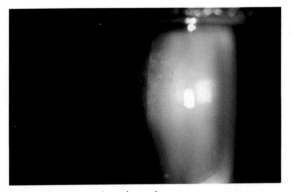

Fig 3.11 Large posterior subcapsular cataract

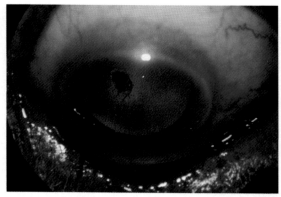

Fig 3.12 Lens puncture as a complication of intravitreal injection

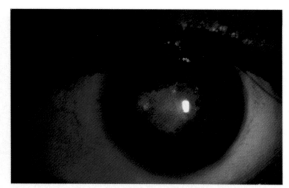

Fig 3.15 Uveitic cataract with posterior synechiae

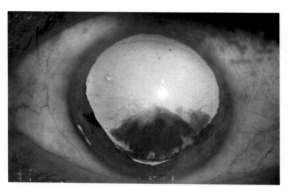

Fig 3.13 Traumatic cataract due to blunt trauma, with associated iris dialysis

Visualized with retroillumination

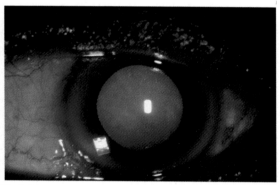

Fig 3.16 Mature white cataract

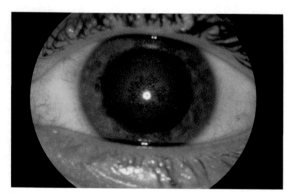

Fig 3.14 Electric cataract caused by lightning strike

Courtesy of S. Rajak

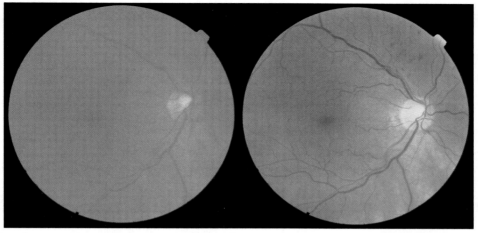

Fig 3.17 Retinal screening photographs for diabetic retinopathy. The same eye is imaged before and after cataract sugery

In clinical practice, most patients are referred with an existing diagnosis of cataract. They may already have expectations that surgery will be arranged following their outpatient visit. Cataract is a clinical diagnosis. The decision to list a patient for surgery is based in most cases on history and examination findings alone.

Cataract surgery involves removal of the opaque crystalline lens and then implantation of an intraocular lens. Most cataract surgery is performed under local anaesthesia as a daycase procedure. Despite this, a thorough medical history should be obtained from all patients, in order to establish any general factors that may increase the risks of cataract surgery (see Table 3.1).

Clinical evaluation

History

- Age
- Previous ophthalmic history (especially history of ocular trauma or amblyopia)
- Previous medical history
- Medications (e.g. tamsulosin and other alpha 1 receptor antagonists, and warfarin).
- Allergies (e.g. sulpha drugs; acetazolamide is routinely used by some surgeons post-operatively)
- Family history of eye disease
- Driving status
- Social history, including occupation and hobbies

Ask about the following cataract symptoms:

- Blurred vision
- Glare (in strong sunlight, or headlights)
- Haloes or starbursts
- Night-driving problems
- Increasing short-sightedness (myopia)
- Yellow/brownish discolouration of vision (more apparent when one eye has been operated)

Examination

Before pupil dilation

- Visual acuity: unaided, best spectacle-corrected and best pinhole visual acuity
- Pupil examination: cataract does not cause a relative afferent pupillary defect. If present, suspect optic nerve or retinal disease.
- Cover test
- Intraocular pressure (IOP)
- Careful slit lamp examination, with attention to ocular factors that may render cataract surgery technically difficult, risky, or limit the visual outcome of surgery (see Table 3.2)

After pupil dilation

- How well does the pupil dilate?
- Assess cataract morphology.
- Fundus examination

General

- Blood pressure
- Blood glucose

Investigations

Investigations are not required to diagnose cataract per se. Dense cataracts may preclude a clear view of the fundus. If no view is possible, a B-scan ultrasound is necessary to exclude posterior segment co-pathology (e.g. retinal detachment). An intraocular lens is implanted during cataract surgery, and the intraocular lens power must be tailored to each eye. The eye is measured preoperatively, in order to calculate the required intraocular lens power. These measurements are known as biometry (see Section 3.9).

Patients taking warfarin should have their international normalized ratio measured, to ensure it does not exceed their therapeutic range. The few patients undergoing cataract surgery under general anaesthesia require appropriate anaesthetic workup.

Indications for cataract surgery

Visual symptoms due to cataract

The presence of a cataract alone is not an indication for surgery; the patient must have visual symptoms which can be attributed to the cataract.

Snellen visual acuity does not directly correlate with cataract symptoms, and therefore no universally agreed visual acuity threshold for cataract surgery exists. Despite this fact, some healthcare providers restrict access to surgery to a Snellen acuity cut-off level (e.g. 6/9 or worse). In general, cataract surgery should aim to achieve an appreciable improvement in measured visual acuity and/or subjective quality of vision.

Acute glaucoma

- **Phacomorphic glaucoma:** an enlarged lens causes shallowing of the anterior chamber, and secondary angle-closure glaucoma.
- **Phacolytic glaucoma:** lens proteins leaked from a hypermature cataract cause inflammation and obstruct the trabecular meshwork, causing secondary open-angle glaucoma.
- **Acute angle closure:** there is a growing body of evidence supporting cataract surgery as a primary treatment for acute angle closure in eyes with coexisting cataracts.

Chronic glaucoma/primary angle closure

- **Primary angle closure/angle-closure glaucoma:** cataract surgery deepens the anterior chamber and widens the angle; this procedure is ideally performed before peripheral anterior synechiae develop.
- **Primary open-angle glaucoma:** cataract surgery may produce a modest reduction in IOP; this procedure may be advantageous in eyes with coexisting cataracts.

Improve retinal visualization

A cataract may obscure the view of the fundus, making clinical evaluation and photographic screening of retinal disease difficult or impossible.

Cosmesis

Cataract extraction is occasionally performed in a blind eye with a white cataract for cosmetic reasons alone.

As with all surgical procedures, the decision to proceed to cataract surgery should follow careful consideration of the risks and benefits involved, with informed consent obtained prior to surgery.

Table 3.1 General factors that may contribute to adverse outcomes of local anaesthetic/daycase cataract surgery

History	Factor/pathology	Risk	Action
Age	Young age	Unable to tolerate local anaesthetic	Consider general anaesthetic
Past medical history	Anxiety	Unable to tolerate local anaesthetic	Consider general anaesthetic
Past medical history	Claustrophobia	Unable to tolerate local anaesthetic and/or lying beneath drape	Consider general anaesthetic, or use a clear drape
Past medical history	Marked tremor	Unable to lie still	Consider general anaesthetic, akinesia can be helpful in these cases
Past medical history	Persistent cough	Unable to lie still	Cautiously consider general anaesthetic
Past medical history	Impaired lung function or heart failure	Unable to lie flat	Cautiously consider general anaesthetic
Past medical history	Uncontrolled hypertension	Suprachoroidal or expulsive haemorrhage	Treat prior to surgery
Medication	Anticoagulants	Suprachoroidal or expulsive haemorrhage	Ensure that the international normalized ratio is in therapeutic range
Medication	Tamsulosin or other alpha 1 receptor antagonists	Intraoperative floppy iris syndrome	Cautious surgery, dispersive viscoelastic, iris hooks, intracameral mydriatic (e.g. phenylephrine)

Table 3.2 Ocular factors that may contribute to adverse outcomes of cataract surgery

Structure	Pathology	Risk	Action/possible surgical strategies
Lids	Blepharitis	Endophthalmitis	Treat blepharitis prior to surgery
Lids	Conjunctivitis	Endophthalmitis	Treat infection prior to surgery
Cornea	Guttata/Fuchs endothelial dystrophy	Corneal decompensation	Counsel preoperatively, shortest possible surgical time, use of dispersive viscoelastic/soft shell technique. Consider phaco-DSAEK if decompensation is established
Cornea	Corneal opacity/scar	Poor visualization during surgery	Stain capsule with trypan blue; consider penetrating keratoplasty if view severely obscured
Cornea	High corneal astigmatism	Residual post-operative astigmatism	Placement of incision along steepest meridian, additional corneal procedure to treat astigmatism, toric IOL
Cornea	Previous laser refractive surgery	Post-operative refractive error if standard formula used	Acquire pre-refractive surgery biometry if available; use appropriate IOL power calculation formula
Anterior chamber	Shallow	Corneal endothelial trauma, iris prolapse, technically difficult surgery	Cautious surgery, use of dispersive viscoelastic
IOP	Uncontrolled IOP	Iris prolapse, suprachoroidal haemorrhage	Treat IOP prior to surgery
Pupil	Posterior synechiae	Poor visualization during surgery	Synechiolysis, sphincterotomy, pupil stretching, iris hooks, or other pupil-expanding device as required
Pupil	Poor pupil dilation	Poor visualization during surgery	Pupil stretching, iris hooks, or other pupil-expanding device
Lens	Instability/phacodonesis (e.g. pseudoexfoliation)	Zonular dehiscence, IOL decentration	Capsular tension ring (or ring segments), capsulorrhexis fixation by iris hooks intraoperatively; sulcus fixation of IOL
Lens	Very dense cataract	High level of phaco power may cause corneal decompensation	Cautious surgery, use of dispersive viscoelastic, phaco chop technique
Lens	Posterior polar cataract	Posterior capsular rupture during hydrodissection	Hydrodelineate; avoid hydrodissection
Vitreous	Previous vitrectomy	Unstable anterior chamber	Cautious surgery, low bottle height, and low vacuum levels
Vitreous	Silicone oil in vitreous cavity	Post-operative refractive error due to incorrect axial length measurement	Use of conversion factor for ultrasound biometry, or appropriate settings on IOL Master
Retina	Visually significant retinal or macular disease (e.g. age-related macular degeneration)	Limited improvement in vision	Preoperative counselling regarding limited visual improvement from surgery
General	Active uveitis	Persistent post-operative uveitis, cystoid macular oedema	Treat uveitis prior to surgery; may require perioperative systemic steroids, intravitreal triamcinolone at time of cataract surgery
General	Heterotropia	Post-operative diplopia	Counsel preoperatively
Axial length	Nanophthalmos/short axial length	Post-operative aqueous misdirection	Suture wound to avoid wound leakage and anterior chamber shallowing; dilate pupil post-operatively
Axial length	High myopia/long axial length	Retinal detachment	Counsel preoperatively; educate regarding symptoms of retinal detachment
Axial length	High myopia/long axial length	Post-operative refractive error	Counsel preoperatively; careful choice of IOL power

CCC, continuous curvilinear capsulorhexis; DSAEK, Descemets stripping automated endothelial keratoplasty; IOL, intraocular lens; IOP, intraocular pressure.

Conservative

Asymptomatic cataracts do not require surgery, unless dictated by other co-pathology (e.g. primary angle-closure glaucoma). In eyes with minimal lens opacity and good corrected visual acuity, the risks of cataract surgery are likely to outweigh its benefits. Patients with asymptomatic cataracts should be advised to seek further review when symptoms develop.

Surgical

The standard treatment for cataracts is phacoemulsification and intraocular lens implantation. Phacoemulsification was first performed in 1967 and has undergone considerable refinement since that time. It has superseded extracapsular cataract extraction (ECCE) in the developed world; ECCE is now rarely performed in the United Kingdom. The majority of cataract surgery is performed under local anaesthesia (see Section 3.12).

Phacoemulsification and intraocular lens implantation

Phakos is Greek for 'lentil', as a lentil approximates the shape of the human crystalline lens. Phacoemulsification involves removal of the crystalline lens using ultrasonic energy. The basic steps that comprise phacoemulsification cataract surgery are reproduced worldwide. However, the techniques utilized for each step vary among individual surgeons.

Step 1: Preparation of skin and the conjunctival sac

Local anaesthetic drops (e.g. tetracaine 1%) are instilled into the conjunctival sac. Povidone iodine 5% is used to wash the lids, lashes, and conjunctival sac, staying in contact with the sac for at least 2 minutes (see Figure 3.18). The area is then carefully dried.

Step 2: Draping

A sterile drape with a transparent, adhesive central window is placed over the eye, care being taken to direct the lashes away from the eye. A small incision is made in the drape, directly over the eye, and a speculum is inserted to keep the lids open. The surgical field should be entirely free of lashes (see Figure 3.19).

The microscope can now be positioned over the eye, and surgery commenced.

Step 3: Primary incision

The main incision into the anterior chamber may be corneal, limbal, or scleral and may be located temporally, superiorly, or along the steepest corneal meridian. It must be sized according to the phaco probe, to achieve a good fit (see Figure 3.20). Corneal wounds are constructed to be self-sealing. The keratome blade penetrates the corneal epithelium peripherally and enters the anterior chamber through the corneal endothelium centrally. It may be constructed to have one, two, or three planes (see Figure 3.21).

Step 4: Secondary incision (side port)

A smaller second incision is made to accommodate the 'second instrument' during phacoemulsification. Two side port incisions may be made if bimanual surgery (e.g. irrigation and aspiration) is to be used (see Figure 3.22).

Step 5: Viscoelastic insertion

The anterior chamber is filled and deepened with a high molecular weight, transparent, viscous gel. This stabilizes the anterior chamber for the subsequent step, capsulorrhexis, and protects the corneal endothelium from mechanical trauma and ultrasound energy during phacoemulsification (see Figure 3.23).

Step 6: Continuous curvilinear capsulorrhexis

The anterior lens capsule is punctured centrally, and a flap of capsule is fashioned. This flap is then carefully advanced, tearing a circular hole in the anterior capsule. The ideal continuous curvilinear capsulorrhexis (CCC) should be circular, centred around the Purkinje reflexes from the operating microscope, and slightly smaller in diameter than the intraocular lens optic (see Figure 3.24).

Step 7: Hydrodissection

Balanced salt solution (BSS) is gently injected beneath the anterior lens capsule, underneath the capsulorrhexis edge. A 'fluid wave' can be seen advancing, dissecting the lens capsule away from its contents. This wave frees the lens matter to rotate within the capsule in preparation for phacoemulsification (see Figure 3.25).

Step 8: Phacoemulsification

The phaco probe is inserted into the eye with the irrigation running. Constant irrigation with BSS maintains anterior chamber depth and intraocular pressure. Aspiration removes soft or emulsified lens matter. Axial (+/− rotational) movement of the phaco needle at ultrasonic frequency results in cavitation of lens matter at the tip of the needle (see Figures 3.25 and 3.26).

A second instrument is then inserted into the eye via the side port incision. Commonly used second instruments include choppers and nucleus rotators. Using both the phaco probe and the second instrument, the lens nucleus is rotated and broken into fragments, which are sequentially emulsified. Common techniques for fragmentation of the nucleus include 'divide and conquer' and 'stop and chop' (see Figures 3.27 and 3.28).

Step 9: Irrigation and aspiration

Residual soft lens matter is aspirated from the lens capsule (see Figure 3.29).

Step 10: Viscoelastic insertion

Further viscoelastic is inserted into the capsular 'bag', reopening the bag and creating space for intraocular lens insertion (see Figure 3.30).

Step 11: Intraocular lens insertion

A foldable intraocular lens is advanced into the eye via an injector, or occasionally forceps. The lens is then placed into the capsular bag, where it unfolds (see Figure 3.31).

Step 12: Viscoelastic removal

Viscoelastic is removed using the irrigation and aspiration probe, taking care to remove all viscoelastic from behind the lens (see Figure 3.32). Centration of the lens can be assessed at this stage.

Step 13: Anterior chamber refilling and intracameral antibiotic

The anterior chamber is refilled with BSS until the globe is firm. Cefuroxime (1 mg in 0.1 mL) is injected into the anterior chamber with a cannula.

Step 14: Wound closure

Corneal oedema is induced at the wound edge by injecting BSS into the corneal stroma. This process results in tight apposition of the wound edges (see Figure 3.33). Incisions should be checked meticulously for leaks. Suturing is rarely required.

Femtosecond laser cataract surgery

Femtosecond lasers, usually utilized for corneal refractive surgery, have recently been applied to several steps of the cataract surgery procedure. They may be utilized for:

• Construction of corneal incisions
• Capsulotomy
• Nuclear segmentation

These steps are performed as separate procedures. The corneal incisions, capsulotomy size and shape, and pattern of nuclear segmentation can be precisely planned and optimized for each patient.

After the initial laser treatment, the eye is prepared as for conventional cataract surgery. The corneal incisions are opened with a blunt instrument, the disc of anterior capsule is removed from the capsulotomy, and phacoemulsification is performed, with or without hydrodissection. The level of ultrasound energy required for femtosecond laser cataract surgery is lower than that for conventional cataract surgery, as the nucleus is already segmented.

ECCE

This technique is still used as the primary technique for cataract surgery in some parts of the developing world. Rarely, it may be useful in cases where the nucleus is deemed too hard for phaco. Phaco cases that are complicated by extensive tearing of the anterior capsule can be 'converted' to ECCE cases. More recently, the technique has been modified to reduce the size of the wound (small incision ECCE). The standard technique is as follows.

1. A large stepped wound is created at the superior limbus (for small incision ECCE, a scleral tunnel is created). The wound needs to be large enough to accommodate the whole lens nucleus.
2. Viscoelastic is inserted.
3. A CCC is made.
4. Two or three small relieving incisions are made in the capsule perpendicular to the CCC edge.
5. The nucleus is 'expressed' using a squint hook placed on the inferior sclera just posterior to the lens. Gentle pressure is applied with the squint hook, and the nucleus is 'delivered' out of the capsular bag, through the wound, and out of the eye.
6. The soft lens matter is aspirated.
7. An intraocular lens is inserted and the viscoelastic is removed.
8. The wound is sutured with continuous or interrupted 10–0 nylon sutures.

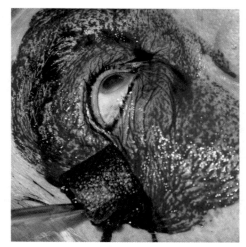

Fig 3.18 Skin preparation with povidone iodine

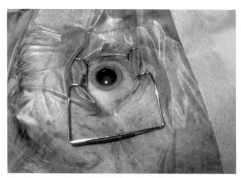

Fig 3.19 Draped eye with speculum in situ

117

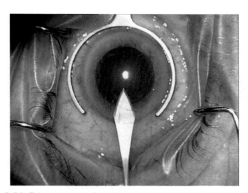

Fig 3.20 Primary corneal incision

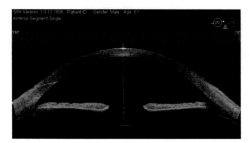

Fig 3.21 Corneal incision visible post-operatively with optical coherence tomography (the incision is on the left side of the cornea)

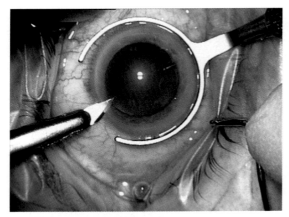

Fig 3.22 Second incision (side port)

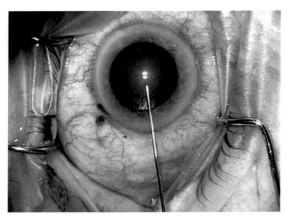

Fig 3.23 The anterior chamber is filled with viscoelastic

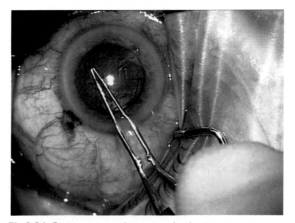

Fig 3.24 Continuous curvilinear capsulorrhexis

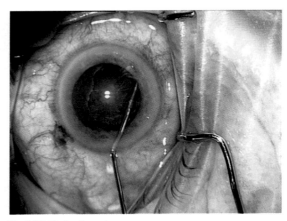

Fig 3.25 Hydrodissection

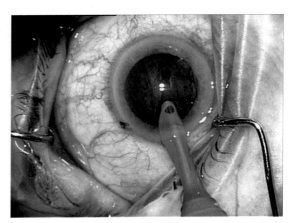

Fig 3.26 Phacoemulsification
Sculpting a central groove in the lens nucleus

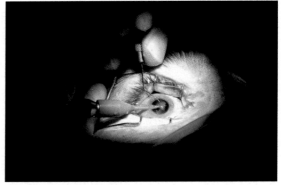

Fig 3.27 Phaco probe and chopper within the eye

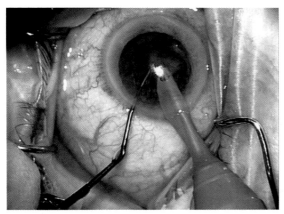

Fig 3.28 Phacoemulsification
Removal of a nuclear segment

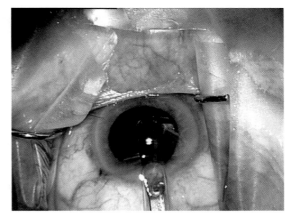

Fig 3.31 Intraocular lens insertion

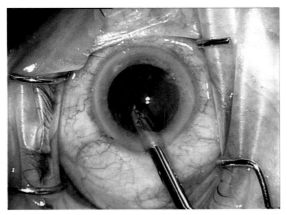

Fig 3.29 Irrigation and aspiration

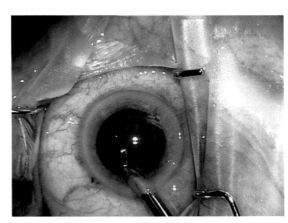

Fig 3.32 Viscoelastic removal

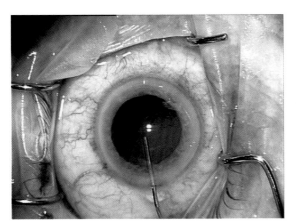

Fig 3.30 Refilling the capsular bag with viscoelastic

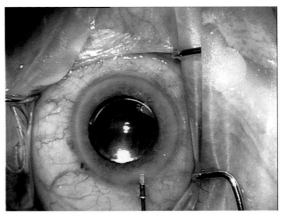

Fig 3.33 Corneal wound hydration

Phacoemulsification cataract surgery yields high success rates. Patient expectations for good visual outcomes are high. Intraoperative complications do occur, with higher rates observed in the hands of trainee surgeons than with experienced surgeons. Rates of posterior capsule rupture and/or vitreous loss are used as benchmarks for operative complications in the United Kingdom. A 2% rate of these complications is acceptable in modern surgical units.

Many potential complications of cataract surgery can be prevented by:

* Careful preoperative assessment
* Surgical planning, including appropriate case selection for trainees
* Meticulous perioperative and intraoperative technique

Loss of the capsulorrhexis

The capsulorrhexis may tear out towards the lens equator, potentially extending posteriorly to involve the posterior capsule. This complication may occur when surgeons are learning the procedure and should be recognized before it becomes irretrievable.

Posterior capsular rupture

Rupture of the posterior capsule occurs when a surgical instrument inadvertently comes into contact with the thin posterior capsule, usually during phacoemulsification or during irrigation and aspiration.

Early signs of posterior capsule rupture include sudden, transient pupil dilation ('pupil snap' sign), sudden deepening of the anterior chamber, and difficulty with nucleus rotation. When posterior capsular rupture is suspected, the anterior chamber pressure must be maintained; viscoelastic should be inserted before withdrawing the phaco needle.

Rupture without vitreous loss

When the posterior capsule defect is small and no vitreous has migrated into the anterior chamber, surgery may proceed relatively normally, with cautious implantation of the intraocular lens in the capsular bag.

Rupture with vitreous loss

When vitreous advances into the anterior chamber through a posterior capsular defect, an anterior vitrectomy is required. Bimanual anterior vitrectomy should be performed through separate side ports, not the main incision. Diluted triamcinolone can be used to visualize vitreous in the anterior chamber. Vitrectomy should be performed at the maximum possible cut rate, in cut-IA mode. All vitreous should be cleared from the anterior chamber.

When lens implantation into the capsular bag is not possible, it may be placed in the ciliary sulcus if adequate capsular support is available. Retinal detachment and cystoid macular oedema rates are higher in eyes in which vitreous is 'lost' than in those undergoing uncomplicated cataract surgery.

Dropped nucleus

If the posterior capsule is breached before phacoemulsification is complete, the nucleus may fall posteriorly into the vitreous cavity, in part or in its entirety (see Figure 3.34). Prompt referral to a vitreoretinal surgeon for vitrectomy and fragment removal is necessary. Retained lens fragments cause intraocular inflammation and raised IOP. Lens fragments may occasionally be retained in the anterior chamber (see Figure 3.35). These fragments also require surgical removal.

Surgical trauma to ocular tissue

Corneal trauma

Direct mechanical contact between surgical instruments or nuclear fragments and the corneal endothelium may occur, particularly if the anterior chamber is very shallow. Corneal wound burns may occur if high phaco energy is utilized; however, this is less common than before owing to improvements in phaco technology.

Iris trauma

The soft, friable iris may be inadvertently aspirated into the phaco tip or the irrigation and aspiration tip. Alternatively, iris tissue may prolapse (see Figure 3.36) into one or both of the surgical wounds. This complication may occur as part of intraoperative floppy iris syndrome (IFIS). This syndrome is observed in some patients taking alpha 1 receptor antagonists, particularly tamsulosin.

The characteristic triad of IFIS is:

* Floppiness and billowing of the iris
* Iris prolapse into one or both of the surgical wounds
* Progressive pupillary constriction

Intraoperative complications due to IFIS may be minimized by careful surgical planning. The pupil may be additionally dilated with intracameral phenylephrine or adrenaline. The length of the surgical incisions should be increased and the incisions should enter the anterior chamber anteriorly. Iris hooks or pupil-expanding devices (see Figure 3.37) may be used to maintain the pupil size. Any prolapsed iris must be repositted into the anterior chamber.

Iris trauma is evident post-operatively as one or more transillumination defects and may cause glare symptoms in some patients.

Zonular dehiscence

Zonular dehiscence is more likely in eyes with underlying zonular instability (e.g. in patients with Marfan syndrome, pseudoexfoliation syndrome, or previous ocular trauma). Lens implantation in the capsular bag may be impossible or result in poor lens centration.

Suprachoroidal haemorrhage

Risk factors for this feared complication include:

* Age
* High myopia
* Glaucoma or raised IOP
* Posterior capsular rupture
* ECCE (vs phacoemulsification)
* Diabetes
* Hypertension

Pathophysiology

Haemorrhage into the suprachoroidal space occurs after rupture of a short or long ciliary artery. In mild cases, the haemorrhage is small and localized. In severe cases, progressive haemorrhage generates high IOP, displacing the intraocular contents from the globe. This form is referred to clinically as an 'expulsive haemorrhage'.

Clinical signs

The globe becomes hard, the anterior chamber shallows, and the posterior capsule bulges anteriorly. A dark shadow may be evident within the pupil, obscuring the red reflex, which may be lost entirely if the haemorrhage progresses. Intraocular contents are extruded from the eye: first the iris and then, in advanced cases, the lens, the vitreous, and the retina.

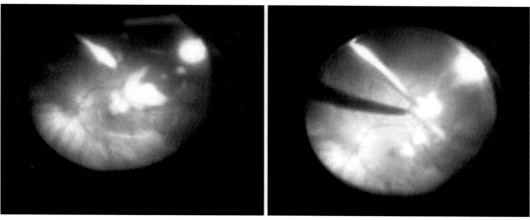

Fig 3.34 Dropped nuclear fragments, seen during the secondary surgical procedure Vitrectomy and fragment remova
Courtesy of R. Wong

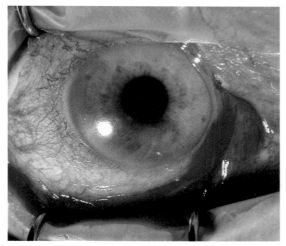

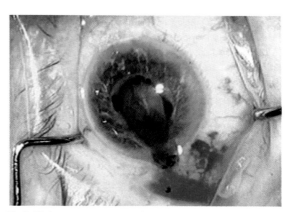

Fig 3.36 Intraoperative iris prolapse

Fig 3.35 Retained nuclear fragment in the anterior chamber
Courtesy of C. Jenkins

Immediate management

Surgical instruments should be withdrawn from the eye, and the wound closed immediately.

Subsequent management

In cases of limited suprachoroidal haemorrhage, the eye may be observed, monitoring reabsorption of the haemorrhage clinically and with B-scan ultrasound. Drainage sclerostomy rarely may be performed to evacuate a clot.

Secondary anterior segment procedures may be required, for example secondary intraocular lens implantation.

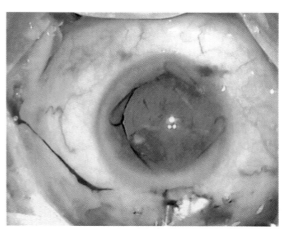

Fig 3.37 Pupil-expanding device (Malyugin ring) used intraoperatively

3.6 Infectious post-operative complications of cataract surgery

Acute post-operative endophthalmitis

Acute post-operative endophthalmitis is a sight-threatening emergency. Treatment with intravitreal antibiotics must be performed without delay once a diagnosis is made.

Incidence

Reports vary: 0.015% to 0.5% of all cataract surgeries. The incidence of endophthalmitis is reduced by the use of intracameral cefuroxime 1 mg in 0.1 ml at the end of cataract surgery (European Society of Cataract and Refractive Surgeons Endophthalmitis Study Group 2007).

Risk factors

* Age
* Non-use of intravitreal cefuroxime
* Vitreous loss/complicated surgery.
* Clear corneal incisions
* Silicone vs acrylic intraocular lens material

Aetiology

Bacteria are inoculated into the eye during (or shortly after) cataract surgery via the surgical wound(s).
The most common causative organisms are Gram positive:
* Coagulase-negative staphylococci
* *Staphylococcus aureus*
* *Streptococcus pneumonia*
* Beta haemolytic streptococci
* Viridans group streptococci
* Enterococci
  The following Gram-negative organisms are occasionally isolated:
* *Haemophilus influenza*
* *Pseudomonas aeruginosa*
* *Escherichia coli*
* *Serratia marcescens*
* *Klebsiella* spp., *Moraxella* spp., and *Proteus* spp.

Pathogenesis

Intraocular bacteria incite a florid intraocular inflammatory response.

Clinical evaluation

History

The following symptoms develop between 1 day and 2 weeks after cataract surgery:
* Pain
* Redness
* Watering
* Photophobia
* Decreased vision
* Discharge

Examination
* Reduced visual acuity
* Relative afferent pupillary defect
* Loss of red reflex
* Lid oedema
* Proptosis
* Chemosis, and conjunctival congestion (see Figure 3.38)
* Corneal oedema, infiltrate, or abscess
* Intense anterior uveitis with cells, hypopyon, keratitic precipitates, and fibrinous membrane on the intraocular lens surface (see Figure 3.39)
* Vitritis
* Hazy or absent fundus view

Differential diagnosis
* **Retained lens matter:** fragments of nuclear material or soft lens matter within the anterior chamber, capsular bag, or vitreous incite post-operative inflammation and require removal
* **Post-operative uveitis:** inflammation may be exaggerated in eyes with previous uveitis, or following lengthy or complicated surgery.
* **Toxic anterior segment syndrome:** this acute, sterile anterior uveitis typically occurs 12–24 hours after surgery. Inflammation is caused by contamination of fluids or instruments used in cataract surgery, and thus cases tend to occur in outbreaks. Endotoxins have been isolated in previous outbreaks. Treatment is with intensive steroid therapy.
* Acute bacterial keratitis

Investigations
* B-scan ultrasound if there is no fundus view
* Microbiological specimens: anterior chamber tap (see Figure 3.40) and vitreous tap. If facilities are available, vitreous samples may be obtained with a vitreous cutter or portable vitrector.
* Urgent Gram stain microscopy is required. Culture, antibiotic sensitivities, and PCR are performed.

Management

Intravitreal antibiotics
The following combination of antibiotics should be administered intravitreally (see Figure 3.41):
* Amikacin 0.4 mg in 0.1 ml (or ceftazidime 2 mg in 0.1 ml)
* Vancomycin 12 mg in 0.1 ml
  Note: Ceftazidime and vancomycin are physicochemically incompatible and should be administered via separate needles and syringes.

Other surgical procedures
* Vitrectomy if visual acuity is perception of light or worse (Endophthalmitis Vitrectomy Study Group 1995)

Post-procedure management
* Admission to hospital in most cases
* Systemic antibiotics: moxifloxacin (or ciprofloxacin and clarithromycin)

- Topical, preservative-free dexamethasone 0.1% hourly
- Topical, preservative-free chloramphenicol four times a day
- A topical, preservative-free mydriatic
- Consider oral prednisolone 1 mg/kg 24 hours after initial treatment.
- Consider repeating intravitreal antibiotics after 48–72 hours if no improvement.

Ongoing antibiotic therapy should be tailored to microscopy, culture, and sensitivity findings.

Prevention of endophthalmitis
Cataract surgery pathways now incorporate steps specifically aimed at endophthalmitis prophylaxis.

Preoperative assessment
Pre-existing blepharitis or conjunctivitis requires treatment before surgery is scheduled.

Operating theatre and surgical instruments
Operating theatres should ideally be equipped with appropriate air flow design. All surgical instruments should be sterile. Single-use instruments are preferable when cost allows.

Skin and conjunctival preparation
The skin and conjunctival sac are sterilized with povidone iodine 5% prior to surgery.

Surgical technique
All lashes must be draped away from the surgical field. Surgical wound construction should generate a self-sealing incision; if the wound leaks, it must be sutured.

Antibiotic prophylaxis
- Intracameral cefuroxime (1 mg in 0.1 ml) at the end of surgery
- Post-operative topical antibiotics (e.g. levofloxacin or tobramycin)

Chronic post-operative endophthalmitis

Rarely, endophthalmitis may present weeks or even years after uncomplicated cataract surgery with anterior uveitis and vitritis. Initial response to steroids is good, and so diagnosis of endophthalmitis may be delayed. The clinical course is indolent, as causative organisms are of low virulence. Sequestration of bacteria within the capsular bag also contributes to the chronicity of these infections and to their refractoriness to treatment. Inflammation may develop after Nd:YAG posterior capsulotomy, which 'releases' bacteria from the capsular bag.

Aetiology
- *Proprionobacterium acnes*
- *Staphylococcus epidermidis*
- *Streptococcus viridans*
- Gram-negative rods

Eradication of infection is difficult, and in some cases requires intraocular lens explantation and capsulectomy.

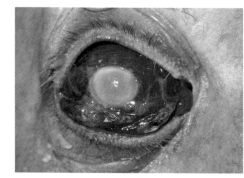

Fig 3.38 Severe post-operative endophthalmitis
Courtesy of B. Dong

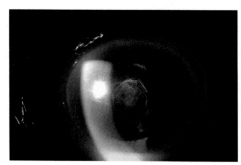

Fig 3.39 Post-operative endophthalmitis, with hypopyon and fibrin deposits on the anterior intraocular lens surface

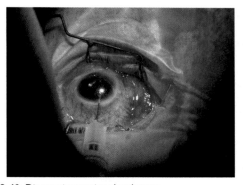

Fig 3.40 Diagnostic anterior chamber tap

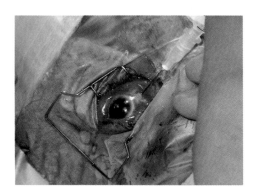

Fig 3.41 Intravitreal antibiotic administration

3.7 Non-infectious post-operative complications of cataract surgery

Corneal decompensation/pseudophakic bullous keratopathy

Corneal clarity is maintained by the corneal endothelium. The endothelium may be compromised during cataract surgery by direct mechanical trauma or by phaco energy, resulting in decompensation.

Factors predisposing to corneal decompensation include:

* Fuchs endothelial dystrophy
* Corneal guttata
* Age (endothelial cell density declines with age)
* Prolonged or complicated surgery
* High phaco energy

Pseudophakic cystoid macular oedema

Clinical cystoid macular oedema is the most common cause of unexpected visual loss following cataract surgery, occurring in 0.1%–2.3% of cases. Its incidence peaks at 4–6 weeks post-operatively. Angiographic pseudophakic cystoid macular oedema is found in a much greater proportion of patients; however most of these cases are asymptomatic.

Risk factors

* Pre-existing ocular disease, including uveitis, diabetic maculopathy, epiretinal membrane, retinal vein occlusion, and possibly eyes treated with prostaglandin analogues
* Surgical complications, including posterior capsular rupture, vitreous loss, and iris trauma

Intraocular lens malposition

Intraocular lenses may be decentred, tilted (see Figure 3.42), subluxated (see Figure 3.43), or completely dislocated into the anterior chamber or vitreous cavity. The malposition may result from:

* Incorrect intraoperative lens placement
* Zonular instability or dialysis
* Inadequate capsular support due to poor capsulorrhexis construction, anterior capsule tear, or posterior rupture
  Mild decentration may be asymptomatic. Dislocated intraocular lenses may cause reduced visual acuity, inflammation due to movement and iris chafing, raised IOP, cystoid macular oedema, and retinal detachment. Treatment options include:

* Intraocular lens repositioning (with or without suturing)
* Intraocular lens exchange
* Intraocular lens removal

Retinal detachment

Incidence

The average incidence of rhegmatogenous retinal detachment after cataract surgery is 0.7%.

Risk factors

* **Patient factors:** male sex, age greater than 65 years
* **Ocular factors:** axial length greater than 23 mm, previous retinal detachment in the fellow eye
* **Surgical factors:** posterior capsule tear/vitreous loss, zonular dehiscence

Posterior capsule opacification

Posterior capsule opacification (PCO) is the most common complication of cataract surgery (see Figure 3.44).

Incidence

Incidence rates are highly variable, depending on patient, surgical, and intraocular lens factors.

Nd:YAG capsulotomy rates are often utilized as a proxy measure for PCO, and cumulative incidence rates as high as 33% have been reported. However, these rates have fallen significantly since the introduction of hydrophobic acrylic, square-edged intraocular lenses.

Risk factors

* **Patient factors:** young age, uveitis
* **Surgical factors:** residual cortical lens matter, incomplete overlap of the capsulorrhexis on the intraocular lens optic, sulcus intraocular lens fixation
* **Intraocular lens factors:** intraocular lenses without a square posterior edge are associated with a higher rate of PCO incidence than those with a square posterior edge are; hydrophilic acrylic intraocular lenses are associated with a higher rate of PCO incidence than hydrophobic acrylic intraocular lenses are.

Pathogenesis

PCO results from the proliferation of lens epithelial cells onto the posterior capsule (Fig. 3.44).

Management

Management involves Nd:YAG laser posterior capsulotomy (Section 3.13).

Anterior capsule opacification

In the months following cataract surgery, the anterior capsule may opacifiy, and the capsulorrhexis may contract (anterior capsular phimosis; see Figure 3.45). Contraction of the anterior capsule may adversely affect the position of the intraocular lens, whilst opacification precludes a complete view of the retina.

Risk factors

* High myopia
* Pseudoexfoliation
* Uveitis
* Retinitis pigmentosa
* Diabetes mellitus

Management

Management involves Nd:YAG laser anterior capsulotomy.

Post-operative refractive error

In a European study of 523 921 eyes, 91.5% achieved a post-operative refraction within 1 D of their target refraction. Intraocular lens power calculation formulae are limited by their inability to precisely predict post-operative anterior chamber depth, which determines the effective lens power of the intraocular lens.

Post-operative ametropia may be due to:

* Insertion of the wrong lens; this error should be avoided by performing meticulous preoperative checks
* Using the wrong A-constant for the lens

- Inaccurate biometry (e.g. posterior staphyloma; underestimation of axial length, due to corneal indentation during A-scan ultrasound; systematic errors with measurements)
- Previous corneal refractive surgery
- Results in eyes with extreme biometry (e.g. highly hypermetropic or myopic eyes) are less predictable than those in eyes for which the biometry is not extreme.

Management

- Conservative: glasses or contact lens correction of residual refractive error
- Corneal refractive surgery
- Intraocular lens exchange or implantation of an additional sulcus-fixated intraocular lens ('piggyback intraocular lens')

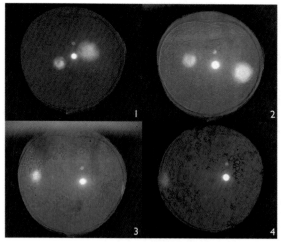

Fig 3.44 Progression of posterior capsule opacification

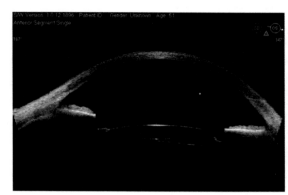

Fig 3.42 Tilted intraocular lens, demonstrated with optical coherence tomography

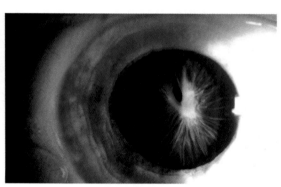

Fig 3.45 Severe anterior capsule opacification and fibrosis
Courtesy of E. Hughes

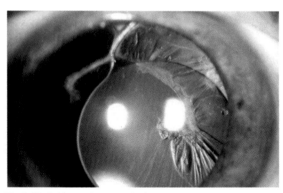

Fig 3.43 Subluxated intraocular lens

3.8 Lens dislocation

Lens dislocation

Displacement of the crystalline lens from its normal location within the eye is also known as ectopia lentis. It may be incomplete (subluxation) or complete (luxation).

Aetiology

- Congenital:
  - Marfan syndrome
  - Familial ectopia lentis
  - Ectopia lentis et pupillae
  - Homocystinuria
  - Weill–Marchesani syndrome
  - Spherophakia
  - Ehlers–Danlos syndrome
  - Hyperlysinaemia
  - Aniridia
  - Stickler syndrome
- Acquired:
  - Trauma
  - Pseudoexfoliation
  - Uveal tumours
- Idiopathic

Pathogenesis

Loss of zonular support for the crystalline lens results in dislocation.

Clinical evaluation

Subluxed lens

- Visual acuity may be normal or reduced.
- The lens equator and zonular fibres, usually obscured by the iris, are visible through a dilated pupil.
- With progressive subluxation, the lens equator approaches the optical axis and may be visible through an undilated pupil.
- Phacodonesis and iridodonesis are present.
- The direction of subluxation varies with aetiology:
  - **Marfan syndrome:** typically supero-temporal (see Figure 3.46)
  - **Homocystinuria:** infero-nasal
  - **Familial ectopia lentis:** supero-temporal

Luxated (dislocated) lens

- **Anterior chamber dislocation:** the entire lens is located anterior to the iris. There may be associated corneal decompensation due to endothelial touch, uveitis, and raised IOP. Incarceration in the pupillary aperture may cause pupil block and acute glaucoma.
- **Posterior chamber dislocation:** the crystalline lens may be visualized free in the vitreous cavity, either directly or with indirect ophthalmoscopy. There may be associated uveitis, retinal tears, or retinal detachment.

Management

Management is determined by the degree of subluxation and visual acuity. There is a risk of ametropic or meridional amblyopia in children with subluxed lenses, and these cases require close observation and early intervention when visual acuity is impaired.

Mild subluxation with normal visual acuity

In the case of mild subluxation with normal visual acuity, only observation is required.

Moderate-to-severe subluxation

With progressive displacement, the lens periphery and equator approach the optical axis, causing refractive error, aberrations, edge effects, and reduced visual acuity. The lens may dislocate beyond the visual axis, rendering the eye optically aphakic.

- **Conservative management:** refractive correction with contact lenses or spectacles
- **Surgical management:** usually involves extraction of the crystalline lens, and intraocular lens implantation. Compared to the case with standard cataract surgery, additional measures are required to stabilize the lens implant within the capsular bag:
  - Capsular tension ring insertion (+/− scleral ring fixation).
  - Scleral intraocular lens fixation
  - Anterior chamber intraocular lens implantation

Luxation

- **Anterior chamber dislocation:** pupillary dilation and supine posturing can return the lens to the posterior chamber. Endothelial touch, uveitis, and acute glaucoma are indications for lens extraction.
- Posterior capsule dislocation requires a vitreoretinal referral for pars plana vitrectomy and lens extraction.
- As there is no capsular support, any intraocular lens must be fixated in the anterior chamber, iris fixated or scleral fixated.

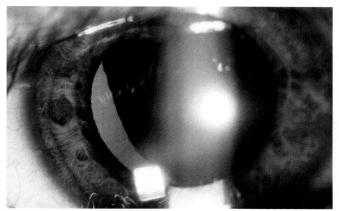

Fig 3.46 Subluxated crystalline lens in a patient with Marfan syndrome
The zonules are visible

3.9 Biometry

Precise measurements of corneal curvature and axial length are required prior to cataract surgery. These biometric data will determine the optimal intraocular lens power required to achieve the desired refractive outcome in each eye.

Intraocular lens power calculations

The original SRK formula (after Sanders, Retzlaff, and Kraff) describes the approximate relationship between lens power, refractive outcome, axial length, and keratometry. The SRK is a regression formula, generated by analysing large series of biometric and refractive outcome data retrospectively:

$$P = A - B(AL) - C(K),$$

where P is the lens power (in dioptres); A is the A-constant, which is unique for each intraocular lens design and is influenced by post-operative anterior chamber depth; B is a multiplication constant for axial length measurement; AL is axial length (mm); C is a multiplication constant for keratometry measurement; and K is the average keratometry measurement (in dioptres).

Emmetropia

In emmetropia,

$$P = A - 2.5(AL) - 0.9(K).$$

Non-emmetropic refractive targets

In the case of non-emmetropic refractive targets,

$$P = A - 2.5(AL) - 0.9(K) - D(R),$$

where D is a multiplication constant for target refraction, and R is the target refraction (in dioptres).

Note that errors in axial length measurement are multiplied by a factor of 2.5, and therefore have an important effect on refractive outcome.

The SRK and other regression formulae are no longer in use; they have been superseded by more accurate theoretical formulae which are based on geometrical optics. These include:

* SRK/T
* Holladay
* Hoffer-Q
* Haigis (also requires anterior chamber depth)

Obtaining measurements for intraocular lens power calculation

IOL Master

The IOL Master is the most widely used biometry device in the United Kingdom (see Figures 3.47, 3.48, and 3.49).

Principle used

Axial length is measured with partial coherence interferometry. Keratometry is measured by analysing reflection patterns off the central 2.5 mm anterior corneal surface; the light to be reflected is generated by six light-emitting diodes. Anterior chamber depth measurements use a photographic slit technique.

Advantages

* Rapid and easy to use
* High accuracy (+/− 0.01 mm) and reproducibility
* Non-contact
* Measures parallel to the optical axis
* One device for all measurements

Disadvantages

* Unable to obtain axial length measurements in eyes with very dense cataracts, and with some posterior subcapsular cataracts. Anterior chamber depth measurements are less accurate than those obtained with other methods.

Applanation A-scan ultrasound

Principle used

This method utilizes 10 MHz ultrasound; the probe contacts (and slightly indents) the cornea (see Figures 3.50 and 3.51).

Advantages

* Measures axial length and anterior chamber depth in the presence of dense cataracts or corneal opacity

Disadvantages

* Highly operator dependent
* Low accuracy (+/−0.10–0.12 mm)
* Contact technique; requires topical anaesthesia
* Risk of corneal epithelial trauma and contamination
* Corneal indentation during applanation may result in underestimation of axial length.
* Measurement is not necessarily along the visual axis but wherever the operator directs the probe.
* Risk of axial length overestimation in the presence of posterior staphyloma
* Correction factor required when the vitreous cavity is filled with silicone oil

Immersion ultrasound

Principle used

In immersion ultrasound, 10 MHz ultrasound is used and the probe contacts the eye via a coupling fluid. The patient views a fixation target.

Advantages

* Measures axial length and anterior chamber depth in the presence of dense cataract or corneal opacity
* Measures along the visual axis
* Contacts via a coupling fluid and therefore does not indent the cornea
* Immersion vector A-scans and B-scans can be combined to image the eye in two dimensions; this approach is useful when posterior staphyloma is present.

Disadvantages

* Low accuracy (+/−0.10–0.12 mm)
* Does not measure keratometry
* Correction factor required when the vitreous cavity is filled with silicone oil

Lenstar

The biometric principles of a Lenstar are similar to those of the IOL Master; it utilizes optical low-coherence reflectometry for axial length measurements.

Pentacam

The Scheimpflug technique images the anterior segment by capturing multiple cross-sectional images with a rotating camera. This procedure measures both anterior and posterior corneal surfaces, thus calculating the 'true net power' of the cornea. Pentacam keratometry is useful for intraocular lens power calculations in eyes post refractive surgery (see Box 3.1).

Box 3.1 Checklist for selecting intraocular lens power

Is the patient being examined the correct patient?

Is the eye being examined the correct eye?

Keratometry:
Do the three measurements agree?
Select location for on-axis corneal incisions if appropriate.

Axial length:
Is the signal curve valid?
Signal-to-noise ratio (SNR): SNR >2, clear signal; SNR >10, very good signal
Morphology of signal curves: clear peaks (maxima) on a low baseline

Are the axial lengths of the two eyes similar (within 0.5 mm)?
If not, is the difference supported clinically by anisometropia?

What intraocular lens type will be implanted?
Is the A-constant correct?

For second eye surgery:
What intraocular lens was implanted into the first eye?
Was the refractive target met?
If not, why not?

What is the refractive target?

Pitfalls:
Is there silicone oil in the vitreous cavity?
Is there a history of corneal refractive surgery?

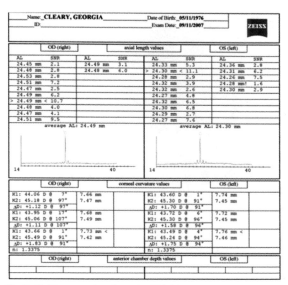

Fig 3.48 Biometry data from the IOL Master

Courtesy of Carl Zeiss Limited

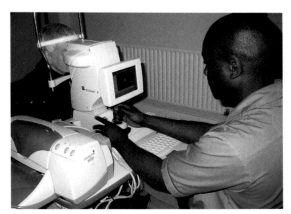

Fig 3.47 Biometry measurements with the IOL Master

Courtesy of Carl Zeiss Limited

Name: **CLEARY, GEORGIA**   ID:
Date of Birth: **05/11/1976**   Eye Surgeon: **St. Thomas'**
Exam Date: **09/11/2007**   Formula: **SRK/T**

Preoperative Data:

AL: **24.49 mm**   Refraction:
K1: **43.66 D @ 1°**   Visual Acuity:
K2: **45.49 D @ 91°**   Eye Status: **phakic**
opt. ACD: Target. Ref.: **plano**

OD right

acrysof SA60		si40		acrysof SA60		acrysof ma30ac	
A Const:	118.8	A Const:	118.4	A Const:	118.8	A Const:	118.9
IOL (D)	REF (D)	IOL (D)	REF (D)	IOL (D)	REF (D)	IOL (D)	REF (D)
18.5	−1.11	18.0	−1.05	18.5	−1.11	18.5	−1.03
18.0	−0.77	17.5	−0.71	18.0	−0.77	18.0	−0.70
17.5	−0.44	17.0	−0.38	17.5	−0.44	17.5	−0.37
17.0	**−0.12**	**16.5**	**−0.05**	**17.0**	**−0.12**	**17.0**	**−0.05**
16.5	0.21	16.0	0.28	16.5	0.21	16.5	0.27
16.0	0.52	15.5	0.61	16.0	0.52	16.0	0.58
15.5	0.84	15.0	0.93	15.5	0.84	15.5	0.90

Preoperative Data:

AL: **24.30 mm**   Refraction:
K1: **43.49 D @ 4°**   Visual Acuity:
K2: **45.24 D @ 94°**   Eye Status: **phakic**
opt. ACD: Target. Ref.: **plano**

OS left

acrysof SA60		si40		acrysof SA60		acrysof ma30ac	
A Const:	118.8	A Const:	118.4	A Const:	118.8	A Const:	118.9
IOL (D)	REF (D)	IOL (D)	REF (D)	IOL (D)	REF (D)	IOL (D)	REF (D)
19.0	−0.88	19.0	−1.18	19.0	−0.88	19.5	−1.14
18.5	−0.54	18.5	−0.83	18.5	−0.54	19.0	−0.80
18.0	−0.21	18.0	−0.49	18.0	−0.21	18.5	−0.47
17.5	**0.11**	**17.5**	**−0.16**	**17.5**	**0.11**	**18.0**	**−0.14**
17.0	0.44	17.0	0.18	17.0	0.44	17.5	0.18
16.5	0.76	16.5	0.51	16.5	0.76	17.0	0.50
16.0	1.07	16.0	0.83	16.0	1.07	16.5	0.82

Fig 3.49 Intraocular lens calculations from the IOL Master

Courtesy of Carl Zeiss Limited

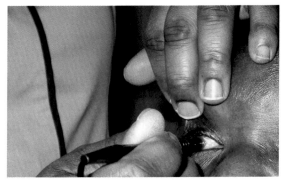

Fig 3.50 Axial length measurement with applanation ultrasound

LEFT

AUTO2   Dense Cataract
Velocity :Avg   1548 m/s
Velocity :LENS 1629 m/s
Gain   :   7

Avg AXIAL: **24.24 mm**
SD : 0.04 mm RANGE : 0.11 mm
Avg ACD   : 3.71 mm
Avg LENS : 5.60 mm

NO. 10   AXIAL :24.19 mm
            ACD   : 3.66 mm
            LENS : 3.65 mm

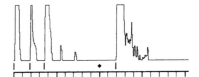

SRK/T

Input Parameters
AXIAL : 24.19 mm
K1   : 43.37 D
K2   : 45.00 D
Ds Ref : 0.00 D

	A	B	C
A-const.	118.40	118.80	115.30
Power	17.80	16.22	14.98

A		B	
IOL	Ref.	IOL	Ref.
16.50	0.86	16.50	1.11
17.00	0.53	17.00	0.79
17.50	0.20	17.50	0.47
18.00	**−0.14**	**18.00**	**0.14**
18.50	−0.48	18.50	−0.19
19.00	−0.82	19.00	−0.52
19.50	−1.17	19.50	−0.86

C	
IOL	Ref.
13.50	1.13
14.00	0.75
14.50	0.37
15.00	**−0.02**
15.50	−0.41
16.00	−0.80
16.50	−1.21

Fig 3.51 An A-scan axial length trace

3.10 Local anaesthesia

Around 95% of cataract surgery in the United Kingdom is performed under local anaesthesia. The use of general anaesthesia for cataract surgery has fallen dramatically over the past two decades. Indications for general anaesthesia include:

* Young age
* Anxiety
* Claustrophobia
* Inability to lie flat
* Inability to lie still
* Dementia, and learning difficulties
* Patient preference

The use of sharp needle techniques such as retrobulbar and peribulbar anaesthesia is declining. These techniques achieve effective anaesthesia and akinesia but carry greater risks of serious anaesthetic complications than blunt cannula sub-Tenon's anaesthesia.

The use of topical and topical–intracameral anaesthesia is increasing. Whilst a mobile eye may be considered problematic by inexperienced cataract surgeons, it can also be of benefit, as changes in ocular position can make some surgical manoeuvres easier.

Topical anaesthesia

Technique

Local anaesthetic drops, usually tetracaine 1%, are administered into the conjunctival fornix preoperatively.

Advantages

* Fast
* Rapid visual recovery
* No post-operative diplopia

Disadvantages

* Ocular motility preserved
* Suboptimal intraocular anaesthesia (e.g. of the iris).

Topical–intracameral anaesthesia

In topical–intracameral anaesthesia, the topical anaesthetic technique is supplemented with intracameral anaesthetic solution.

Technique

Preservative-free lignocaine 1% is injected into the anterior chamber at the start of surgery, or during hydrodissection.

Advantages

* Fast
* Rapid visual recovery
* No post-operative diplopia
* Good anaesthesia of intraocular structures

Disadvantages

* Ocular motility preserved

Sub-Tenon's anaesthesia

The sub-Tenon's block may be administered before or after prepping and draping the eye.

Technique

Local anaesthetic drops are inserted; then, the conjunctival sac is irrigated with povidone iodine. A lid speculum is inserted. The conjunctiva and Tenon's capsule are grasped with forceps, and a small infero-nasal incision is made with curved spring scissors,

5 mm from the limbus. A local anaesthetic solution is injected into the sub-Tenon's space with a flat, blunt-tipped cannula (see Figure 3.52). The solution may comprise a mixture of agents, including lignocaine, bupivacaine, and Hyalase.

Advantages

* Good anaesthesia
* Provides effective post-operative analgesia if a long-acting local anaesthetic (e.g. bupivacaine) is utilized

Disadvantages

* Subconjunctival haemorrhage common
* Chemosis is common and may impair the surgical view owing to the pooling of fluid over the cornea.
* Variable akinesia

Peribulbar anaesthesia

In peribulbar anaesthesia, anaesthetic is injected into the orbit, outside the extraocular muscle cone.

Technique

A 25 mm needle is inserted below the globe at the junction between the outer third and the inner two-thirds of the inferior orbital rim. The needle is initially directed posteriorly and then angled superiorly once half of the needle is inserted. The solution may contain a mixture of agents, like the sub-Tenons mixture.

Advantages

* Effective analgesia and akinesia
* Useful for complex or combined cases of long duration, e.g. cataract and vitreoretinal surgery

Disadvantages

* Slower than topical anaesthesia, topical–intracameral anaesthesia, or sub-Tenons anaesthesia, as the anaesthetic solution requires time to diffuse
* Slower visual recovery
* Chemosis in some cases
* Post-operative diplopia and ptosis
* Risk of retrobulbar haemorrhage
* Risk of globe perforation
* Risk of brainstem anaesthesia

Retrobulbar anaesthesia

Retrobulbar blocks are now rarely used.

Technique

With the use of a long, 38 mm needle, local anaesthetic solution is injected behind the globe, within the extraocular muscle cone.

Advantages

* Very effective analgesia and akinesia

Disadvantages

* Slower visual recovery due to post-operative diplopia, ptosis, and optic nerve anaesthesia
* Risk of direct optic nerve trauma
* Risk of intravascular injection
* Risk of retrobulbar haemorrhage
* Risk of globe perforation
* Risk of brainstem anaesthesia
* Contraindicated in high myopes (long axial length)

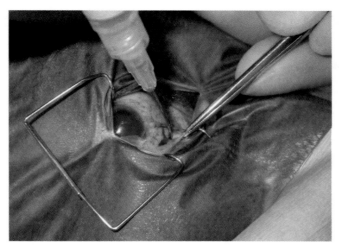

Fig 3.52 Sub-Tenon's anaesthetic administration

Operating microscope

All intraocular surgery is performed with an operating microscope (see Figure 3.53). The use of the microscope facilitates:

- A binocular, stereoscopic view of the surgical field
- Good illumination, producing a bright red reflex
- Variable magnification (zoom)
- Variable focus
- Hands-free motorized control of magnification, focal plane, and X–Y position.

Both hands are utilized for the phacoemulsification surgical procedure; control of the microscope is via a foot pedal (see Figure 3.54). Microscopes may be floor standing or ceiling mounted.

A beam splitter within the device allows attachment of a co-observation (assistant's) eyepiece. This is essential for teaching and supervising intraocular surgery.

Video cameras are coupled to the microscope, allowing real-time viewing of the surgical procedure on a monitor within the operating theatre. This process allows the scrub nurse to view the progression of the procedure.

Phacodynamics

Safe and effective phacoemulsification cataract surgery requires a stable anterior chamber. Stabilization of the anterior chamber is achieved by:

- Precise fit of surgical instruments into the eye, avoiding wound leak
- Balanced flow of fluid into and out of the eye by the phaco machine, thereby maintaining the anterior chamber volume and pressure

The exact parameters for fluid inflow and outflow, vacuum, and ultrasound power can be preset on all phaco machines. The settings can be optimized to suit individual surgeons and individual cataracts.

Phacoemulsification handpiece

Most phaco surgery is performed with a coaxial handpiece. The tip of the handpiece comprises a hollow needle surrounded by an irrigating sleeve (see Figure 3.55). The soft irrigating sleeve is deformed by the shape of the incision, reducing wound leak, and provides a heat-insulating layer around the phaco needle, thus preventing corneal wound burns. Fluid and lens matter are evacuated through the hollow centre of the needle

The cataract is emulsified by ultrasonic movements of the needle; movements are classically axial but also may be rotational or transverse. Oscillations are generated by piezoelectric or magnetostrictive systems within the handpiece.

Ultrasonic movement of the phaco needle emulsifies the cataract by several physical mechanisms:

- A mechanical jackhammer effect of the tip of the needle against the cataract
- An acoustic wave in front of the needle tip
- Cavitation at the needle tip

Phaco power

The power generated by the phaco tip is determined by:

- Oscillation frequency: this is preset to a constant frequency for each phaco machine, usually in the range of 35–45 kHz.
- Stroke length: this is the axial excursion of the phaco tip with each oscillation. Most phaco machines have maximum stroke lengths in the range of 0.05–0.10 mm. Stroke length can be modified; when set to 100% phaco power, the tip travels through the full stroke length with each oscillation. When set to 60% phaco power, the tip travels through up to 60% of its stroke length.

Irrigation

Irrigation via the phaco sleeve is primarily gravity dependent and is determined by the bottle height relative to the patient' eye height. The flow of irrigating fluid into the eye is equal to the rate of fluid leaving the eye:

irrigation = aspiration + leakage from wounds.

The irrigation fluid bottle is suspended above the phaco machine, producing a pressure gradient. The bottle height is the distance between the phaco pump and the bottle; the pump should be level with the eye. Raising the bottle deepens the anterior chamber and raises the intraocular pressure.

Aspiration and vacuum

Fluid and lens matter is withdrawn from the eye under the influence of two factors:

- Aspiration rate: the rate at which fluid and lens matter are evacuated from the eye through the unoccluded phaco tip (ml/min)
- Vacuum: this is a negative suction force exerted at the phaco tip; it allows nuclear fragments to be engaged and subsequently phacoemulsified. Vacuum is generated by the phaco pump. Maximum vacuum limits can be specified ($mmHg/mm^2$).

Aspiration rate and vacuum are linked in Venturi pumps and diaphragmatic pumps (vacuum transfer pumps). In peristaltic pumps, they are independent.

Venturi pumps

With a Venturi pump, a vacuum is generated within the phaco machine and then transferred to the handpiece tubing. The vacuum draws fluid from the eye, down a pressure gradient, and into the cassette. Because flow is generated by the vacuum, the aspiration rate cannot be changed independently.

Peristaltic pumps

Tubing originating from the phaco handpiece is stretched over rollers. The rollers within the pump softly roll over and compress the flexible tubing, pushing fluid away from the handpiece and generating negative pressure. This pressure draws fluid from the eye through the phaco tip. Increasing the speed of rotation increases the aspiration rate.

Rise time

Rise time is the time taken for the vacuum to reach its maximum setting in the presence of tip occlusion.

Foot pedal control of phacoemulsification

Phacoemulsification is controlled by a foot pedal, on which there are three sequential positions:

* Position 1: irrigation
* Position 2: irrigation plus aspiration
* Position 3: irrigation, plus aspiration, plus ultrasound

Sound generated by the phaco machine provides feedback to indicate the foot position in use.

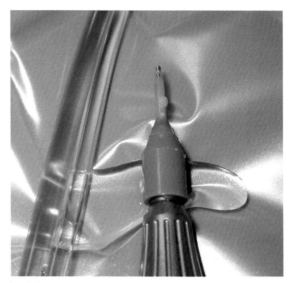

Fig 3.55 Phaco handpiece

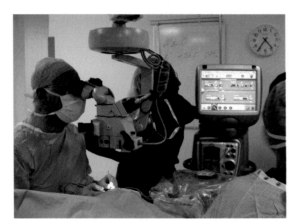

Fig 3.53 Operating microscope

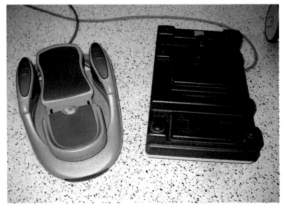

Fig 3.54 Phaco machine and operating microscope foot pedals

3.12 Intraocular lenses

The first intraocular lens was implanted in 1949. Prior to this, patients were left aphakic after cataract extraction, and required contact lenses or thick aphakic spectacles for refractive correction.

Intraocular lenses achieve better optical correction, compared to contact lenses or spectacles. They are now routinely implanted at the time of cataract extraction in adults and in children.

Intraocular lens design

The basic design of an intraocular lens comprises a central circular optic which is fixed and centred in the eye by its haptics.

Optic

* Delivers the optical power of the intraocular lens
* Optical power may be built into the anterior or posterior surface of the intraocular lens, or both.
* Most implanted intraocular lenses have a monofocal optic.
* Additional refractive correction may be built into the optic, e.g. toricity or multifocality.

Haptics

* Haptics fix the intraocular lens in its desired position within the eye. The haptics should centre the optic along the visual axis.
* Most intraocular lenses have two or four haptics.
* Haptics may lie in the plane of the optic or be angulated, pushing the optic anteriorly or posteriorly.

Common optic–haptic configurations

Single-piece intraocular lens

The intraocular lens is manufactured in one piece (see Figure 3.56); thus, the optic and the haptics are composed of identical material.

Multiple-piece intraocular lens

The optic and the haptics are manufactured separately and are composed of different materials (see Figure 3.57).

Intraocular lens biomaterial

Acrylic

Acrylic is the most common intraocular lens material in use in the developed world. Acrylic intraocular lenses are soft and foldable and can be injected into the eye via a small incision. They unfold slowly within the eye after insertion and are easy to position.

Acrylic intraocular lenses may be:

* Hydrophobic
* Hydrophilic

Hydrophobic acrylic intraocular lenses are associated with low rates of PCO.

Silicone

Silicone intraocular lenses are also foldable. They unfold rapidly within the eye after injection. They are also associated with low PCO rates.

Polymethylmethacrylate

Polymethylmethacrylate is hard and brittle and therefore not foldable. Polymethylmethacrylate intraocular lenses must be inserted through a large incision but have proven biocompatibility and are cheap to manufacture. They were widely utilized until the turn of the century, when soft, foldable intraocular lenses gained popularity. They remain in widespread use in the developing world.

A UV filter is usually incorporated into the intraocular lens optic material. Blue light filtering intraocular lenses are favoured by some surgeons, for the purpose of retinal photoprotection. These intraocular lenses are yellow due to the incorporation of a blue light filtering chromophore.

Site of implantation

Posterior chamber intraocular lenses

The vast majority of intraocular lenses are implanted into the posterior chamber.

* 'In-the-bag' implantation, into the intact capsule, is the ideal and most physiological location for intraocular lens placement.
* Sulcus implantation is usually performed in the context of complicated cataract surgery, when the posterior capsule has ruptured or zonular support is questionable. The haptics rest in the ciliary sulcus between the iris and ciliary body.
* Posterior chamber intraocular lenses are occasionally sutured into the iris or the sclera when capsular support is insufficient.

Anterior chamber intraocular lenses

* Iris-fixated intraocular lenses utilize 'claws' which enclavate iris tissue and thus hold the intraocular lens in place (see Figure 3.58).
* Angle-supported intraocular lenses are stabilized by haptics which rest in the iridocorneal angle (see Figure 3.59).

Presbyopia-correcting intraocular lenses

Standard cataract surgery with monofocal intraocular lens implantation typically results in good unaided distance vision; however, glasses are required for reading. Many intraocular lenses have been designed to achieve good unaided visual acuity for both distance and near, allowing patients (in theory) to be spectacle free. Presbyopia-correcting intraocular lenses are the subject of much research effort and commercial interest.

Multifocal intraocular lenses

The optics of these intraocular lenses have two focal lengths: distance and near. Concentric optical zones alternate between the two focal lengths, and light entering the eye is divided between the two optical zones.

Problems reported with these intraocular lenses include:

* Loss of contrast sensitivity
* Poor intermediate visual acuity (e.g. for computer use)
* Haloes
* Glare

Accommodating intraocular lenses

Accommodation is the ability of the youthful crystalline lens to change focus from distance to near. Hardening of the crystalline lens results in loss of accommodation with age. However, the ciliary muscles, which facilitate accommodation, continue to function.

Accommodating intraocular lenses are designed to shift forwards within the eye with accommodative effort. Forwards movement of the intraocular lens within the eye would produce a myopic refractive status, thus facilitating near vision. Thus far, no accommodating intraocular lenses have demonstrated clinically meaningful pseudophakic accommodation.

Phakic intraocular lenses

Intraocular lenses are occasionally inserted into the eye in the presence of the crystalline lens. They are usually inserted for the treatment of high refractive error, usually myopia. See refractive surgery chapter.

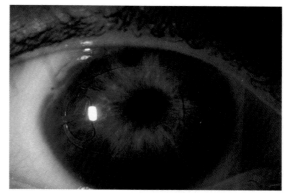

Fig 3.58 Iris-fixated anterior chamber intraocular lens

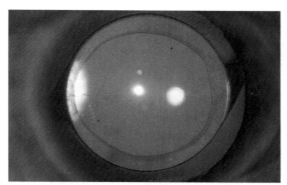

Fig 3.56 Single piece intraocular lens

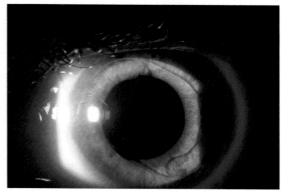

Fig 3.59 Angle-supported anterior chamber intraocular lens

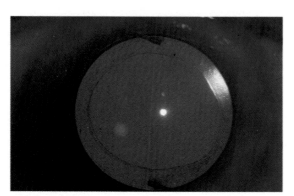

Fig 3.57 Three-piece intraocular lens

3.13 Nd:YAG laser capsulotomy

Nd:YAG laser capsulotomy is a common, elective procedure. Indications include:

- PCO (see Figure 3.60)
- Posterior capsule distension syndrome (retained viscoelastic)
- Anterior capsule opacification
- Anterior capsular phimosis

The Nd:YAG laser

In Nd:YAG laser capsulotomy, 1064 nm infrared radiation is generated from neodymium suspended in a yttrium-aluminium-garnet crystal. Pulsed laser radiation strips electrons from atoms, forming a gaseous state of ions and electrons called plasma. Plasma expands rapidly, creating shock and acoustic waves, which together cause mechanical disruption to adjacent tissues, creating a defect or hole. Because the 1064 nm wavelength is invisible, the laser device is also fitted with a red helium–neon aiming beam.

Indications for Nd:YAG laser posterior capsulotomy

Visual impairment

- Reduced visual acuity
- Glare
- Monocular diplopia

The threshold for Nd:YAG posterior capsulotomy may be lower with multifocal intraocular lenses than with monofocal intraocular lenses.

To improve retinal visualization

- For use e.g. in diabetic retinopathy screening

Performing Nd:YAG posterior capsulotomy

After obtaining informed consent:

- The pupil is dilated.
- Local anaesthetic drops are administered.
- Initial laser settings are confirmed:
  - Posterior focus
  - Approximately 1.0 mJ per pulse (may be increased)
- The patient is instructed to look towards a fixation light with his/her fellow eye.
- A capsulotomy contact lens is held against the cornea, using a viscous coupling fluid (e.g. Viscotears) in most cases.
- Through use of the aiming beam, the laser is focused on or immediately posterior to the posterior capsule.
- The laser is fired.

Various configurations for constructing the capsulotomy have been described (e.g. cross, spiral, inverted 'U'). Adjacent capsular defects created by the laser coalesce to form an opening in the posterior capsule; the opening should be at least 3–4 mm in diameter (see Figure 3.61).

Additional management varies among centres but may include:

- Immediate iopidine eye drops, 1.0%, pre- or post-laser
- A short course of steroid, e.g. prednisolone eye drops, 0.5%, three times a day for 1 week
- Review in clinic to evaluate visual acuity and assess for complications

Complications

- Raised IOP
- Uveitis
- Lens trauma:
  - Pitting
  - Cracking
  - Posterior movement
  - Dislocation
- Cystoid macular oedema
- Posterior vitreous detachment
- Possibly retinal breaks or detachment
- Chronic endophthalmitis

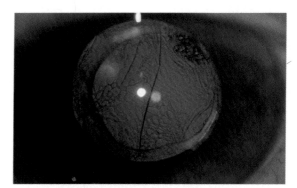

Fig 3.60 Posterior capsule opacification

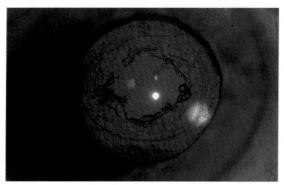

Fig 3.61 Posterior capsule following Nd:YAG laser capsulotomy

Chapter 4

Refractive surgery

Georgia Cleary, Allon Barsam, and Eric Donnenfeld

Basic science

Clinical assessment

Clinical knowledge

Practical skills

4.1 Refractive error, aberrations, and presbyopia

In a perfect optical system, a point source of light is focused onto a single point on the image plane; in the eye, light is focused on the retina. Optical aberrations are caused by imaging system imperfections which cause deviations in the transmission of light, preventing the convergence of light to a single point of focus. A wavefront of light travelling through an aberrated optical system will be distorted, producing a 'wavefront profile' which can be analysed mathematically.

The eye is not a perfect optical system and has low levels of inherent optical aberrations. Despite this, an emmetropic eye achieves a high level of resolution when a distant object is focused on the retina.

The resolving power of the eye, and therefore visual acuity, is degraded when the magnitude of aberrations increase. Low-order refractive errors such as defocus (myopia/hyperopia) and cylindrical refractive errors (astigmatism) are the most clinically important aberrations. However, in recent years an increased understanding of higher-order wavefront aberrations has allowed improvements in both the measurement and treatment of refractive error.

The Zernike model of aberrations

The Zernike model of aberrations is a mathematical method of classifying and measuring aberrations in optical systems. Individual aberrations can be identified from complex wavefront profiles by mathematical curve fitting. Each particular type of aberration has a characteristic shape and is identified by a polynomial ordering number and/or Zernike mode. Individual aberrations can be measured using aberrometry (see Table 4.1 and Figure 4.1).

Lower-order aberrations

Lower-order aberrations, notably defocus (spherical refractive error, Z^0_2) and astigmatism (Z^{-2}_2 and Z^2_2), have the greatest influence on visual function.

Higher-order aberrations

There are an infinite number of possible higher-order aberrations. However, these have a lesser effect on visual function than lower-order aberrations do. Spherical and coma aberration are the most significant visually and are associated with halo and glare, respectively.

Measuring aberrations

It can be useful to measure aberrations in patients with unexplained visual symptoms known as dysphotopsias. These phenomena include glare, starbursts, arcs, and rings of light.

Ocular aberrations are measured with an aberrometer. This device is essentially a complex autorefracting device, capable of analysing a wavefront profile which is deviated during its transmission through the eye. A range of optical methods are used to measure ocular aberrations. These methods include ray tracing and Hartmann–Shack aberrometry (see Figure 4.2).

Accommodation

Emmetropic eyes have good uncorrected distance visual acuity. Near vision requires an increase in the refractive power of the eye. This increase is achieved by increasing the optical power of the crystalline lens, thus producing a net myopic shift which allows the image of a close-up object to be focused onto the retina. Accompanying pupillary miosis enhances depth of focus, further optimizing near visual function.

During accommodation, there are multiple changes that occur within the eye:

- The ciliary muscle contracts, producing anterior and centripetal movement (towards the lens equator) of the ciliary processes.
- Tension on the zonules relaxes, allowing the crystalline lens to assume a more spherical shape under the elastic forces of the lens capsule.
- An overall increase in the optical power of the crystalline lens occurs as a result of:
  — Steepening the anterior lens surface
  — Steepening the posterior lens surface
  — Increased axial thickness
  — Net anterior movement, increasing the effective lens power

Table 4.1 Summary of the first 12 Zernike polynomials (this list continues infinitely)			
	J (polynomial ordering number)	Zernike term/mode	Description
Lower-order aberrations	0	Z^0_0	Piston
	1	Z^{-1}_1	Vertical tilt
	2	Z^1_1	Horizontal tilt
	3	Z^{-2}_2	Oblique astigmatism
	4	Z^2_2	Defocus
	5	Z^2_2	Vertical astigmatism
Higher-order aberrations	6	Z^{-3}_3	Vertical trefoil
	7	Z^{-1}_3	Vertical coma
	8	Z^1_3	Horizontal coma
	9	Z^3_3	Oblique trefoil
	10	Z^{-4}_4	Oblique quadrifoil
	11	Z^{-2}_4	Oblique secondary astigmatism
	12	Z^0_4	Primary spherical

Presbyopia

Accommodative function, and therefore near visual ability, reduces with age and is primarily due to stiffening of the crystalline lens. Presbyopia is *not* due to a loss of ciliary muscle contractile function.

Subjective amplitude of accommodation is measured with the RAF rule. Amplitude (measured in dioptres (D)) falls with age (from Donders table):

- 10 years: 14.0 D
- 20 years: 10.0 D
- 30 years: 7.0 D
- 40 years: 4.5 D
- 50 years: 2.5 D
- 60 years: 1.0 D

These subjective accommodative measurements are also influenced by other optical factors, including pupillary miosis, uncorrected astigmatism, and some aberrations; these factors can contribute to enhanced depth of focus and improved near visual function (pseudoaccommodation).

Correction of refractive error

Myopia

To correct myopia, the overall refractive power of the eye must be reduced. This effect can be achieved by flattening the cornea or inserting an appropriate intraocular lens.

Hypermetropia

In the case of hypermetropia, the refractive power of the eye must be increased, either by steepening the cornea or by inserting an intraocular lens.

Astigmatism

The refractive power of the eye is not the same in all meridians. Correction involves flattening the cornea along its steepest meridian and/or steepening the cornea along its flattest meridian. These corrections can be accomplished via relaxing corneal incisions or through excimer laser vision correction. Astigmatism may also be corrected by inserting an intraocular lens with an astigmatic (toric) correction.

Presbyopia

Presbyopia correction is discussed in Section 4.7.

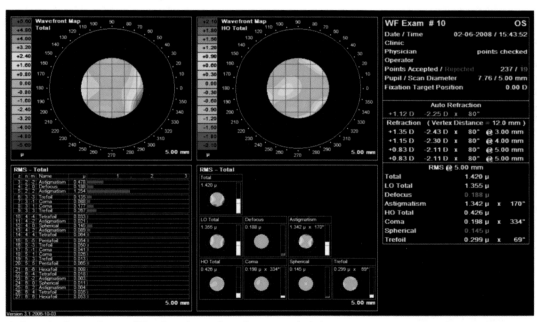

Fig 4.1 Example of a wavefront and Zernike polynomial map from a pseudophakic eye

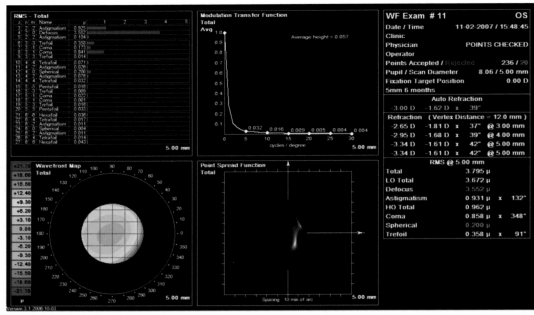

Fig 4.2 Higher-order aberrations

4.2 Preoperative evaluation for refractive surgery

Introduction

The single most important aspect in the preoperative evaluation of refractive surgery patients is understanding and managing their visual expectations. Unrealistic expectations must be identified and addressed before considering surgery. It is also very important for patients to undergo a thorough safety evaluation in order to exclude patients who are at particular risk of complications. Appropriate patient selection is critical.

Examples

- A pre-presbyopic patient undergoing laser refractive surgery to achieve good uncorrected distance visual acuity may require reading glasses some years after surgery; this development may be a cause of discontent if not properly explained to them preoperatively.
- Multifocal intraocular lenses may not deliver the same quality of vision as monofocal intraocular lenses in certain lighting conditions. Visual symptoms such as glare and haloes must be discussed preoperatively as they may affect night-driving ability.

History

- Work/leisure/sports vision requirements: establish any particular requirement for distance versus near vision
- Lifestyle risks (e.g. flap injury post LASIK in martial arts)
- Previous ocular history (amblyopia, previous refractive procedures, keratoconus, dry eye)
- Past medical history (certain connective tissue diseases can compromise healing after corneal surgery)
- Family history (keratoconus)

Examination

- Subjective refraction
- Slit lamp examination: particularly lid margin, tear film, corneal dystrophies, corneal degeneration, lens opacities, macular disease
- Intraocular pressure (IOP; may be underestimated after laser treatment because of decreased corneal thickness)
- Anterior chamber depth (for phakic intraocular lenses)
- Mesopic pupil diameter (to determine the optimal width of the laser treatment zone)

Investigations

Investigations are performed after contact lenses have been removed (soft lenses, 1 week; rigid gas permeable lenses, 3 weeks; hard lenses, 4 weeks). Some surgeons recommend removal of rigid or gas permeable contact lenses for 1 month for every decade of wear. When in doubt, two consecutive topographies that are similar document refractive stability. Recent contact lens wear may affect the subjective refraction, corneal thickness, keratometry, and topography.

It is crucial to identify patients with early keratoconus because of the risk of post-operative corneal ectasia with photoablative procedures.

Investigations include:

- Corneal topography (ideally using a system that measures both the anterior and posterior cornea; this approach increases the detection rate of manifest and forme fruste keratoconus)
- Pachymetry to confirm sufficient depth available for laser treatment, or placement of intracorneal ring segments. A minimum residual stromal bed thickness of 250 μm is recommended by the US FDA but many surgeons consider a 300 μm bed after LASIK to be optimal to prevent future corneal ectasia.
- Keratometry
- Endothelial cell count (for phakic intraocular lenses)
- Aberrometry/wavefront analysis

Corneal topography

Background

- Corneal topography provides a three-dimensional map of the cornea, including its anterior surface contour, refractive power, thickness, and posterior surface contour (see Figure 4.3).
- Colour-coded maps of various indices (power, thickness, etc.) are produced.

Indication

- Diagnosis and monitoring of keratoconus. Keratoconus is a contraindication to refractive surgery and must be excluded prior to surgery.
- Diagnosis of other forms of corneal ectasia (pellucid marginal degeneration)
- Monitoring of corneal thinning in cases of infective or inflammatory corneal disease
- Pre-/post-operative assessment of astigmatism for cataract surgery (to corroborate IOL Master keratometry and distinguish corneal astigmatism from lenticular astigmatism)
- Post-operative assessment of corneal shape and power after corneal surgery
- Pre-/post-operative assessment for refractive surgery. As well as being useful for screening patients at risk of ectasia, the corneal thickness calculation is important for determining which patients can be safely treated.
- Complex contact lens fitting

Technique

- Scheimpflug imaging (Pentacam) uses a rotating camera which captures multiple radial cross-sectional photographs of the anterior segment. These images are analysed to produce a three-dimensional map of the anterior segment, including the cornea, anterior chamber, anterior iris surface, and anterior lens surface within the pupillary aperture. Provides data for both anterior and posterior cornea, corneal thickness, and anterior chamber depth.
- Placido-based systems were initially utilized; these devices project rings on the cornea and analyse the reflected image. This system assesses only the anterior corneal surface and is extremely accurate for assessing the anterior corneal surface but does not give any information regarding the corneal pachymetry or posterior corneal surface and alone may be less able to detect early keratoconus. It is also prone to artefacts from tear-film abnormalities.
- Elevation-based scanning slit devices (e.g. Orbscan) also provide anterior and posterior corneal measurements, although the measurements are not as accurate as those provided by Scheimpflug systems.

OCULUS - PENTACAM

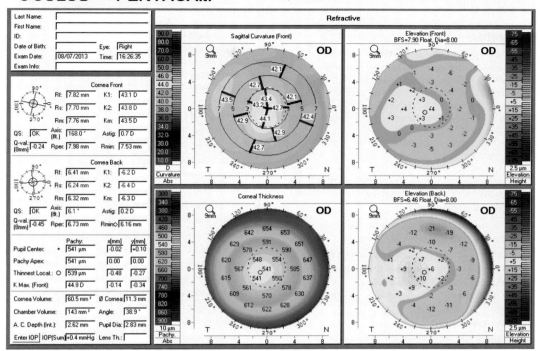

Fig 4.3 Pentacam corneal topography showing anterior corneal curvature, corneal thickness measurements, and anterior and posterior corneal elevation

4.3 Laser refractive surgery

Introduction

The cornea is responsible for approximately two-thirds of the refractive power of the eye, and its most important refractive interface is its anterior surface. Laser refractive surgery reshapes the anterior corneal surface, altering its refractive power.

Corneal reshaping is achieved by ablating corneal stromal tissue. Removal of 12–18 μm of corneal stroma corrects roughly 1 D of refractive error.

Laser refractive surgery is the most common type of refractive surgery procedure, and millions of treatments have now been safely carried out worldwide. In the hands of properly trained consultant surgeons and with appropriate patient selection, it is associated with very high rates of patient satisfaction.

Laser refractive procedures

* LASIK (laser-assisted stromal in situ keratomileusis)
* PRK (photorefractive keratectomy)
* LASEK (laser-assisted subepithelial keratomileusis)
* Epi-LASIK (epithelial laser-assisted in situkeratomileusis)
* ReLEx (refractive laser lenticule extraction)

PRK, LASEK, and epi-LASIK can be broadly categorized as surface treatments.

Myopic laser treatment

* Ablates the central corneal stroma
* Flattens the central cornea, reducing refractive power

Hyperopic laser treatment

* Ablates corneal stroma at the periphery of the treatment zone
* Steepens the central cornea, increasing refractive power

Wavefront-guided treatment

* Pre-existing higher-order aberrations are treated during the ablation procedure, in addition to refractive error.

Lasers utilized for refractive surgery

Excimer laser

An excimer (excited dimer) laser reshapes the cornea by photoablation of corneal tissue. The laser utilizes light in the UV range (usually 193 nm).

Femtosecond laser

Femtosecond lasers (1040 nm) are photodisruptive, using extremely short duration pulses (10^{-15} s) to produce multiple small cavitation bubbles within the corneal stroma. Adjacent bubbles create a surgical plane.

General risks of laser refractive surgery

* Visual loss
* Undercorrection/overcorrection of refractive error; re-treatments can be performed and are often referred to as 'enhancements'
* Corneal haze, haloes, glare, night-vision problems
* Rare complications include recurrent erosions, corneal infiltrates, infectious keratitis, and corneal ectasia.

LASIK

LASIK is now the most common form of laser refractive surgery. A flap is cut into the superficial corneal stroma, then reflected back to expose the underlying stromal bed (see Figure 4.4 and 4.5). The thickness of the flap ranges from around 80 μm to 160 μm. Flaps were initially created with a mechanical blade (microkeratome), but femtosecond lasers are increasingly used with a higher degree of precision and the ability to create thinner flaps. The stromal bed is treated with an excimer laser to modify its anterior curvature, and the flap is replaced.

Advantages of LASIK

* Relatively painless
* Reduced risk of infection
* Rapid visual recovery
* Associated with lower rates of post-operative corneal haze than surface treatments are

Disadvantages of LASIK

* Greater risk of ectasia compared with surface treatments, as the residual stromal bed is thinner
* Complications related to the perioperative flap, including incomplete or torn flaps, free flaps, or buttonholing, particularly with mechanical microkeratomes. Post-operative problems include folds and striae, dislocation, and epithelial ingrowth (see Figure 4.6).
* Diffuse lamellar keratitis: interface inflammatory process normally occurs within 1 week of LASIK, characterized by a fine granular opacification at the interface ('sands of the Sahara'). Treatment is with early intensive topical steroids.
* Corneal nerves are cut when the flap is created, predisposing to dry eye.

PRK

PRK was the first method of laser refractive surgery to be used. The corneal epithelium may be loosened with 20% alcohol and then debrided and discarded. The denuded corneal stromal surface is treated with an excimer laser. A contact lens is worn for several days after the procedure to minimize post-operative pain and promote re-epithelialization.

Advantages of PRK

* Lower risk of ectasia than LASIK, as the residual stromal bed is thicker
* No flap-related complications
* More suitable for patients who participate in contact sports (e.g. boxing) who are at risk of flap dislocations with ocular trauma

Disadvantages of PRK

* Painful, large epithelial defect post procedure
* Slower visual recovery
* Greater risk of infection
* Greater risk of post-operative corneal haze; mitomycin C may be used to minimize haze

LASEK

LASEK is similar to PRK; however, the epithelium is not discarded. Instead, it is loosened with alcohol and then swept aside to allow the excimer laser procedure to be performed. The epithelial flap is then replaced over the treated stromal bed.

Epi-LASIK

Epi-LASIK is similar to LASEK, but alcohol is not utilized. Instead, an epithelial flap is cut with a microkeratome (epikeratome) prior to the excimer laser treatment.

ReLEx

This procedure, also known as SMILE (small incision lenticule extraction), requires a femtosecond laser to cut a disc-shaped lenticule from the corneal stroma. The lenticule is then extracted manually. No excimer laser photoablation is required for this procedure.

Other considerations after corneal refractive procedures

IOP measurement

Corneal refractive surgery decreases the corneal thickness and hysteresis. This may influence the accuracy of IOP measurements post-operatively.

Intraocular lens power calculations after refractive surgery

Conventional intraocular lens power calculation formulae are not valid after corneal refractive surgery (see Chapter 3, Section 3.9). Post-operative refractive surprises, usually hyperopia, occur if standard intraocular lens power calculations are used. Special intraocular lens power calculations, such as the American Society of Cataract and Refractive Surgery online intraocular lens calculator, are needed.

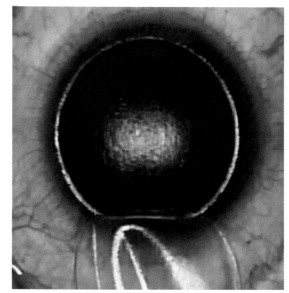

Fig 4.5 LASIK flap being reflected back to expose the underlying stromal bed

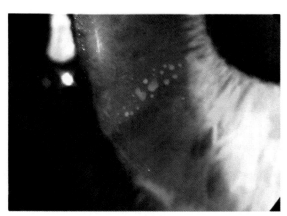

Fig 4.6 Epithelial ingrowth post LASIK

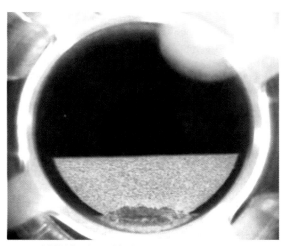

Fig 4.4 LASIK flap being lifted

In addition to laser refractive surgery, various other methods can be utilized to modify the curvature of the anterior surface of the cornea, thus correcting refractive error. Incisional corneal procedures (e.g. limbal relaxing incisions) are often used as an adjunct to cataract surgery to correct astigmatism at the time of the procedure.

When planning treatment to reduce corneal astigmatism, it is essential to mark the eye preoperatively, with the patient in the upright position, prior to local anaesthesia, because the eye is likely to rotate when the patient is supine and after sub-Tenons anaesthesia. Typically, the limbus is marked with an indelible marker pen, either at the meridian requiring treatment or at the horizontal and/or vertical meridians. Various devices are available to assist with marking.

Corneal relaxation procedures

These procedures flatten the cornea along the treated meridian.

Limbal relaxing incisions

Deep limbal incisions of varying arc are used during cataract surgery to reduce pre-existing corneal astigmatism. A guarded blade, usually with a depth of 600 μm, is used. Curved incisions, parallel to the limbus, are made along the steepest meridian. The arc length (in clock hours) and number of incisions (one incision or two paired incisions) are determined by the amount of preoperative corneal astigmatism, the patient's age, and the location of the steepest axis. Nomograms are available for guidance (e.g. see http://www.lricalculator.com; see Figure 4.7).

Opposite clear corneal incisions

Standard clear corneal incisions used during cataract surgery have a small astigmatic effect; this result is surgeon dependent and is influenced by the incision diameter and incision architecture. An additional identical clear corneal incision can be made opposite the primary incision to enhance its astigmatic effect.

Arcuate keratotomy

Similar to limbal relaxing incisions, arcuate keratotomy is performed more centrally in clear corneas and therefore has a greater astigmatic effect. It is most often used to treat astigmatism after corneal graft surgery. Incisions can be created with diamond knives, and now femtosecond lasers are being used to create these incisions.

Wedge resections

Wedge resections are used to treat high levels of astigmatism (generally above 8 D of cylinder), which can be seen following penetrating keratoplasty. A wedge of corneal tissue is removed from the flat axis, and sutures are used to close the stromal defect. The sutures are left in place for at least 3 months and, when removed, result in a steepening of the cornea in that axis.

Radial keratotomy

Multiple deep radial stromal incisions are made in the clear cornea to achieve flattening (see Figure 4.8). This procedure was widely used in the 1980s and early 1990s for the treatment of myopia and astigmatism but has largely been abandoned.

Corneal addition procedures

Intracorneal ring segments

Usually used to treat keratoconus, semicircular ring segments are inserted into the corneal stroma after channels are pre-cut manually or with a femtosecond laser. The central cornea that lies within the segments is flattened. This treatment may not restore good uncorrected acuity but may improve contact lens fit (see Figure 4.9).

Compression sutures

Sutures are placed along the flattest meridian to reduce astigmatism. They are often used in eyes with astigmatism after corneal graft surgery.

Other rarely used procedures

- **Epikeratophakia:** the removal of epithelium and placement of a donor lenticule made of Bowmans layer and anterior stroma
- **Keratophakia:** intrastromal placement of a donor lenticule made of corneal stroma after raising a microkeratome flap or by creating a stromal pocket by lamellar dissection
- **Intracorneal lens:** placement of a hydrogel lens inside the corneal stroma

Other refractive procedures

Corneal thermocoagulation

Thermokeratoplasty (heating the peripheral cornea to shrink collagen and steepen the central corneal curvature) can be used to treat hyperopia and presbyopia.

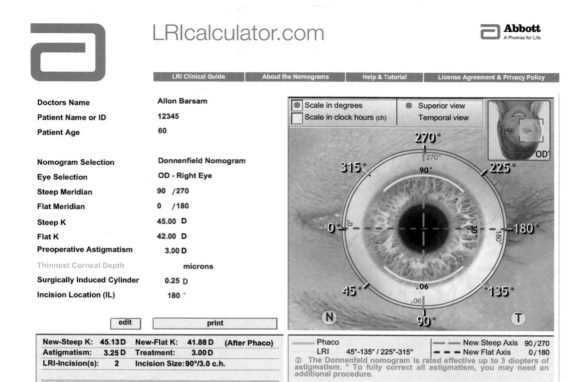

Fig 4.7 Abbot Medical Optics LRI Calculator to show planning of placement and arc length for limbal relaxing incisions

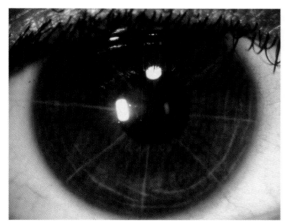

Fig 4.8 Radial keratotomy scars

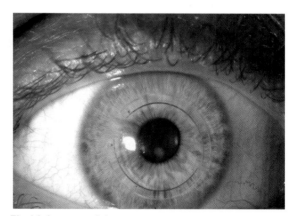

Fig 4.9 Intracorneal ring segments
Courtesy of Saj Khan

4.5 Refractive lens surgery and 'premium' intraocular lenses

Removal of the crystalline lens and implantation of an intraocular lens into the capsular bag affords the opportunity to correct pre-existing refractive error. This procedure is most commonly performed in the context of conventional cataract surgery, when opacification of the crystalline lens causes visual symptoms and a reduction in best-corrected visual acuity. However, refractive lens exchange can be used in the absence of cataract when laser vision correction is not suitable.

Clear lens extraction/Refractive lens exchange

Clear lens extraction/refractive lens exchange entails a surgical procedure that is identical to that used for cataract surgery; however, it is performed in eyes with a clear crystalline lens. Preoperative best-corrected visual acuity is good; the aim is thus to eliminate refractive error and improve uncorrected visual acuity.

'Premium' intraocular lenses

Historically, conventional intraocular lenses corrected only spherical refractive error (myopia and hyperopia) and introduced some degree of spherical aberration to the eye. So-called premium intraocular lenses possess additional refractive properties above those found in conventional monofocal intraocular lenses. These intraocular lenses typically utilize the same 'platform' (i.e. biomaterial, optic size, and haptic design) as conventional monofocal intraocular lenses, and the additional refractive properties are built onto one surface of the intraocular lens optic.

Aspheric intraocular lenses

The average cornea has 27 μm of positive spherical aberration. Implanting a conventional intraocular lens (which may also have positive spherical aberration) increases the total ocular spherical aberration. Aspheric intraocular lenses have zero or negative spherical aberration (depending on the manufacturer), thus counteracting corneal spherical aberration.

Multifocal intraocular lenses

Multifocal intraocular lens optics are divided into zones which are focused for distance and near, respectively (see Figure 4.10).

Advantages

After bilateral implantation, there is a high rate of spectacle independence.

Disadvantages

- Dividing incoming light between two focal lengths means that the quality of vision for some patients can be affected.
- Glare, haloes, and reduced contrast sensitivity are well described side effects. Night-driving may be difficult. These symptoms are intolerable in some patients, and occasionally intraocular lens exchange is required.
- Unsuitable in patients with macular disease, because of reduced contrast sensitivity

Light-adjustable intraocular lenses

Light-sensitive macromers are incorporated into the intraocular lens optic material. Following implantation, any residual refractive error (up to 2 D of sphere and/or cylinder) can be corrected by exposing the intraocular lens to UVA irradiation, which causes a predictable change in intraocular lens shape and therefore refractive power. The final desired intraocular lens power is 'locked-in' permanently by further exposure to UVA radiation.

Accommodating intraocular lenses

Most accommodating intraocular lenses have a monofocal optic which is designed to shift anteriorly on its flexible haptics (via the 'focus shift' principle) as a result of ciliary muscle forces exerted during near visual effort. Thus far, these intraocular lenses have failed to demonstrate clinically significant objective accommodation and have been associated with very high rates of posterior capsule opacification.

More complex accommodating intraocular lens designs include dual optic systems and lens refilling techniques; these intraocular lenses remain investigational.

Piggyback intraocular lenses

Occasionally, it may be necessary to implant more than one intraocular lens into the eye following removal of the crystalline lens in order to achieve the desired refractive outcome (polypseudophakia).

Primary polypseudophakia

Implantation of two intraocular lenses is planned at the time of lens extraction. This may be required in highly hyperopic/nanophthalmic eyes in which a single intraocular lens of sufficient power is unavailable (e.g. >40.0 D). Both intraocular lenses may be implanted into the capsular bag; however, this technique may be complicated by growth of lens epithelial cells between the two lenses (termed interlenticular opacification). Therefore, the favoured approach is to implant one intraocular lens into the capsular bag, and one into the ciliary sulcus.

Secondary polypseudophakia

A secondary, sulcus-fixated intraocular lens is implanted as a secondary procedure, usually to correct refractive error following cataract surgery when laser vision correction is not indicated. Implantation of a monofocal, sulcus-fixated intraocular lens will correct spherical refractive error; toric and multifocal intraocular lenses are also available.

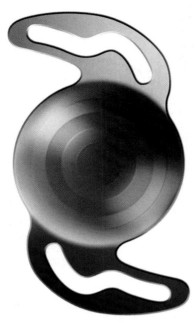

Fig 4.10 Diffractive optical rings of a multifocal intraocular lens

4.6 Phakic intraocular lenses

Phakic intraocular lenses are inserted into the phakic eye to correct refractive error. They are a useful option in patients who are unsuitable for laser refractive surgery (e.g. those with extreme myopia) or those in whom clear lens extraction is not considered appropriate (e.g. pre-presbyopes).

Not all patients are eligible for phakic intraocular lenses. For the most part, phakic intraocular lenses are primarily used for myopia and are less commonly used with hyperopia. Eyes with very shallow anterior chambers are unsuitable because of the risk of endothelial trauma and pupil block glaucoma. Anterior chamber depth must be assessed preoperatively.

The main advantages of phakic intraocular lenses over other forms of refractive correction (laser refractive surgery and refractive lens exchange) are reversibility, and preservation of accommodation.

The first generation of phakic intraocular lenses required a laser peripheral iridotomy to reduce the risk of pupil block and secondary angle-closure glaucoma. However, there are now new versions available with central holes to allow the passage of aqueous humour.

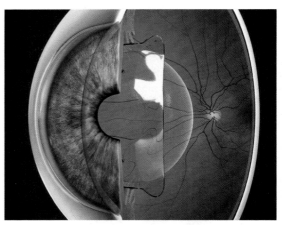

Fig 4.11 Posterior chamber phakic intraocular lens

Phakic intraocular lens fixation

Posterior chamber: Sulcus fixation
A thin, flexible, anteriorly vaulted intraocular lens is inserted into the ciliary sulcus. There should be no contact between the posterior intraocular lens surface and the underlying crystalline lens; otherwise, a cataract is likely to develop (see Figure 4.11).

Anterior chamber: Iris fixation
The intraocular lens is fixed in the anterior chamber by attaching it to the anterior iris surface via two claw-like haptics. Iris tissue is enclavated into the claws to secure the intraocular lens (see Figure 4.12).

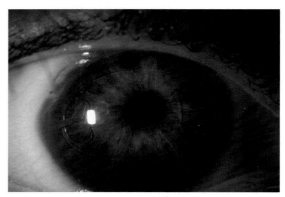

Fig 4.12 Anterior Chamber Phakic Intraocular Lens

Complications

* General risks of intraocular surgery (including bacterial endophthalmitis)
* Cataract
* Pigment dispersion
* Chronic uveitis
* Pupillary block glaucoma
* Corneal endothelial cell loss, risk of corneal decompensation

4.7 Presbyopia correction

Accommodative function declines with age. As accommodative amplitude falls, near vision becomes increasingly difficult, requiring near refractive correction.

Presbyopic symptoms usually begin in the fifth decade and may manifest as difficulty focusing on small print, eyestrain, and headaches. These symptoms are relieved by spectacle correction for near vision.

Surgical presbyopia treatments aim to achieve good distance and near acuity without glasses. Currently, there are no surgical methods available to restore accommodation. However, good near vision can be achieved without glasses using other optical methods ('pseudoaccommodation').

Monovision

Emmetropia is planned for the dominant eye to facilitate distance vision, and a myopic refractive outcome is planned for the non-dominant eye for near vision. Up to 2.5 D of anisometropia is acceptable. Monovision is generally well tolerated but requires a short period of neuroadaptation.

Monovision can be achieved using various methods:

- Contact lenses
- Laser refractive surgery
- Monofocal intraocular lens implantation after cataract surgery or clear lens extraction

It is desirable to trial monovision with contact lenses before a permanent surgical correction is made.

Multifocality

Bilateral implantation of multifocal intraocular lenses is the most common multifocal procedure. This approach is generally best tolerated in hyperopes who present with bilateral cataracts. Multifocal intraocular lenses are discussed in Section 4.5.

Multifocal contact lenses have been available for many years prior to the introduction of multifocal intraocular lenses. Multifocal corneal refractive procedures may also be performed; however, this approach is uncommon.

Enhanced depth of focus

Corneal inlays (e.g. the AcuFocus KAMRA inlay) may be inserted into the central corneal stroma. These small, disc-shaped inlays have a central aperture which produces a pinhole effect, simulating a reduced pupillary aperture and increasing depth of focus. This procedure has the advantage of reversibility (see Figure 4.13).

Accommodating intraocular lenses

A true accommodating intraocular lens (one that is able to produce a clinically significant objective change in the refractive status of the eye with near visual effort) is considered the holy grail of contemporary cataract surgery. Currently available accommodating intraocular lenses do not deliver true pseudophakic accommodation. However, some do achieve relative spectacle independence by employing other adjunctive optical techniques. These techniques include 'mini-monovision' (approximately 0.75 D of anisometropia between eyes) and inclusion of modifications to the intraocular lens optic (e.g. the Crystalens HD contains an anterior surface modification that enhances depth of focus). Accommodating intraocular lenses are discussed in Section 4.5.

153

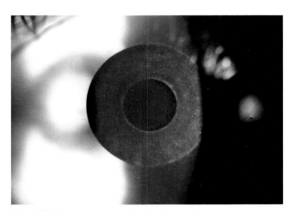

Fig 4.13 Kamra intracorneal inlay for presbyopia
Courtesy of David Allamby

Chapter 5

Vitreoretinal surgery

Sidath E. Liyanage, Fred K. Chen, and James W. Bainbridge

5.1 Retinal anatomy and physiology

Retinal anatomy

Embryology

The neurosensory retina (NSR) and retinal pigment epithelium (RPE) are derived from neuroectodermal cells in the forebrain region of the neural plate. They form the inner and outer layers of the optic cup. The hyaloid vascular system nourishes the lens and inner layer of the optic cup, later regressing and leading to formation of the vitreous gel. Condensation of mesodermal and neural crest-derived cells around the optic cup forms the choroid and sclera. The distal edge of the optic cup becomes the pupillary border of the iris. Therefore, the RPE and NSR are continuous with the epithelium of the ciliary body and iris.

The vitreous

The vitreous, located between the lens and the retina, occupies the majority (80%, or 4 ml) of the globe volume. Although 99% of the vitreous is composed of water, collagen (type 2) fibrils and associated hyaluronan impart a gel-like consistency. The patellar fossa is a depression, located in the anterior vitreous gel, which accommodates the lens. The vitreous base straddles the ora serrata and is strongly adherent to the posterior 2 mm of the pars plana epithelium and 1–4 mm of the anterior retina. Other areas of firm vitreoretinal attachment include the optic disc margin, the major retinal vessels, the fovea, and the parafoveal regions. Regression of the hyaloid vessel leaves an empty Cloquet canal, extending from the posterior pole of the lens to the optic disc. Incomplete regression of the hyaloid vasculature can result in remnants evident at the posterior lens capsule (Mittendorf dot) or optic disc (Bergmeister papilla).

The neurosensory retina

The NSR is a thin (200 μm) neural tissue that extends from the ora serrata to the optic disc margin. The NSR has three layers of cells separated by the inner and outer plexiform layers. The outer nuclear layer contains the photoreceptor cell bodies and nuclei. The middle layer of cells, confusingly called the inner nuclear layer, comprises the cell bodies of bipolar, horizontal, and amacrine cells. The innermost layer of cells forms the ganglion cell layer. The unmyelinated nerve fibres of the ganglion cells extend along the inner retinal surface towards the optic nerve head, forming the nerve fibre layer. Müller cells extend across the entire thickness of the NSR, with their apical sides extending to the photoreceptor inner segments and their foot processes (basal sides) forming the internal limiting membrane, a basement membrane separating the NSR from the vitreous.

The macula lutea (also called the macula, posterior pole, or area centralis) is an oval retinal area containing yellow xanthophyll pigments and two or more layers of ganglion cells. It measures 5–6 mm in diameter and is located between the temporal retinal vascular arcades. The fovea is a central depression in the macula, measuring 1.5 mm in diameter. The foveola lies at the centre of the fovea, measures 0.35 mm in diameter, and contains a single layer of NSR consisting of only photoreceptors. The foveal avascular zone, within which retinal capillaries are absent, is located in the central fovea and is 250–600 μm wide. The NSR is thickest in the rim of retina around the central fovea; this area is called the perifoveal zone and is 500 μm wide. The remaining rim of macula outside the perifoveal zone is the parafoveal zone (see Figure 5.1).

The extramacular retina is divided into near, mid-, and far peripheral retina. The mid-peripheral retina is a band that is 3 mm wide and straddles the equator. The near periphery is a 1.5 mm band, between the arcades and the mid-periphery,

whilst the far periphery extends 6 mm from the mid-periphery to the ora serrata. The posterior limit of the vitreous base and the majority of tractional retinal tears are located in the far periphery.

The RPE–choroid complex

The RPE is a monolayer of hexagonal cuboidal cells that extends from the ora serrata to the optic disc. The apical side of the RPE is in contact with the photoreceptor outer segments via villous processes. A potential sub-NSR space lies between the photoreceptors and the RPE. The basal side of the RPE is attached to Bruchs membrane, which is a five-layer structure. The RPE basement membrane and the choriocapillaris endothelium form the inner- and outermost layers, respectively. The inner three layers are composed of a middle layer of elastic fibres sandwiched between an inner and an outer layer of collagen. The choriocapillaris is a fenestrated capillary network fed by choroidal arterioles and drained by venules located in the outer layer of the choroidal stroma. The venules converge to form four to six vortex veins, which are usually located in the mid-periphery of each quadrant. These can often be visualized in pale fundi as small, dark-brown swellings in continuation with choroidal vasculature. The choroid is loosely attached to the sclera by connective tissue. A potential suprachoroidal space lies between the choroid and sclera.

Submacular RPE cells are taller than those in the periphery, which are flat and may contain two nuclei. Specialized proteins found on the apical and basal surfaces of RPE cells have important metabolic and transport functions. Tight, adherens, and gap junctions found at the lateral membrane of the RPE cells are important components of the outer blood–retinal barrier. Adult RPE cells contain melanin and lipofuscin granules. Fundus autofluorescence imaging utilizes the autofluorescent properties of lipofuscin to image the RPE.

Retinal physiology

The primary functions of the NSR include phototransduction and the initial neural processing of visual information. Prerequisites for normal photoreceptor function include delivery of oxygen and nutrients from choroidal blood flow, metabolic support for the photoreceptor outer segments from the RPE, and outer segment contact with the RPE.

Visual function

The photoreceptors convert photon energy into a cell membrane potential that leads to reduced release of the neurotransmitter glutamate, in the bipolar and horizontal cell synapses in the outer plexiform layer. Visual information is then conveyed to ganglion cells via synapses in the inner plexiform layer and onwards by ganglion cell axons to the lateral geniculate nucleus. Neuromodulation occurs at each synapse, involving cells such as horizontal and amacrine cells.

Cone photoreceptors are concentrated in the fovea, whereas rod photoreceptors are concentrated in the parafoveal region. The ratio of cones to rods overall is 1 : 20. The photoreceptors contain visual pigments (rhodopsin in rods, and iodopsin in cones) that capture photons with varying efficacy dependent upon the energy state of the photon (e.g. green wavelengths in green-sensitive cones). The pigments are localized in the discs of the outer segments for optimal light capture.

Light-sensitive visual pigments contain the 11-*cis* conformation of retinal (an aldehyde of vitamin A) in complex with the opsin protein. Upon stimulation by a photon, the retinal converts into the all-*trans* conformation, separates from the opsin, and binds to a protein to be transported back to the RPE. The RPE stores the retinal and reconverts it to the 11-*cis* form for use by the rod outer segment opsins. Metabolism of retinal in cones may be dependent upon the Müller cells. Photoreceptor outer segments are constantly regenerated, whilst their distal tips are shed cyclically (rods at dawn, and cones at dusk). Photoreceptor survival depends upon a balance between these two processes.

A light-induced conformational change in the retinal–opsin complex leads to a reduction in cyclic GMP in the cytosol via an amplification cascade involving transducin and phosphodiesterase. In rods, this process leads to a reduction in cytosolic calcium concentration and hyperpolarization of the photoreceptor cell. The activation process is rapidly switched off by arrestin in conjunction with rhodopsin kinase, and is switched on again when cyclic GMP levels are restored through the action of guanylate cyclase.

Retinal and choroidal circulation

The retina is supplied by a dual circulation arising from the central retinal artery and the short posterior ciliary arteries. The central retinal artery and its branches are located in the nerve fibre layer. It feeds into superficial (ganglion cell layer) and deep (inner nuclear layer) capillary networks, with endothelial tight junctions forming the inner blood–retinal barrier. The metabolic requirements of the inner two-thirds of the NSR are supplied by the central retinal artery. The outer third is supplied by the choriocapillaris capillary network from the short posterior ciliary arteries (see Figure 5.2). The outer blood–retinal barrier is formed by intracellular tight junctions in the RPE. Up to 75% of retinal oxygen and glucose requirements are supplied by the choroidal circulation, reflecting the high metabolic demand of the outer retina and the RPE.

Retinal circulation is autoregulated. Retinal capillary pericytes interact with vascular endothelial cells, providing structural support, assisting in autoregulation, and inhibiting endothelial cell proliferation. These pericytes and their associated basement membranes are damaged in diabetic retinopathy. The choroidal vasculature is controlled by the autonomic nervous system. The RPE provides trophic support for the choriocapillaris. In age-related macular degeneration (AMD), RPE atrophy is associated with choriocapillaris loss and outer retinal atrophy.

RPE

Functions of the RPE include maintenance of the outer blood–retinal barrier, vitamin A (retinal) metabolism, outer segment phagocytosis, and trophic support for the choriocapillaris. RPE also synthesizes melanin, which absorbs radiant energy, binds redox-active metal ions, and sequesters reactive chemicals; these properties underlie the RPE response to laser photocoagulation, siderosis, and drug toxicity. Melanin may have a role in retinal development, and its absence in ocular albinism is associated with a lack of foveal development. The RPE expresses Class 1 major histocompatibility complex (MHC) antigens. However, RPE expression of Class 2 MHC antigens can be induced by interferon gamma, suggesting that the RPE may play a role in autoimmune diseases and contribute to the relative immune privilege of the subretinal space. Through secretion of a variety of cytokines, the RPE can also modulate the function of macrophages, lymphocytes, and vascular endothelial cells. In addition to secreting vascular endothelial growth factor (VEGF), which acts on the choriocapillaris, the RPE also secretes other growth factors which have autocrine or paracrine trophic effects on the NSR. RPE cells may dedifferentiate, detach from Bruchs membrane, migrate, and transform into fibroblast-like and phagocytic cells in response to mechanical, chemical, thermal, or anoxic injury. The RPE may also produce extracellular matrix and metalloproteinases.

Retinal attachment

Attachment of the NSR to the RPE is a complex physiological process involving RPE metabolic activity (the RPE pump), ionic environment modulation by energy-dependent membrane ion channels, specific physico-chemical conditions in the interphotoreceptor matrix, and fluid movement from the vitreous to the choroid. The interdigitation between the tips of the outer segment microvilli and the RPE microvilli, in combination with adhesive components of the interphotoreceptor matrix, contributes to the strength of retinal adhesion.

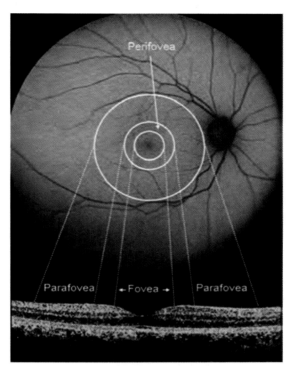

Fig 5.1 Fundus autofluorescence image showing absence of autofluorescence at the optic disc, masked autofluorescence along the vascular arcades, and reduced autofluorescence in the macula lutea resulting from masking by xanthophyll pigments in the neuroretina. Three zones of the macula are indicated and correlated with an optical coherence tomography scan through the foveal centre

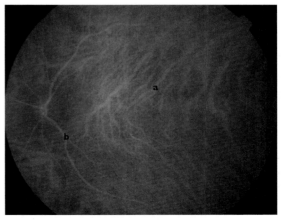

Fig 5.2 Fundus indocyanine angiography demonstrating normal patterns of (a) choroidal and (b) retinal vascular structures

History taking

Conditions affecting the posterior segment can present with a variety of symptoms, which can overlap with those of optic nerve and other neurological conditions. Careful history taking is therefore important to establish an accurate diagnosis.

Ocular symptoms

Central visual disturbance

* Central visual blurring may occur in a wide variety of macular disorders, particularly AMD, central serous chorioretinopathy (CSCR), and macular dystrophies.
* A hypermetropic shift may be seen in association with CSCR, pigment epithelial detachments, or posterior sclerochoroidal mass lesions.
* Distortion or metamorphopsia is highly suggestive of macular disease and may occur with choroidal neovascularization (CNV), CSCR, epiretinal membranes, or vitreomacular traction.
* Paracentral scotomata occur when areas of photoreceptor loss occur in the macular region, sparing the foveal centre.
* Charles Bonnet syndrome is characterized by visual hallucinations (varying from vague unformed images to distinct images of faces or objects). It may occur in association with any cause of visual loss but is most often noticed in advanced AMD.

Peripheral visual disturbance

* Visual field defects may result from CNS or optic nerve disease, retinoschisis, retinal vascular occlusion, or retinal detachment.
* Concentric visual field defects may occur in advanced glaucoma, advanced uveitis, retinal dystrophies, and certain drug toxicities.

Floaters

* Causes include a Weiss ring following posterior vitreous detachment, vitreous condensations, vitreous haemorrhage, liberated pigment cells associated with retinal tears, inflammatory cells, tumour cells, and asteroid hyalosis.

Flashing lights

* Photopsia refers to the perception of light in the absence of a light stimulus. Monocular photopsia is typically due to vitreoretinal pathology, whereas binocular photopsia is usually a cortical phenomenon. Causes include:
  1. Mechanical retinal stimulation by retinal traction (posterior vitreous detachment, retinal tears, flick phosphene), retinal impaction (Moores streak), or external compression (pressure phosphenes)
  2. Subretinal pathology: CNV, uveitis (white dot syndromes), choroidal tumours
  3. Cortical ischaemia (migraine or transient ischaemic attack: scintillations, accompanied by neurological symptoms) or visual hallucinations (Charles Bonnet syndrome)

Pain and photophobia

* Posterior segment pathology does not typically produce pain unless associated with anterior segment inflammation, ischaemia, raised intraocular pressure, or scleritis.

Redness

* Redness is due to conjunctival or scleral vascular engorgement or inflammation, or subconjunctival haemorrhage.

Leucocoria

* Leucocoria may be due to lenticular or vitreous opacities, retinal detachment, extensive retinal exudation, or a tumour. When leucocoria occurs in a child, the diagnosis of retinoblastoma must be excluded.

Colour vision abnormalities

* Colour vision loss is often a feature of optic nerve disease but it can also be due to certain types of maculopathy or dystrophy.
* Congenital red–green colour discrimination deficiency is found in 5%–8% of males.
* Blue–yellow deficiency is rarely due to congenital colour deficiency. In acquired cases, a cause must be sought.

Photoaversion and nyctalopia

* Photoaversion in combination with reduced colour vision and visual acuity may occur in cone dystrophies.
* Nyctalopia with concentric visual field constriction is characteristic of rod–cone dystrophies and end-stage glaucoma.

Past ocular history

* Refractive error: myopia is associated with a risk of rhegmatogenous retinal detachment (RRD), certain retinal dystrophies, and white dot syndromes. Hypermetropia is more common in patients with retinoschisis and can be associated with uveal effusions. Significant oblique astigmatism can be associated with posterior staphyloma and tilted disc syndrome.
* Previous ocular conditions, surgery, or trauma should be noted.

Past medical history

* Retinal vascular disease may be a presenting feature of diabetes mellitus, hypertension, hyperlipidaemia, sickle cell anaemia, and prothrombotic states.
* Posterior uveitis, retinal vasculitis, scleritis, and endophthalmitis may be manifestations of systemic infection, systemic autoimmune disease, or malignancy.
* Posterior segment tumours may occur in association with neurophakomatoses, hereditary cancer syndromes, or systemic malignancies.
* Inherited vitreoretinopathies, retinal dystrophies, and choroidal dystrophies may be associated with systemic connective tissue or metabolic disorders.
* A history of medication and drug allergy should be documented.

Social history

* Smoking, alcohol, and drug use
* Recreational and occupational visual tasks, e.g. reading, driving, flying, and work requiring colour discrimination

Family history

* Important in inherited vitreoretinopathies, retinal dystrophies, and choroidal dystrophies

- May help to distinguish between X-linked, autosomal dominant, recessive, and mitochondrial inheritance patterns

Review of systems
- If an associated systemic condition is thought to be relevant, a full review of systems should be conducted.

Examination

A methodical and thorough examination of the eye is key to formulating a diagnosis upon which to base further investigations and treatment. Accurate documentation supplemented by imaging investigations provides a baseline for future comparisons. It is important to record both the presence and absence of important clinical signs (see Figure 5.3).

Visual function
- Unaided, spectacle-corrected, and pinhole distance visual acuity is commonly measured using a Snellen chart, although in some clinical settings distance best-corrected visual acuity is more appropriately determined using a logMAR-style acuity chart such as the Early Treatment Diabetic Retinopathy Study (ETDRS) chart.
- Near visual acuity should be documented using a near-vision chart.
- Other parameters of visual function may be measured depending upon the clinical situations, e.g. central visual field (the Amsler grid, microperimetry), colour vision (the Ishihara chart), reading speed (the MNRead chart), and contrast sensitivity (the Pelli–Robson chart).

External exam
- Note signs of previous periocular disease and treatment (e.g. cancer, trauma, radiation).
- Abnormalities of globe size and ocular alignment
- Check pupil reflexes, pupil shape, and iris colour.

Anterior segment
- A small peripheral corneal laceration and a peripheral iris defect in combination with a history of hammering point to the possibility of an intraocular foreign body.
- Adequate conjunctival covering of any scleral buckle, its sutures, and its sponge should be noted.
- Absence of anterior chamber cells and the presence of intracameral silicone oil may be relevant. Note the absence or presence of iris or angle neovascularization in ischaemic retinopathy.
- Lens stability (phakic or pseudophakic) is relevant in planning vitreous surgery and may be symptomatic of an associated underlying systemic disease. Vitreous in the anterior chamber is a sign of zonular defect. Presence and location of iridotomy in aphakic eyes filled with silicone oil should be noted.

Vitreous
- The anterior vitreous is best visualized with dynamic slit lamp biomicroscopy of the retrolental vitreous gel (ask the patient to generate saccadic eye movements before looking into the primary position).
- Document the presence or absence and severity of vitreous cells (inflammatory cells, neoplastic cells, pigmented cells, or red blood cells) or vitreous opacities (asteroid hyalosis, synchysis scintillans, vitreous haemorrhage, foreign body).

- Look for signs of a posterior vitreous detachment (Weiss ring, visible posterior hyaloid membrane).
- Qualitative assessment of vitreous anatomy and fibrillar pattern may provide clues to the presence of hereditary vitreoretinopathies, e.g. Stickler syndrome.

Optic nerve head
- Glaucoma is associated with central retinal vein occlusion. Glaucoma can also result from various vitreoretinal procedures such as silicone oil injection.
- Disc swelling should be documented, and buried optic nerve head drusen should not be confused with papilloedema, papillitis, or ischaemic, hereditary, or toxic optic neuropathies.
- Myopic eyes and posterior staphyloma are associated with large, oval, or tilted discs with large areas of peripapillary atrophy. These disc features should be noted as they can have associated macular complications such as foveoschisis, macular hole, choroidal neovascularization, and serous macular detachment.
- Document important negatives such as the absence of disc neovascularization in diabetics, and pale discs in unexplained visual loss.

Retinal vasculature
- Note the appearance of the retinal vessels in terms of vessel calibre, colour, changes at arteriovenous crossings, and presence of micro or macro aneurysms.
- Arteriolar narrowing may be seen in association with systemic hypertension, vascular occlusions, retinal dystrophies, or drug toxicities.

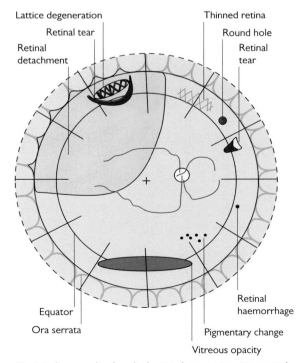

Fig 5.3 An example of medical notes documenting vitreous and retinal findings

- Venous dilatation, beading, and loops are commonly seen in severe pre-proliferative and proliferative diabetic retinopathy.
- Arteriovenous nipping may occur with chronic hypertension and arteriosclerosis.
- Retinal neovascularization typically occurs at the junction between non-perfused and perfused retina. Neovascularization may be flat or elevated.
- Intraretinal microvascular abnormalities (IRMA) are shunts between retinal arteries and veins found at the junction of non-perfused and perfused retina, and are a feature of severe non-proliferative diabetic retinopathy.
- A variety of arteriolar emboli may be observed, including calcium emboli, cholesterol emboli, platelet emboli, talc emboli, or septic emboli.
- Retinal vasculitis is characterized by a white or yellowish sheathing of the vessels. The type of vessel involvement (periarteritis or periphlebitis) should be noted.

Macula

- Note the presence and quality of the foveal reflex. A red dot can indicate an outer lamellar macular defect or 'microhole'. A yellow dot can indicate a Stage 1A pre-macular hole lesion.
- Look for epiretinal membranes and associated changes (retinal vascular distortion, retinal thickening, pseudoholes).
- Retinal thickening and oedema may be assessed with oblique slit beam illumination and high-magnification contact lens examination. The location (in relation to the fovea) and extent of retina thickening should be documented. Associated features such as microaneurysms and retinal exudates should also be noted.
- Subretinal neovascularization may be evident as a greyish subretinal membrane. Associated features may include intraretinal haemorrhage and retinochoroidal anastomosis as seen in retinal angiomatous proliferation. Deep orange nodules are seen in polypoidal choroidal vasculopathy. Retinal thickening, subretinal fluid, retinal exudates, or haemorrhage are signs of an active membrane. For drusen, note the number, size, location, and type (hard/soft), and the presence or absence of RPE changes.
- Other macular signs include non-specific RPE pigment hyperplasia, pigment epithelial detachments, RPE rip, geographic atrophy, Bulls eye maculopathy, vitelliform lesions, pattern dystrophy, telangiectasia, and serous detachment.
- Location and stability of fixation may also be determined.

Peripheral retina

- The peripheral retina may be visualized using slit lamp non-contact biomicroscopy (e.g. with a 90-dioptre (D) lens), contact biomicroscopy (e.g. with a Goldmann three-mirror contact lens), or binocular indirect ophthalmoscopy with scleral indentation (e.g. with a 20 or 28 D lens).
- Detailed assessment of the peripheral retina is important to detect peripheral retinal lesions such as a retinal break (horseshoe tear, atrophic hole, retinal dialysis), retinal detachment, peripheral retina degeneration (e.g. lattice degeneration), a tumour (e.g. choroidal melanoma), or inflammation (e.g. snow banking associated with pars planitis).

Choroid and sclera

- Choroidal lesions include tumours (e.g. choroidal melanoma, choroidal haemangioma) and inflammatory lesions (choroiditis, granulomas). In addition to the size, shape, and location of choroidal lesions, the presence or absence of associated overlying RPE and/or retinal changes should be documented.
- Posterior scleritis may be associated with an exudative retinal detachment or choroidal folds.

5.3 Diagnostic lenses

Diagnostic lenses (see Figure 5.4 and Table 5.1) enable visualization of the fundus by neutralizing the optical power of the eye (direct lenses) or increasing the refractive power of the eye to create an inverted real image of the fundus anterior to the eye (indirect lenses).

Direct lenses

Direct lenses are plano-concave with negative power. The image produced is upright and not inverted.

Non-contact lens

The non-contact Hruby lens enables examination of the posterior pole. The concave surface faces the patient. The −58.6 D power of the lens neutralizes the optical power of the eye. The lens is mounted on a slit lamp and aligned with the patient's visual axis in the primary position. The slit lamp illumination is aligned with the slit lamp microscope. Through the lens and a dilated pupil, an upright fundus image (5°–8° field) is produced as the distance between the lens and the eye is adjusted. The small limited field of view and reflections within the lens are its main disadvantages, and this lens has largely been superseded by indirect lenses (see 'Indirect lenses').

Contact lens

The Goldmann three-mirror lens is a contact lens commonly used during slit lamp examination and laser treatment of the posterior pole, peripheral retina, and the anterior chamber angle. It consists of a central 64 D plano-concave lens which neutralizes the optical power of the eye at the cornea. Three internal mirrors tilted at 59° (thumbnail shape), 66° (or 67°, dependent on manufacturer; barrel shape), and 73° (trapezoid) are used to visualize the angle/far peripheral retina, mid-peripheral retina/equator, and posterior pole to equator, respectively.

After instillation of topical anaesthetic and filling of the lens concavity with a coupling agent (e.g. methylcellulose), the lens is placed on the cornea. A 30° field of the posterior pole is visible through the central lens.

Table 5.1 Summary of lens specifications				
Lens	Static/Dynamic FOV	M/LSM	WD	Uses
Indirect BIO lenses				
Ocular 20 D	50°	2.97×/0.34×	47 mm	PP, PR
Volk 20 D	46°/60°	3.13×/0.32×	50 mm	PP, PR
Ocular 22 D	60°	2.73×/0.37×	39 mm	PP, PR
Volk Pan Retinal® 2.2	56°/73°	2.68×/0.37×	40 mm	PP, PR
Ocular 28 D	58°	2.11×/0.47×	27 mm	PR, SP, P
Volk 28 D	53°/69°	2.27×/0.44×	33 mm	PR, SP, P
Ocular 30 D	63°	1.97×/0.51×	26 mm	PR, SP, P
Volk 30 D	58°/75°	2.10×/0.44×	30 mm	PR, SP, P
Volk Digital ClearField™	55°/72°	2.79×/0.36×	37 mm	PR
Volk Digital ClearMag™	38°/49°	3.89×/0.26×	60 mm	PP
Indirect slit lamp examination lenses				
Ocular 60 D	85°/154°	1.00×/1.00×	10 mm	PP
Volk 60 D	68°/81°	1.15×/0.87×	13 mm	PP
Ocular 78 D	88°/154°	0.98×/1.02×	10 mm	PP
Volk 78 D	81°/97°	0.93×/1.08×	8 mm	PP
Ocular 90 D	94°/153°	0.75×/1.34×	5 mm	PR, SP
Volk 90 D	74°/89°	0.76×/1.32×	7 mm	PR, SP
Volk Super 66®	80°/96°	1.00×/1.00×	11 mm	PP
Volk Super Field®	95°/116°	0.76×/1.30×	7 mm	PR, SP
Volk Digital 1.0™	60°/72°	1.00×/1.00×	12 mm	PP
Volk Digital High Mag™	57°/70°	1.30×/0.77×	13 mm	PP
Volk Digital Wide Field™	103°/124°	0.72×/1.39×	4–5 mm	PR
Indirect contact lenses				
Volk Area Centralis®	70°/84°	1.06×/0.94×	0	PP
Volk TransEquator®	110°/132°	0.70×/1.44×	0	PP, SP
Volk QuadrAspheric®	120°/144°	0.51×/1.97×	0	PR
Volk Super Quad® 160	160°/165°	0.50×/2.00×	0	PR

D, dioptre; FOV, field of view; LSM, laser spot magnification; M, magnification; P, paediatric; PP, posterior pole; PR, peripheral retina; SP, small pupil; WD, working distance.

Indirect lenses

Indirect lenses are double aspheric convex lenses with positive power. The images produced are vertically and horizontally inverted.

Non-contact lenses

Non-contact lenses range in power from +10 D to greater than +100 D. Lenses of power greater than +40 D are combined with slit lamp examination, whereas lower-power lenses are used with binocular indirect ophthalmoscopy (BIO). The most commonly used lenses for slit lamp examination are the +78 D and the +90 D lenses, whereas the +20 D and the +28 D lenses are used for BIO. Improvements in lens design, manufacturing, and lens coatings have enabled high-resolution, wide-field viewing of the retina, with reduced glare and reflections.

During slit lamp examination, the +78 or +90 D lens is held approximately 8 or 7 mm anterior to the cornea, respectively (see Figure 5.5). An inverted fundus image is brought into focus as the slit lamp is pulled away from the eye. To visualize the peripheral retina, the patient is directed to look in the direction of the area to be examined. The +78 D lens is best suited for examination of the posterior pole, and the +90 D lens is better for peripheral retinal viewing. A wide variety of recently developed indirect viewing lenses provide superior depth perception, resolution, and fewer reflections.

During BIO, the +20 or +28 D lens is held approximately 5 or 3.3 cm anterior to the cornea, respectively (see Figure 5.6). The lens should be orientated with the white or silver ring towards the patient. An inverted fundus image is brought into focus as the BIO (attached to the examiner's head) moves away from the lens. As with slit lamp examination, the peripheral retina is visualized by asking the patient to look in the direction of the area to be examined. The examiner needs to maintain a position in which the centres of the lens, the BIO, and the pupil are aligned with the fundus area being examined. Scleral depression is required to examine the pre-equatorial retina. The +20 D lens is adequate for visualizing the peripheral retina in adults whereas the +28 D lens is better suited for peripheral retinal examination in infants and patients with small pupils.

Contact lenses

Indirect contact lenses are commonly used during laser treatment of the fundus because they provide better image resolution and fewer troublesome reflections, and help to stabilize the eye by restricting ocular movements.

Various types of indirect contact lenses are available, ranging from those with image magnification (up to 1.5×) and a narrow field of view (up to 60°) and which are suitable for macular assessment and laser treatment, to those with image minification (up to 0.5×) and a wide field of view (up to 160°) and which are suited for peripheral laser treatment. The lenses may be coated to reduce reflections during laser treatment. Lenses with redesigned contact surfaces are also available, to avoid the need for a coupling agent.

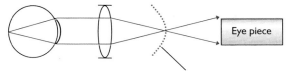

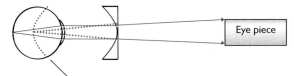

Inverted real image of retina formed by convex lens

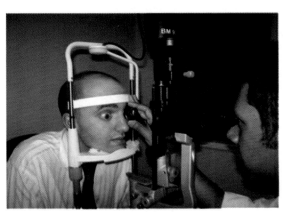

Upright virtual image of retina formed by concave lens

Fig 5.4 Ray diagrams illustrating the optics of indirect (convex) and direct (concave) non-contact lenses

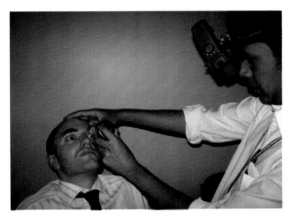

Fig 5.5 Indirect fundus examination on a slit lamp

Fig 5.6 Binocular indirect examination of the fundus

5.4 Optical coherence tomography

Optical coherence tomography (OCT) is a non-contact imaging technique that produces micrometre-resolution, cross-sectional images of the retina and vitreoretinal interface. Macular OCT is commonly used for the evaluation of AMD, diabetic macular oedema, and diseases of the vitreoretinal interface.

Principles and technology

- OCT is based on the principle of low-coherence optical interferometry.
- In conventional time-domain OCT design, a light source (super luminescent diode) emits low-coherence near-infrared light (820 nm) with bandwidth of 20 nm directed via a beam splitter into the eye and a reference mirror.
- The light reflected from different retinal layers contains signals of varying amplitudes and latencies. This light interacts with light reflected from the reference mirror to produce an interference pattern.

- The depth information is provided by the position of a movable reference mirror in time-domain OCT. The rate at which this mirror moves is the limiting factor for scanning speed (400 A-scans per second) in time-domain OCT.
- As the light source moves across the retina, a two-dimensional image (B-scan) is constructed and displayed in grey or colour scales (see Figure 5.7). White represents areas of high reflectivity, whereas black represents areas of low reflectivity.
- Time-domain technology is now superseded by frequency-domain OCT. Two types of frequency-domain design are commercially available: spatially encoded (also called spectral domain; see Figure 5.8) and time encoded (also called swept source).
- In spectral domain OCT (SD-OCT), interference formed by a diffraction grating is analysed by Fourier transformation to give the depth information. The scanning speed for SD-OCT ranges from 20 000–50 000 A-scans per second. The light source in commercial SD-OCT also has broader bandwidth (up to 150 nm), providing improved depth resolution. The main drawback of this design is the drop-off of the signal-to-noise ratio along the depth of the scanned image.
- In swept source OCT (SS-OCT), a narrowband laser (1050 nm) is rapidly tuned through a broad optical bandwidth (~100 nm). The main advantages of SS-OCT are a faster scanning speed of over 100 000 A-scans per second; deeper light penetration, which enables choroidoscleral imaging; and the lack of significant signal-to-noise ratio drop-off.
- Axial resolution is 6–10 μm, depending on the bandwidth of the light source, and horizontal resolution is 20 μm, limited by the optics of the eye.

Macular OCT images

- Reconstruction of serial A-scans produces tomographic (cross-sectional; i.e. B-scan) images of the macula.
- A three-dimensional image of the macula can be reconstructed by using closed-space B-scans obtained in a raster pattern (see Figure 5.9).

- A normal time-domain OCT scan shows a highly reflective external band composed of an outer layer derived from the RPE–Bruchs–choriocapillaris complex and an inner layer representing the boundary between the inner and outer segments of the photoreceptors. The nerve fibre and plexiform layers are moderately backscattering, whereas the outer/inner nuclear and ganglion cell layers are weakly backscattering. The vitreous has no reflectivity, whereas the choroid reflectivity is masked by the RPE backscatter.
- A macular topography map demonstrates the foveal depression in blue (100–200 μm thick) and perifoveal elevation in green (200–300 μm thick). Computer software can automatically detect an inner boundary at the vitreoretinal interface and the inner and outer segments. The retinal thickness is calculated from the distance between the two boundary lines and plotted as a topographic map.

Vitreoretinal interface pathology

- Epiretinal membrane may be evident as a highly reflective layer on the retinal surface; it is often associated with a loss of the normal foveal contour and the development of intraretinal cystic spaces, both of which occur in response to retinal oedema. An epiretinal membrane which simulates a macular hole (a macular pseudohole) is characterized by steepening of the slope surrounding the foveal depression on OCT.
- Vitreomacular traction is typically evident as a reflective posterior vitreous face exerting focal vitreoretinal traction on the retina, with associated distortion of the normal retinal contour.
- Macular holes are evident as full-thickness defects in the NSR, involving the fovea and with or without attachment of the posterior vitreous face to the edge of the hole. The edges of a full-thickness macular hole are typically elevated from the RPE and demonstrate intraretinal cystic changes.
- Lamellar holes have defects in the inner retinal layers at the fovea, with continuous outer retinal layers. There is usually an overhanging inner retinal tissue which may represent part of the roof of an intraretinal cyst.

Intraretinal pathology

- In retinal oedema, cystic spaces of varying sizes are seen in the outer nuclear and plexiform layers. Foveal involvement may be associated with a loss of the foveal contour and an increased foveal thickness.
- Intraretinal changes may be accompanied by hyporeflective spaces between the NSR and the RPE, representing subretinal fluid.
- Retinal atrophy may manifest as a reduced retinal thickness. Loss of the outer retinal layers and the RPE gives rise to increased backscattering of the choroid.
- Hard exudates are observed as spots of high reflectivity in the inner or outer retina, casting shadows of low reflectivity posteriorly.

- In type 2 idiopathic juxtafoveal telangiectasia, characteristic localized inner or outer retinal cystic defects involving the temporal foveal or juxtafoveal retina may be present, with an absence of retinal thickening. Other features may include an extension of the highly reflective band into the retina (representing intraretinal pigment plaques) and a loss of the outer retinal band (due to focal loss of photoreceptors).

Subretinal pathology

- Pigment epithelial detachments are seen as focal, dome-shaped elevations of the highly reflective outer band. Intraretinal and subretinal fluid can often be seen extending beyond the boundaries of the pigment epithelial detachment.
- In RPE rips, the highly reflective band is broken. One edge of the RPE displays a steep ripple-like pattern. As the RPE folds upon itself, the thickened highly reflective band blocks light penetration into the choroid, creating a shadow defect.
- Occult CNV typically shows well-defined irregular elevation of the highly reflective RPE layer, with mild choroidal

backscattering. Classic CNV typically shows fusiform enlargement, irregularity, and duplication of the highly reflective external band. Actively leaking CNV can be detected by the presence of adjacent subretinal or intraretinal spaces and retinal thickening, representing subretinal fluid and intraretinal oedema.

- Enhanced depth imaging is a modality that enables high-definition OCT imaging of the external retinal layers, choroid, and lamina cribosa. This technology has been used to highlight choroidal thinning associated with age and increasing myopia, as well as choroidal thickening due to CSCR, Vogt–Koyanagi–Harada syndrome, and polypoidal choroidal vasculopathy.

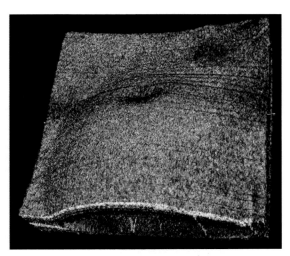

Fig 5.9 Three-dimensional reconstruction of raster scans acquired by spectral domain optical coherence tomography, showing serous retinal detachment in the macular region

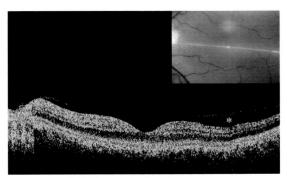

Fig 5.7 Image of normal macula on time-domain optical coherence tomography
Perifoveal vitreous separation from the retina is indicated by the asterisk

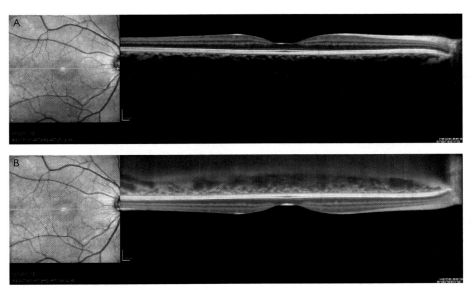

Fig 5.8 Image of normal macula with spectral domain optical coherence tomography
Top of the optical coherence tomography viewing screen has the best signal-to-noise ratio. To visualize the choroidal structures, the image can be inverted using the technique of enhanced depth imaging.

5.5 Ultrasonography

For posterior segment ultrasound imaging, sound frequencies in the range of 8–10 MHz are used. These high frequencies allow visualization of the vitreous, the posterior hyaloid face, the sub-hyaloid space, the retina, the choroid, and the sclera, with a resolution of approximately 150 μm.

Indications for posterior segment ultrasound

- Inability to visualize the posterior segment: small pupil; media opacities such as corneal lesions; hyphaema; cataract; vitreous haemorrhage; or inflammation
- Measurement of axial length or size and height of intraocular lesions: iris, ciliary body, or choroidal tumours
- To provide diagnostic information: detect fluid in Tenons capsule and thickening of posterior coats in posterior scleritis, detect vitreous attachment to a fibrovascular complex, outline posterior staphylomas, identify choroidal effusions, evaluate calcified optic disc drusen or sclerochoroidal calcification, and detect haemolysis of suprachoroidal haemorrhages.

Principles and technology

- Based on the reflection of acoustic waves at the interface between tissues of different acoustic impedances
- Ultrasound waves produced by a piezoelectric transducer
- Echoes reflected from each intraocular interface (e.g. aqueous–lens or vitreous–retina) return to the transducer. The strength of each echo is dependent on the magnitude of the impedance difference, the shape of the interface, and the extent of sound scattering, absorption, and refraction. The time delay of each echo depends upon the velocity of sound in the different ocular tissues.
- The piezoelectric transducer also detects the reflected sound waves and processes the information to produce a graph of intensity versus time (A-scan). The distance travelled by the sound waves is calculated from the time delay of the echoes.
- Two-dimensional images (B-scans) are reconstructed from multiple A-scans performed at different angles. The echo intensity at each time point is displayed as a dot in grey scale, and the location, derived from the time delay and direction of echo, is displayed in two dimensions.
- Doppler technology may be incorporated into the two-dimensional scan (duplex scans) to determine lesion vascularity.

Technique of posterior segment ultrasound

- A- and B-scans should be used concurrently to provide maximal information.
- Screening: set the B-scan on high gain initially (to detect vitreous opacities or gross retinal lesions) and then low gain (for flat retinal lesions). The fundus is imaged with the patient looking away from the probe, in the direction of the fundal area to be examined. The probe is orientated transversely (parallel to the limbus) at the limbus to examine the posterior pole. The probe is then shifted from the limbus towards the fornix to screen progressively more peripheral fundus. This process is repeated in all four quadrants before horizontal and vertical axial scans are performed with the patient gazing in the primary position and the probe held in line with the visual axis.
- Topography: the meridional extent (number of clock hours) of a lesion can be determined on transverse scanning. The anteroposterior extent of a lesion can be assessed with longitudinal scanning (probe held perpendicular to limbus). Axial scans with the probe held over the cornea demonstrate the relationship of the lesion to macula or optic disc. Lesion size and thickness should be measured.
- Quantitative echography: internal reflectivity is best assessed with A-scans. Low internal reflectivity is typically seen in choroidal melanomas because of their regular homogenous cellular structure. High internal reflectivity occurs in choroidal haemangiomas associated with multiple intralesional vascular spaces. Ultrasound attenuation by intraocular calcium or foreign bodies casts an acoustic shadow on the B-scan posteriorly.
- Kinetic echography: differences in the movement and attachment of the hyaloid face and detached retina may aid in the differential diagnosis. Internal vascularity can be assessed with Doppler ultrasound techniques.

Posterior vitreous detachment, vitreous haemorrhage, and retinal detachment

- Posterior vitreous detachment (PVD) is typically evident as a mobile, fine, hyperechoic linear density which is separate from the optic disc.
- Vitreous haemorrhage is visualized as opacities that move within the vitreous body and range in size and reflectivity depending on age and severity. These opacities may layer because of gravity.
- In contrast to PVD, a retinal detachment appears as a mobile, prominent hyperechoic linear density (see Figure 5.10) which is continuous with the optic disc. This tethering causes a funnel appearance in total retinal detachments. The mobility of the retinal detachment decreases with the presence of proliferative vitreoretinopathy, with the retinal detachment becoming fixed in advanced cases. The retinal detachment may appear splinted, taut, or concave in tractional cases (see Figure 5.11). Coexisting PVDs, retinal breaks, and vitreous haemorrhages may be visualized.
- A choroidal detachment appears as a smooth, thick, and immobile convexity. When extensive, separate choroidal detachments may extend towards each other and make contact ('kiss').

Intraocular mass lesions

- Typical features of choroidal melanomas (see Figure 5.12) include thickness greater than 3 mm, homogenous appearance with low-to-medium internal reflectivity (acoustic hollowness), internal vascularity, choroidal excavation, and associated serous retinal detachment. A bumpy irregular surface is more typical of metastatic tumours. High internal reflectivity is a feature of choroidal haemangiomas. Subretinal disciform lesions associated with AMD typically have two or more spikes and may reduce in height with time. Posterior scleritis is characterized by thickened sclera, and fluid in Tenons capsule (visible as a T-sign on the B-scan).

- In children with media opacity, ultrasound is often performed to evaluate the possible presence of a retinoblastoma. Typical features of this tumour include a solid mass lesion arising from the retina, with highly reflective internal lesions due to calcification. Stage 5 retinopathy of prematurity (ROP) is characterized by a dense retrolental vitreous opacity associated with a funnel-shaped retinal detachment. Persistent fetal vasculature is associated with a small globe and a band extended between the lens and the optic disc of varying severity. In Coats syndrome, a multifocal or large bullous retinal detachment may be associated with subretinal cholesterol deposits.

Ocular trauma and suprachoroidal haemorrhage

- Posterior scleral rupture should be suspected when the scleral contour is irregular, often with lower reflectivity detectable at the rupture site. Associated features such as PVD, vitreous or retinal incarceration, retinochoroid thickening, and intraocular haemorrhage may also be detected. Intraocular foreign bodies can be precisely localized by ultrasound.

- A traumatic or iatrogenic suprachoroidal haemorrhage initially demonstrates a dome-shaped choroidal detachment with irregular internal reflectivity. The vortex veins may be visualized as linear structures traversing the detachment. As the clot liquefies, the height of the lesion reduces and the internal reflectivity reduces. This feature is useful for guiding the timing of surgical drainage of the suprachoroidal haemorrhage, if indicated.

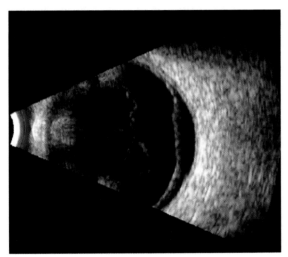

Fig 5.10 B-scan of a patient with vitreous haemorrhage and rhegmatogenous retinal detachment due to posterior vitreous detachment

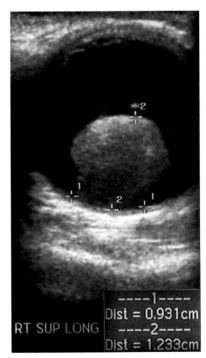

Fig 5.12 Typical features of choroidal melanoma are shown: mushroom shape, low internal reflectivity, and measuring 9 mm at base and 12 mm in height

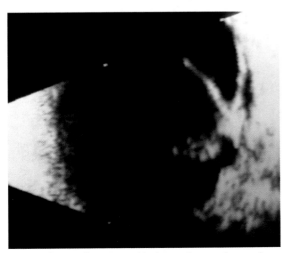

Fig 5.11 B-scan of a patient with vitreous haemorrhage and tractional retinal detachment due to proliferative diabetic retinopathy

5.6 Retinal photocoagulation

168

Light from a laser (which stands for 'light amplification by stimulated emission of radiation') is monochromatic, directional, parallel, and coherent. Argon and diode lasers are the most commonly used types for retinal treatment. Laser is delivered using a slit lamp or binocular indirect ophthalmoscope system, transcleral devices, or endoscopic probes.

Thermally induced necrosis occurs with intraocular tissue temperatures above 65°C. The temperature correlates directly with the amount of light absorbed by tissues. The retina is vulnerable to light of wavelengths between 400 and 1400 nm. The cornea and lens absorb the majority of UV light (<400 nm). The high water content of the ocular media absorbs the majority of infrared light (>750 nm). In the retina, three pigments are important in the absorption of light:

* Melanin (present in the RPE and the choroid) has a broad light-absorption range that spans the visual spectrum.
* Oxyhaemoglobin (present in retinal capillaries) absorbs light with wavelengths of less than 600 nm.
* Xanthophylls (present in the macula) have moderate absorption of light with wavelengths in the range of 400–500 nm.

The extent of tissue injury is also dependent upon the burn duration, laser spot size, and power. Light from an argon green laser (514 nm) or frequency-doubled Nd:YAG laser (532 nm) is absorbed by both melanin and oxyhaemoglobin but less so by xanthophylls. However, thermal damage may extend from the RPE into the retina and the choroid as the power and duration of laser delivery is increased. Thus, light from a diode laser (810 nm) may also cause thermal retinal and choroidal damage, despite its poor absorption by haemoglobin or xanthophylls.

Pan-retinal photocoagulation

Pan-retinal photocoagulation (PRP) involves laser ablation of the peripheral retina in patients with severe retinal ischaemia and retinal neovascularization. The resultant reduction in VEGF levels usually leads to a regression of retinal and optic disc neovascularization.

Approach

* Anaesthesia: optional pretreatment oral analgesia may be given. Topical anaesthetic is usually sufficient. Periocular or general anaesthesia may be appropriate in selected patients. Larger burns of longer duration are typically associated with greater discomfort.
* Laser settings vary depending upon the model of laser used and should be titrated to produce a light grey-white burn.
* Typical settings for single spot slit lamp delivery are:
  — Spot size: 200–500 μm (depending on lens laser spot magnification)
  — Duration: 0.05–0.20 seconds
  — Power (variable depending on fundus pigmentation): 100–300 mW.
* Typical settings for multi-spot slit lamp delivery are:
  — Spot size: 200–500 μm (depending on lens laser spot magnification)
  — Duration: 0.01 seconds
  — Power (variable depending on fundus pigmentation): 300–800 mW

* Laser application:
  1. Laser spots are placed one to three burn widths apart. The inferior retina should be treated first in case subsequent vitreous haemorrhage precludes treatment of the inferior retina. The nasal, temporal, and superior retina is then treated, leaving a clear margin of at least three disc diameters temporal to the fovea, and one disc diameter nasal to the optic disc.
  2. Great care should constantly be taken to ensure awareness of the location of the macula in relation to the laser aiming beam to avoid inadvertent foveal burns.
  3. Depending upon the severity of the underlying retinal disease severity, two to four treatment sessions are typically required to complete a full PRP (400–800 visible burns per session).
  4. Fluorescein angiograms should be reviewed to guide the area and extent of treatment.
* Post-laser care: corneal exposure following peribulbar anaesthesia should be avoided via the use of an eye pad
* Follow-up: review in 2–3 weeks to assess the response and consider further laser treatment

Macular focal and grid photocoagulation

Focal and grid macular laser treatments are most commonly performed for the treatment of macular oedema associated with diabetic maculopathy and branch retinal vein occlusions. Direct ablation of leaky microaneurysms (focal treatment) and mild thermal injury of the RPE to stimulate pumping of subretinal fluid (grid treatment) are thought to be the mechanisms of macular photocoagulation in reducing intraretinal oedema. Although several trials have demonstrated superior visual acuity outcome with anti-VEGF therapy, macular laser still has a role in patients with non-centre-involving diabetic macular oedema or in cases where anti-VEGF therapy is contraindicated.

Approach

* Anaesthesia: topical anaesthesia is usually sufficient. Periocular anaesthesia is occasionally required for selected patients.
* Laser settings vary depending upon the model of laser used and should be titrated to produce a faint grey-white burn (see Figure 5.13).
* Typical settings for slit lamp delivery are:
  — Spot size: 50–200 μm (depending on lens laser spot magnification)
  — Duration: 0.05–0.1 seconds
  — Power (variable depending of retinal thickness and subretinal fluid): 50–150 mW
* Laser application:
  1. Review fluorescein angiograms to determine location and areas of leakage, extent of capillary dropout, and margins of the foveal avascular zone.
  2. Identify the patient's fixation point to avoid foveal burn.
  3. The original ETDRS technique (1985) consists of (1) focal treatment which aims to directly coagulate (whitening or

darkening) all leaking microaneurysms, IRMA, or short capillary segments between 500 and 3000 µm from the centre of the macula, avoiding burns within 500 µm of the optic disc; (2) grid treatment to areas of thickening showing diffuse leakage or capillary dropout: treat all areas with oedema 500–3000 µm from the centre of the macula, avoiding treating within 500 µm of the optic disc. Space burns at least one spot's width apart; and (3) focal retreatment using 50 µm spot of 0.05 second duration within 500 µm of foveal centre is allowed.

4. Modified ETDRS technique (2003; DRCR.net): similar to the original ETDRS technique except that (1) the laser burn size is no greater than 50 µm, (2) coagulation of the leaking lesion is not required as merely a mild grey-white burn of the underlying RPE will suffice, (3) never treat within 500 µm of the foveal centre, and (4) space grid laser burns at least two spots' width apart.

• Follow-up: review at 3–4 months to assess regression of retinal thickening. Earlier review is required if concurrent retinal ischaemia or proliferative disease requiring PRP is present.

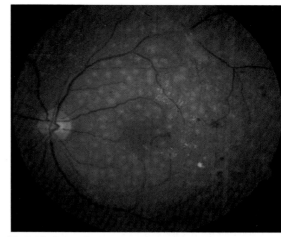

Fig 5.13 Colour fundus photography of posterior pole showing macular grid for treatment of diffuse macular oedema

Micropulse and nanopulse macular lasers

The end point of conventional macular laser application is a light grey burn. This phenomenon is due to the conduction of thermal energy, which is absorbed by the RPE, to the adjacent neuroretina. It is this rise in temperature that causes the loss of photoreceptors and paracentral scotoma associated with macular laser. It has been suggested that NSR damage is not required for resolution of macular oedema and that sublethal injury to the RPE alone may be adequate for modifying angiogenic growth factors for repairing blood–retinal barrier. Two types of sub-threshold lasers have been used in the treatment of macular oedema and early AMD.

Micropulse

• Uses a 532 nm, 577 nm, 660 nm, or 810 nm diode laser to cause a selective photothermal effect in the RPE layer and 30 µm above and below the RPE layer

• The laser is delivered as short repetitive pulses (0.05–1.0 milliseconds) separated by 1.0–10.0 millisecond gaps over a 10.0–3000.0 millisecond envelope.

• Confluent application and retreatment over the same area is possible.

• No visible lesion on angiography or autofluorescence imaging

Nanopulse

• Uses a 532 nm Q-switched Nd:YAG laser to cause (1) bubble formation within the RPE melanin granules and (2) the release of active metalloproteinases

• The laser is delivered as a single 3-nanosecond pulse with a beam profile that finely distributes laser energy over a treatment spot size of 400 µm and causes a barely discernible retinal reaction (damaging <20% of irradiated RPE cells).

• Apply the laser in a grid pattern, with burns at one spot's width apart, over the thickened retina.

• Lesions are visible on angiography and autofluorescence imaging.

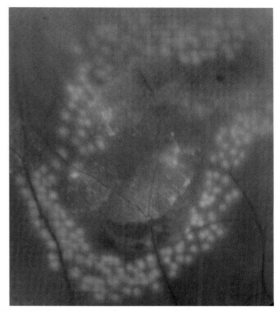

Fig 5.14 Confluent laser burns surrounding a retinal horseshoe tear

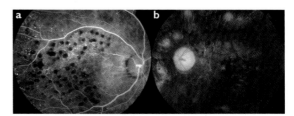

Fig 5.15 Complications of laser photocoagulation include (a) accidental foveal burn during macular laser and (b) progressive enlargement of laser scars due to heavy laser burns

Laser retinopexy

Laser retinopexy is performed for the treatment of retinal tears. Formation of a chorioretinal scar is induced with a consequent increased adhesion of the retina to the RPE; this adhesion prevents the extension of subretinal fluid.

Approach

- Anaesthesia: topical anaesthesia is usually sufficient. Periocular or general anaesthesia may be necessary in selected patients, particularly when treatment of anterior retinal pathology involving scleral indentation is required.
- Laser settings vary depending upon the model of laser used and should be titrated to produce confluent white burns. Typical laser settings for slit lamp or binocular indirect ophthalmoscopic delivery are:
  - Spot size: 200–1000 μm
  - Duration: 0.2–0.5 seconds
  - Power (variable between lasers): 100–300 mW
- Laser application:
  1. Retinal tears: two or three confluent rows of laser burns are placed around the retinal tear and any associated subretinal fluid (see Figure 5.14).
  2. Retinal dialyses and selected retinal detachments: three confluent rows of laser burns are placed immediately posterior to the dialysis or detached retina, extending from the ora serrata from one border of the affected area to the other border in order to surround the area.
  3. Multiple small anterior retinal tears: two or three confluent rows of laser burns are placed around the entire circumference of the peripheral retina, creating a 360° barrier between the anterior breaks and posterior retina. This method limits any retinal detachment from an unseen and untreated retinal tear. In addition, 360° laser retinopexy by endolaser photocoagulation is used in complex retinal detachment surgery. Some authorities support its use as prophylaxis in conditions such as Stickler syndrome.
- Post-laser care: patients should be advised to seek urgent attention if new floaters or a visual field defect develops.
- Follow-up: review in 1 week to detect progression of subretinal fluid or development of new retinal tears and assess the adequacy of the chorioretinal adhesion.

Complications of laser treatment

Anterior segment

- Corneal epithelial toxicity from anaesthesia, abrasion from contact lens, and oedema from scleral depression
- Inadvertent corneal, iris, and lenticular laser burns
- Neuropathic keratopathy; poor pupillary dilatation and accommodation resulting from damage to the long ciliary nerves (heavy laser should be avoided in the 3 and 9 o'clock meridians to prevent such damage)

Posterior segment

- Foveal burn (see Figure 5.15a)
- Haemorrhage: subretinal, preretinal, or vitreous haemorrhage may result from laser-induced vessel-wall rupture.
- Epiretinal membrane
- CNV: rupture of Bruchs membrane may lead to CNV
- Extension of RPE atrophy: progressive RPE atrophy associated with juxtafoveal burns may lead to foveal involvement (see Figure 5.15b).
- RPE rip may occur following laser treatment over a pigment epithelial detachment.
- Macular oedema may progress following PRP.
- Exudative retinal or choroidal detachment may cause angle closure and raised intraocular pressure (IOP) following PRP.

5.7 Vitreous disorders

The vitreous is a transparent extracellular matrix made up of 99% water and 1% collagen and hyaluronic acid. Occupying 80% (4 ml) of the ocular volume, the vitreous plays important roles during ocular development and in the pathogenesis of many vitreoretinal disorders, including retinal tears, retinal detachments, vitreomacular traction syndrome, idiopathic macular holes, epiretinal membranes, and fibrovascular proliferation associated with ischaemic retinopathies. Genetic and environmental factors which modify normal collagen formation and retinovascular development can affect the vitreous structure.

Posterior vitreous detachment (PVD)

Pathophysiology

- During aging, photochemically generated free radicals lead to dissociation between hyaluronan and collagen, causing vitreous liquefaction (synchysis) and collapse (syneresis). These are accompanied by partial separation of the posterior vitreous cortex from the internal limiting membrane of the retina.
- Liquefied vitreous enters the retrohyaloid space through a prepapillary hole (Weiss ring; see Figure 5.16) in the posterior vitreous cortex, and saccadic eye movements facilitate further separation of the posterior hyaloid from the retina.
- PVD typically begins in the perifoveal retina, extending to the fovea, optic disc, and peripheral retina to the vitreous base.
- Conditions predisposing to early PVD include myopia, hereditary vitreoretinopathies, trauma, uveitis, vitreous haemorrhage, diabetes, aphakia, and pseudophakia.

Anomalous PVD: Complications

- Anomalous PVD with incomplete anterior separation due to areas of strong vitreoretinal adhesion: horseshoe retinal tears and retinal detachment. In 10% of cases, vitreous haemorrhage occurs because of avulsion of retinal vessels.
- Anomalous PVD with incomplete posterior separation due to persistent vitreous adhesion to the macula (vitreomacular traction syndrome, foveoschisis, macular hole) or optic disc (vitreopapillary traction syndrome)

Clinical evaluation

History and examination

- Often asymptomatic
- Floaters and flashing lights (photopsia), located in the temporal visual field
- Weiss ring: peripapillary glial tissue that remains attached to the posterior vitreous cortex following PVD
- Posterior hyaloid membrane, visible as a crinkled membrane immediately posterior to the lens on slit lamp examination or with a 90 D lens; located posteriorly in the vitreous cavity
- Vitreous pigment deposits (Shafers sign) indicate a high likelihood of a retinal tear being present.
- Peripheral retinal tears, best detected using BIO with scleral indentation

Differential diagnosis

- **Photopsia:** migraine, dysphotopsia associated with the intraocular lens (IOL), white dot syndrome, uveal melanoma
- **Floaters:** vitreous haemorrhage or vitritis

Management

- No treatment is required for uncomplicated PVD.
- Educate the patient regarding symptoms of retinal detachment.
- Laser retinopexy or cryotherapy if retinal tear is present
- Retinal detachment surgery if retinal detachment is present

Complications

- Retinal break in 10%–15% of symptomatic PVDs and higher in those associated with vitreous haemorrhage or vitreous pigment
- Vitreous haemorrhage
- Retinal detachment

Prognosis

- Up to 4% of eyes with initially uncomplicated PVD may develop subsequent retinal tears over 6 weeks follow-up.
- If not already present, PVD commonly develops in the fellow eye within 3 years.

Vitreous haemorrhage

Aetiology

- PVD related: with and without retinal tear
- Vascular: proliferative diabetic retinopathy (see Figure 5.17), retinal vein occlusion, macroaneurysm, proliferative sickle cell retinopathy, central retinal artery occlusion
- Inflammation: sarcoidosis-related posterior uveitis, Behcets disease
- Iatrogenic: retinal laser photocoagulation, vitrectomy, trabeculectomy
- Trauma: direct ocular trauma, Terson syndrome
- Tumour: choroidal melanoma
- Degenerative: choroidal neovascular membrane secondary to AMD, idiopathic polypoidal choroidal vasculopathy
- Blood dyscrasia: leukaemia
- Valsalva retinopathy
- Paediatric conditions: ROP, familial exudative vitreoretinopathy, shaken baby syndrome, juvenile X-linked retinoschisis

Clinical evaluation

History and examination

- Decreased visual acuity depending on severity of vitreous haemorrhage
- History, symptoms, and signs associated with causative pathology, particularly signs of retinal vascular disease evident in the unaffected eye

Differential diagnosis

- Floaters: vitritis

Management

- Mild vitreous haemorrhage can be managed conservatively if the fundal view allows exclusion of pathology requiring urgent intervention. A conservative approach may be adopted in selected cases of proliferative diabetic retinopathy, sickle cell retinopathy, and retinal vein occlusion.

- B-scan ultrasonography to exclude retinal tears or detachment if the fundal view is poor. Ultrasonography may aid diagnosis by identifying PVD, choroidal neovascular membrane, and tumours.
- Follow up if vitreous haemorrhage or risk factors present for retinal tears (high myopia, family history, retinal detachment in fellow eye).
- Early vitrectomy may be appropriate where the likelihood of retinal tear is considered greater than the sequela of retinal vascular disease.
- Vitrectomy is indicated for non-clearing vitreous haemorrhage, for vitreous haemorrhage affecting quality of life, or if there is a high suspicion of underlying pathology requiring urgent treatment (e.g. retinal detachment).

Complications
- Haemosiderosis bulbi, and retinal damage following the liberation of iron during the catabolism of haemoglobin. This condition can occur in extensive, long-standing vitreous haemorrhage.
- Ghost cell glaucoma

Prognosis
- Natural history and prognosis dependent on underlying cause
- Retinal detachment associated with vitreous haemorrhage carries a poor prognosis if surgery is delayed.

Asteroid hyalosis

Pathophysiology
- A degenerative process resulting in deposition of calcium hydroxyapatite or calcium phosphate and phospholipid complexes in the vitreous gel

Clinical evaluation

History
- Asymptomatic, incidental finding
- Floaters and reduced visual acuity are rare.

Examination
- Yellow-white spherical opacities in vitreous gel (see Figure 5.18)
- Suspended opacities move with vitreous motion.
- Usually an attached posterior vitreous cortex
- Obscured retinal view

Differential diagnosis
- Synchysis scintillans (cholesterol crystal accumulation in the vitreous, appearing as flat angular crystals which settle with gravity)

Management
- No treatment is usually required.
- Retinal imaging with ultrasound, with fundus fluorescein angiography (FFA), or with OCT if the fundal view is limited and retinal pathology is suspected
- Vitrectomy is rarely indicated if there is reduced visual acuity.

Complications
- Late dystrophic calcification of silicone plate IOLs

Prognosis
- No long-term sequelae

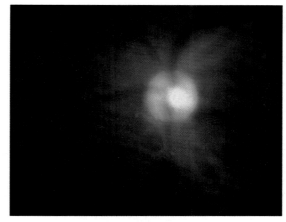

Fig 5.16 Weiss ring as seen on slit lamp

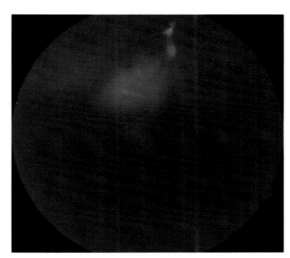

Fig 5.17 Vitreous haemorrhage due to proliferative diabetic retinopathy

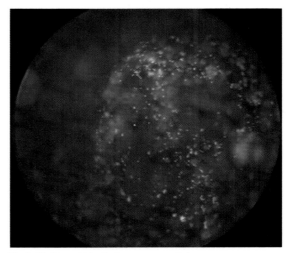

Fig 5.18 Asteroid hyalosis as seen on slit lamp

A retinal detachment is the separation of the NSR from the RPE. The disruption in the normal apposition of the NSR and the RPE impairs the survival and function of the retinal photoreceptors (see Section 5.1).

Pathogenesis

Retinal detachment occurs when the physiological forces maintaining normal apposition of the NSR to the RPE (see Section 5.1) are overcome by one or more of the following processes: (1) fluid flow from the vitreous cavity into the subretinal space via a retinal break held open by vitreoretinal traction; (2) exudation or haemorrhage in the subretinal space due to a compromised blood–retinal barrier associated with inflammation, retinochoroidal vascular abnormalities, or fluid leakage from an optic disc pit; and (3) traction from proliferating membranes on the surface of the retina or associated with an anomalous PVD.

Pathophysiology

Retinal detachment leads to proliferation and migration of the RPE, recruitment of macrophages into the subretinal space, degeneration of photoreceptors, and secondary inner retinal changes. The degree of visual loss depends upon the duration and the extent of separation of the NSR from the RPE (area and height). Significant visual recovery may occur if timely reattachment of the NSR to the RPE is achieved.

Rhegmatogenous retinal detachment (RRD)

The Greek word *rhegma* means 'break'. Approximately 6% of all eyes have a retinal break, but less than 0.1% of the population will develop RRD during their lifetime. Factors important in the development of RRD include:

- Vitreous liquefaction (associated with aging, inflammation, intraocular surgery, myopia, hereditary vitreoretinopathies)
- Full-thickness breaks in the NSR
- Vitreoretinal traction on retinal breaks
- Fluid flow from the vitreous cavity into the subretinal space stimulated by saccadic eye movements

Types of retinal break causing RRD

- **Two types of breaks occur in the presence of PVD:** (1) localized horseshoe tears and operculated tears (when the flap of retina is avulsed) and (2) giant retinal tears, when the circumferential extent of the break is 3 clock hours or greater (see Figure 5.19). These tears are due to abnormally strong vitreoretinal adhesion.
- **Two types of breaks occur in the absence of PVD:** (1) atrophic round holes, which are sometimes related to lattice degeneration or myopia, and (2) retinal dialysis, which can be spontaneous or traumatic through vitreous base avulsion
- **Myopic macular holes:** breaks in the central macular area; associated with abnormal vitreomacular traction and elongation of posterior staphyloma
- **Combined mechanisms:** (1) tractional tears near fibrovascular complexes in proliferative diabetic retinopathy or sickle cell retinopathy and (2) retinal necrosis in viral retinitis

Risk factors for RRD

- **Ocular:** myopia (40% of RRDs), cataract surgery (40% of RRDs), ocular trauma (10% of RRDs), infective necrotizing retinitis, miotic eye drops, senile retinoschisis, chorioretinal coloboma
- **Systemic:** Stickler syndrome, Marfan syndrome, Goldmann–Favre syndrome, Ehlers–Danlos syndrome

Clinical evaluation

History

- Photopsia
- Floaters
- Visual field defect
- Ocular and systemic risk factors
- Family history of RRD

Examination

- Visual acuity, normal (if macula attached) or reduced (if macula detached)
- Peripheral visual field defect
- Relative afferent papillary defect if extensive retinal detachment
- Reduced IOP
- Anterior chamber or vitreous pigment deposits
- Vitreous haemorrhage
- PVD (absent or partial, with retinal detachment due to retinal dialysis, atrophic round holes, myopic macular hole, acute retinal necrosis, and proliferative diabetic retinopathy)
- One or more retinal breaks: in primary RRD, the shape of the retinal detachment (RD) is determined by gravity, retinal anatomy, and the location of the break. Lincoffs rules state that, for supero-temporal or supero-nasal RDs, the break is within 1.5 clock hours of the high side of the RD; if the superior detachment crosses the vertical midline, then the break lies between the 10.30 and 1.30 meridians; in inferior RDs, if the borders are unequal, the high border indicates the side of the break whereas, if the borders are equal, the break is on the 6.00 meridian; if an inferior RD is bullous, the break lies above the horizontal meridian on the high side
- Detached retina: elevated, mobile, and corrugated appearance (see Figures 5.20 and 5.21)
- Signs of chronicity or slow progression: retinal pigment demarcation line (tide mark), retinal cysts

Investigations

- B-scan ultrasound, if dense vitreous haemorrhage

Differential diagnosis

- PVD
- Tractional retinal detachment (see Figures 5.22 and 5.23)
- Exudative retinal detachment
- Retinoschisis/tractional schisis (see Figures 5.24)
- Choroidal detachment

Management

Treatment varies depending upon the clinical features of the retinal detachment, the medical facilities available, and surgeon preference. Surgical repair is recommended for the vast majority of symptomatic RRDs and involves localization and closure of all retinal breaks by scleral indentation or intraocular tamponade. Permanent closure of the breaks is accomplished with cryotherapy or laser retinopexy (see Figure 5.25).

Observation

* Appropriate for selected asymptomatic retinal detachments with signs of chronicity or spontaneous reattachment
* Most suitable for shallow, inferior, and peripheral retinal detachments in patients with easy access to vitreoretinal services

Laser demarcation

* Used in selected asymptomatic macular-sparing retinal detachments, usually associated with atrophic round holes, retinoschisis, or retinal dialysis
* Two to three rows of confluent laser burns are applied along the posterior border of the retinal detachment up to the ora serrata, using an indirect ophthalmoscopic delivery system.
* Maximum chorioretinal adhesion may take up to 2 weeks.

Pneumatic retinopexy

* Most often used for superior RRD associated with small breaks confined to one quadrant, located within the superior third of the retina, and without significant vitreoretinal traction or proliferative vitreoretinopathy (PVR) or inferior retinal pathology
* Typically performed under local anaesthesia
* Cryotherapy of the retinal breaks is followed by intravitreal injection of an expansile gas (100% SF_6 or C_3F_8). An alternative approach is to perform an initial intravitreal gas injection followed by laser retinopexy of the retinal breaks the following day, after reattachment of the retina.
* Post-operative posturing may be advised to ensure adequate tamponade and closure of the retinal breaks.

Scleral buckling

* Suitable for most types of RRD without advanced PVR
* Particularly indicated in young phakic patients with RRD and attached vitreous (e.g. RRD associated with atrophic round holes or retinal dialysis)
* General anaesthesia is usually used, although local anaesthesia is possible for selected patients.
* Involves conjunctival peritomy, muscle sling, search for scleral thinning, localization of all retinal breaks, cryotherapy, external drainage of subretinal fluid in selected cases, and application of a local or encircling scleral explant to indent the retinal breaks

Pars plana vitrectomy

* Increasingly used for all varieties of retinal detachment associated with a PVD
* Particularly indicated for pseudophakic RRD and for RRD associated with PVR
* Local or general anaesthesia used
* Currently, 20-, 23-, and 25-gauge vitrectomy systems are available.
* Vitrectomy to relieve vitreoretinal traction, fluid–air exchange with internal drainage of subretinal fluid (via retinal breaks or a retinotomy) to reattach the retina, and laser retinopexy or cryotherapy of retinal breaks followed by

exchange of air with an non-expansile concentration of inert gas (12%–14% C_3F_8 or 18%–20% SF_6, lasting approximately 6 weeks and 2 weeks, respectively) for post-operative tamponade of retinal breaks. An expansile concentration (>14% C_3F_8 or >20% SF_6) may be used in certain situations.

* Post-operative posturing to facilitate gas tamponade of retinal breaks whilst retinopexy takes effect

Combined vitrectomy and scleral buckling

* Typically used to treat RRD associated with inferior retinal tears
* Particularly indicated for complex RRD (e.g. advanced PVR) and significant retinal shortening as an alternative to retinectomy

Adjunctive agents and procedures

* Various densities of silicone oil for intraocular tamponade, commonly used for complex RRD associated with PVR
* Heavy liquids (e.g. perfluoro-*n*-octane and perfluoroperhydrophenanthrene) used to facilitate subretinal fluid drainage via peripheral retinal breaks, stabilize the retina during retinectomies, aid in localization of occult retinal tears using subretinal trypan blue, unfold giant retinal tears, and act as a temporary tamponade for inferior retinal detachment surgery

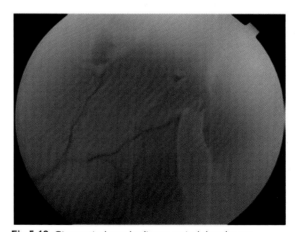

Fig 5.19 Giant retinal tear leading to retinal detachment

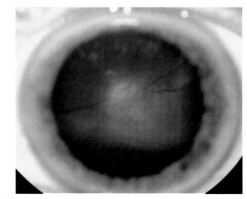

Fig 5.20 Bullous superior retinal detachment seen behind the lens

- Epiretinal membrane peeling and retinectomy used for PVR cases; subretinal trypan blue injection used for finding small retinal breaks

Complications

- PVR, epiretinal membrane, and failure of retina to reattach

Observation and laser demarcation

- Progression of retinal detachment

Scleral buckling

- **Explant related:** infection, intrusion, or extrusion; strabismus; ptosis; induced refractive error; intraoperative perforation whilst suturing explant
- **Subretinal fluid drainage related:** retinal incarceration, choroidal and subretinal haemorrhage, endophthalmitis

Vitrectomy

- Cataract
- Endophthalmitis (see Figure 5.26)
- Gas-related: increased IOP due to expansile gas concentrations; transient posterior subcapsular cataract; central retinal artery occlusion; angle closure
- Air travel and nitrous oxide anaesthesia are contraindicated prior to absorption of gas.

- Silicone oil related: glaucoma, cataract, band keratopathy, emulsification, or unexplained visual loss
- Sympathetic ophthalmia related to multiple procedures

Prognosis

- The visual acuity outcome after successful retinal reattachment is strongly influenced by involvement of the macula.
- Macula-on retinal detachment: 90% will retain preoperative visual acuity; 10% may have suboptimal visual acuity due to macular oedema, persistent subretinal fluid, or epiretinal membrane formation
- Macula-off retinal detachment: 50% achieve visual acuity of 6/12 or better. Reduced visual acuity is associated with a longer duration and greater height of macular detachment.
- The risk of retinal detachment in the fellow eye increases incrementally with a history of myopic retinal detachment, aphakic retinal detachment, or pseudophakic retinal detachment. The highest risk of fellow eye retinal detachment is associated with a giant retinal tear (up to 48%).

5.9 Retinal detachment II

Exudative retinal detachment

Aetiology

* **Ocular:** primary retinal/choroidal tumours, CNV, central serous chorioretinopathy (CSCR), optic disc pit/coloboma, Coats syndrome, sympathetic ophthalmia, posterior scleritis, cryotherapy, PRP, uveal effusion syndrome
* **Systemic:** Vogt–Koyanagi–Harada syndrome, metastatic retinal/choroidal tumours, malignant hypertension, eclampsia, hypoproteinaemia

Clinical evaluation

* Associated with underlying ocular or systemic disease
* Vitreous usually clear except in uveitis
* Retinal detachment: gravity-dependent, convex, elevated bullae, and no retinal break. Exudative retinal detachments can masquerade as RRD and must be excluded if no retinal break is seen.
* Subretinal fluid: turbid and shifting to dependent position

Management

* Treat underlying systemic condition
* CSCR laser or photodynamic therapy (PDT) to leakage areas
* Optic disc pit/coloboma: barrier laser around disc or coloboma and vitrectomy/gas
* Coats syndrome: cryotherapy/laser
* Uveal effusion syndrome: sclerectomy and drainage

Prognosis

* Visual outcome determined by the effect of underlying condition on macular and optic nerve function

Tractional retinal detachment

Aetiology

* **Ocular:** proliferative vitreoretinopathy, penetrating injury, vitreomacular traction syndrome, pars planitis, retinitis
* **Systemic:** ischaemic retinopathies associated with retinal neovascularization; e.g. diabetic retinopathy, ROP, sickle cell retinopathy, radiation retinopathy

Clinical evaluation

* Characteristic features associated with underlying ocular or systemic disease, as listed under 'Aetiology'
* Epiretinal and fibrovascular membranes
* Retinal detachment: immobile retina, concave retina, areas of visible vitreoretinal traction; may be associated with tractional retinal breaks

Management

* Treat underlying ocular or systemic condition (e.g. PRP for ischaemic retinopathies).
* Observation for non-progressive extramacular retinal detachment
* Vitrectomy surgery is indicated if progressive retinal detachment, or if macula is threatened. Preoperative anti-VEGF agents have been advocated as a means of controlling intraoperative haemorrhage but may promote tractional detachment.

Complication and prognosis

* Progressive retinal traction may cause retinal breaks leading to combined tractional and RRD.
* Visual outcome determined by the effect of the underlying condition on macular and optic nerve function

Choroidal effusion/detachment

Pathophysiology

* A choroidal effusion is the accumulation of fluid within the potential space between the choroid and sclera. The fluid may be a transudate or an exudate, depending on the protein concentration and aetiology.

Aetiology

* Hypotony
* Trauma
* Inflammation
* Suprachoroidal haemorrhage (usually painful with high IOP)
* Nanophthalmos
* Uveal effusion syndrome

Clinical evaluation

* Characteristic features associated with underlying ocular disease, as listed in 'Aetiology'
* Usually painless with variable visual loss
* Choroidal elevation which is dark brown, convex, smooth, and immobile. The elevation may be shallow or annular. If the effusion extends under the pars plana, the ora serrata will be visible without indenting. If severe, 'kissing choroidals' may develop.
* A shallow anterior chamber, low intraocular pressure, and myopic shift may be present.
* An accompanying exudative detachment dependent on severity and pathology

Management

* Treat underlying ocular condition, which may include topical corticosteroid use and cycloplegia.
* Observation for shallow or mild choroidal effusions
* Anterior chamber reformation may be performed if the anterior chamber is flat.
* If painful, chronic, or persistent iridocorneal touch is present, drainage by posterior sclerostomies may be performed.

Prognosis

* The prognosis is dependent on the severity of the choroidal effusion as well as the aetiology.

Proliferative vitreoretinopathy (PVR)

Pathophysiology

* When open retinal breaks are present, migration and proliferation of RPE, glial, inflammatory, and fibroblastic cells, with extracellular matrix deposition on the subretinal and epiretinal surfaces, may occur, leading to PVR (see Table 5.2).

Risk factors

* Multiple or large retinal breaks
* Vitreous haemorrhage
* Accompanying choroidal detachment

Table 5.2 Grading of proliferative vitreoretinopathy

Grade	Features
A	Vitreous haze, vitreous pigment clumps, pigment clusters on inferior retina
B	Wrinkling of inner retinal surface, retinal stiffness, vessel tortuosity, rolled and irregular edge of retinal break, decreased mobility of vitreous
C (A or P)	Focal, diffuse, or circumferential full-thickness folds,* subretinal strands,* anterior displacement,*† condensed vitreous with strands†

*Expressed in number of clock hours involved.
†Applies only to anterior proliferative vitreoretinopathy.
A, anterior; P, posterior.

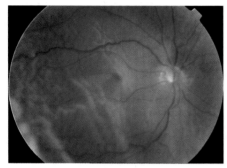

Fig 5.21 Temporal retinal detachment extending under the fovea; macula-off retinal detachment

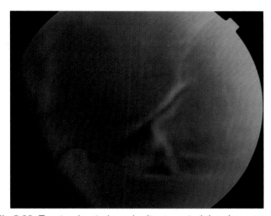

Fig 5.22 Tractional retinal tear leading to retinal detachment

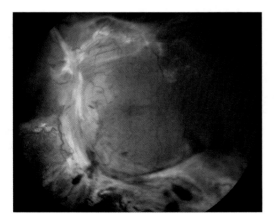

Fig 5.23 Colour fundus photograph of tractional retinal detachment in proliferative diabetic retinopathy

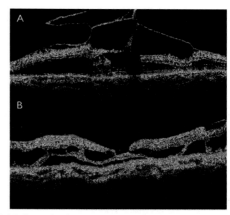

Fig 5.24 Optical coherence tomography showing (a) dense preretinal fibrous membrane and (b) tractional schisis

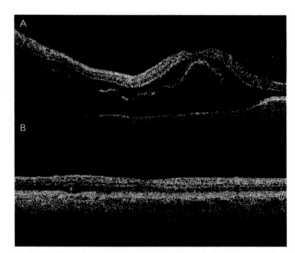

Fig 5.25 Optical coherence tomography (a) before and (b) after macula-off retinal detachment repair

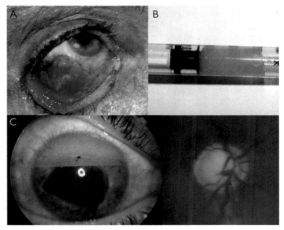

Fig 5.26 Complications of vitreoretinal surgery: (a) suture granuloma after scleral buckling, (b) endophthalmitis (vitreous biopsy sample of *Haemophilus* endophthalmitis), (c) silicone oil emulsification (inverse hypopyon), and (d) raised intraocular pressure (glaucomatous cupping of disc)

5.10 Peripheral retinal abnormalities

Retinal abnormalities are commonly detected during examination of the peripheral retina with scleral indentation. The majority of peripheral retinal abnormalities are clinically insignificant but lattice degeneration, degenerative retinoschisis, and peripheral retinal tufts are associated with an increased risk of RRD. However, prophylactic treatment of these changes is generally not indicated except in rare, high-risk cases.

Developmental changes

During embryonic development, the NSR terminates at the ciliary processes. As the eye enlarges, the sensory retina recedes posteriorly from the pars plicata, forming a boundary with multiple tooth-like (dentate) indentations called the ora serrata. Abnormal recession of the ora serrata leads to formation of meridional folds, meridional complexes, enclosed oral bays, and peripheral retinal tufts.

Meridional complexes

Meridional complexes are seen in 16% of autopsy eyes and are formed by elongated dentate process with ciliary process in the same meridian. Over half are bilateral and usually at the nasal ora. They are not associated with retinal breaks.

Enclosed oral bays

Enclosed oral bays are oval islands of pars plana epithelium located posterior to the ora serrata and separated from the pars plana by sensory retina. If incompletely separated, they are called partially enclosed oral bays. They are found in 4% of the general population and associated with 17% of meridionally aligned retinal tears occurring at the posterior border of the vitreous base following PVD.

Meridional folds

Meridional folds are radial folds of retina and are usually found in the supero-nasal retina aligned with dentate processes, meridional complexes, or ora bays. They are found in 26% of autopsy eyes, and over half are bilateral. PVD can induce a tear at the posterior border of the fold.

Peripheral retinal tufts

These small peripheral retinal elevations are formed by focal vitreous or zonular traction. Tufts associated with cystic retinal changes or contiguous with a thickened zonule at its apex may predispose to a retinal break secondary to PVD.

Degenerative changes

Cobblestone or pavingstone degeneration

Cobblestone or pavingstone degeneration appears as well-defined areas of chorioretinal atrophy located between the equator and the ora serrate (see Figure 5.27). It is found in 22% of adults and has no predisposition to retinal break formation.

Ora serrata pearls

These opalescent spheres are located at dentate process and are thought to be analogous to giant drusen. They are found in 20% of autopsy eyes and do not predispose to retinal breaks.

Pars plana cysts

Pars plana cysts are cystic lesions located anterior to the ora serrata. They may arise from vitreous base or zonular traction but are not associated with retinal breaks. They occur in 18% of autopsy eyes.

Peripheral cystoid degeneration

Peripheral cystoid degeneration is characterized by areas of microscopic intraretinal spaces located immediately posterior to the ora serrata. Histologically, the anterior zone has spaces in the mid-retinal layers (typical), whereas the posterior zone, if present, has spaces in the nerve fibre layer (reticular). These changes are found in all eyes by 8 years of age, progressing posteriorly and circumferentially with time. Both typical and reticular microcystic spaces may coalesce to form a schisis cavity.

Degenerative retinoschisis

Degenerative retinoschisis is a splitting of the NSR, is found in 7% of people over 40 years of age, and typically occurs in hypermetropes. It most frequently involves the infero-temporal retina and is often bilateral. Histologically, cavities filled with acid mucopolysaccharides split the peripheral retina at the outer plexiform layer (typical retinoschisis) or the nerve fibre layer (reticular retinoschisis) into inner and outer leaves. Retinoschisis results in a loss of retinal function and an absolute visual field defect (see Table 5.3). Breaks in the inner or outer leaf may occur. Potential complications include posterior extension of the retinoschisis cavity, and retinal detachment. Treatment for retinoschisis should be limited to patients who develop symptomatic, progressive retinal detachments. Prophylactic treatment is not recommended for asymptomatic patients with or without outer retinal leaf breaks.

Posterior extension

Despite producing an absolute visual field defect, posterior extension of a retinoschisis is usually asymptomatic. Routine treatment of asymptomatic patients with posterior progression is not recommended because this posterior extension frequently stops spontaneously, macular involvement is extremely rare, and demarcation laser treatment may be associated with severe complications.

Retinal detachment

Retinal detachment occurs in 0.05% of eyes with retinoschisis and occurs in two forms: a more common, localized, relatively stable form with outer leaf breaks only, and a rarer, symptomatic, rapidly progressive form with retinal breaks in both inner and outer leaves. Treatment is usually required only for the rapidly progressive form of retinal detachment.

Table 5.3 Differential features of retinal detachment and retinoschisis

Clinical feature	Retinal detachment	Schisis
Presentation	Visual field defect	Usually asymptomatic
Surface	Corrugated	Smooth
Blood or pigment	Present	Absent
Subretinal fluid	Variable shifting	Not shifting
Fields defect	Relative	Absolute
Reaction to laser	Absent	Present if no subretinal fluid
OCT findings	Elevation of NSR	Attached NSR with splitting within plexiform layers

Lattice degeneration

Lattice degeneration is found in 6%–10% of autopsy eyes and is characterized by well-demarcated, circumferentially orientated, oval areas of retinal thinning with overlying vitreous liquefaction and exaggerated vitreoretinal attachments along its posterior margin. Other features include lattice-like fine white lines in the crossing retinal vessels, alterations of retinal pigment (see Figure 5.28), small white particles at the margin or surface of the lesion, punched-out areas of retinal thinning, or excavations and atrophic retinal holes or retinal breaks (see Figure 5.29). Lattice lesions are commonly located near the vertical meridians between 11 and 1 o'clock and between 5 and 7 o'clock. The lesions are usually anterior to the equator but can be present posterior to the equator, where they are frequently radially orientated. They are bilateral in up to 50% of cases and are more common in myopic patients.

Atrophic holes and tractional tears

Atrophic retinal holes occur in 20% of eyes with lattice degeneration and are typically small and round. They may lead to an asymptomatic localized retinal detachment and, rarely, a progressive retinal detachment during the second and third decades. Tractional horseshoe-shaped retinal tears develop at the posterior or lateral margins of lattice lesions from vitreous traction following PVD after the fifth decade.

Retinal detachment

Lattice degeneration is the most important peripheral retinal degeneration that predisposes to RRD and occurs in 1% of eyes with lattice changes followed for 10 years. Most RRDs associated with lattice degeneration are due to tractional retinal tears following PVD. Although lattice degeneration is a risk factor for RRD, only a small minority of affected eyes develop RRD, and 80% of RRDs are not associated with lattice degeneration. Laser retinopexy of lattice for prophylaxis against RRD is unproven and may cause harm by causing RRD or stimulating the development of epiretinal membrane.

Further reading

1. Byer NE: Long-term natural history of lattice degeneration of the retina. *Ophthalmology* 1989 Sept; **96**(9): 1396–1402

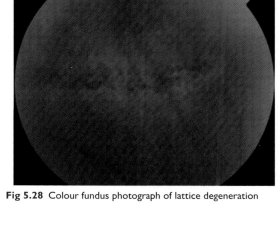

Fig 5.28 Colour fundus photograph of lattice degeneration

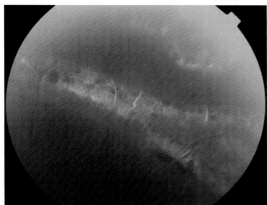

Fig 5.29 Colour fundus photograph of lattice degeneration with retinal breaks

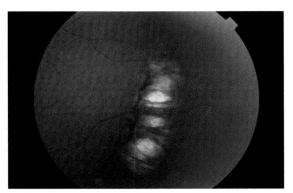

Fig 5.27 Pavingstone degeneration

5.11 Macular surgery

Macular surgery is often performed to relieve traction from the macular surface in conditions such as epiretinal membrane, macular hole, tractional macular detachment, and vitreomacular traction syndrome (see Figures 5.30 and 5.31). Less frequently, macular surgery is performed to remove subhyaloid or submacular haemorrhage, choroidal neovascular membrane, or scar tissue associated with a variety of aetiologies.

Epiretinal membrane

Epiretinal membrane (also called macular pucker, epimacular proliferation, preretinal macular fibrosis, and cellophane maculopathy) is an avascular, fibrocellular membrane that proliferates on the inner surface of the retina and produces varying degrees of visual impairment. The prevalence of macular epiretinal membrane is 2% in individuals under the age of 60 years and 12% in those over 70 years. Bilateral involvement occurs in 31% of cases.

Aetiology

The majority of epiretinal membranes are idiopathic and occur in otherwise normal eyes. Defects in the inner limiting membrane are thought to allow migration of glial cells to the retinal surface. Secondary causes include trauma, retinal breaks, retinal venous occlusions, diabetic retinopathy, uveitis, some congenital conditions, retinal laser treatment, cryotherapy, and intraocular surgery. Epiretinal membranes variably comprise glial cells, RPE cells, macrophages, fibrocytes, and collagen fibres. Different proportions of these components are associated with different aetiologies.

Clinical evaluation

Most patients are asymptomatic. The commonest symptoms are decreased visual acuity and metamorphopsia. Less common symptoms include micropsia, macropsia, and monocular diplopia. The severity of symptoms is related to the area of involvement and the thickness of epiretinal membrane. Contracture of the epiretinal membrane causes retinal distortion and may induce macular oedema and a tractional retinal detachment in advanced cases. The peripheral retina should be examined to exclude the presence of retinal breaks. Amsler grid testing can document the degree of metamorphopsia present. FFA may show distortion of retinal vessels and fluorescein leakage. It may help to exclude an underlying retinal vein occlusion. OCT demonstrates a hyper-reflective membrane on the inner retinal surface often associated with retinal thickening, intraretinal oedema, and tractional elevation of the retina.

Management

Asymptomatic epiretinal membranes do not require treatment. Patients with severe metamorphopsia due to epiretinal membrane benefit most from vitrectomy and surgical peeling of the epiretinal membrane. In many cases, improvement in metamorphopsia is more marked than visual acuity.

Prognosis

Epiretinal membranes follow a variable course. Most will be static or slowly progress. Rarely, the epiretinal membrane may spontaneously detach from the retina with symptomatic improvement. Without surgery, a quarter of cases will experience loss of two lines of visual acuity. Uncomplicated vitrectomy and epiretinal membrane peeling typically result in a gradual improvement in metamorphopsia and acuity.

Vitreomacular traction syndrome

Vitreomacular traction (VMT) is characterized by persistent vitreous attachment and anteroposterior traction in the macula. Associated findings may include epiretinal membrane, varying degrees of macular oedema, and tractional macular detachment. The symptoms of metamorphopsia and central scotoma may be progressive but they usually stabilize after 1–2 years.

Aetiology

VMT arises from an incomplete and anomalous PVD which leads to persistent vitreoretinal adhesion in the peripapillary and macular regions.

Clinical evaluation

VMT may cause reduced visual acuity because of retinal distortion, tractional retinal detachment, and macular oedema or macular schisis. FFA may demonstrate leakage from the optic disc and macular region. OCT typically shows adhesion of the posterior hyaloid in the macular region; the adhesion is often associated with focal elevation of the retina at points of vitreoretinal attachment. Associated epiretinal membrane and intraretinal cystic spaces may also be visible.

Management

If symptomatic, vitrectomy may restore normal foveal anatomy with visual acuity improvement in 70% of cases. A Phase 3 double-blinded randomized controlled trial (MIVI-TRUST) showed that intravitreal ocriplasmin resolved vitreomacular adhesion in approximately 25% of eyes. The National Institute for Health and Care Excellence (NICE) has approved ocriplasmin use in patients who are symptomatic but without the presence of an epiretinal membrane.

Prognosis

Spontaneous separation of the posterior hyaloid can occur with resolution of macular oedema and improvement in visual acuity in 11% of cases. Without complete PVD, acuity may deteriorate in 70% of cases.

Full-thickness macular hole

The majority of full-thickness macular holes are classified as idiopathic, typically occurring in the sixth to eighth decades. Females are affected more frequently than males, and bilateral involvement eventually occurs in up to 13% of cases. Full-thickness macular holes associated with high myopia tend to occur in patients 10–20 years younger than those with idiopathic macular holes and may be associated with epiretinal membranes, foveoschisis, and retinal detachment.

Aetiology

Idiopathic and myopic full-thickness macular holes are caused by a combination of anteroposterior, oblique, and tangential traction associated with an anomalous perifoveal PVD. Full-thickness macular holes due to ocular trauma may be caused by contusion necrosis or vitreoretinal traction. Full-thickness macular holes associated with certain types of laser injury may be caused by vaporization of retinal tissue.

Clinical evaluation

Stage 1 impending macular holes are characterized by foveal detachment and a visible yellow spot (Stage 1A) or ring at the fovea (Stage 1B). These may progress to a Stage 2 full-thickness macular hole with a central round or crescent-shaped full-thickness foveal defect (<400 μm) associated with persistent vitreofoveal traction. Further enlargement of the defect to >400 μm leads to a Stage 3 full-thickness macular hole, usually associated with further visual loss. A pre-foveal opacity formed by vitreous condensation with variable amounts of retinal tissue may be visible as the hyaloid separates from the edge of the hole. A Stage 4 full-thickness macular hole occurs when a complete PVD is present. The Watzke–Allen test may be useful in confirming the presence of a full-thickness macular hole. It is performed by placing a thin slit beam of light on the macular hole. A positive Watzke–Allen sign occurs when the patients perceives a break in the light beam. An uninterrupted or narrowed beam is negative. FFA demonstrates localized hyperfluorescence at the fovea owing to a window defect caused by the macular hole. OCT demonstrates a full-thickness central retinal defect with a surrounding cuff of subretinal fluid and intraretinal cystic spaces at the margins of the hole.

Partial-thickness defects of the inner retina occur in lamellar holes. The differential diagnosis includes a pseudohole (due to a focal defect in an epiretinal membrane). These may be differentiated on OCT, as lamellar holes are associated with sloping or undermined edges whilst a more vertical edge is noted in pseudoholes. Partial-thickness defects of the outer retina at the fovea are noted in solar retinopathy, achromatopsia, alkyl nitrite retinopathy, microholes, and after spontaneous resolution or surgical repair of idiopathic full-thickness macular holes.

Management

No treatment is indicated for Stage 1 'holes' because of the high rate of spontaneous resolution. Stage 2–Stage 4 full-thickness macular holes can usually be closed using vitrectomy and gas tamponade with or without a variable period of post-operative prone positioning. Internal limiting membrane peeling with or without indocyanine green (ICG) or trypan blue-assisted staining is a commonly performed adjuvant technique and may increase hole closure rates, particularly in large and chronic holes. There is a general shift away from using ICG because of reported retinal toxicity. A randomized controlled trial (FILMS) found that peeling 1–2 disc diameters of internal limiting membrane around the macular hole was associated with significantly higher levels of closure of Stage 2 and Stage 3 holes. The MIVI trials also showed that intravitreal ocriplasmin can result in full-thickness macular hole closure in approximately 40% patients. NICE has approved the use of ocriplasmin in patients who have a full-thickness macular hole of <400 μm,

with associated VMT and who do not have an epiretinal membrane.

Prognosis

Spontaneous resolution occurs in up to 50% of Stage 1 'holes' owing to vitreous separation from the macula. Spontaneous closure of Stage 2–Stage 4 holes is rare. Unoperated full-thickness macular holes typically have a stable visual acuity of approximately 6/60. Surgical treatment results in anatomical closure in over 80% of cases and an improvement in visual acuity in over 60% of cases. Factors associated with less favourable anatomic and visual results include macular holes of long duration, absent subretinal fluid, intraretinal oedema at the edge of the hole, and large hole diameter. If no PVD is present, the risk of developing a macular hole in the fellow eye is 15% in a 5-year period. The presence of an incomplete perifoveal PVD (Stage 0 'hole') on OCT is associated with up to 54% risk of developing a macular hole compared to 4% without a perifoveal PVD. The risk of developing a full-thickness macular hole in an eye with a complete PVD is negligible.

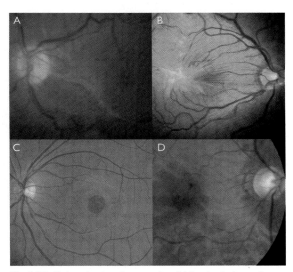

Fig 5.30 Colour fundus photographs of (a) epiretinal membrane, (b) vitreomacular traction syndrome, (c) full-thickness macular hole, and (d) lamellar macular hole

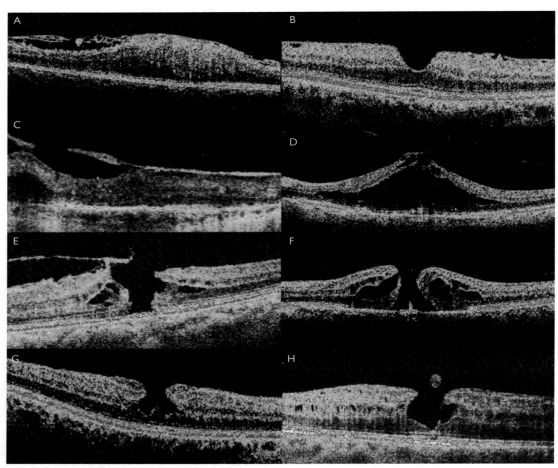

Fig 5.31 Optical coherence tomography images of (a) epiretinal membrane causing diffuse retinal thickening, (b) mild epiretinal membrane causing steepened foveal depression, (c) broad macular attachment, (d) focal foveal attachment of posterior hyaloid in vitreomacular traction syndrome, (e) full-thickness macular hole with and (f) without hyaloid attachment to the hole, and (g and h) lamellar macular holes

5.12 Submacular surgery

Surgical removal of submacular haemorrhage (see Figure 5.32) or CNV with associated blood and scar tissue may stabilize or improve visual acuity in selected cases.

Submacular CNV removal

The visual outcome following submacular surgery depends upon the viability of photoreceptors and the integrity of the underlying RPE. Surgical removal is best suited for Type 2 CNV (located in the subretinal space, above the RPE) because CNV removal may be associated with preservation of the underlying RPE. Type 2 CNV occurs in localized disease with focal RPE and Bruchs membrane involvement, such as in ocular histoplasmosis syndrome, punctate inner choroidopathy, idiopathic, or iatrogenic causes. CNV with extrafoveal ingrowth sites is associated with better visual results, compared to CNV without such sites. Surgical removal of Type I CNV (located beneath the RPE) is not recommended because of the risks of removing the overlying RPE. Type I CNV occurs in the presence of diffuse RPE and Bruchs membrane pathology and is commonly associated with AMD. The visual results of submacular surgery are often poor, even after successful CNV removal.

The technique of CNV removal involves a pars plana vitrectomy with separation of the posterior hyaloid, followed by a retinotomy to access the subretinal space and allow removal of the CNV by using subretinal forceps. A partial fluid–air exchange is performed and the patient postured post-operatively to close the retinotomy. In addition to the usual complications of vitrectomy surgery, submacular surgery carries the risk of perioperative submacular haemorrhage and post-operative recurrence of the CNV. Careful post-operative follow-up is required to detect CNV recurrence.

Submacular haemorrhage

Submacular haemorrhage is toxic to the outer retinal layers, and the visual prognosis is worse when the haemorrhage is extensive and thick. Submacular haemorrhage with AMD carries a poor prognosis, particularly if associated with CNV. Submacular haemorrhage associated with trauma and retinal arterial macroaneurysms carries a more favourable course, with spontaneous improvement being common. The surgical technique of submacular haemorrhage removal is similar to that used for CNV removal. After vitrectomy and the creation of a PVD, an access retinotomy is made, followed by injection of tissue plasminogen activator (tPA) subretinally into the area of haemorrhage. After 20–45 minutes, the tPA and liquefied submacular haemorrhage are irrigated out of the subretinal space. A fluid–air exchange is performed and the patient postured post-operatively to close the retinotomy and displace any residual submacular haemorrhage. A less invasive surgical approach suitable for thin submacular haemorrhages is the use of an intravitreal injection of expansile gas, often combined with intravitreal tPA and prone positioning to pneumatically displace the submacular haemorrhage.

The results of submacular haemorrhage removal are variable and the ultimate visual acuity is determined by the aetiology. Patients with good pre-haemorrhage visual acuity have a better prognosis. The timing of surgery is important, as photoreceptor damage can occur within 1 hour after subretinal haemorrhage, progressing to full-thickness retinal degeneration within 2 weeks.

Submacular RPE reconstruction

Laser, PDT, or anti-VEGF therapies will not affect visual outcome in RPE rip and geographic atrophy. Diseased submacular RPE can be replaced by foveal relocation to an area of extramacular RPE or by submacular RPE transplantation. Macular translocation with 360° retinotomy followed by counter-rotation extraocular muscle surgery may restore visual acuity in selected patients. Post-operative complications are common, however, and can result in severe visual loss. Autologous equatorial RPE–choroid patch graft to the submacular space has been performed but remains experimental. In both procedures, CNV recurrence can occur in 10%–20% of cases, typically within the first 2 years.

185

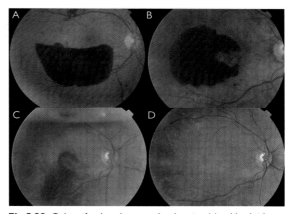

Fig 5.32 Colour fundus photographs showing (a) subhyaloid haemorrhage from macroaneurysm; this condition is distinguished from (b) submacular haemorrhage by the blood level and preretinal location of the blood in (a); (c) gas displacement of submacular haemorrhage, and (d) its resolution

Retinal vascular tumours

Retinal vascular tumours can be classified into four types: (1) retinal capillary haemangioma, (2) retinal cavernous haemangioma, (3) retinal arteriovenous communications (Wyburn–Mason syndrome), and (4) retinal vasoproliferative tumour. The first three lesions are vascular hamartomas (benign neoplasms consisting of tissue normally found at the site).

Capillary haemangioma

Forty per cent of these benign congenital vascular tumours are associated with von Hippel–Lindau syndrome. Clinically, the vascular tumour starts as a red dot which enlarges to form a vascular mass, typically located in the periphery or adjacent to the optic disc (approximately 15% of cases). Peripheral capillary haemangiomas have dilated retinal feeder and draining vessels. These lesions can result in subretinal exudates (see Figure 5.33) or epiretinal membranes and vitreous bands. Macular exudates and exudative or tractional retinal detachment may lead to symptoms in the second or third decade of life. FFA shows diffuse mid- and late-phase leakage from the angioma. Systemic assessment for evidence of von Hippel–Lindau syndrome is indicated. If present, annual fundal examination is necessary. Conservative management is considered for small and asymptomatic lesions which may spontaneously fibrose. Laser photocoagulation and cryotherapy are performed for small posterior and larger anterior lesions, respectively. PDT, radiotherapy, and anti-VEGF therapies have also been used. Vitrectomy is indicated to treat rhegmatogenous/tractional detachment.

Cavernous haemangioma

This benign congenital vascular tumour is occasionally associated with CNS and skin haemangiomas. Clinically, a purplish retinal mass resembling a bunch of grapes may be seen in the peripheral retina or at the optic disc (see Figure 5.34). No feeder vessels are present. Vitreous haemorrhage can occur in 10% of cases. FFA typically reveals early hypofluorescence with late pooling of dye and a meniscus visible at the fluorescein–blood interface within each lobule of the haemangioma. Neurological examination is indicated owing to an association with cerebral aneurysms. Treatment is not required in the majority of cases.

Retinal arteriovenous malformation

Retinal arteriovenous malformation is a benign congenital vascular lesion, also called a racemose haemangioma, characterized by an abnormal arteriovenous communication. Group 1 retinal arteriovenous malformation is usually asymptomatic with an abnormal capillary plexus between the major vessels. Group 2 retinal arteriovenous malformation has direct arteriovenous communication without intervening capillaries, and Group 3 retinal arteriovenous malformation has a more extensive complex arteriovenous communication often associated with visual loss. Although ocular complications (e.g. branch retinal vein occlusion) are rare, an association with midbrain lesions (Wyburn–Mason syndrome) is more common in Groups 2 and 3. In some cases, vascular malformations in the mandible or the maxilla may complicate routine dental procedures. FFA typically shows no evidence of vascular leakage. Management is generally conservative.

Retinal vasoproliferative tumours

These acquired vascular tumours may be primary (idiopathic) or secondary to ocular conditions diseases such as uveitis, retinal detachment, retinitis pigmentosa, toxoplasmosis, and Coats syndrome. Clinically, single or multiple yellow or pink retinal nodules are seen in the pre-equatorial retina, and typically in the infero-temporal retina. Visual loss due to macular exudates, oedema, epiretinal membrane, exudative retinal detachment, vitreous haemorrhage, and rubeotic glaucoma may prompt presentation, usually in patients between 40–60 years of age. FFA demonstrates profuse leakage from capillary or telangiectatic vessels within the tumour. The differential diagnosis includes eccentric choroidal neovascularization, capillary haemangioma, choroidal melanoma, and choroidal haemangioma. The management is conservative for small, asymptomatic, peripheral lesions. Cryotherapy, brachytherapy, and PDT have been used with some success. Vitrectomy may be indicated for recurrent vitreous haemorrhage and epiretinal membrane.

Hamartoma of the RPE and retina

These benign lesions are sometimes associated with a systemic cancer syndrome or phacomatosis.

Typical congenital hypertrophy of RPE

Typical congenital hypertrophy of RPE (CHRPE) typically appears as a solitary, round, flat, well-defined, deeply pigmented lesion (see Figure 5.35a). With time, depigmentation around or within the lesion may appear, forming a halo or lacunae, respectively. Although the overlying retina appears normal clinically, histology shows loss of photoreceptors in the area of CHRPE. A 'bear tracks' arrangement of multiple typical CHRPE lesions is not uncommon. Typical CHRPE lesions are not associated with systemic disease.

Atypical CHRPE

Atypical CHRPE or 'multiple RPE hamartomas' usually have four or more variably sized lesions (see Figure 5.35b) in one or both eyes (as small as 50 μm) and are of variable shape (round, oval, comet-shaped, irregular). Larger lesions with depigmented haloes and RPE mottling may be accompanied by small satellite lesions. Atypical CHRPE can occur as an extracolonic manifestation of Gardner syndrome, which is caused by a germline mutation of APC (5q21). Similar to retinoblastoma, the inheritance of this condition is dominant but its molecular mechanism is recessive. Other extracolonic features may include bone and soft tissue hamartomas or dental abnormalities.

Combined hamartoma of RPE and retina

These lesions may be associated with neurofibromatosis type 1 or type 2. This tumour is composed of RPE, vascular, and glial tissues forming a solitary elevated lesion in the posterior pole, around the disc or mid-peripheral retina. Varying pigmentation, vascular tortuosity, and epiretinal membranes are characteristic. Visual loss may be due to direct involvement of the fovea, the papillomacular bundle, or the optic disc. It may also be secondary to associated epiretinal membrane, vitreous haemorrhage, or CNV.

Astrocytic hamartoma

Astrocytic hamartomas occur in patients with tuberous sclerosis. It is usually located at or near the optic disc, appearing as a white, calcified, endophytic nodular mass or a flat, translucent, smooth intraretinal tumour. Visual loss can occur because of vitreous haemorrhage from the tumour or retinal neovascularization. Systemic workup should include a CT head scan and renal ultrasound. Two genes responsible for tuberous sclerosis are TSC1 (Chromosome 9q34) and TSC2 (Chromosome 16p13).

Posterior segment and paraneoplastic syndromes

Cancer-associated retinopathy

Over half of cancer-associated retinopathies are associated with lung carcinomas. Development of anti-recoverin and other anti-retinal autoantibodies may account for the features of photoreceptor loss, progressive visual loss (typically ring scotoma and nyctalopia), vascular attenuation, pigmentary changes, minimal vitritis, and extinguished response on electroretinography (ERG). In melanoma-associated retinopathy, anti-bipolar cell autoantibodies may cause non-progressive central visual loss, nyctalopia, and an electronegative ERG. Visual prognosis is generally poor, with treatment of the primary tumour not appearing to alter the final visual acuity.

Bilateral diffuse uveal melanocytic proliferation

Bilateral diffuse uveal melanocytic proliferation is characterized by diffuse uveal thickening, multiple, slightly elevated uveal melanocytic lesions, multiple round or oval red patches at the level of RPE, with corresponding angiographic leakage, exudative retinal detachment, and progressive cataract. The onset of these features may predate the discovery of malignancy (e.g. ovarian or pancreatic carcinoma) by 3–12 months.

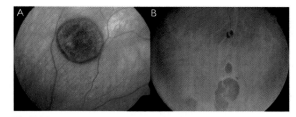

Fig 5.35 Colour fundus photographs of (a) solitary typical and (b) multifocal atypical congenital hypertrophy of retinal pigment epithelium

CHAPTER 5 **Vitreoretinal surgery**

187

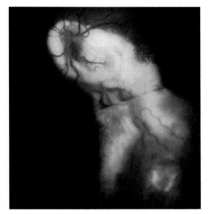

Fig 5.33 Composite colour fundus photograph showing capillary haemangioma with extensive exudation in a patient with von Hippel–Lindau syndrome

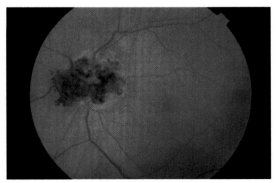

Fig 5.34 Colour fundus photograph showing cavernous haemangioma at the optic disc

Primary tumours of the choroid may originate from melanocytic, vascular, neural, or connective tissues cells. Many are benign tumours (neoplasms of tissue normally found at the site, e.g. melanocytic naevi and haemangioma) or choristomas (neoplasms of tissue not normally found at the site, e.g. choroidal osteoma). Neoplastic infiltration of the choroid from systemic malignancy may occur in lymphoma, leukaemia, carcinoma, and melanoma.

Choroidal naevus

A choroidal naevus is a melanocytic hamartoma composed of naevus cells with limited growth potential. Naevi may rarely transform into melanomas.

- **Age:** >30 years
- **Sex:** M = F
- **Ethnic group:** Caucasian
- **Prevalence:** 1%–8%

A melanocytoma is a special subtype of choroidal naevus with distinct epidemiological, clinical, and histological features.

Aetiology

There is an increased rate of choroidal naevi in patients with neurofibromatosis and dysplastic naevus syndrome.

Pathology

Naevus cells are classified into four types: (1) plump polyhedral naevus cells, (2) slender spindle naevus cells, (3) intermediate naevus cells (with features in-between those of the first two types of cells), and (4) balloon cells (thought to be due to an autoimmune reaction). Melanocytomas are composed exclusively of plump polyhedral naevus cells. Not to be confused with a naevus, ocular melanocytosis is characterized by an increased number of uveal melanocytes rather than naevus cells. Secondary degenerative changes in the choriocapillaris, Bruchs membrane, and the RPE are commonly seen overlying the naevus.

Clinical evaluation

- Will this lesion grow (i.e. is it a small melanoma)?
- Is this lesion sight-threatening (i.e. retinal complication)?

History

- Field defect
- Photopsia (consider the possibility of melanoma)

Examination

- Flat or slightly elevated greyish lesion with well-defined borders (see Figure 5.36a)
- Low-risk factors for tumour for growth: small size, overlying drusen, RPE degenerative changes, location greater than two disc diameters from the optic disc
- High-risk factors for tumour for growth: large diameter, orange pigment (lipofuscin), less than two disc diameters from the optic disc, subretinal fluid without CNV (see Figures 5.36b and 5.36c)

Investigations

- **Ultrasound:** less than 2 mm thickness, no internal blood flow
- **Fundus photography:** linear dimensions under seven disc diameters

- **FFA:** hyperfluorescence associated with RPE defect, RPE leak, CNV, or drusen; hypofluorescence associated with choriocapillary closure or pigment masking
- **OCT:** subretinal fluid or retinal oedema

Differential diagnosis

- Small melanoma
- RPE hypertrophy (CHRPE) or hamartoma
- Choroidal metastasis or haemangioma

Management

Low risk of growth

- Observation with annual fundus exam or photography

High risk of growth

- Observation with examinations every 4–6 months
- Consider ultrasound or FFA.

Complicated: CNV

- Laser photocoagulation, PDT

Complications and prognosis

- Misdiagnosing early melanoma as a naevus
- CNV formation with subretinal fluid and haemorrhage
- Optic disc melanocytomas (see Figure 5.36d) may rarely cause central retinal vein occlusion or anterior ischaemic optic neuropathy.

Choroidal haemangioma

Choroidal haemangioma is a vascular hamartoma occurring in two distinct forms: (1) circumscribed and (2) diffuse. The latter type is associated with Sturge–Weber syndrome.

Clinical evaluation

Visual loss due to a circumscribed choroidal haemangioma may be associated with macular oedema or a serous retinal detachment. It is typically found posterior to the equator, usually temporal to the optic disc, with a yellowish or orange-red colour, slight elevation, and associated RPE changes. Subretinal fluid and epiretinal membrane may also occur. Investigation with FFA, ICG angiography, and ultrasound can usually distinguish a choroidal haemangioma from a choroidal melanoma. Diffuse choroidal haemangioma is typically found when screening patients with Sturge–Weber syndrome.

Management

Asymptomatic lesions do not need treatment. Serous retinal detachment may respond to treatment with radiation (external beam or brachytherapy), laser photocoagulation, transpupillary thermotherapy, or PDT.

Complications and prognosis

Rarely, significant growth of the lesion can occur, especially during pregnancy. In addition to causing serous retinal detachment, CNV may complicate circumscribed choroidal haemangioma.

Choroidal osteoma

Choroidal osteoma is typically found in healthy females in their 20s–30s. Familial and bilateral cases have been described. Pathological features suggest an osseous choristoma, although similar ossification may occur following intraocular inflammation.

Clinical evaluation

Visual symptoms may result from an epiretinal membrane or CNV. Typical lesions appear as an oval, placoid, yellow or orange choroidal mass adjacent to the disc. FFA, ultrasound, and CT scanning of the orbit may differentiate this lesion from melanoma, metastasis, haemangioma, AMD, sclerochoroidal calcification, and posterior scleritis.

Management and prognosis

The risk of CNV is greater than 50% over 20 years, and visual acuity is greater than 6/60 in 40% of patients. Laser, PDT, and surgical excision may be used to treat secondary CNV.

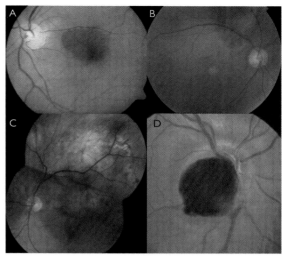

Fig 5.36 Colour fundus photography of (a) a submacular choroidal naevus, (b) a high-risk choroidal naevus with orange pigmentation, (c) a diffuse choroidal melanoma developed from a choroidal naevus with orange pigmentation, and (d) an optic disc melanocytoma composed of plump polyhedral naevus cells with no malignant potential

5.15 Choroidal tumours II

Choroidal melanoma

Choroidal melanoma is the most common intraocular malignancy. Its incidence is one-eighth that of cutaneous melanoma.

- **Age:** median = 55 years
- **Sex:** M = F
- **Ethnic group:** Caucasian
- **Incidence:** 6 per million per year

Aetiology

The risk of melanoma is increased in ocular or oculodermal melanocytosis (lifetime risk of 26 per 10 000), and dysplastic naevus syndrome. Familial cases have rarely been reported. UV exposure may play a role. Assuming all melanomas arise from choroidal naevi, 1 in 5000 naevi per year will transform into melanomas.

Pathology

Melanoma cells are derived from neural crest cells. Histological examination of choroidal melanomas shows spindle cells, clear cells, balloon cells, epithelioid cells, and areas of necrosis. The presence of the latter two is associated with a high mortality rate. Other features that correlate with high mortality are an increased epithelioid cell density, nuclear or nucleolar size, aneuploidy, Monosomy 3, duplication of Chromosome 8, lymphocytes, and certain extracellular matrix patterns. Secondary RPE transformation to lipofuscin-filled macrophages and migration to the subretinal space gives rise to orange pigment. Exudative retinal detachment is common. Tumour extension through Bruchs membrane gives rise to a mushroom-shaped appearance. Extension through the retina may result in vitreous seeding and melanomalytic glaucoma. Extrascleral extension may account for orbital recurrence after enucleation.

Clinical evaluation

- Can it be benign (e.g. melanocytoma/disciform scar)?
- Does it have extra/intraocular extension?
- Risk factors for metastasis?

History

- Visual field defect (associated with the tumour mass or associated exudative retinal detachment)
- Photopsia
- Painful red eye (acute rise in IOP)

Examination

- Elevated dome-shaped lesion with variable pigmentation and vascularity (see Figure 5.37)
- Exudative retinal detachment, macular oedema
- Low-risk features for metastasis: small size
- High-risk features: large diameter (>16 mm), orange pigment, anterior location, subretinal fluid without CNV

Investigations

- Fundus photography
- Ultrasound: tumour height >2 mm, with medium internal reflectivity and internal blood flow (high risk of metastasis if >8–10 mm in height)
- FFA and ICG angiography are usually not required
- Systemic workup for metastasis (liver function test with or without liver ultrasound)

Management

- **Patient characteristics:** age, systemic metastasis, health
- **Tumour characteristics:** size and location, intraocular or extraocular extension, cytogenetic risk factors (if biopsy sample available)
- **Contralateral visual function:** need to conserve vision?

Indeterminate melanocytic lesion

- Observation every 4–6 months with photography and ultrasound
- High-risk lesions may be treated with transpupillary thermal therapy (<3 mm thick, >3 mm from fovea), or laser.

Small-sized melanoma (documented growth)

- Observation (risk of early occult metastasis)
- Transpupillary thermotherapy or laser photocoagulation

Medium-sized melanoma

- Brachytherapy (^{106}Ru up to 5 mm or ^{125}I up to 10 mm; see Figure 5.38)
- Charged particle irradiation
- Lamellar sclerouvectomy (>6 mm thick, <16 mm at the base)
- Vitrectomy and endoresection
- Combination of above

Large-sized melanoma (with or without vitreous seeding, glaucoma)

- Enucleation

Melanoma with extrascleral or optic nerve extension

- Enucleation, with or without pre-enucleation external beam radiotherapy
- Limited exenteration plus pre-enucleation external beam radiotherapy

Melanoma with systemic metastasis

- Enucleation
- Chemoemoblization or resection of solitary hepatic foci

Recurrence from failed-eye-conserving treatment

- Enucleation

Complications and prognosis

- Cataract, vitreous haemorrhage, retinal detachment, radiation retinopathy, optic neuropathy, strabismus, CNV
- Local tumour recurrence: 5%–15% (brachytherapy), 6% (resection), 4% (proton beam)
- Visual function: 50% >6/60, and 30% >6/12 (radiation)
- Metastasis: monitor with a liver function test every 6 months; clinical metastasis manifests in 3–5 years, as predicted by tumour histology and cytogenetics.
- Mortality: 10% at 5 years and 20% at 10 years

Posterior segment metastasis

Ten per cent of patients who die from cancer may have intraocular metastases. Carcinomatous metastases in the choroid are much more common than retinal, vitreal, ciliary body, or iris metastases. Multiple tissue sites may be involved concurrently. In females, two-thirds of choroidal metastases are associated with breast carcinoma and, in males, 40% are associated with lung carcinoma. Despite systemic workup, 1 in 6 may have no detectable primary malignancy. Leukaemia, CNS lymphoma, and systemic/cutaneous lymphoma may affect the eye in 30%–80%, 15%–25%, and 7% of patients, respectively. These haematological malignancies may present with a masquerade syndrome mimicking pan-uveitis or opportunistic infections.

Clinical evaluation

Carcinoma and melanoma

- **Carcinoma:** multiple cream or yellow choroidal lesions with minimal elevation, some RPE clumping, and subretinal fluid
- **Melanoma:** retinal infiltrates with cells extending into the vitreous, forming golden-brown clumps or sheets

Leukaemia and lymphoma

- **Leukaemia:** retinal and optic disc infiltrates with haemorrhage (see Figure 5.39), vitreous cells, and pseudohypopyon
- **Lymphoma:** sub-RPE/choroid yellow infiltrates (leopard spots) with vitreous and anterior chamber cells, and retinal vascular occlusion (see Figure 5.40)

Diagnosis and management

- Systemic workup (tailored to symptoms and risk factors)
- Tissue diagnosis (vitreous, retinal, or choroidal biopsy)
- Systemic or CNS treatment of primary malignancy
- Ocular treatment: systemic chemotherapy, radiation, intraocular methotrextate, and rituximab (lymphoma)

Further reading

1. Singh AD, Kivela T: The collaborative ocular melanoma study. *Ophthalmol Clin N Am* 2005 Mar; **18**(1): 129–142

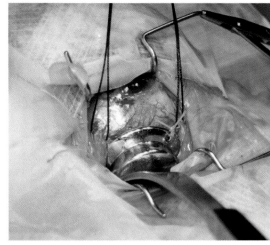

Fig 5.38 Iodine-seeded plaque being sutured to sclera for brachytherapy of choroidal melanoma

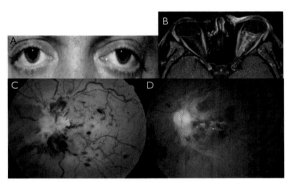

Fig 5.39 Ocular leukaemia: (a) left proptosis with perception of light vision, (b) optic nerve thickening, on a T1-weighted MRI scan of the orbit and brain, and (c) optic nerve head and retinal infiltrates, with combined central retinal vein and artery occlusions. (d) After further chemotherapy, vision did not improve owing to severe optic neuropathy

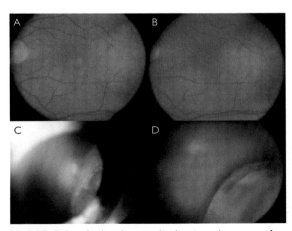

Fig 5.37 Colour fundus photographs showing enlargement of a choroidal melanoma over a 2-year period from (a) to (b) with development of cystoid macular oedema and macular pigmentary changes and a patient with large anterior choroidal-ciliary body melanoma seen on (c) slit lamp and (d) fundoscopy

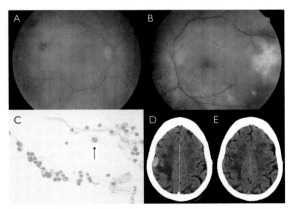

Fig 5.40 Primary CNS lymphoma: subretinal pigment epithelium infiltrates, vascular occlusion, retinal haemorrhage, and vitreous cells (a, b). (c) Vitreous biopsy showed atypical lymphocytes (arrow). Three months after onset of vitritis, the patient presented with (d) complex partial seizure due to (d) cerebral lymphoma; contrast-enhancing cortical lesion on head CT. (e) After radiotherapy, the cortical lesion reduced in size. Ocular lesions resolved with orbital radiotherapy

5.16 Vitreoretinopathies

Vitreoretinopathy describes a number of pathological processes which have a common association with retinal detachment.

1. Proliferative vitreoretinopathy: a growth and contraction of cellular membranes within the vitreous cavity and on both retinal surfaces leading to traction following RRD
2. Hereditary vasculoretinopathies, or proliferative retinopathies, are a group of disorders characterized by an arrest of retinal vasculogenesis, leading to retinal neovascularization, fibrous tissue proliferation, and tractional retinal detachment. Associated systemic manifestations may be present.
3. Hereditary vitreoretinopathies, or hyaloideoretinal degenerations, refer to a group of disorders characterized by fibrillar or membranous vitreous changes which may lead to an optically empty vitreous, varying degrees of chorioretinal atrophy, myopia, cataract, a risk of RRD, orofacial malformation, skeletal abnormalities, and hearing loss.

Hereditary vasculoretinopathies

These disorders are distinguished from one another by inheritance patterns, ophthalmic features, and systemic manifestations.

Familial exudative vitreoretinopathy

Familial exudative vitreoretinopathy may be inherited via autosomal dominant, autosomal recessive, or X-linked recessive patterns. Mutation in the *FZD4* or *LRP5* genes have been found in affected individuals. Clinical features vary from asymptomatic temporal retinal vascular insufficiency demonstrable with FFA to bilateral severe fibrovascular proliferation and retinal detachment (in 20% of cases) due to a combination of retinal vascular exudation, vitreoretinal traction, and retinal breaks. Non-progressive falciform retinal folds (typically extending from the optic disc to the inferotemporal retina) are seen in up to 40% of eyes. There are no associated systemic features. Treatment is directed towards reducing VEGF production by laser or cryoablation of avascular retina.

Norrie syndrome

This X-linked recessive condition is associated with a mutation in the norrin gene, which plays a role in retinal vasculogenesis. Affected males are blind at birth because of retinal dysplasia. The presenting feature is often leucocoria caused by bilateral retinal detachments or retrolental masses. Developmental delay and cognitive disability occur in up to 50% of cases and during adolescence over 50% of cases develop severe hearing loss. Although no treatment is available, genetic counselling and prenatal diagnosis may be helpful.

Incontinentia pigmenti (Bloch–Sulzberger syndrome)

This X-linked dominant condition is due to a mutation in the nuclear factor kappa B essential modulator (NEMO) gene. The condition is lethal in most but not all males. Affected females may develop hyperpigmented skin lesions at around 6 months of age, and later develop alopecia, hypodontia, dystrophic nails, cognitive delay, and retinal vascular abnormalities. Visual loss may occur because of retinal neovascularization, tractional retinal detachment, or macular or occipital lobe infarction.

Hereditary vitreoretinopathies

These disorders are characterized by vitreous degeneration associated with mutations in genes coding for collagen, versican, or potassium channels.

Stickler syndrome

Stickler syndrome, which is an autosomal dominant condition, is due to a mutation in genes coding for collagen type 2 (*COL2A1*) or type 11 (*COL11A1*). Diagnostic clinical criteria include a congenital vitreous anomaly (seen on slit lamp examination as a membranous vitreous structure visible behind the lens or as aggregations of beaded vitreous fibrils), and any three of the following: (1) onset of myopia before 6 years of age, (2) RRD or paravascular pigmented lattice changes, (3) joint hypermobility with an abnormal Beighton score, (4) sensorineural hearing loss, and (5) midline clefting. Other ocular findings may include non-progressive cataract, ectopia lentis, glaucoma, and giant retinal tears.

Hyaloideoretinal degenerations (Wagner syndrome, Jansen syndrome)

Wagner syndrome and Jansen syndrome are autosomal dominant ocular conditions affecting the vitreous and retina. Wagner syndrome is due to a mutation in the *CSPG2/versican* gene and is characterized by an optically empty vitreous cavity with thickened and incompletely separated posterior vitreous cortex. Other features include nyctalopia, ring scotoma, mild-to-moderate myopia, early-onset cataract, peripheral tractional retinal detachment (55%), ectopic fovea, progressive loss of rod and cone ERG responses, and chorioretinal atrophy.

Goldmann–Favre syndrome

This autosomal recessive condition is characterized by nyctalopia in early childhood, vitreous syneresis with veils and membranes, macular and peripheral retinoschisis, pigmentary retinopathy, hypermetropia, an electronegative ERG, and an abnormal electrooculogram. Mutations in the *NR2E3* gene may affect photoreceptor function, leading to increased sensitivity of S cones.

Snowflake vitreoretinal degeneration

This autosomal dominant condition, linked to mutations in the *KCNJ13* gene, is characterized by early-onset cataract, fibrillar vitreous degeneration, granular and minute crystalline deposits near the equatorial retina, corneal guttae, and optic nerve head dysplasia. Retinal detachment can occur in 20% of cases, but systemic features are absent. The condition progresses from extensive white-with-pressure to the snowflake features, chorioretinal pigmentary changes and vascular sheathing, and then finally the disappearance of peripheral retinal vessels. In the late stages, the ERG is reduced, with visual field constriction.

Collagen disorders associated with retinal detachment

Other systemic disorders associated with vitreous syneresis, myopia, and an increased risk of RRD include Marfan syndrome, Weill–Marchesani syndrome, spondyloepiphyseal dysplasia, Kniest dysplasia, and Knobloch syndrome.

The posterior segment may be involved in both ocular and systemic injuries. Direct ocular trauma is the cause of a significant proportion of blindness in young adults.

Aetiology

Ocular injuries involving the posterior segment

- Mechanical trauma:
  - Closed-globe injury: contusion, lamellar laceration with or without a superficial foreign body
  - Open-globe injury: penetrating (full-thickness entry wound) or perforating (full-thickness entry and exit wounds) injury with or without an intraocular foreign body; globe rupture (full-thickness wound from blunt force)
- Electromagnetic radiation:
  - Radiation retinopathy and optic neuropathy
  - Retinal laser burns
  - Solar maculopathy
  - Lightning retinopathy

Systemic injuries affecting the posterior segment

- Shaken baby syndrome
- Terson syndrome
- Purtscher retinopathy

Pathophysiology

Blunt ocular injury

Blunt globe trauma may cause a rupture of the sclera at its weakest locations (rectus muscle insertions, optic nerve head, or previous surgical wound). Even in the absence of a scleral rupture, vitreoretinal traction induced by compression and decompression of the globe can cause a retinal dialysis (disinsertion of retina at ora serrata), avulsion of vitreous base, retinal tears, or a macular hole (see Figure 5.41). The choroid may rupture, typically in a circumferential pattern around the optic nerve head. The photoreceptor–RPE complex can be sheared, in which case commotio retinae may result. With severe trauma, the retina and choroid can undergo contusional necrosis (retinitis sclopetaria).

Penetrating ocular injury

A sharp object may penetrate or perforate the globe, causing a retinal break, retinal detachment, or vitreous haemorrhage. Intraocular foreign bodies with a significant copper or iron content can cause chalcosis or siderosis, respectively (see Table 5.4). The risk of endophthalmitis is 10% and the onset is usually acute.

Systemic trauma

In shaken baby syndrome, increased intracranial pressure and vitreoretinal traction may lead to multiple retinal haemorrhages, vitreous haemorrhage, and circular retinal folds. In Terson syndrome, a subarachnoid haemorrhage causes an acute rise in intracranial pressure with a resultant acute reduction in retinal venous outflow, damage to peripapillary tissues, rupture of retinal capillaries, and vitreous haemorrhage. Purtscher retinopathy is due to embolic occlusion of the pre-capillary arterioles, typically occurring following visceral or orthopaedic injury. A

Table 5.4 Comparison between siderosis and chalcosis

Ocular features	Chalcosis	Siderosis
Acute reaction	Pan-ophthalmitis	Non-specific inflammation
Affinity for tissue	Basement membrane	Neuro-epithelial cells
Cornea	Descemet membrane deposit, Kayser–Fleischer ring	Deposit in corneal endothelium and stroma, angle damage
Iris	None	Deposit in iris stroma and epithelium causing brown iris and tonic pupil
Lens	Lenticular capsule deposit forming sun flower cataract	Deposit in lens epithelium forming yellow cataract
Vitreous	Fibrotic mass encapsulating intraocular foreign body	Metallic intraocular foreign body
Retina–RPE	Internal limiting membrane deposit	Deposit in RPE causing atrophy and visual field loss; reduction in B-wave may be reversible

similar Purtscher-like retinopathy may occur in association with pancreatitis.

Clinical evaluation of ocular injuries

History

- Timing and mechanism of injury (nature of object, infection, or likelihood of retained foreign body)
- Circumstance of the injury (compensation claim)
- Eye protection worn at the time of injury
- Immediate ophthalmic treatment
- Previous ocular surgery (see Figure 5.42)
- Associated maxillofacial, neurologic, and systemic injuries (see Figure 5.43)

Examination

- Inspection of periocular skin for puncture wounds
- Document visual acuity and pupil responses.
- Careful inspection to identify corneal, limbal, or scleral wounds which may be small and self-sealing
- Deep anterior chamber with very low IOP: suspect posterior rupture
- Visualize the posterior segment.
- Need to distinguish between closed- and open-globe injuries
- Exclude intraocular foreign body and endophthalmitis in open-globe injuries.

Investigations

- Document injuries with photographs (important in cases of subsequent medico-legal action).
- A B-scan is useful in detecting posterior scleral rupture, retinal detachment, choroidal detachment, and intraocular

foreign body when associated anterior segment pathology or vitreous haemorrhage prevents fundal visualization.

* A CT scan and a facial X-ray may be indicated to assess for orbital injuries and may detect an intraocular foreign body.

Management

Initial management

* **If endophthalmitis is suspected or present:** systemic and intravitreal (during globe repair) antibiotics; need to cover *Bacillus cereus* (25% of cases) with vancomycin
* **Intraocular foreign body:** systemic antibiotics and removal of intraocular foreign body
* **Open-globe injury:** examination under anaesthetic with primary repair, disinsert rectus muscles if unable to visualize posterior limit of scleral wounds. A primary enucleation or evisceration is generally avoided unless primary repair is impossible.
* **Closed-globe injury:** no immediate specific treatment required for choroidal rupture, sclopetaria, or macular hole. Laser retinopexy is required for new retinal tears.

Review

* After open-globe repair, monitor daily for any wound leak, onset of infection, or retinal detachment.
* Secondary repair, if required, is usually performed 4–10 days after initial injury.
* In closed-globe injury, monitor for raised IOP, cataract, lens dislocation, and PVD-induced retinal tear.
* Delayed complications: macular pigmentary changes from commotio retinae, epiretinal membrane, retinal detachment, sympathetic ophthalmia, CNV, traumatic macular hole, non-clearing vitreous haemorrhage, siderosis, chalcosis

Complications

* Failure to diagnose an open-globe injury, especially when the entry wound is small or imaging is not performed in the presence of a poor fundal view
* A missed intraocular foreign body may lead years later to chronic siderosis, which may cause irreversible visual loss despite the removal of the intraocular foreign body.
* **Retinal dialysis and retinal detachment:** scleral buckling or vitrectomy surgery
* **Non-clearing vitreous haemorrhage and persistent macular hole:** vitrectomy. The timing of surgery is controversial.

Prognosis

* **Closed-globe injury:** prognosis depends upon the macular status; poor outcome associated with choroidal rupture underlying the fovea
* **Open-globe injury:** posterior limit of scleral wound determines visual outcome. A high rate of proliferative vitreoretinopathy limits the success of retinal detachment surgery.

Further reading

1. Pieramici DJ, Sternberg P Jr, Aaberg TM Sr, et al.: A system for classifying mechanical injuries of the eye (globe). The Ocular Trauma Classification Group. *Am J Ophthalmol* 1997 Jun; **123**(6): 820–883

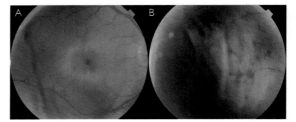

Fig 5.41 Blunt ocular injury resulting in (a) macular hole and (b) retinal detachment secondary to retinal dialysis

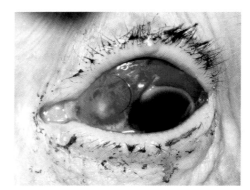

Fig 5.42 Blunt ocular injury resulting in globe rupture and extrusion of intraocular lens

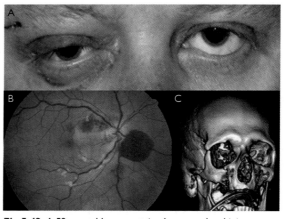

Fig 5.43 A 53-year-old man sustained a severe head injury resulting in (a) right traumatic oculomotor nerve palsy, (b) Purtscher retinopathy, with cotton wool spots, retinal and preretinal haemorrhages, and macular branch retinal artery occlusion, and (c) severe craniofacial fractures complicated by intracranial haemorrhage

Venki Sundaram and Michel Michaelides

Clinical assessment

Clinical knowledge

6.1 Fundus fluorescein angiography

Anatomy

Fundus fluorescein angiography (FFA) is type of fundus photography in which a series of images taken in rapid sequence is obtained following an intravenous injection of fluorescein sodium. FFA is done to image both retinal and choroidal circulation.

General principles

Fluorescence is the property of certain molecules to emit light energy of a longer wavelength when stimulated by light of a shorter wavelength. Fluorescein sodium is an orange, water-soluble dye that, when injected intravenously, remains largely intravascular and circulates in the bloodstream. About 70%–85% of injected fluorescein binds to serum proteins (bound fluorescein), and the remainder remains unbound (free fluorescein). The choriocapillaris allows free fluorescein to pass through it (the walls of the choriocapillaris contain multiple fenestrations) whereas the inner blood–retinal barrier does not allow any physiological fluorescein leakage. The excitation peak for fluorescein is 490 nm and the emission is at 530 nm.

Purpose of the test

* To aid diagnosis and assess disease severity in many common diseases, e.g. diabetic retinopathy, macular oedema, central serous chorioretinopathy, age-related macular degeneration, and vascular occlusive disease
* To help guide laser procedures

Contraindications

* Known allergy to fluorescein
* Severe renal impairment

Procedure

* Check which eye to start imaging in the first instance.
* Patient preparation:
  - Explain procedure.
  - Discuss risks and benefits.
  - Obtain formal consent.
  - Dilate pupils.
  - Obtain intravenous access.
  - Make sure a resuscitation trolley is available.
  - Seat patient comfortably and align camera.
  - Ask patient to focus on fixation target in camera.
* Take colour and 'red-free' fundus photographs.
* Inject intravenous fluorescein (5 ml of a 20% solution) rapidly, then follow with a saline flush through the cannula.
* Initially, take a series of rapid-sequence photographs (1-second intervals, for 25–30 seconds).
* Take images at a lower frequency between 5 and 10 minutes after injection.
* Take late images at 10–20 minutes after injection.

Side effects

* Mild:
  - Yellow discolouration of the skin (common)
  - Yellow discolouration of the urine (common)
  - Nausea (not infrequent) and vomiting (uncommon)
* Moderate:
  - Urticaria (1 : 82)
  - Syncope (1 : 340)
* Severe:
  - Severe anaphylaxis (1 : 1900)
  - Seizures (1 : 14 000)
  - Fatal anaphylaxis (1 : 220 000)

Phases of the normal angiogram

Fluorescein enters the eye through the ophthalmic artery, passing into the choroidal circulation through the short posterior ciliary arteries and into the retinal circulation through the central retinal artery. The choroidal circulation is filled 1 second earlier than the retinal circulation because the route to the retinal vasculature is longer than that to the choroidal vasculature. Angiograms are best read sequentially according to their phases, as follows:

Comment on the red-free photograph

Ensure that the red-free photograph is assessed prior to proceeding to comment upon the rest of the examination.

Choroidal (pre-arterial) phase

* Occurs 8–12 seconds after injection
* Patchy filling of the choroid, because of leakage of free fluorescein through the fenestrated choriocapillaris. A cilioretinal artery, if present (present in ~20% of the population), will fill at this time because it is derived from the posterior ciliary circulation.

Arterial phase

* The retinal arteries start filling with fluorescein whilst choroidal filling continues (see Figure 6.1).

Arteriovenous (capillary) phase

* This phase is characterized by complete filling of the arteries and capillaries with early lamellar flow in the veins (dye seen along walls of veins; see Figure 6.2).
* Choroidal filling continues; choroidal fluorescence increases as free fluorescein leaks from the choriocapillaris.

Venous phase

* **Early venous:** complete arterial and capillary filling, more marked lamellar venous flow
* **Mid-venous:** almost complete venous filling
* **Late venous:** complete venous filling with reduced arterial concentration of dye (see Figure 6.3).

Late (elimination) phase

* Dilution and elimination of the dye
* Late staining of the optic disc is normal.
* Fluorescein is normally absent from the angiogram after 10–15 minutes.

Why is the fovea dark?

* Avascularity of the foveal avascular zone
* Blockage of background choroidal fluorescence due to an increased density of xanthophyll pigment at the fovea
* Retinal pigment epithelium (RPE) cells are larger and contain more melanin at the fovea than elsewhere in the retina.

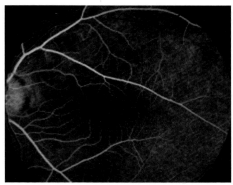

Fig 6.1 Arterial phase of a fluorescein angiogram showing arterial filling

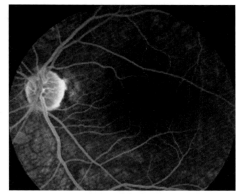

Fig 6.3 Late venous phase

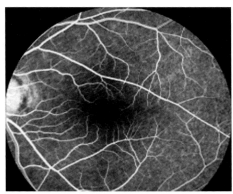

Fig 6.2 Arteriovenous phase showing filling of arteries and early filling of veins

6.2 Abnormal fluorescein angiography

Whilst reporting an angiogram, it is important to recognize areas of abnormal fluorescence and determine whether they are hyperfluorescent or hypofluorescent.

Hyperfluorescence

Increased fluorescence is seen as a result of pseudofluorescence, autofluorescence, RPE window defects, or leakage, pooling, or staining of dye.

Preinjection fluorescence

* **Pseudofluorescence:** occurs when the blue exciter filter and the green barrier filter overlap; the overlapping light passes through the system, reflects off highly reflective surfaces, and stimulates the film; e.g. in scar tissues and exudates.
* **Autofluorescence:** emission of fluorescent light from ocular structures in the absence of fluorescein sodium; e.g. in optic nerve head drusen and astrocytic hamartomas

Transmitted fluorescence (RPE window defect)

* RPE atrophy causes unmasking of normal background choroidal fluorescence.
* Characterized by early hyperfluorescence, which increases in intensity and then fades without changing in size or shape
* Examples: macular hole and geographic age-related macular degeneration

Leakage of dye

* Dye leaking into the extravascular space
* May occur because of:
  - Abnormal retinal or disc vasculature (see Figure 6.4), e.g. proliferative diabetic retinopathy (PDR)
  - Abnormal choroidal vasculature, e.g. choroidal neovascular membrane
  - Breakdown in the inner blood–retinal barrier, e.g. macular oedema
* Normally fluorescein empties almost completely from the retinal and choroidal circulations in about 10–15 minutes after injection. Any fluorescence that remains in the fundus after the retinal and the choroidal vessels have emptied of fluorescein is extravascular fluorescence and thereby represents leakage.

* Abnormalities in either or both of the two vascular systems can produce abnormal late fluorescence, which is accompanied by leakage if defects are present in the barrier to fluorescein:
  - The retinal vascular system barrier is formed by the tight junctions between retinal vessel endothelial cells.
  - The barrier to the choroidal circulation is the integrity of the RPE.
* Characterized by hyperfluorescence that increases in intensity and size

Pooling of dye

* Defined as leakage of fluorescein into a distinct anatomic space; due to a breakdown of the outer blood–retinal barrier
* In the sub-RPE space: as in pigment epithelial detachment, is characterized by early hyperfluorescence that increases in intensity but not in size

Staining of dye

* Defined as leakage of fluorescein into tissue or material
* Characterized by late hyperfluorescence which does not increase in size, has clear margins, and does not fade in comparison to window defects
* Examples: disciform scars and drusen (see Figure 6.5)

Hypofluorescence

* Reduction or absence of fluorescence may be due to blockage (masking) of a normal quantity of fluorescein or due to filling defects.
* **Blocked fluorescence:** fluorescence can be blocked by lesions at various anatomical levels; appearing dark throughout the angiogram:
  - Pre-choroidal lesions: subretinal blood (see Figure 6.6), pigment (choroidal naevi), lipid
  - Intraretinal lesions: haemorrhages, lipid
  - Preretinal lesions: media opacity, haemorrhage
* **Filling defects** may result from:
  - Vascular occlusion (see Figure 6.4); may involve the retinal or the choroidal vasculature, e.g. retinal artery occlusions, capillary dropout seen in diabetic retinopathy, choroidal infarcts secondary to accelerated hypertension

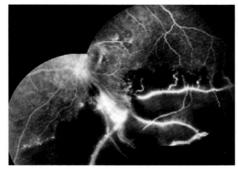

Fig 6.4 Angiogram showing areas of hypofluorescence due to filling defects, and areas of hyperfluorescence due to leakage from retinal neovascularization

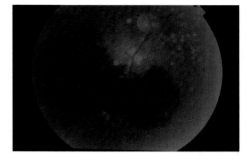

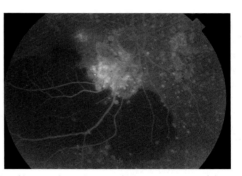

Fig 6.6 Above: colour photograph showing an area of dense retinal haemorrhage. Below: blocked fluorescence

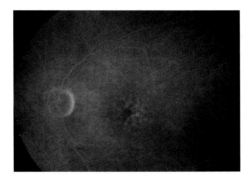

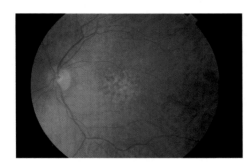

Fig 6.5 Above: colour photograph showing multiple confluent soft drusen. Below: angiogram showing staining of drusen

6.3 Indocyanine green angiography

Indocyanine green (ICG) is a dye which was first used in ophthalmology by Flower and Hochheimer in the early 1970s to image the choroidal circulation, but it was only in the early 1990s that it became an established method of investigation. The fluorescence efficiency of ICG is 25 times less that of fluorescein sodium. ICG dye is 98% protein bound and, as a result, the amount of leakage through the fenestrated choriocapillaris is minimized, so that there is an enhanced delineation of the choroidal circulation.

Technique

ICG, a tricarbocyanine dye, is injected intravenously and is imaged as it passes through ocular vessels. An excitation filter with a peak at 805 nm, and a barrier filter with a transmission peak of 835 nm, which corresponds to the maximum fluorescence emitted by the dye in whole blood, are required. The standard technique is to slowly inject 25 mg of ICG dye dissolved in 5 ml of water. The circulating dye is rapidly excreted by the biliary system. In addition to early photographs, late images at 5, 10, 15, and 20 minutes are taken.

Normal angiogram

* Early phase: 1 minute after injection
  - Dye in larger and middle-sized choroidal vessels
* Middle phase: 5–15 minutes after injection
  - Diffuse homogenous choroidal fluorescence
* Late phase: after 15 minutes
  - No details of retinal or choroidal circulation
  - Choroidal neovascularization (CNV) is seen as a hyperfluorescent lesion in the late phase.

Adverse reactions

* Safe and well tolerated; adverse reaction less common than with FFA
* Minor (1 : 666): nausea, vomiting, sneezing, transient itching, discomfort, dye extravasation
* More severe: urticaria, syncope, fainting, pyrexia
* Severe (1 : 1900): hypotensive shock, anaphylaxis

Contraindications

* Known allergy to the dye
* Iodine allergy
* Significant liver disease
* Seafood allergies
* Uraemia
* Pregnancy

Main indications and features

* Patient allergic to fluorescein
* Choroidal lesions (see Figure 6.7)
* Inflammatory choroidal disorders
* When large haemorrhagic lesions of retina preclude view of the choroid (see Figure 6.8)

Birdshot chorioretinopathy

* Multiple widespread hypofluorescent lesions

Multifocal choroiditis

* Hypopigmented lesions in the late stages of the angiogram
* Zone of peripapillary hypofluorescence may be seen

Multiple evanescent white dot syndrome

* Dots and spots configuration: small hypofluorescent spots on larger hypofluorescent areas

Acute zonal occult outer retinopathy

* Well-demarcated zonal abnormalities
* Multiple hypofluorescent spots
* Serpiginous choroiditis
* Occult satellite lesions

Vogt–Koyanagi–Harada syndrome

* Exudative detachments

Idiopathic polypoidal choroidal vasculopathy

* ICG shows small hyperfluorescent 'polyps' in regions of aneurysmal dilatation (see Figure 6.7).

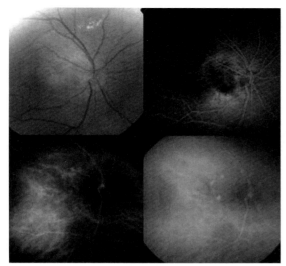

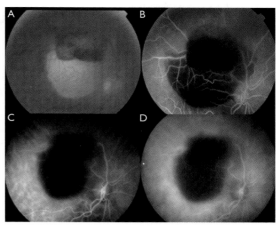

Fig 6.7 Idiopathic polypoidal choroidal vasculopathy
Top left: a red-free image showing a pale lesion adjacent to the disc. Top right: a fluorescein angiogram shows a non-specific hypofluorescent lesion with surrounding areas of hyperfluorescence. Bottom left: an early indocyanine green image showing choroidal vessels and early filling of polyps. Bottom right: a late indocyanine green image showing vascular choroidal polyps

Fig 6.8 (a) Colour fundus photograph showing a trilaminar submacular haemorrhage extending to the superior arcade. (b) Fluorescein angiography showing an area of hypofluorescence corresponding to the haemorrhage. (c, d) Indocyanine green angiograms showing an area of hypofluorescence corresponding to the haemorrhage but no underlying choroidal neovascularization

6.4 Fundus autofluorescence imaging

Principles

Fundus autofluorescence (FAF) imaging is a diagnostic technique for documenting the presence of fluorophores in the human eye. Fluorophores are chemicals that possess fluorescent properties when exposed to light of an appropriate wavelength. Fluorescence occurs when these molecules absorb electromagnetic energy, which excites them to a higher energy state and triggers the emission of light at wavelengths longer than the excitation source. FAF imaging is used to record fluorescence that may occur naturally in the eye or accumulate as a by-product of a disease process. The term 'autofluorescence' is used to differentiate this type of fluorescence from that which occurs from the administration of fluorescent dyes such as fluorescein or ICG.

Abnormalities

FAF imaging is currently used to evaluate the deposition of lipofuscin in the RPE. Lipofuscin is a fluorescent pigment that accumulates in the RPE as a metabolic by-product of cell function. Lipofuscin deposition normally increases with age but may also occur because of RPE cell dysfunction or an abnormal metabolic load on the RPE. The dominant fluorophore in lipofuscin is believed to be A2-E, a compound that possesses toxic properties that may interfere with normal RPE cell function. When excited with short-to-medium wavelength illumination, lipofuscin granules autofluoresce, exhibiting a broad emission spectrum from 500 to 750 nm, with peak emission at about 630 nm. FAF imaging has the potential to provide useful information in conditions where the RPE plays a key role in underlying pathophysiology. Increased autofluorescence is a sign of lipofuscin accumulation due to increased outer segment shedding or reduced RPE clearance and may represent areas at high risk for subsequent RPE and photoreceptor cell loss (see Figure 6.9). Areas of reduced autofluorescence represent either loss of RPE cells or reduced photoreceptor outer segment shedding (see Figures 6.10 and 6.11).

Uses

Potential applications of FAF imaging have been explored in a variety of retinal diseases, including age-related macular degeneration and inherited retinal degeneration. Focal areas of increased FAF are often present in a junctional zone adjacent to existing areas of RPE and photoreceptor loss (see Figure 6.9). Longitudinal FAF imaging allows evaluation of the rate and extent of progression of outer retinal/RPE cell loss.

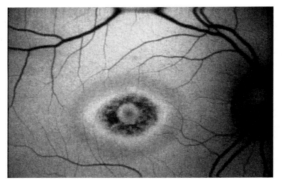 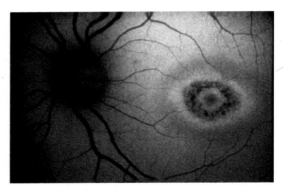

Fig 6.9 Images of a perifoveal area of irregular and reduced autofluorescence, surrounded peripherally and centrally by rings of increased autofluorescence, in a bull's-eye maculopathy-like appearance, in a patient with Stargardt disease

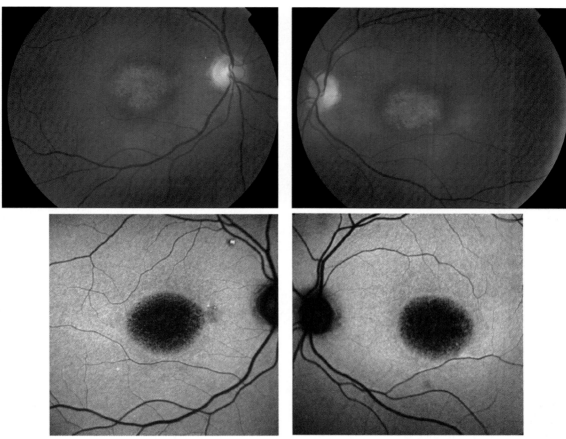

Fig 6.10 Above: colour fundus photo showing macular atrophy in a patient with a cone dystrophy. Below: corresponding area of reduced autofluorescence

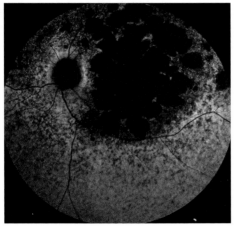

Fig 6.11 Widespread multifocal areas of markedly reduced autofluorescence in a patient with advanced electrophysiological Group 3 (macular and generalized cone and rod dysfunction) Stargardt disease

6.5 Electrophysiology

Electrophysiological examination of the visual system provides objective information in relation to the function of the visual pathways. It can help in establishing the level of any abnormality (e.g. photoreceptor/RPE or inner retina), and also the extent in terms of macular and/or peripheral dysfunction. The standard electrophysiological tests performed include the full-field electroretinogram (ERG), the pattern ERG, and the electro-oculogram (EOG). In addition, the visual evoked potential (VEP) is an assessment of cortical activity in response to a visual stimulus.

ERG

Full-field ERG

A full-field ERG records the massed electrical response of the retina and allows assessment of generalized retinal function under light-adapted (photopic) and dark-adapted (scotopic) states, using a Ganzfeld bowl flash stimulus. The recording is made between a corneal electrode and a reference electrode placed on the patient's forehead.

Components of a normal ERG
- Initial negative a wave: photoreceptor cell activity
- Subsequent positive b wave: bipolar and horizontal cells
- Final prolonged positive c wave: RPE cells
- Electrical events within the ganglion cells or optic nerve fibres do not contribute to the ERG. Thus, disorders such as glaucoma and various types of optic atrophy, which selectively affect ganglion cells or optic nerve, do not necessarily decrease the ERG response.
- Any retinal disorder which prevents generation of the normal a wave will also affect development of the b wave, e.g. retinitis pigmentosa, retinal detachment, and ophthalmic artery occlusion.
- Disorders that cause diffuse degeneration or dysfunction of cells in the inner nuclear layer (Müller or bipolar cells) can selectively decrease the ERG b wave without affecting the a wave, e.g. central retinal artery occlusion (CRAO).
- To reduce a and b wave amplitudes, the disorder must involve a large retinal area.

Standard recording protocol
Recordings should be done according to standards set by the International Society for Clinical Electrophysiology of Vision (see Figure 6.12):
- Pupil dilatation and dark adaptation for 20 minutes:
  1. Rod response: very dim flash of white light
  2. Standard combined: bright white flash to elicit the combined rod and cone response (maximal response); driven primarily by rods, given their far greater number. Oscillations on the upper limb of the b wave are called oscillatory potentials, which are reduced in diabetic retinopathy or vigabatrin toxicity.
  3. High intensity: a high-intensity stimulus can be used to better assess photoreceptor function.

- Light-adapted for 10 minutes
  1. Single flash cone response: a single bright light on a rod-suppressing background elicits cone responses
  2. Thirty-hertz flicker: this frequency of flickering light suppresses rod function further and elicits a pure cone response.

Interpreting ERG results
- Reduced a and b wave:
  - Retinitis pigmentosa
  - Ophthalmic artery occlusion
  - Cancer- and melanoma-associated retinopathy
- Reduced b:a wave ratio ('electronegative ERG'):
  - Congenital stationary night blindness
  - X-linked retinoschisis
- Abnormal photopic, normal scotopic ERG:
  - Cone dystrophy
  - Achromatopsia
- Reduced oscillatory potentials:
  - Diabetic patients with an increased risk of proliferative changes

Pattern ERG
- Retinal response to a structured stimulus, such as a reversing black and white chequerboard or a grating covering 16° of the central visual field
- Generated primarily in the macular region
- Allows objective evaluation of macular function and retinal ganglion cell function
- As it is a small response, recording is technically more difficult.
- Main waveforms: P50 and N95 (see Figure 6.13)
- Selective reduction of P50 indicates macular dysfunction, whereas a normal P50 with a reduced N95 indicates retinal ganglion cell/optic nerve pathology.

Multifocal ERG
- Useful for revealing the degree and extent of central retinal dysfunction
- Simultaneous stimulation of multiple retinal areas (see Figure 6.14)
- Fast stimulation rates (75 Hz) through the use of a rapid random stimulator
- Both eyes are tested simultaneously.
- Takes time and is demanding for the patient; requires good fixation and concentration
- Applications:
  - Retinal dystrophies
  - Macular disease
  - Inflammatory disorders
  - Toxic retinopathies

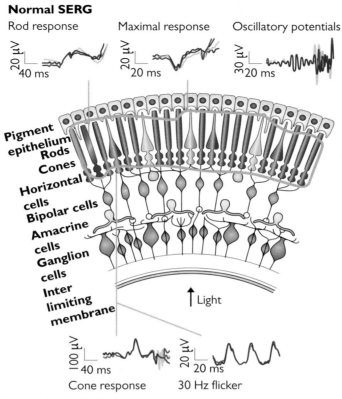

Normal SERG

Rod response   Maximal response   Oscillatory potentials

Pigment
epithelium
Rods
Cones
Horizontal
cells
Bipolar cells
Amacrine
cells
Ganglion
cells
Inter
limiting
membrane

↑ Light

Cone response   30 Hz flicker

Fig 6.12 Normal electroretinogram showing the five components

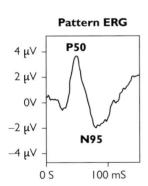

Pattern ERG

4 μV
2 μV
0V
−2 μV
−4 μV

P50

N95

0 S   100 mS

Fig 6.13 Normal pattern electroretinogram
Courtesy of Anthony Robson

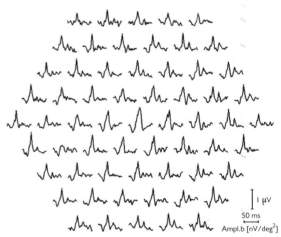

1 μV

50 ms
Ampl.b [nV/deg²]

Fig 6.14 Normal multifocal electroretinogram
Courtesy of Anthony Robson

EOG

An EOG measures the standing potential between the electrically negative back of the eye and the electrically positive cornea. It reflects the activity of the RPE and the photoreceptors. Diffuse and extensive disease of the RPE is needed to affect the EOG response significantly. An eye blinded by lesions distal to the photoreceptors (e.g. optic nerve pathology) will have a normal EOG. An example of a condition that would produce an abnormal EOG is Bests disease.

Technique

* An EOG is performed in both dark- and light-adapted states.
* Electrodes are attached to the skin near the medial and lateral canthi.
* The patient is asked to look rhythmically from side to side. Each time the eye moves, the cornea makes the nearest electrode positive with respect to the other one.
* The potential difference between the two electrodes is amplified and recorded.

* The data are analysed by dividing the height of the potential in the light (light peak) by the height obtained in the dark (dark peak) and expressed as the Arden ratio (percentage). The normal value is over 1.85 (185%; see Figure 6.15).

VEP

A VEP is a gross electrical response recorded from the visual cortex in response to a changing visual stimulus, such as multiple flashes (flash VEP) or chequerboard pattern (pattern-onset/-reversal VEP) stimuli (see Figure 6.16). Pattern-reversal VEP requires good fixation and concentration by the patient. If the patient is unable to fixate well, then pattern-onset VEP is preferred.

Indications

* Optic nerve disease, including demyelination
* Chiasmal and retrochiasmal dysfunction
* Non-organic visual loss

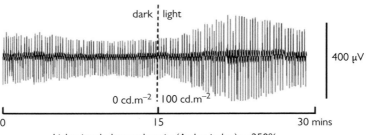

Light rise:dark trough ratio (Arden index) = 250%

Fig 6.15 Normal electroretinogram

Courtesy of Anthony Robson

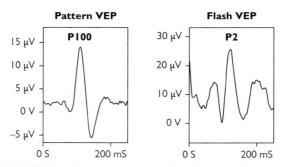

Fig 6.16 Normal pattern-reversal and flash visual evoked potential

Courtesy of Anthony Robson

Diabetes mellitus is estimated to affect 200 million people worldwide and is the commonest cause of blindness in the working population. Diabetes mellitus is divided into type 1 (insulin dependent) and type 2 (insulin independent). The onset of type 1 diabetes is usually during childhood, adolescence, or early adulthood and is due to insulin deficiency, whereas type 2 diabetes typically occurs in adults and is due to acquired insulin resistance. The best predictors of diabetic retinopathy are duration of disease, and glycaemic control. It is very rare to develop diabetic retinopathy before puberty.

Prevalence of diabetic retinopathy

* **Type 1:** rare at diagnosis, and 90% at 15 years
* **Type 2:** 20% at diagnosis, and 60% at 15 years

Risk of retinopathy

* Increased duration of diabetes
* Poor glycaemic control, relevant to both development and progression
* Hypertension, if poorly controlled, is associated with worsening of retinopathy.
* Hypercholesterolaemia
* Nephropathy is associated with worsening of retinopathy.
* Pregnancy may be associated with rapid progression that is often difficult to manage.
* Obesity

Pathogenesis

Diabetic retinopathy is a microangiopathy primarily affecting pre-capillary arterioles, capillaries, and post-capillary venules. Features are of microvascular occlusion and leakage.

* Microvascular occlusion: loss of pericytes, thickening of the basement membrane, damage to and proliferation of endothelial cells, deformation of red blood cells, and increased platelet stickiness and aggregation lead to occlusion with subsequent non-perfusion and hypoxia, which in turn leads to the formation of arteriovenous shunts and neovascularization.
* Microvascular leakage: due to a breakdown of the inner blood–retinal barrier and the resulting formation of microaneurysms, haemorrhages, exudates, and oedema
* Microaneurysms: ischaemia causes weakening of the walls of the capillaries by inducing necrosis of the supporting cells (pericytes); the consequent out-pouching in the capillary wall can be seen as white dots on FFA images. With time, these microaneurysms may fill with basement membrane deposits and consequently may no longer be visualized via FFA.
* Hard exudates: poor perfusion of the vascular bed and damage to the endothelium of the deep capillaries leads to plasma leakage into the outer plexiform layer; this leakage appears as yellow and well-circumscribed deposits. Histologically, 'hard' exudates are eosinophilic masses and contain foamy macrophages that have lipid in their cytoplasm.

* Haemorrhage: breakdown of vessel walls, leading to leakage of red blood cells; can take several forms in the retina:
  — Flame haemorrhages occur in the nerve fibre layer.
  — Dot haemorrhages are in the outer plexiform layer.
  — Blot haemorrhages are larger than dot haemorrhages and represent bleeding from capillaries, with tracking between the photoreceptors and the RPE.
  — Intraretinal microvascular abnormalities are flat new vessels growing from the venous side of the capillary bed within an area of arteriolar non-perfusion.
* Cotton wool spots are fluffy white areas of swelling in the retina and represent micro-infarctions of the nerve fibre layer.

Stages of diabetic retinopathy

The staging of diabetic retinopathy is important in understanding its severity, in order to stratify patients who are at low/moderate/high risk of visual loss. Staging thus helps in the tailoring of appropriate management and follow-up. A classification system used in the Early Treatment Diabetic Retinopathy Study (ETDRS) is widely accepted. In addition, the NHS Diabetic Eye Screening Program has an alternative grading system to guide graders on appropriate referral (see Table 6.1).

Non-proliferative diabetic retinopathy

* Mild non-proliferative diabetic retinopathy (NPDR): microaneurysms only
* Moderate NPDR: microaneurysms, dot and blot haemorrhages (see Figure 6.17), hard exudates, cotton wool spots
* Severe NPDR: one feature of the 4–2–1 rule **(**see Figure 6.18)
  — Intraretinal haemorrhages in all **four** quadrants
  — Venous beading in **two** quadrants
  — Intraretinal microvascular abnormalities in **one** quadrant
* Very severe NPDR: presence of two of the conditions described in the 4–2–1 rule

PDR

* Low risk:
  — Neovascularization of the optic disc (NVD), occurring in less than one-quarter to one-third of the disc area, with no vitreous haemorrhage
  — New vessels elsewhere (NVE), occurring in less than one-half of the disc area and without vitreous haemorrhage (see Figure 6.19)
* High risk:
  — Mild NVD with vitreous haemorrhage (see Figure 6.20)
  — Moderate-to-severe NVD (more than one-quarter to one-third of the disc area)
  — New vessels elsewhere (NVE) in more than one-half of the disc area with vitreous haemorrhage

Diabetic maculopathy

* Macular oedema with hard exudates and/or ischaemia is the most common cause of visual impairment (see Figures 6.21 and 6.22).

Table 6.1 Revised English Diabetic Eye Screening Programme Grading Classification, screening action, and comparative Early Treatment Diabetic Retinopathy Study grading

Grade	Description	Retinopathy	Screening action	ETDRS grading
R0	No retinopathy		Annual recall in screening	No apparent retinopathy
R1	Background	Microaneurysm(s) Retinal haemorrhage(s) Venous loop Any exudate in the presence of other non-referable features of DR Any number of cotton wool spots in the presence of other non-referable features of DR	Annual recall in screening	Mild non-proliferative
R2	Pre-proliferative	Venous beading Venous reduplication Multiple blot haemorrhages Intraretinal microvascular abnormality	Referral and to be seen in clinic within 13 weeks	Moderate non-proliferative Moderately severe non-proliferative
R3a	Active proliferative retinopathy	All newly occurring R3 patients with: • New vessels on disc • New vessels elsewhere • Preretinal or vitreous haemorrhage • Preretinal fibrosis ± tractional retinal detachment	Referral and to be seen in clinic within 2 weeks	Proliferative
R3s	Treated proliferative retinopathy	Evidence of peripheral retinal laser treatment and no active lesions		
M0	No maculopathy		Annual recall in screening	
M1	Maculopathy	Exudate within one disc diameter of the centre of the fovea Group of exudates within the macula Retinal thickening within one disc diameter of the centre of the fovea (if stereo available) Any microaneurysm or haemorrhage within one disc diameter of the centre of the fovea, only if associated with a best visual acuity of ≤6/12 (if no stereo)	Referral and to be seen in clinic with 13 weeks	Clinically significant macular oedema
P	Photocoagulation	Evidence of focal/grid to macula or peripheral scatter		
U	Unclassifiable	An image set that is inadequate for grading		

DR, diabetic retinopathy; ETDRS, Early Treatment Diabetic Retinopathy Study.
Adapted from NHS diabetic eye screening (DES) programme. This information is licenced under the terms of the Open Government Licence v3.0 (https://www.nationalarchives.gov.uk/doc/open-government-licence/version/3/)

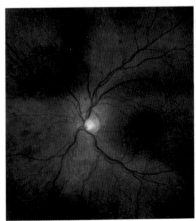

Fig 6.17 Colour fundus photograph of left eye showing microaneurysms and dot and blot haemorrhages

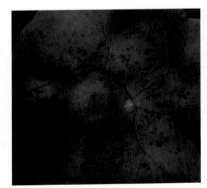

Fig 6.18 Colour fundus photograph of right eye showing severe non-proliferative diabetic retinopathy and maculopathy

Classification

- Focal oedema: well-circumscribed retinal leakage associated with complete or incomplete rings of perifoveal hard exudates; FFA shows late, focal hyperfluorescence due to leakage
- Diffuse oedema: diffuse retinal thickening; FFA shows widespread early hyperfluorescence, microaneurysms, and late diffuse hyperfluorescence due to diffuse leakage
- Ischaemic: macula may clinically appear 'featureless'; capillary non-perfusion on FFA; enlarged foveal avascular zone, perifoveal capillary loss, and a broken irregular foveal capillary ring
- Mixed: features of oedema and ischaemia at the macula
- Clinically significant diabetic macular oedema:
  - Thickening of the retina at or within 500 μm of the centre of the macula
  - Hard exudates at or within 500 μm of the centre of the macula, if associated with thickening of adjacent retina
  - A single zone or multiple zones of retinal thickening one disc area or larger, any part of which is within one disc diameter of the centre of the macula

Systemic complications of diabetes mellitus

- **Microvascular:** peripheral and autonomic neuropathy, nephropathy
- **Macrovascular:** stroke, myocardial infarction, peripheral vascular disease

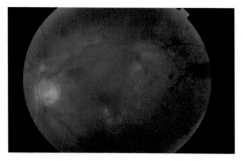

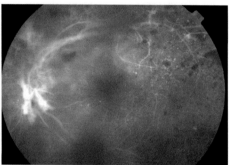

Fig 6.20 Above: colour fundus photograph of the left eye showing new vessels at the optic disc with vitreous haemorrhage. Below: corresponding fluorescein angiogram showing leakage from these new vessels

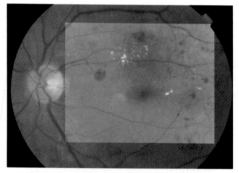

Fig 6.21 Colour fundus photograph showing diabetic maculopathy with hard exudates and dot and blot haemorrhages

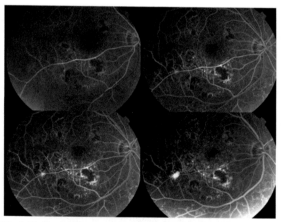

Fig 6.19 Fundus fluorescein angiography showing areas of capillary dropout (non-perfusion) and leaking new vessels elsewhere (increasing area and intensity of hyperfluorescence)

6.7 Diabetic retinopathy II

Management

Optimal diabetic care is best achieved by a multidisciplinary approach comprising a primary care physician, a diabetologist, a nephrologist, an ophthalmologist, and other specialists as needed. Patient education and self-management are critical.

General measures

Lifestyle changes

* Cessation of smoking
* Regular exercise, more than 30 min/day
* Weight control

Glycaemia control

* Aim for HbA1c of 6.5–7.5% (48–58 mmol/mol).

Blood pressure control

* Aim for blood pressure less than 130/80 mmHg, or 125/75 mmHg in patients with proteinuria.

Cholesterol control

* Statin is the first choice, with recent evidence suggesting additional benefit with fenofibrate.

Support of renal function

* Angiotensin-converting enzyme (ACE) inhibitors preferred
* Microalbuminuria is indicative of early nephropathy.

Ophthalmic management

Retinopathy

* No retinopathy: discharge to community screening service for annual review
* Mild NPDR: discharge to community screening service for annual review, or 9–12 month hospital review if severe systemic disease
* Moderate NPDR: review at 6 months, disease progression is common; one study showed 16% progression to PDR over 4 years in type 1 diabetes; laser treatment and FFA are not indicated for this group
* Severe NPDR: review at 4-month intervals, as risk of progression to PDR is high; 50% will develop low-risk PDR, and 15% will develop high-risk PDR in 1 year
* Very severe NPDR: review at 3-month intervals, as 75% will develop PDR, and 45% will develop high-risk PDR in 1 year
* The ETDRS suggested that there should be no laser treatment for mild-to-moderate NPDR; that laser photocoagulation should be considered for use in treating severe or very severe NPDR if follow-up cannot be maintained; and that pan-retinal photocoagulation (PRP) should definitely be used for high-risk PDR.
* High-risk PDR:
  - PRP divided in two or more sessions: 2500–3500 burns in a scatter pattern, extending from the posterior fundus to cover the peripheral retina. Further laser may be required depending on response.
  - Adjust laser power and duration to get a pale white burn (see Figure 6.23); review 4–6 weeks later.
* Regressed PDR: review every 4–6 months

Maculopathy

* Standard therapy for clinically significant diabetic macular oedema (CSMO) has been laser treatment, with ETDRS showing that appropriate macular laser photocoagulation reduces the risk of visual loss of 15 letters by more than 50% when compared with no treatment at all. The goal of laser treatment is to stabilize vision, although vision improves in a minority of patients.
* Macular oedema, which is not clinically significant, should be closely monitored for progression.
* Multiple studies (DRCR.net, READ-2, RESOLVE, RESTORE, RISE, and RIDE) have shown superior results with both intra-vitreal ranibizumab and intravitreal bevacizumab compared to laser therapy, with visual gains of approximately 7–10 letters.
* Adjunctive laser therapy may reduce the number of anti-VEGF required.
* The National Institute for Health and Care Excellence (NICE) has approved ranibizumab and aflibercept in cases where central retinal thickness is ≥400 µm. For other cases, laser treatment according to ETDRS guidelines is indicated.
* In pseudophakic cases that have not responded to non-corticosteroid therapy, or when such treatment is not suitable for them, NICE has approved the use of Ozurdex.
* Intravitreal fluocinolone acetonide (Iluvien) is a long-acting steroid implant that has been approved by NICE for use in chronic (>3 years) pseudophakic cases.

Focal leakage

* Focal argon laser photocoagulation to the centre of leakage or to individual microaneurysms
* Use 50–100 µm spot size × 0.05–0.1 second duration; adjust power to achieve mild slow blanching.
* Review every 3–4 months.

Diffuse leakage

* Grid argon laser photocoagulation to areas of diffuse retinal thickening located more than 500 µm from centre of fovea
* Use 100–200 µm spot size × 0.1 second duration; adjust power to achieve mild, slow blanching.
* Review every 3–4 months.

Ischaemia

* FFA to confirm diagnosis
* Laser photocoagulation is not indicated.

Persistent maculopathy

* Consider repeat laser therapy.
* Consider anti-vascular endothelial growth factor (VEGF) agents.

Resolved maculopathy

* Watch every 4–6 months.

Rubeosis (iris neovascularization)

* With clear media: urgent PRP
* With vitreous haemorrhage: vitrectomy plus endolaser

- Rubeotic glaucoma:urgent PRP with or without procedures to decrease intraocular pressure (IOP). Adjunctive treatment with intravitreal anti-VEGF can aid rapid resolution of new iris vessels and thereby control IOP.

Vitreous haemorrhage

- Adequate view of fundus: PRP
- No view of fundus: repeated ultrasounds to ensure no retinal detachment
- Persistent(1 month in type 1 diabetes and 3–6 months in type 2 diabetes): consideration of vitrectomy plus endolaser

Pars plana vitrectomy: Indications

- Persistent or recurrent vitreous haemorrhage
- Tractional retinal detachment threatening or involving the macula
- Combined tractional and rhegmatogenous retinal detachment
- Premacular subhyaloid haemorrhage
- Uncontrolled PDR despite full PRP

Complications of laser photocoagulation
PRP

- Pain and discomfort, loss of peripheral visual field; with possible loss of driving licence, temporary worsening of central vision, decreased contrast sensitivity, decreased night vision, vitreous haemorrhage

Macular/focal laser

- Extension of laser scar under fovea, inadvertent laser injury to fovea, small paracentral scotoma

Clinical trials

Diabetes Control and Complication Trial

- Purpose: to determine whether intensive blood glucose control (vs standard control) slows the progression of diabetic eye, kidney, and nerve disease in type 1 diabetes
- Conclusions: tight control (HbA1c 7.2% vs 9.0%) was associated with a 76% reduction in retinopathy incidence and a 54% reduction in retinopathy progression, 60% reduction in neuropathy, and 54% reduction in nephropathy.

United Kingdom Prospective Diabetic Study

- Purpose:
  1. To determine whether intensive blood glucose control reduced the risk of complications in type 2 diabetes
  2. To determine whether tight blood pressure control reduced the risk of complications in type 2 diabetes
- Conclusions:
  1. Tight glycaemic control (HbA1c 7.0% vs 7.9%) reduces the risk of major diabetic eye disease by a quarter and early kidney damage by a third.
  2. Tight blood pressure control reduces the risk of strokes, serious visual loss, and death from long-term complications of diabetes by a third.

Direct Retinopathy Candesartan Trials (DIRECT)

- Purpose: three randomized controlled trials to investigate the effects of candesartan on:
  1. DIRECT-Prevent 1: prevent onset of DR in type 1 diabetes
  2. DIRECT-Protect 1: prevent progression or promote DR regression in type 1 diabetes
  3. DIRECT-Protect 2: prevent progression or promote DR regression in type 2 diabetes
- Conclusions:
  1. Prevent 1 showed a 35% reduction in onset of retinopathy.
  2. Protect 1 did not show prevention of progression or promote regression in type 1 diabetes.
  3. Protect 2 showed no significant reduction in progression, but a 34% increase in probability of DR regression in mild-to-moderately severe NPDR. This was the first study to show DR regression induced by a drug.

Action to Control Cardiovascular Risk in Diabetes

- Purpose: to determine whether treatment with fenofibrate (a PPAR alpha agonist) plus simvastatin reduced the progression of mild-to-moderate NPDR in type 2 diabetes
- Conclusions: 40% reduction in progression in patients treated with dual therapy instead on simvastatin alone

Fenofibrate Intervention and Event Lowering in Diabetes

- Purpose: to determine whether treatment with fenofibrate alone reduced the progression of mild-to-moderate NPDR in type 2 diabetes
- Conclusions: approximately 30% reduction in need for laser for CSMO or PDR

Diabetic Retinopathy Study

- Purpose: to determine whether photocoagulation helps prevent severe visual loss from PDR and also to determine whether there was any difference in the efficacy and safety of argon lasers versus xenon lasers
- Conclusions: in patients with high-risk PDR, both argon laser and xenon laser photocoagulation reduced the risk of severe visual loss by more than 50%.

ETDRS

- Purpose:
  1. Is photocoagulation beneficial for diabetic macular oedema?
  2. When in the course of the disease is the best time to begin photocoagulation for diabetic retinopathy?
  3. Does aspirin treatment alter the progress of diabetic retinopathy?
- Conclusions:
  1. Focal photocoagulation for macular oedema reduces the risk of moderate visual loss and should be considered for eyes with clinically significant macular oedema.

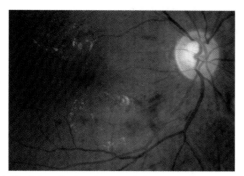

Fig 6.22 Colour fundus photograph showing diabetic maculopathy with hard exudates and dot haemorrhages

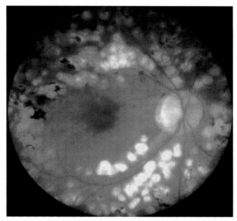

Fig 6.23 Colour fundus photograph showing pan-retinal photocoagulation laser treatment for proliferative diabetic retinopathy

2. Scatter photocoagulation reduces the risk of severe visual loss. Provided adequate follow-up can be managed, it is safe to defer scatter photocoagulation until retinopathy reaches the high-risk stage.
3. Aspirin (650 mg/day) has no significant effect on diabetic retinopathy progression.

Diabetic Retinopathy Vitrectomy Study

* Purpose: to compare early vitrectomy with conventional management (vitrectomy if vitreous haemorrhage fails to clear in 6–12 months) of recent severe vitreous haemorrhage secondary to diabetic retinopathy
* Conclusions:
  — The early vitrectomy group did better (visual acuity 6/12 or better) than the conventional group did (25% vs 15%).
  — The benefit of early vitrectomy was greater in type 1 diabetes (36% vs 12%).
  — At the 4-year follow-up, the conclusions were similar.

6.8 Hypertensive retinopathy

Systemic hypertension is the leading cause of morbidity and mortality worldwide. It affects 60% of people over 60 years of age in the Western world. Hypertensive retinopathy represents the ophthalmic findings of end-organ damage secondary to systemic arterial hypertension.

Risk factors

* Increasing age
* Gender (males > females)
* Ethnicity (blacks > Caucasians)
* Society (industrialized > agricultural)

Types

* Chronic 'essential' hypertension is by far the commonest type; it causes both sclerosis and narrowing of retinal as well as choroidal arterioles.
* Acute or 'accelerated'/'malignant' hypertension accounts for about 1% of cases; it causes fibrinoid necrosis of arterioles and accelerated end-organ damage.

Essential hypertension

* Unknown cause
* Diagnosed when blood pressure over 140 mmHg systolic and/or over 90 mmHg diastolic on two or more occasions

Systemic features

* Usually asymptomatic
* End-organ damage: cardiovascular, cerebrovascular, renal, peripheral vascular

Ophthalmic features

* Narrowing of arterioles (see Figure 6.24)
* Arteriovenous crossing changes (nipping)
* Flame haemorrhages
* Cotton wool spots: small yellowish-white areas in the retina; caused by localized nerve fibre layer infarcts (see Figure 6.25)
* Complications: retinal vein occlusions, macroaneurysms, non-arteritic anterior ischaemic optic neuropathy, retinal artery occlusions, diabetic retinopathy development and progression, glaucoma risk factor

Investigations and treatment

* Liaise with physicians for monitoring and lowering of blood pressure.
* Lifestyle changes:
  — Cessation of smoking
  — Exercise
  — Weight control

Accelerated or malignant hypertension

Systemic features

* Severe raised blood pressure (>220 mmHg systolic or >120 mmHg diastolic)
* Headache
* End-organ damage: myocardial infarction, stroke, encephalopathy, cardiac failure, renal failure

Ophthalmic

* Dimness in vision, double vision, photopsia
* Retinopathy (see Table 6.2):
  — Focal arteriolar narrowing
  — Cotton wool spots
  — Hard exudates
  — Macular oedema
  — Retinal haemorrhages: flame shaped
* Choroidopathy:
  — **Elschnigs spots:** punctate, tan-white lesions that leak on FFA and ICG angiography; represent necrosis and atrophy of RPE due to focal occlusion of choriocapillaries
  — **Siegrists streaks:** linear pigmentation along the choroidal arteries; serous retinal detachments
  — **Hypertensive optic neuropathy:** disc swelling with or without macular oedema (see Figure 6.26)

Investigations and treatment

* Accelerated or malignant hypertension is a medical emergency: refer to a medical team for admission and cautious lowering of blood pressure.

Classification

Table 6.2 Keith–Wagner–Barker classification: Combines findings of arteriosclerosis and hypertension	
Grade 1	Mild-to-moderate arteriolar narrowing
Grade 2	Moderate-to-severe arteriolar narrowing; exaggerated light reflex; arteriovenous crossing changes
Grade 3	Retinal arteriolar narrowing and focal constriction
	Retinal oedema
	Retinal haemorrhage
	Cotton-wool spots
Grade 4	All the above with optic disc swelling

Reproduced with permission from Keith, N. et al, 'Some Different Types of Essential Hypertension: Their Course And Prognosis', *The American Journal of the Medical Sciences*, 197.3. Copyright (1939) with permission from Wolters Kluwer Health, Inc.

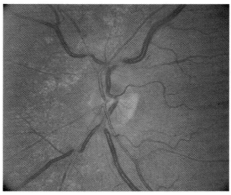

Fig 6.24 Colour photograph showing arteriolar narrowing and arteriovenous crossing changes

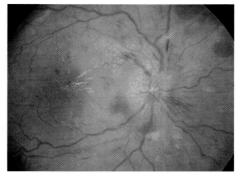

Fig 6.26 Colour photograph showing arteriolar narrowing, cotton wool spots, blot and flame-shaped haemorrhages, partial 'macular star' (exudates), and optic disc swelling

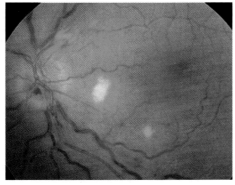

Fig 6.25 Colour photograph showing cotton wool spots

6.9 Retinal vein occlusion I

Retinal vein occlusions are relatively common, second only to diabetic retinopathy in incidence. They occur at any age, but typically affect patients older than 50 years.

Classification

Retinal venous occlusions are classified according to whether the central retinal vein or one of its branches is occluded, and whether it is ischaemic or non-ischaemic. Central retinal vein and branch retinal vein occlusion differ with respect to pathophysiology, underlying systemic associations, clinical course, and therapy.

* Central retinal vein occlusion (CRVO)
* Branch retinal vein occlusion (BRVO)
* Hemispheric retinal vein occlusion

CRVO

CRVO is found most commonly in individuals over 50 years old. Diabetes mellitus, systemic hypertension, and atherosclerotic cardiovascular disease are the most common systemic associations. Completely normal medical and laboratory findings are found in about a quarter of patients with CRVO. Patients with primary open-angle glaucoma (POAG) are five times more likely to sustain a CRVO than those who do not.

The pathogenesis of CRVO is believed to be due to in situ thrombosis in the central retinal vein. Arteriosclerosis of the neighbouring central retinal artery, causing turbulent venous flow and endothelial cell damage, is thought to be contributory. The retinal venous circulation is a relatively high-resistance, low-flow system; thus, it is particularly sensitive to prothrombotic factors.

CRVO is divided into non-ischaemic and ischaemic variants. This division is important because nearly two-thirds of those who have an ischaemic CRVO develop complications such as iris neovascularization and neovascular glaucoma. CRVO can occur in young people, in which case the underlying pathogenesis is uncertain and often no cause(s)/risk factors are identified; the prognosis, however, is often good.

Non-ischaemic CRVO

* More common than ischaemic (75%–80% of all CRVOs)
* Painless, mild-to-moderate vision loss (usually better than
* 6/60), intermittent blurring, or transient visual obscuration
* Normal pupil responses
* Variable number of retinal haemorrhages present in all four quadrants
* (see Figure 6.27), engorgement and tortuosity of retinal veins, mild optic nerve head swelling, a few cotton wool spots, and/or macular oedema
* Most retinal findings may resolve in 6–12 months.
* Neovascularization of anterior or posterior segment is rare in true non-ischaemic CRVO (<2% incidence).
* Thirty per cent of cases convert to the ischaemic form; such cases are usually associated with further visual deterioration.

* Recovery to normal vision is seen in fewer than 10% of cases.

Ischaemic CRVO

* Less common than non-ischaemic CRVO (20%–25% of all CRVOs)
* Acute, marked, painless decrease in vision (usually <6/60)
* Relative afferent pupillary defect
* Extensive retinal haemorrhages in all four quadrants; widespread cotton wool spots; rarely, breakthrough vitreous haemorrhage; serous retinal detachment; massive lipid exudation; severe macular oedema; oedematous optic disc
* Progression to rubeosis (iris neovascularization) is high: 37% by 4 months (so-called 100 day glaucoma)

Associations of CRVO

Atherosclerosis

* Hypertension
* Diabetes mellitus
* Raised cholesterol
* Smoking

Inflammatory conditions

* Sarcoidosis
* Behcets disease
* Systemic lupus erythematosus
* Wegeners granulomatosis
* Polyarteritis nodosa

Blood dyscrasias

* Protein S deficiency
* Protein C deficiency
* Antithrombin deficiency
* Antiphospholipid syndrome
* Hyperhomocysteinaemia
* Factor V Leiden
* Multiple myeloma

Ophthalmic

* POAG
* Orbital pathology

Other

* Oral contraceptives

Investigations

* Check blood pressure.
* Full blood count (FBC), erythrocyte sedimentation rate (ESR), iron/B12/folate, glucose, lipid profile, urea and electrolytes, thyroid function tests, protein electrophoresis, electrocardiogram

- Further investigation may be directed by clinical indications; especially worth undertaking in young people. Such investigation includes a thrombophilia screen, a C-reactive protein (CRP) test, an ACE test, an autoantibodies test, an anti-cardiolipin antibody test, a lupus anticoagulant test, and a test to determine the fasting homocysteine level.
- FFA: to determine the extent of capillary non-perfusion if in doubt; >10 disc areas in ischaemic CRVO
- Optical coherence tomography (OCT): for objective diagnosis and monitoring of macular oedema

Treatment

- Lifestyle changes: cessation of smoking, control of systemic and ocular risk factors
- Lower IOP if raised
- Watch non-ischaemic CRVO for ischaemic transformation.
- Close observation of ischaemic CRVO: look for evidence of rubeosis (gonioscopy is essential to look for new angle vessels) and dilated fundoscopy

Central Retinal Vein Occlusion Study

- Purpose:
  1. To determine whether photocoagulation therapy could prevent iris neovascularization in eyes with CRVO and evidence of retinal ischaemia
  2. To assess whether macular grid laser photocoagulation would reduce central visual loss due to macular oedema secondary to CRVO
- Conclusions:
  1. Prophylactic PRP for ischaemic CRVO (ten or more disc areas of retinal capillary non-perfusion on FFA) did not prevent the development of iris neovascularization. This result suggests that, with careful follow-up, it is safe to wait for the development of early iris neovascularization and then apply PRP.
  2. Macular grid photocoagulation was effective in reducing angiographic evidence of macular oedema but did not improve visual acuity in eyes with reduced vision due to macular oedema from CRVO.

Anterior segment neovascularization

- PRP is indicated when iris or angle new vessels are visible.
- Adjunctive intravitreal anti-VEGF with PRP can reduce neovascularization more quickly, with repeat injections if new vessels recur.
- PRP is also indicated for NVD and NVE.

Macular oedema

- Ozurdex (dexamethasone) biodegradable implant: approved by NICE; the GENEVA study has shown improvements in visual acuity (mean gain of ten letters at Day 60) and macular oedema reduction. Retreatment after 4-6 months may be required. Regular monitoring of IOP is required. There was a moderate rise in IOP in 15% of cases, peaking at 2 months following implant. Cataract formation is often accelerated.
- Intravitreal ranibizumab: the CRUISE study showed visual gains of 14.9 letters at 6 months in patients receiving monthly injections. Vision can be maintained at 12 months, with a reduced number of injections in the latter 6 months. Treatment has been approved by NICE.
- VEGF trap-eye (Eylea, aflibercept): a VEGF receptor fusion protein; Phase 3 trials (COPERNICUS, GALILEO) showed that it had beneficial effects on visual acuity and retinal thickness.
- Intravitreal bevacizumab: many uncontrolled case series have reported improvement in visual acuity and macular oedema when this treatment is used.
- Intravitreal triamcinolone: the SCORE study used a specific preparation of triamcinolone (Trivaris) and showed anatomical and functional improvement, albeit not maintained, with this therapy, with the 1 mg dose having a better safety profile than the others. However, Trivaris is not available in the United Kingdom. Numerous other studies/reports show other preparations of intravitreal triamcinolone (e.g. Kenalog) to be effective in reducing macular oedema and improving visual acuity, but the effect is transient, and repeat injections may be necessary. Also, the risks of glaucoma and of cataract development are significant with all preparations.

Other treatments

- Isovolaemic haemodilution, radial optic neurotomy, and laser chorioretinal anastomosis have no proven efficacy.

Complications

- Chronic macular oedema
- Neovascular glaucoma
- Blind, painful, or phthisical eye

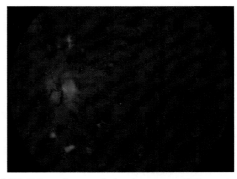

Fig 6.27 Colour photograph showing venous dilation and tortuosity, and retinal haemorrhages in all four quadrants: central retinal vein occlusion

BRVO

BRVO is a common retinal vascular disorder of the elderly and occurs when one of the branches of the central retinal vein is obstructed. It is three times more common than CRVO. Men and women are equally affected, with the age of onset often over 60 years. BRVO almost always occurs at arteriovenous crossings, where the artery and vein share a common adventitial sheath. It is postulated that the rigid artery compresses the retinal vein, which results in turbulent flow and endothelial damage, followed by thrombosis and obstruction of the retinal vein. BRVO is supero-temporal in more than 60% of cases; this characteristic is suggested to be due to the increased number of arteriovenous crossings in that quadrant. Hypertension is the most common association of BRVO. Macular oedema and retinal/disc neovascularization are the major complications requiring intervention, with rubeosis much less common compared with CRVO.

Clinical evaluation

History

- May be asymptomatic, dependent upon location of occlusion; variable decrease in vision; distortion; visual field defect/positive scotoma

Examination

- **Acute stage (in the affected quadrant):** dot, blot, or flame-shaped retinal haemorrhages; dilated and tortuous veins with retinal oedema; cotton wool spots (see Figure 6.28); with or without macular oedema (which occurs in approximately 15% of cases)
- **Chronic:** venous sheathing, retinal exudation, pigment disturbance, collateral vessel formation, with or without macular oedema. The fundus may eventually look normal.

Investigations

- As for CRVO
- FFA: at 3 months if vision is less than 6/12 or if uncertain of diagnosis; can also assess extent of retinal ischaemia (see Figure 6.29)
- OCT: for objective detection and monitoring of macular oedema

Branch Vein Occlusion Study

- Purpose:
  1. Can macular argon laser photocoagulation improve visual acuity in eyes with macular oedema reducing vision to 6/12 or worse?
  2. Can peripheral scatter argon laser photocoagulation prevent the development of retinal neovascularization and vitreous haemorrhage?
- Conclusions:
  1. Macular grid laser photocoagulation is effective for macular oedema and improves visual acuity in eyes with visual acuity of 6/12–6/60.
  2. Scatter laser photocoagulation could prevent the development of both neovascularization and vitreous haemorrhage to a significant degree. The data suggest that peripheral scatter laser treatment should be applied after, rather than before, the development of neovascularization.

Treatment

General

- Lifestyle changes: smoking, exercise, weight control
- Blood pressure control

Macular oedema

- **Macular grid laser:** as per the Branch Vein Occlusion Study. Consider in cases where vision is less than 6/12 and no macular ischaemia is present on FFA.
- **Ozurdex implant:** approved by NICE and indicated if laser treatment has not been beneficial or is not possible because of the extent of macular haemorrhage. The GENEVA study has shown improvements in visual acuity (30% achieving 15 letter improvement, and 52% gaining 10 letters) and macular oedema reduction. Retreatment after 4-6 months may be required. Regular monitoring of IOP required. Moderate IOP rise in 15% of cases, peaking at 2 months following implant. Cataract formation often accelerated.
- **Intravitreal ranibizumab:** The BRAVO study showed a visual gain of 18.3 letters at 6 months in patients receiving monthly injections, with 20% of patients receiving adjunctive laser treatment after 3 months. Treatment has been approved by NICE in cases in which laser treatment has not been effective or is not possible owing to the extent of macular haemorrhage.

Retinal/disc neovascularization

- Retinal neovascularization occurs in approximately 40% of cases with >5 disc areas of non-perfusion on FFA. Sector PRP (see Figure 6.30) is indicated as per the Branch Vein Occlusion Study.
- Persistent vitreous haemorrhage: vitrectomy plus endolaser

Other treatments

- **Intravitreal triamcinolone:** reports suggest that it reduces macular oedema and improves visual acuity, but the effect is transient, and repeat injections may be required; glaucoma is a significant problem. The SCORE study showed that Trivaris was not more effective than laser therapy and carried a higher adverse effect profile than laser therapy did.
- **Arteriovenous sheathotomy:** no definite efficacy demonstrated

Prognosis

- In BRVO, overall 50%–60% of cases retain a visual acuity of 6/12 or better at 1 year.
- Rubeosis in 1% of BRVO cases
- Fellow eye involvement in 10% of cases over time

Hemispheric retinal vein occlusion

Hemispheric retinal vein occlusion is generally regarded as a variant of CRVO. Similarly, it can be ischaemic or non-ischaemic. It is often managed as per a BRVO.

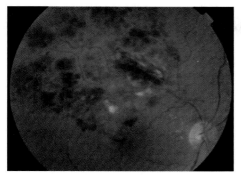

Fig 6.28 Colour photograph showing retinal haemorrhages and cotton wool spots in the supero-temporal quadrant in branch retinal vein occlusion

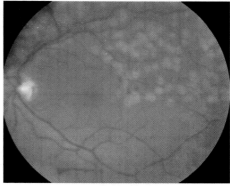

Fig 6.30 Colour photograph showing sector pan-retinal photo-coagulation for retinal neovascularization in branch retinal vein occlusion

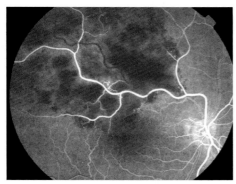

Fig 6.29 Fluorescein angiogram showing blocked fluorescence with capillary dropout

6.11 Retinal artery occlusions

Retinal artery obstructions are categorized as central (CRAO) or branch (branch retinal artery occlusion (BRAO)), depending on the site of obstruction.

CRAO

In CRAO, there is an abrupt reduction in the blood flow through the central retinal artery, severe enough to cause ischaemia of the inner retina (the outer retina receives its blood supply from the choriocapillaris). The most common site of obstruction of the central retinal artery is behind the lamina cribrosa; thus, the precise site of the occlusion is generally not visible on ophthalmoscopy. Men are more commonly affected than women. The mean age of onset is 60 years, and bilateral involvement occurs rarely (in 1%–2% of cases). CRAO is primarily due to thrombosis (atherosclerosis) within the central retinal artery, whilst embolic causes are far less common. In patients younger than 60 years old, the likely causes include migraine, trauma, and coagulation disorders. The critical period after which irreversible retinal damage occurs is 90–100 minutes of non-perfusion.

Causes

Atherosclerosis

- Hypertension
- Diabetes mellitus
- Smoking
- Raised serum cholesterol

Embolic sources

- Carotid artery disease
- Aortic artery disease
- Cardiac valve vegetations
- Cardiac tumours

Haematological

- Protein S/Protein C deficiency
- Antiphospholipid syndrome
- Lymphoma, leukaemia

Inflammatory

- Giant cell arteritis (GCA)
- Polyarteritis nodosa
- Systemic lupus erythematosus
- Wegeners granulomatosis

Infective

- Syphilis
- Toxoplasmosis

Medications

- Oral contraceptives

Other causes

- Trauma
- Migraine
- Optic disc drusen

Clinical evaluation

History

- Abrupt, painless loss of vision
- Amaurosis fugax precedes loss of vision in 10% of patients.
- Ask for symptoms of GCA: temple tenderness, jaw claudication, muscle weakness, weight loss, loss of appetite, fever

Examination

- Typically, visual acuity 6/240 or worse
- Swollen pale retina with a cherry-red spot (see Figure 6.31), arteriolar attenuation
- A patent cilioretinal artery results in a small area of central retina that appears normal, with or without preserved central vision.
- Four to six weeks after obstruction, retinal whitening usually resolves, and the optic disc develops pallor.

Investigations

- The urgent priority is to rule out GCA:
  - Raised ESR, CRP, plasma viscosity
  - Temporal artery biopsy
- Other investigations; e.g.:
  - Check blood pressure
  - Blood tests: FBC, blood sugar, lipid profile (for atherosclerosis); clotting screen, antiphospholipid antibodies; serum protein electrophoresis (for coagulopathies)
  - Carotid ultrasound imaging
  - Cardiac investigation: electrocardiogram, echocardiogram

Treatment

- Decrease IOP with intravenous acetazolamide 500 mg, with or without anterior chamber paracentesis.
- Ocular massage: for at least 15 minutes, intermittent direct ocular pressure
- Rebreathing into a bag (CO_2 retention resulting in vasodilation)
- Treat underlying GCA urgently.

Complications

- Neovascular glaucoma
- Optic atrophy

Prognosis

- Thirty-five per cent of cases achieve 6/60 or better; 20% achieve 6/12 or better.

BRAO

BRAO is defined as an abrupt reduction of blood flow through a branch of the central artery, severe enough to cause ischaemia of the inner retina in the territory of the affected vessel. It is less common than CRAO. Overall, men are more commonly affected than women are. The temporal circulation is more often affected than nasal circulation is. Most BRAOs are due to emboli (see Figure 6.32), and three main types have been identified clinically:

- **Cholesterol (Hollenhorst plaque):** small, yellow-orange, refractile, does not always result in blockage, typically arises from atheromatous carotid plaques
- **Fibrinoplatelet:** long, smooth, white, intraretinal plugs that may be mobile or may break up in time, usually seen with cardiac and carotid thrombosis
- **Calcific:** solid, white, non-refractile plugs associated with calcification of heart valves or the aorta

Clinical features

History and examination

- Sudden, painless, unilateral altitudinal field defect

- White swollen retina in the area of the arterial supply; branch arteriolar attenuation (see Figure 6.33) with 'cattle tracking'; visible emboli in over 60% of cases

Investigations

- Identify underlying cause (as for CRAO).

Treatment

- There is no proven treatment for BRAO.
- Try ocular massage or paracentesis.

Prognosis

- Eighty per cent of cases recover to 6/12 or better.
- Retinal new vessels are rare.

Ophthalmic artery occlusion

Ophthalmic artery occlusion is characterized by acute, simultaneous occlusion of retinal and choroidal circulations. It can be differentiated clinically from CRAO by the following features:

- Severe visual loss, barely any or no light perception
- Intense ischaemic retinal whitening extending beyond the macular area
- Mild or no cherry-red spot
- Marked choroidal perfusion defects on FFA
- Non-recordable ERG
- Late RPE alterations

Cilioretinal artery occlusion

A cilioretinal artery exists in about 30% of individuals; it arises directly from the posterior ciliary circulation and not from the central retinal artery. Occlusion of the cilioretinal artery (see Figure 6.34) occurs in three clinical situations:

- Isolated, at a young age, associated with systemic vasculitis; good prognosis
- With CRVO, at a young age; prognosis like that of non-ischaemic CRVO
- With anterior ischaemic optic neuropathy, in elderly patients, usually associated with GCA; poor prognosis

---

Ocular ischaemic syndrome

Ocular ischaemic syndrome occurs as a result of chronic ocular hypoperfusion secondary to severe carotid artery obstruction (atherosclerosis).

- Mean age of onset is 65 years; men > women
- Unilateral in 80% of cases
- Five per cent of patients who have haemodynamically significant carotid artery disease develop ocular ischaemic syndrome.
- Variable loss of vision; dull ache on eye or brow ('ocular angina').
- Corneal striae and oedema, neovascular glaucoma, anterior chamber flare and cells, anterior uveitis, retinal arterial narrowing, venous dilatation without tortuosity, mid-peripheral blot retinal haemorrhages, microaneurysms, NVD/NVE, cherry-red spot, cotton wool spots, ischaemic optic neuropathy
- FFA: delay of ocular perfusion

221

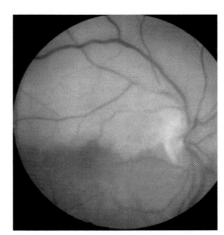

Fig 6.33 Colour photograph showing pale, oedematous superior retina in branch retinal artery occlusion

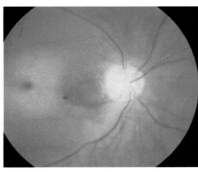

Fig 6.31 Colour photograph showing a 'cherry-red spot' with a pale retina (oedema) in central retinal artery occlusion

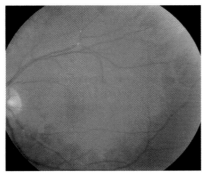

Fig 6.32 Colour photograph showing arterial emboli

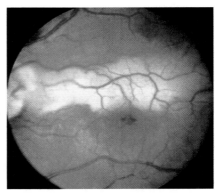

Fig 6.34 Colour photograph showing cilioretinal artery occlusion

Age-related macular degeneration is the most common cause of blindness in the Western world. It is a degenerative process predominantly limited to the macula. Two main forms of age-related macular degeneration (ARMD) occur: dry and wet.

Risk factors

- Increasing age is the main risk factor for ARMD; 0.2% of women and 0.3% of men have ARMD at ages 50–54, compared with 1.5% of women and 2.0% of men in the 70–74 year age group.
- Tobacco smoking is the main modifiable risk factor. Current smokers have a two-to-threefold increased risk of developing ARMD and there is a dose–response relationship with pack-years of smoking.
- Genetic risk factors: consistent with an inflammatory basis to ARMD, as the Complement factor H gene and the Complement component 3 genes are implicated in the pathogenesis of ARMD. Non-complement factor associated genes include *ARMS2/HTRA1*.
- Family history of ARMD (odds ratio = 3.95, confidence interval = 1.35–11.54)
- Race: ARMD is more common in Caucasians than in other ethnic groups.
- Moderate associations with ARMD include high BMI; cardiovascular disease; hypertension; gender; serum lipid levels; and cataract surgery.

Dry (non-neovascular) ARMD

Dry ARMD accounts for 90% of ARMD.

Pathogenesis

Current understanding suggests that oxidative stress and inflammation play an important role in pathogenesis. Retinal waste products including lipofuscin and A2-E accumulate in the RPE, impairing its function and resulting in photoreceptor and choriocapillaris damage. A2-E also activates the complement system, thus leading to localized chronic inflammation and further impairment of RPE function. Specific retinal changes include:

- Loss of RPE/photoreceptors
- Thinning of the outer plexiform layer
- Thickening of Bruchs membrane
- Atrophy of the choriocapillaris

Clinical evaluation

History

- Gradual-onset decreasing central vision
- Inability to read and recognize faces
- Central scotoma

Examination

- Drusen: yellow, round deposits predominantly found at the macula. Asymptomatic patients in the early stages of ARMD have evidence of drusen, which consist of an abnormal thickening of the inner aspect of Bruchs membrane and subretinal deposits. Hard drusen (well-defined borders) do not appear to increase with age and do not appear to predispose an

eye to advanced ARMD. Soft drusen (ill-defined borders of variable size and shape; see Figure 6.35) often increase in size and number with increasing age. Soft drusen are a significant risk factor for the development of advanced ARMD.
- Focal hyperpigmentation: clumps of pigmented cells at the level of the RPE
- Geographic atrophy (GA): late stages of dry ARMD, areas of RPE atrophy (see Figure 6.36); can progress by approximately 2 mm^2/year

Classification

The Age-Related Eye Disease Study (AREDS) has identified four stages of ARMD:

- **Stage 1 (no ARMD):** no or few small drusen (<63 μm in diameter)
- **Stage 2 (early ARMD):** multiple small drusen, a few intermediate drusen (63–124 μm in diameter), or RPE abnormalities
- **Stage 3 (intermediate ARMD):** extensive intermediate drusen, 1 large druse (≥124 μm), or GA not involving the fovea
- **Stage 4 (advanced ARMD):** GA involving fovea and/or neovascular ARMD

Investigations

- FFA is usually not necessary unless there is doubt about the presence of a choroidal neovascular membrane.
- OCT and fundus autofluorescence imaging (FAF) can help document baseline disease severity and monitor progression.

Treatment

- Supportive:
  - Counselling
  - Linking to support groups/social services
- Amsler grid: regular use allows the patient to detect new or progressive distortion in vision, prompting urgent ophthalmic review.
- Lifestyle changes:
  - Cessation of smoking
  - Protect eyes from excessive bright sunlight.
  - Healthy lifestyle with weight reduction
  - Well-balanced diet high in natural antioxidants and leafy green vegetables
  - Nutritional supplementation: the AREDS study showed that high levels of antioxidants and zinc reduced the risk of developing advanced ARMD by 25% in patients with intermediate or advanced ARMD in one eye. The AREDS supplements comprised vitamin C 500 mg, vitamin E 400 IU, beta-carotene 15 mg, zinc oxide 80 mg, and beta carotene. The AREDS2 study showed that supplementation with lutein and zeaxanthin can affect progression to advanced AMD. It also showed that a no beta-carotene formulae worked as well as the original formulation.
- Low-vision assessment, use of low-vision aids

- Registration(e.g. Certificate of Visual Impairment):
  – Sight-impaired patients
  – Severely sight-impaired patients

Future therapies
Several therapeutic strategies are being investigated to slow the progression of dry ARMD. These strategies include the use of:

- **Neuroprotective agents:** e.g. ciliary neurotrophic factor, brimonidine tartrate; this approach aims to prevent apoptosis in viable RPE cells and photoreceptors
- **Complement system inhibitors:** Phase 2 trials of Complement component 3 and Complement component 5 are underway.
- **Visual cycle modification:** e.g. oral fenretinide; this approach aims to slow down photoreceptor activity and reduce metabolic load on these cells
- **Corticosteroids:** A Phase 2 trial of a sustained release intravitreal implant of fluocinolone acetonide is underway, aimed at reducing retinal neuroinflammation and degeneration.

- **Stem cell therapy:** Subretinal administration of RPE cells derived from human embryonic stem cells is being investigated in patients with GA.

Amsler grid
Amsler grid testing subjectively evaluates the central 10° of the visual field surrounding fixation and is useful for both screening and monitoring macular disease. The test involves a series of charts, each consisting of a 10 cm square (see Table 6.3). Chart 1 is suitable for most patients. It consists of a 20 × 20 grid of 5 mm squares, each representing 1° of central field (viewed at a distance of 33 cm).

Procedure
- Have the patient view the chart from 33 cm away (reading distance) and with reading glasses.
- Ask the patient to occlude one eye, fixate on the central dot, and comment on whether any of the small squares are missing or distorted. Chart 2 helps those who find it difficult to fixate.

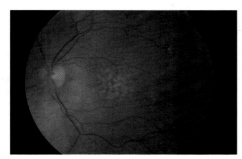

Fig 6.35 Colour fundus photograph of the left macula showing multiple confluent soft drusen

Table 6.3 Amsler charts

Chart	Design	Use
1	Standard grid Black on white	Most patients
2	Grid with diagonals Black on white	Diagonal lines aid in fixation in patients unable to see central dot
3	Red on black	Red squares helpful in detecting colour desaturation in optic nerve lesions or early toxic maculopathy
4	Random dots White on black	Tests scotoma only
5	Horizontal lines White on black	Detect metamorphopsia in specific meridian

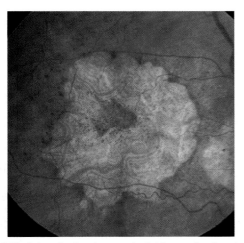

Fig 6.36 Colour fundus photograph of right eye showing a large area of geographical atrophy at the macula

Wet (neovascular) ARMD

Wet macular degeneration is less common than dry and accounts for 10%–15% of all ARMD. It tends to develop quickly and is also known as neovascular ARMD. It is characterized by CNV, which is an ingrowth of permeable and fragile new vessels from the choroid into the RPE and the subretinal spaces. It is thought to be stimulated by the pathological secretion of VEGF. These vessels can bleed, eventually causing macular scarring resulting in profound loss of central vision (disciform scars). In the United Kingdom, CNV causes severe visual impairment or blindness in around 3.5% of people aged 75 or more.

Clinical evaluation

History

- Usually with sudden onset, with a rapid decrease in central vision
- Metamorphopsia (distorted vision)
- Central scotoma

Examination

- Grey or yellow-green plaque-like membrane
- Retinal, subretinal, or sub-RPE haemorrhage
- Subretinal fluid
- Macular oedema
- Retinal or subretinal lipid exudates
- Retinal pigment epithelial detachment
- RPE tear
- Subretinal fibrosis or disciform scar
- Associated features of non-neovascular ARMD

Investigations

- FFA: vital for diagnosis and assessment for treatment, identifying type of CNV, and monitoring progress
- OCT: detects macular oedema, subretinal fluid, pigment epithelial detachment
- ICG angiography: primarily used in diagnosis of idiopathic polypoidal choroidal vasculopathy and has a role in the diagnosis of retinal angiomatous proliferation
- Classification of CNV based on position:
  - Extrafoveal: lesion located 200–2500 μm from the centre of the foveal avascular zone, as per the Macular Photocoagulation Study
  - Juxtafoveal: lesion located 1–199 μm from the centre of the foveal avascular zone, as per the Macular Photocoagulation Study
  - Subfoveal: lesion located under the fovea
- Based on type:
  - Classic: early, well-demarcated, lacy hyperfluorescence with progressive leakage in the middle and late frames and which obscures the boundaries of the lesion (see Figure 6.37)
  - Predominantly classic: an area of classic CNV occupying >50% of the total area of the lesion at baseline
  - Minimally classic: an area of classic CNV occupying less than 50% but more than 0% of the area of the entire lesion at baseline
  - Occult: no classic CNV (see Figures 6.38 and 6.39)

There are two types of occult CNV:

1. Fibrovascular pigment epithelial detachment (PED; see Figure 6.40)
2. Late leakage of indeterminate origin: poorly demarcated boundaries, fluorescein leakage from undetermined source in the late phase of the angiogram

Supportive

- Counselling
- Linking to support groups/social services
- Low-vision assessment, use of low-vision aids
- Registration (e.g. Certificate of Visual Impairment)
- Lifestyle changes: smoking cessation, vitamin supplementation

Historical treatment of wet ARMD

Before the year 2000, treatment for neovascular ARMD was limited to laser photocoagulation, based on the Macular Photocoagulation Study; however, laser treatment reduced severe visual acuity loss in extrafoveal or juxtafoveal CNV only. Photodynamic therapy (PDT) with verteporfin (introduced in 2000) was the first treatment proven to reduce risk of visual loss in subfoveal CNV. Verteporfin is a photoactivated dye which becomes concentrated in the proliferating vascular bed of the CNV. When activated by an 83-second pulse of laser light with a wavelength of 689 nm, it forms free-radical singlet oxygen, which causes local endothelial cell death and occlusion of the blood supply to the CNV. However, its modest efficacy was limited to classic or small CNV and it failed to improve vision in clinical trials.

Intravitreal anti-VEGF agents are now the mainstay of treatment (see Section 6.14).

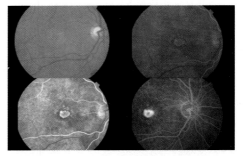

Fig 6.37 Colour fundus photograph lesion in right fovea and three progressive frames of fundus fluorescein angiography, showing early well-localized hyperfluorescence with late leakage: classic choroidal neovascularization

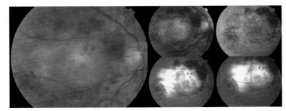

Fig 6.38 Left: colour fundus photograph showing a large, elevated, yellow lesion with haemorrhage. Right: four frames of fundus fluorescein angiography, showing occult choroidal neovascularization

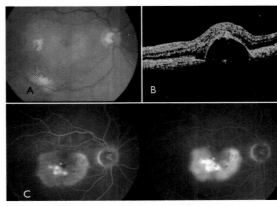

Fig 6.40 (A) Colour fundus photograph, (B) optical coherence tomography image, and (C) fundus fluorescein angiography of fibrovascular pigment epithelial detachment: occult choroidal neovascularization

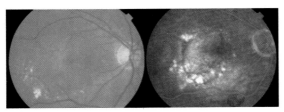

Fig 6.39 Left: colour photograph showing a large, macular, elevated lesion with exudation. Right: fundus fluorescein angiography shows late stippled hyperfluorescence: occult choroidal neovascularization

VEGF has been strongly implicated in pathological ocular neo-vascularization, including the process of CNV formation. Intravitreal injection of anti-VEGF agents has been shown to effectively block the effects of VEGF and effectively treat CNV. This finding has been a major breakthrough in the management of neovascular ARMD. This section describes the anti-VEGF agents currently in use.

Pegaptanib sodium (Macugen)

Pegaptanib sodium (Macugen) was the first anti-VEGF agent shown to be beneficial in treating neovascular ARMD. It is a synthetic pegylated anti-VEGF aptamer (a single-stranded DNA or RNA molecule constructed to bind a ligand), with a molecular weight of 20 kDa. It specifically binds to isoform 165 of VEGF and is usually administered every 6 weeks via intravitreal injection. In the United States, the FDA approved it in December 2004, whereas the European Medicines Agency licensed it in February 2006 at a 0.3 mg dose. It was launched in the United Kingdom in May 2006. The VISION trial showed that Macugen was effective in preventing moderate visual loss, but only 6% of patients showed visual gain, with superior results achieved with ranibizumab and bevacizumab; therefore, it is rarely used now.

Ranibizumab (Lucentis)

Ranibizumab is a humanized recombinant antibody fragment designed to recognize all five human isoforms of VEGF (i.e. it is non-selective). It has a molecular weight of 48 kDa and is licensed for intravitreal use in ARMD. In the United States, it was licensed in 2006 and, in the European Union and the United Kingdom, it was licensed in February 2007.

NICE has approved treatment in cases where the following criteria are met:

* Best-corrected visual acuity is between 6/12 and 6/96
* No permanent structural damage to central fovea
* Lesion size is ≤12 disc areas in the greatest linear dimension.
* There is evidence of recent disease progression (blood vessel growth, as indicated by FFA or recent visual acuity worsening).

Continuous dosing regime

The ANCHOR trial was pivotal in demonstrating superiority over PDT, with 95% of patients who were receiving monthly Lucentis injections losing fewer than 15 letters, compared to 64% receiving PDT. In addition, visual gain was found in 36%–40% of patients receiving Lucentis, versus 6% in the PDT group. The MARINA study compared monthly Lucentis injections versus sham injections, with the Lucentis group having significantly more patients who lost fewer letters, and gained vision.

Treat as required regime

The PRONTO study showed that a variable dosing regimen of Lucentis, guided by OCT, can show results similar to those obtained with monthly administration. After 12 and 24 months, the visual results in this study were similar to those from the MARINA and ANCHOR studies, and patients needed an average of five injections per year for 2 years.

Reinjection was performed if:

* OCT showed an increase in central macular thickness by 100 μm or more
* OCT showed persistent or recurrent fluid in or under the retina
* OCT showed an increase in height or breadth of RPE detachment
* There had been a loss of ≥5 letters since the previous visit
* A new haemorrhage was observed

Treat and extend regime

The treat and extend regime involves injection at every visit but extends the interval between retreatments once stable visual acuity and absence of macular haemorrhage have been achieved (there may or may not be fluid on OCT). If there is renewed disease activity (e.g. worsening of visual acuity/increasing fluid on OCT), the interval between injections is shortened until stability is achieved again.

The aim of this regime is to reduce the treatment burden on patients.

Bevacizumab (Avastin)

Bevacizumab is a humanized monoclonal antibody with a size (149 kDa) three times that of ranibizumab and which, like ranibizumab, also binds all isoforms of VEGF. It is licensed for systemic use in colorectal and renal cancers; however, ophthalmic use remains off-label. It contains no preservative and so has a limited shelf life. The half-life of Avastin is longer than that of Lucentis, and Avastin clears 100 times more slowly than Lucentis does. However, Avastin is much cheaper than Lucentis.

The ABC trial compared the effect of three loading doses of Avastin followed by as-needed treatment at 6 week intervals to alternate treatments (PDT, Macugen, sham). Mean visual acuity improved by seven letters in the Avastin group, as compared to a decrease of nine letters in the standard care group. Also, 32% of patients receiving Avastin gained ≥15 letters, compared to only 3% in the standard care group.

Comparative ranibizumab and bevacizumab trials

The CATT and IVAN studies are two large trials that compared the efficacy of Lucentis and Avastin, as well as continuous versus variable dosing regimes. In the CATT trial, patients were randomized into four groups to receive either Lucentis or Avastin, with either monthly or as-needed administration (without a 3-month loading dose). After 1 year, the patients receiving monthly injections were re-randomized to continue receiving monthly injections or switch to as-needed injections. At 2 years, there was no significant difference between the Lucentis and Avastin groups in terms of letters gained; however, patients receiving monthly injections gained approximately 2.5 more letters than those in the as-needed group did. In addition, patients who switched from monthly injections to as-needed injections after Year 1 lost more letters at Year 2 than those who were on an as-needed regimen throughout. Development of GA (mostly extrafoveal) was greater with the monthly regimen. No differences in death rates or arteriothrombotic events were found between the two drugs.

In the IVAN trial, patients were randomized to receive monthly Lucentis or Avastin, with either a monthly regime or an as-needed regime which involved a loading dose of three monthly injections and then a further course of three injections if reactivation was detected. No significant difference in visual gain was found between drugs or treatment regimes. Arteriothrombotic events or heart failure occurred more commonly in patients receiving Lucentis, but there was no difference between the two drugs in terms of death rates.

Aflibercept (Eylea)

Aflibercept (Eylea, formerly known as VEGF trap-eye) is a soluble fusion protein consisting of two extracellular cytokine receptor domains and a human Fc region of IgG. It binds to all forms of VEGF-A and VEGF-B, as well as to placental growth factor. The binding ability of Eylea is greater than previous anti-VEGF agents, and has a greater half-life than Lucentis does (48–83 days vs 30 days).

Comparative Eylea versus Lucentis trials

VIEW 1 and 2 are two large Phase 3 trials where patients were randomized to monthly 0.5 mg Lucentis, monthly 0.5 mg or 2 mg Eylea, or 2 mg of Eylea after a loading dose of three monthly injections. All Eylea doses and treatment regimes were non-inferior to the Lucentis regime, and the FDA has approved Eylea for wet ARMD at the dose of 2 mg monthly for the first 3 months, followed by 2 mg every 2 months.

Other therapies

Radiotherapy

The rationale for radiotherapy is to selectively target proliferating endothelial cells and decrease scar formation by the inhibition of rapid fibroblast formation. Two delivery approaches are being investigated in clinical trials. Intraocular brachytherapy involves the introduction of an irradiating probe via a vitrectomy procedure. The probe is placed directly above the CNV lesion for several minutes. An alternative delivery system uses stereotactic radiotherapy applied through the sclera, to the macula region. Current trials are investigating whether radiotherapy combined with anti-VEGF injections can reduce the number of future injections required. Risks include radiation retinopathy and cataract.

Combination treatment

Ongoing trials are looking at combinations of anti-VEGF, PDT, and corticosteroid therapy.

Future therapies

Clinical trials are ongoing in several new areas, including:
* Topical VEGF receptor tyrosine kinase inhibitors
* Sustained delivery agents (DARPins)
* Encapsulated cell technology, allowing continuous release of therapeutic agents
* Gene therapy using viral vectors to provide long-term delivery of angiostatic agents

The use of anti-VEGF agents in treating myopic choroidal neovascularization

Myopic choroidal neovascularization is a common cause of visual loss in people with pathological myopia (PM). PM is characterized by an axial length of >26 mm, a refractive error of <6 dioptres, and degenerative changes involving the sclera, the choroid, and the retina.

Clinical evaluation
* Symptoms include an acute decrease in vision, and metamorphopsia.
* Myopic CNVs are usually small (1 disc diameter) and may be associated with subretinal haemorrhage and hyperpigmented borders.
* Other features of PM include tigroid/tessellated fundus; lacquer cracks; patchy atrophy; and peripheral degenerative changes.

Treatment
* Anti-VEGF therapy is now the treatment of choice for this condition.
* The RADIANCE study showed a 13.8 letter gain at 12 months with a mean of 4.6 ranibizumab injections. NICE has approved the use of ranibizumab in this condition. The MYRROR study has also shown beneficial effects with aflibercept therapy. Myopic CNV is generally more self-limited and less aggressive compared to CNV associated with ARMD, requiring fewer injections.

6.15 Central serous chorioretinopathy

Central serous chorioretinopathy (CSCR) is a disease in which a serous detachment of the neurosensory retina occurs over an area of leakage from the choriocapillaris. CSCR may be categorized as acute, recurrent, and chronic, with acute CSCR self-resolving over a few months with mild residual retinal changes. With chronic CSCR, RPE atrophic areas/widespread pigment epithelial changes are present.

Risk factors

* Young adult male (6 : 1, M : F), typically 20–50 years old
* Type A personality
* Stress
* Pregnancy
* Cushings disease
* Medications, mainly corticosteroids in any form, including inhalers and skin creams

Clinical evaluation

History

* Unilateral sudden painless decrease in central visual acuity
* Metamorphopsia (distortion)
* Micropsia
* Increased hypermetropia
* Positive scotoma

Examination

* Shallow detachment of sensory retina at the posterior pole
* May have RPE detachments
* Pigmentary changes suggest chronicity or recurrence.
* Chronic CSCR occurs in 5% of cases, mostly in older patients.
* Recurrent episodes occur in 45% of cases.

Investigations

* **OCT:** shows subretinal fluid/detachment of sensory retina (see Figure 6.41). PED can be present in both active and inactive CSCR and may be located inside or outside areas of serous detachment. Choroidal thickness is increased.
* **FFA:** leakage in 'smokestack' or 'ink-blot' fashion (see Figure 6.42). Multiple/more diffuse leaks may be seen in chronic CSCR.
* **FAF:** hyperautofluorescence corresponding with area of serous detachment in acute CSCR. Areas of increased and decreased FAF in chronic cases.
* **ICG angiography:** shows bilateral multifocal hyperfluorescence

Treatment

* Reduce or stop corticosteroids if possible.
* Lifestyle modification to reduce stress levels
* Eighty per cent of cases show spontaneous resolution by about 6 months, although subtle metamorphopsia/dyschromatopsia may persist.
* Focal photocoagulation to areas of leakage identified with FFA; risk of scotoma and CNV development. Relative indications for argon laser treatment are:
* Persistence: more than 6 months
* Multiple recurrences
* Occupational needs
* PDT: can be considered for chronic CSCR and often (in approximately 60% of patients) can result in improved visual acuity and retinal architecture. Half- and full-dose/half- and full-fluence have all been investigated, with no clear proven difference demonstrated. Complications are rare, with a 2% risk of acute severe visual loss.
* Anti-VEGF agents: studies have shown mixed results of anatomical and functional resolution.

Morbidity

* Patients with classic CSCR (characterized by focal leaks) have a 40%–50% risk of recurrence in the same eye.
* The risk of CNV from previous CSCR is small (<5%).
* A small percentage of patients (5%–10%) may fail to recover 6/12 or better visual acuity. These patients often have recurrent or chronic serous retinal detachments, resulting in progressive RPE atrophy and permanent visual loss.

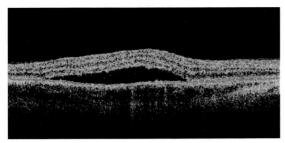

Fig 6.41 Optical coherence tomography showing subretinal fluid (fluid between the neurosensory retina and the retinal pigment epithelium)

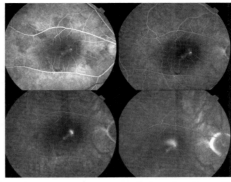

Fig 6.42 Four frames of progressive leakage ('smokestack') on fluorescein angiography

Retinal telangiectasias

Retinal telangiectasias are abnormalities of retinal vasculature in the form of irregular dilatation of the capillary bed, and segmental dilatation of neighbouring arterioles and venules. They can be:

- Congenital or primary, representing a spectrum of disease; e.g.:
  - Coats disease
  - Leber miliary aneurysm
  - Idiopathic juxtafoveal telangiectasia
- Secondary to other retinal disorders, e.g. BRVO and CRVO

Coats disease

Coats disease is an uncommon condition, representing a severe form of retinal telangiectasia. It manifests as multiple saccular out pouches of predominantly the venous and capillary systems. There is no hereditary link and it affects mainly males (in a male/female ratio of 3 : 1). The usual age of onset is 8–16 years but it may remain asymptomatic until the 30s. Five per cent of cases are bilateral with the infero-temporal retina most commonly affected. Often a poor visual prognosis but early treatment can preserve some vision/prevent phthisis bulbi and painful NVG.

Clinical evaluation

- Generally progressive
- Decreased vision, leucocoria, strabismus; may be asymptomatic
- Telangiectatic vessels, 'light bulb' aneurysms, capillary dropout, massive intra- or subretinal exudation, scarring
- Complications: exudative retinal detachment, neovascularization, vitreous haemorrhage, rubeosis, cataract, glaucoma, phthisis

Investigations

- FFA: shows abnormal vessels; early hyperfluorescence, extensive leakage and areas of capillary dropout; in the mid-peripheral and peripheral retina (see Figure 6.43)

Treatment

- Observation if little or no exudation and no impending threat to vision
- Consider early argon laser photocoagulation or cryotherapy of leaking vessels; aim to treat these directly and also apply to areas of non-perfusion. Leaking vessels are often more seen on FFA than clinically.
- Consider adjunctive anti-VEGF therapy.
- For significant exudative retinal detachment, consider scleral buckling surgery and drainage of subretinal fluid.

Leber miliary aneurysms

Leber miliary aneurysm is a localized, less severe form of Coats disease, presenting in adults. It presents with a unilateral decrease in visual acuity. Examination reveals fusiform and saccular aneurysmal dilatation of retinal vessels with local exudation. Direct photocoagulation of leaking vessels is beneficial.

Idiopathic juxtafoveal retinal telangiectasia

Originally described by Gass and Oyakawa in 1982, this condition is uncommon and presents in adults as a mild gradual decrease in vision, with a mean visual acuity of 6/12, when not complicated by CNV.

Subtypes

Type 1 (aneurysmal)

- Usually unilateral parafoveal telangiectasia of the temporal macula; usually occurs in males; characterized by aneurysms (anti-VEGF agents beneficial when this condition is complicated by CNV)

Type 2 (telangiectasia)

- Usually bilateral but can be asymmetrical, parafoveal telangiectasia; no aneurysms; can be complicated by CNV, for which anti-VEGF agents are helpful

Type 3 (occlusive)

- Usually bilateral perifoveal telangiectasia (see Figure 6.44) associated with capillary closure

Retinal macroaneurysm

Robertson in 1973 first coined the term macroaneurysm to describe an acquired focal dilatation of a retinal artery within the first three orders of bifurcation. Macroaneurysms vary in size from 100 to 250 μm in diameter, are saccular or fusiform in shape, and are differentiated from retinal microaneurysms, which are usually smaller than 100 μm in diameter. It tends to occur in older people, and in females more than males. It is typically unilateral, and the most consistent association is systemic hypertension.

Clinical evaluation

- Often asymptomatic or decreased vision
- Saccular or fusiform dilatation of the artery (see Figure 6.45), often near an arteriovenous crossing; haemorrhage (trilayered) and exudation

Investigations

- FFA: to confirm diagnosis (see Figure 6.46), although usually diagnosis is clinical

Treatment

- Improve hypertension control.
- High rate of spontaneous resolution; otherwise consider:
  - Laser photocoagulation (direct and around the macroaneurysm)
  - Vitrectomy: for non-clearing vitreous haemorrhage

Idiopathic polypoidal choroidal vasculopathy

Idiopathic polypoidal choroidal vasculopathy is a rare abnormality characterized by polypoidal aneurysmal dilatation of the choroidal vasculature, usually at the posterior pole, including a peripapillary location. It is more commonly seen in hypertensive women and was first described in Afro-Carribeans, but is now recognized to occur in any race and sex. Clinically, it presents as recurrent multiple serous or haemorrhagic retinal detachments in the absence of features of ARMD or intraocular inflammation. Prognosis is variable.

Investigations
- FFA: can be complicated by an occult CNV
- ICG angiography shows small hyperfluorescent 'polyps' in regions of aneurysmal dilatation.

Treatment
- Observation unless progressive exudation centrally
- Laser photocoagulation if there are extra-macular polyps
- PDT
- Anti-VEGF therapy
- PDT combined with anti-VEGF injections has been shown to be superior to either treatment alone.

Sickle cell retinopathy

Sickle cell haemoglobinopathies can cause retinal vascular occlusions resulting in non-proliferative and proliferative retinopathy. Although sickle cell anaemia produces the most systemic manifestations, sickle cell haemoglobin C disease is associated with more severe retinopathy.

Non-proliferative changes include venous tortuosity, silver-wiring of arterioles, salmon patches (pink pre or intraretinal haemorrhages), black sunbursts (patches of peripheral RPE hyperplasia), and macular/peri-macular retinal thinning.

Proliferative retinopathy occurs in approximately 10% of cases and can be divided into five stages:
- **Stage 1:** Peripheral retinal arteriolar occlusions
- **Stage 2:** Peripheral arteriovenous anastomoses
- **Stage 3:** Neovascular 'sea fan' fronds
- **Stage 4:** Vitreous haemorrhage
- **Stage 5:** Fibrovascular proliferation and tractional retinal detachment

Treatment
- Annual follow-up recommended
- Observation of new vessels not causing symptoms or threatening macula, as these have a high rate of spontaneous regression
- Laser photocoagulation to areas of retinal non-perfusion
- Vitrectomy for non-clearing vitreous haemorrhage or tractional retinal detachment; in such cases, there is a poor prognosis, with a high risk of iatrogenic tears

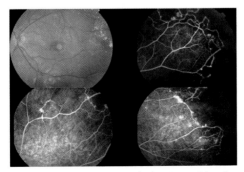

Fig 6.43 Top left: colour photograph showing peripheral exudation. Top right, bottom left, and bottom right: fluorescein angiography showing peripheral capillary closure with light-bulb-like aneurysms and telangiectasia: Coats' disease

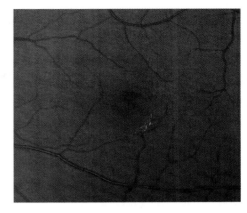

Fig 6.44 Colour photograph showing telangiectasia of perifoveal vessels with exudation

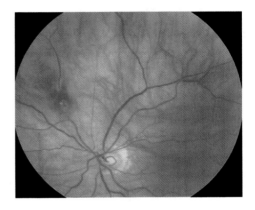

Fig 6.45 Colour photograph showing retinal macroaneurysm in supero-nasal quadrant

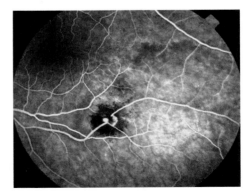

Fig 6.46 Fluorescein angiogram showing retinal macroaneurysm

Retinal dystrophies are a heterogeneous group of disorders in which an underlying gene defect leads to impaired retinal function. They can be classified according to mode of inheritance, principal site of retinal dysfunction (rod, cone, macular, RPE, inner retina), typical age of onset, whether they are progressive or stationary, association with systemic syndromes, and the underlying gene defect. With rod–cone dystrophy, rods are affected first and cones later, whereas with cone–rod dystrophy, cones are affected before rods. Rod–cone dystrophy is characterized by progressive night blindness and tunnel vision initially, with central vision affected in later stages. Cone–rod dystrophy causes day-vision problems of reduced acuity, colour vision deficits, and photophobia in the first instance, with loss of night vision and constricted visual fields over time. Recent advances in molecular genetics have enabled an improved understanding of the mechanisms of inherited retinal dysfunction, facilitating better informed genetic counselling and advice on prognosis. There are increasing numbers of clinical trials of various interventions including gene-directed strategies.

Retinitis pigmentosa

Retinitis pigmentosa (RP) is the most common inherited retinal disorder, affecting about 1 : 3000. It may be sporadic or inherited (autosomal dominant, autosomal recessive, or X-linked). Over 50 different genes have been associated with RP, with autosomal disease being the most common (70%–80% of cases), whereas X-linked RP is the most severe. A number of specific syndromes are known to be associated with RP.

Clinical evaluation

- Age of onset varies; younger age of onset in X-linked and autosomal recessive compared to autosomal dominant; usually diagnosed in young adulthood, with progressive deterioration
- Mid-peripheral 'bone-spicule' retinal pigmentation (see Figure 6.47)
- Waxy pallor of optic disc
- Retinal arteriolar attenuation
- Posterior subcapsular cataract
- Ocular associations: keratoconus, myopia, POAG
- Complication: cystoid macular oedema

Associations of RP

- **Usher syndrome:** accounts for 5% of all cases of deafness in children and is responsible for half of all cases of deafness and blindness. There are two main types:
  - Type 1: congenital profound deafness plus abnormal vestibular function
  - Type 2: associated with less severe deafness in infancy; progressive pigmentary retinopathy develops before puberty
- **Bardet–Beidl syndrome:** developmental delay, polydactyly, obesity, hypogonadism, and renal involvement; often severe cone–rod dystrophy rather than RP
- **Laurence–Moon syndrome:** developmental delay, hypogonadism, spastic paraplegia; less common than Bardet–Beidl syndrome

- **Kearns–Sayre syndrome:** a mitochondrial cytopathy characterized by chronic progressive external ophthalmoplegia, ptosis, and heart block. The condition usually becomes manifest before the age of 20 years and in some cases may be associated with short stature, muscle weakness, cerebellar ataxia, neurosensory deafness, developmental delay, and delayed puberty. Pigmentary retinopathy principally affects the central fundus.
- **Friedreich ataxia:** posterior column disease, ataxia, and nystagmus
- **Refsum disease:** due to defective metabolism of phytanic acid, which affects many tissues, including the eye. Systemic features include peripheral neuropathy, deafness, cerebellar ataxia, ichthyosis, and cardiac arrhythmias. Pigmentary retinopathy causing night blindness is always the presenting feature. The retinal findings are usually of a generalized 'salt-and-pepper' type rather than the classic bone-spicule retinopathy. Cataracts are common. Treatment consists of a phytanic acid-free diet, and plasma exchange.

Variants of RP

- Sectorial or pericentral RP: sectorial or pericentral retinal pigmentation; associated with a better prognosis
- Retinitis punctata albescens: scattered white dots

Investigations

- **Visual fields:** progressive concentric constriction leading to 'tunnel vision'. Monitoring visual fields over time may be used to determine progression.
- **ERG:** scotopic (rod) responses reduced to a greater extent than photopic (cone) responses; may be used for monitoring disease

Treatment

- General supportive:
  - Counselling
  - Low-vision aids
  - Registration as sight impaired or severely sight impaired
  - Lifestyle advice: stop smoking, eat a balanced, healthy diet, and avoid excessive exposure to bright sunlight, including wearing good UV-blocking sunglasses
- Medical: carbonic anhydrase inhibitors (oral or topical) for cystoid macular oedema
- Cataract surgery: reduce operating light, prophylaxis against post-operative cystoid macular oedema
- Treatments under investigation:
  - Retinal prosthesis
  - Neuroprotective agents
  - Gene therapy
  - Stem cell replacement therapy

Congenital stationary night blindness

Congenital stationary night blindness comprises a group of disorders characterized by early-onset, non-progressive night blindness and can be associated with normal or abnormal fundi.

Congenital stationary night blindness with normal fundi

- **Autosomal dominant (rare):** night blindness with near-normal visual acuity, no significant refractive error; ERG shows Riggs abnormality (very small a and b waves)
- **Autosomal recessive and X-linked:** night blindness with poor vision, nystagmus, often high myopia. Electronegative ERG; normal or near-normal a wave and attenuated b wave; reduced b to a ratio. Can be subdivided into complete and incomplete forms on the basis of absent or residual rod ERG, respectively. Sequence variants in *CACNA1F* (incomplete) and *NYX* (complete) are associated with X-linked disease.

Congenital stationary night blindness with abnormal fundi

- **Oguchi disease:** rare autosomal recessive, night blindness, Mizuo–Nakamura phenomenon (abnormal golden-yellow fundus reflex which normalizes after dark adaptation); delay in dark adaptation; abnormal rod function; cone function normal
- **Fundus albipunctatus:** autosomal recessive, multiple tiny white dots involving the posterior pole, sparing the macula, and extending into the mid-periphery; night blindness, delayed dark adaptation, with or without cone dysfunction

Leber congenital amaurosis

Leber congenital amaurosis comprises a group of early-onset, severe retinal dystrophies that are characterized by severe visual impairment from infancy, with an absent or substantially reduced ERG. Other findings can include nystagmus, sluggish pupil reactions, and eye rubbing. Fundus examination may look normal initially, but changes such as retinal pigmentation, vessel attenuation (see Figure 6.48), and macular atrophy can become apparent later, with severity depending on the underlying genotype. In some cases, the underlying genetic defect can be reliably predicted from the retinal phenotype (e.g. Leber congenital amaurosis associated with *CRB1* and *RDH12* mutations). To date, 20 genes have been associated with this condition, with one particular gene, *RPE65*, involved in the visual cycle. This gene is of particular importance, as it was the subject of the first gene replacement therapy trials, with three concomitant trials in the United Kingdom and the United States, all showing evidence of improved retinal function.

Cone–rod dystrophy

Cone–rod dystrophy comprises a group of inherited retinopathies in which reduced visual acuity, photophobia, and colour vision abnormalities occur earlier than rod-derived peripheral and night-vision problems do. There is some overlap in the genes associated with cone–rod dystrophy and other retinal dystrophies, with the more commonly affected genes including *GUCA1A* and *GUCY2D* (autosomal dominant), *ABCA4* (autosomal recessive; see Section 6.18), and *RPGR* (X-linked).

In the early stages, fundus changes may be confined to the macula, ranging from mild RPE changes to bull's-eye maculopathy. Advanced cone–rod dystrophy may be indistinguishable from late-stage RP.

In cone–rod dystrophy, ERG reveals a greater reduction in cone responses than in rod responses.

Achromatopsia

Achromatopsia (ACHM) is an autosomal recessive disorder that is characterized by an absence of functioning cone receptors, with a predominantly stationary natural history. It has an incidence of approximately 1 in 30 000 and presents from birth or early infancy with reduced vision, photophobia, and nystagmus. Visual acuity is typically 6/36 to 6/60 and there is very poor or absent colour vision. ACHM occurs in complete and incomplete forms, with the incomplete form having slightly better visual acuity (6/24–6/36) and some retained colour vision. A hypermetropic refractive error is common and fundus appearance is usually normal, although RPE abnormalities and atrophy may be present.

Recent high-resolution retinal imaging with OCT has revealed a range of abnormalities in outer retinal structure, from normal lamination to complete loss of outer retinal architecture. It remains uncertain whether these changes are truly age dependent or whether they vary independent of age; nevertheless, visual symptoms remain stable in the vast majority of cases.

To date, mutations in five genes have been identified as underlying ACHM: *CNGA3*, *CNGB3*, *GNAT2*, *PDE6C*, and *PDE6H*, all of which encode components of the cone phototransduction cascade.

Several studies have shown that gene therapy can be effective in restoring cone function in animal models of ACHM, with human trials planned.

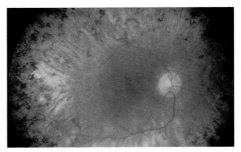

Fig 6.47 Colour photograph showing arteriolar attenuation, bone spicules, and a pale optic disc

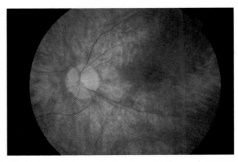

Fig 6.48 Colour photograph showing retinal vessel attenuation and retinal and optic disc pallor in *RPE65* Leber congenital amaurosis

6.18 Macular dystrophies

Macular dystrophies are a group of disorders in which cone function in the macular region is predominantly affected. Although fundus changes may be restricted to the macula, in many conditions there is electrophysiological, psychophysical, or histopathological evidence of more widespread involvement. Best disease and Stargardt disease (STGD) are the two most common macular dystrophies.

Best disease

Best disease is an autosomal dominantly inherited disorder that shows variable clinical expression. Mutations have been found in the bestrophin (*BEST1*) gene, which plays a role in chloride conductance and fluid transport across the RPE.

Onset is often in childhood, in the first or second decades. It is usually asymptomatic in the early stages but manifests as decreased central vision as the disease progresses. Usually, there is bilateral, relatively symmetrical involvement. Lesions evolve through several stages over many years, associated with worsening vision.

Stages

1. Previtelliform: visual acuity 6/6; normal macula; EOG abnormal
2. Vitelliform: well-circumscribed, 0.5–5 mm, round, yellow or orange, egg-yolk-like macular lesion (see Figure 6.49), usually centred on the fovea; can be multifocal; visual acuity often normal
3. Pseudohypopyon: symptoms often benign; part of the subretinal yellow material is resorbed, leaving a fluid level; the material can shift with extended (60–90 minutes) changes in position
4. Vitelliruptive: scrambled-egg appearance due to further resorption of the vitelliform material; pigment clumping and early atrophic changes may be seen.
5. Atrophic stage: yellow material disappears over time; RPE atrophy remains
6. Subretinal fibrosis and/or CNV can develop

Investigations

* The hallmark of Bests disease is an abnormal EOG; reduced Arden ratio (<150%)
* Full-field ERG normal
* Pattern ERG and multifocal ERG are abnormal.

Treatment

* CNV: intravitreal anti-VEGF injections

Prognosis

* Variable but often good
* Some carriers will never phenotypically express their disorder
* Some will not progress beyond the earliest stages and will maintain visual acuity better than 6/12 in both eyes.
* In general, most people will maintain reading vision in at least one eye until the fifth or sixth decade.
* In one study, 88% of patients retained visual acuity of 6/12 or better, and only 4% had visual acuity of 6/60 or worse, in the better eye.

Adult vitelliform macular dystrophy

* Associated with *PRPH2* and *BEST1* mutations in some patients
* Adult onset
* Minimal symptoms
* Smaller vitelliform lesions (see Figure 6.50) than seen in Best disease; the lesions do not progress through stages
* Normal EOG

STGD

STGD is the most common inherited macular dystrophy. It affects approximately 1 in 10 000 and is inherited as an autosomal recessive trait, with mutations identified in the gene *ABCA4*.

Clinical evaluation

* Onset either in childhood (often early teens) or in early adulthood
* Reduced visual acuity (often to 6/60–3/60)
* Characterized by macular atrophy, including bull's-eye maculopathy, and yellow-white lipofuscin-related flecks at the level of the RPE (see Figure 6.51). Flecks are often not present at presentation in childhood; nevertheless, there is wide phenotypic variability in STGD.
* STGD can be classified into three functional ERG phenotypes:
  — Group 1: dysfunction confined to the macula
  — Group 2: macular and generalized cone ERG abnormalities
  — Group 3: macular and both generalized cone and rod ERG abnormalities
  — Based on longitudinal data, patients in Group 1 have the most favourable prognosis, and patients in Group 3, the worst prognosis.
* Fundus flavimaculatus:
  — Usually in adults
  — Yellow-white flecks without macular atrophy, which will develop over time
  — Mutations in *ABCA4* also underlie this form of STGD.

Investigations

* **FAF:** central reduced autofluorescence consistent with macular atrophy, with a characteristic pattern of areas of increased and decreased autofluorescence
* **FFA:** dark choroid (due to blockage of choroidal fluorescence by lipofuscin-laden RPE)

Treatment

* Supportive; low-vision aids
* Avoid vitamin A supplements, which may increase the rate of progression
* Reduce light exposure (e.g. via the use of UV-protective sunglasses)
* A trial of stem-cell-derived RPE cells is currently underway in the United States and the United Kingdom.

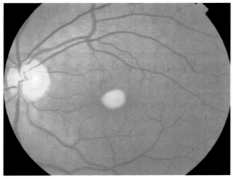

Fig 6.49 Colour photograph showing an egg-yolk-like lesion in Best disease

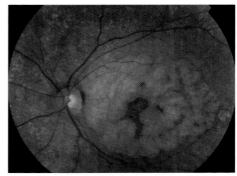

Fig 6.52 Colour photograph showing severe macular atrophy in Sorsby dystrophy

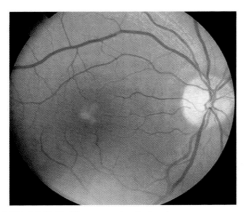

Fig 6.50 Adult vitelliform macular dystrophy

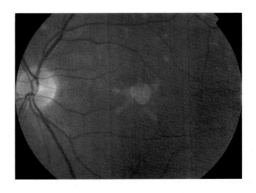

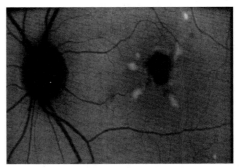

Fig 6.53 Top: colour photograph showing pattern dystrophy in left eye. Bottom: fundus autofluorescence showing the pattern of macular deposits

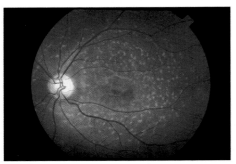

Fig 6.51 Colour photograph showing yellow flecks at the posterior pole in Stargardt disease

Sorsby macular dystrophy

- Rare, autosomal dominant
- Due to mutations in a regulator of the extracellular matrix (*TIMP3*)
- Onset of night blindness in the third decade, and loss of central vision from macular atrophy (see Figure 6.52) or CNV by the fifth decade

North Carolina macular dystrophy

- Rare, autosomal dominant; initially described in North Carolina
- Links to *MCDR1*, Chromosome 6q
- Onset is at birth.
- Non-progressive but variable phenotype from 6/6 visual acuity with few drusen to 6/60 with macular coloboma or CNV

Familial drusen

- Autosomal dominant with variable expression
- Associated with mutations in *EFEMP1*
- Onset in third to fourth decades
- Minimal symptoms of decreased vision at presentation
- Yellow-white drusen at the posterior pole, often confluent
- Later on, macular atrophy and infrequently CNV

Pattern dystrophy

- Group of disorders
- Autosomal dominant
- Bilateral, symmetrical, yellow-orange deposits at the level of the RPE in various distributions, including butterfly or reticular-like patterns (see Figure 6.53)
- Can have an appearance similar to that of STGD
- Usually mild symptoms
- Associated with mutations in *PRPH2*

Progressive bifocal chorioretinal atrophy

- Rare, autosomal dominant, links to Chromosome 6q
- Onset at birth
- Nystagmus
- Severe visual loss
- Progressive chorioretinal atrophy, which spreads from two foci which are temporal and nasal to the optic disc

- Marked photopsia in early/middle age, and retinal detachment extending from the posterior pole, are recognized complications.

Maternally inherited diabetes and deafness

- May present with diabetes mellitus, neurosensory hearing loss, and retinal dystrophy
- Caused by the mitochondrial DNA point mutation A3243G; the same mutation has been linked to MELAS (**m**itochondrial **e**ncephalomyopathy with **l**actic **a**cidosis, and **s**troke-like episodes)
- Found in 1%–2% of the diabetic population; first reported in 1992
- Characterized by RPE hyperpigmentation that can surround the macula or be more extensive and also encompass the optic disc
- In advanced cases, areas of RPE atrophy encircling the macula can be seen; these may coalesce and involve the fovea at a late stage.
- However, prognosis is generally good.

Juvenile X-linked retinoschisis

- X-linked; associated with mutations in *RS1*, which is involved in retinal cellular adhesion and structural stability.
- Affects only males
- Females are carriers
- Ocular features:
- Stellate, cystic foveal schisis
- Peripheral retinoschisis: bilateral in 40% of cases
- Diagnosis:
  - Clinical appearance
  - Electronegative ERG: a wave has a larger amplitude than the b wave does
  - OCT can show foveal schisis.
- No systemic associations
- Treatment:
  - Combined retinoschisis/retinal detachment is rare and needs treatment.
  - Topical carbonic anhydrases may help improve macular schisis.
  - Genetic counselling
- Visual prognosis is generally good unless complicated by retinal detachment or vitreous haemorrhage.

6.19 Choroidal dystrophies

Choroidal dystrophies are a group of progressive, hereditary disorders that are characterized by clinically apparent retinal pigment epithelial and choroidal atrophy.

Choroideraemia

Choroideraemia is an X-linked recessive disorder that affects young males (in the first decade). It is caused by mutations in the *REP-1* gene and results in progressive degeneration of the choroid, RPE, and photoreceptors. It is usually asymptomatic in female carriers, resulting in a 'moth-eaten' mid-peripheral pigmentary disturbance.

Clinical evaluation

- Progressive night blindness
- Mid-peripheral visual field loss (ring scotoma)
- Central visual loss by the fifth decade or later
- RPE/choroidal atrophy: initially mid-peripheral; later on, central and diffuse (see Figure 6.54)
- Macula spared until late stages
- Cataract (posterior subcapsular)
- Lack of both vascular attenuation and optic disc pallor is characteristic.

Investigations

- ERG: rod responses affected more than cone responses
- EOG: abnormal
- Dark adaptation shows elevated thresholds.

Treatment

- No treatment; invariably progressive
- A gene therapy trial is currently underway in the United Kingdom.
- Supportive
- Genetic counselling.

Gyrate atrophy

- Autosomal recessive; slowly progressive chorioretinal atrophy
- Due to mutations in the *OAT* gene, which encodes ornithine aminotransferase, which with vitamin B_6 catalyses the conversion of ornithine to glutamic-g-semialdehyde, and thence to proline
- Two clinical subtypes:
  - Vitamin B_6 responders
  - Vitamin B_6 non-responders
- Onset is in the second or third decade.

Clinical evaluation

- Slowly progressive night blindness
- Decrease in visual acuity
- Peripheral field loss

- Starts with sharply demarcated scalloped areas of chorioretinal atrophy in the mid-peripheral and peripheral retina in a garland-shaped fashion, which then progresses centrally and peripherally, ultimately involving the entire fundus (see Figure 6.55)
- Relative sparing of the macula till late stages
- Myopia, cataract, cystoid macular oedema, epiretinal membrane

Investigations

- **ERG:** rod responses reduced to a greater extent than cone responses in the early stages and become undetectable over time
- **Plasma ornithine level:** 10–20 times the normal level; also elevated in urine and cerebrospinal fluid

Treatment

- Low-protein diet with arginine elimination
- Vitamin B_6 for the responders

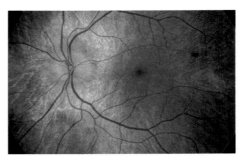

Fig 6.54 Colour fundus photograph showing diffuse retinal pigment epithelium/choroidal atrophy in choroideraemia

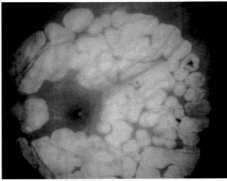

Fig 6.55 Colour photograph sharply demarcated scalloped areas of chorioretinal atrophy in gyrate atrophy

Radiation retinopathy

Radiation retinopathy is a complication following any type of radiation but particularly can occur following external beam radiation therapy for nasopharyngeal, paranasal sinus and orbital tumours, and brachytherapy for choroidal/retinal tumours. It typically occurs between 6 months and 3 years following radiation but has been reported to occur up to 15 years following radiation exposure. Radiation causes damage to vascular endothelial cells, leading to occlusion of capillary beds, microaneurysm formation, and retinal ischaemia.

Clinical evaluation

- Retinal microaneurysms, telangiectasia, and haemorrhage (see Figure 6.56)
- Hard exudates, and macular oedema
- Cotton wool spots
- Retinal and iris neovascularization
- Vitreous haemorrhage
- Tractional retinal detachment
- Optic disc oedema
- Optic atrophy in late stages
- Cataract

Treatment

- Prevention, with shielding of ocular structures
- PRP to areas of retinal ischaemia for severe non-proliferative or proliferative disease
- Macular focal/grid laser
- Anti-VEGF therapy
- Vitrectomy, for non-clearing vitreous haemorrhage or retinal detachment

Solar retinopathy

Solar retinopathy is a form of macular damage that occurs after intense exposure to solar radiation. It has been described following solar eclipse viewing, religious sun gazing, sunbathing, telescopic solar viewing, psychotropic drug use, and in psychiatric disorders. Damage is thought to be caused by short wavelengths (400–500 nm) in the visible spectrum; these wavelengths cause both photochemical and thermal damage.

Clinical evaluation

- Symptoms typically occur 4–6 hours following exposure.
- Reduced visual acuity, metamorphopsia, central/paracentral scotoma, dyschromatopsia
- Small yellow spot within an oedematous retina; the spot often fades after 10–14 days
- The lesion may be replaced by a lamellar inner retinal foveal hole.
- OCT shows a characteristic defect at the inner segment–outer segment photoreceptor junction (see Figure 6.57).

- No specific treatment is required, with most cases showing good recovery with visual acuities of 6/6 or 6/9 within a few weeks.

Toxic retinopathies

Toxic retinopathies are caused by a range of systemic medications that can result in RPE and/or photoreceptor damage and in some cases may be irreversible.

Chloroquine and hydroxychloroquine

Chloroquine and hydroxychloroquine are used as antimalarials and for rheumatoid arthritis and SLE. Retinal toxicity can cause bilateral paracentral scotomas, and macular pigmentary changes can progress to a characteristic 'bull's eye' maculopathy. Doses above 3.5 mg/kg/day for chloroquine and 6.5 mg/kg/day for hydroxychloroquine are likely to cause retinopathy. However, retinopathy is less common with hydroxychloroquine. Vision loss may be reversible if the drug is stopped early enough, but some cases may progress despite stopping medication. Routine screening is not currently recommended by the Royal College of Ophthalmologists, but referral is warranted if visual impairment is detected at baseline, or if visual disturbance occurs after commencement of treatment. Recent findings suggest that toxicity may develop despite daily doses below the recommended maximum, and that a normal retinal appearance may be associated with profound abnormalities on multifocal ERG and visual field testing.

Thioridazine

Thioridazine is a dopamine receptor antagonist used in schizophrenia. Doses above 800 mg/day can cause irreversible visual loss due to pigmentary retinopathy and chorioretinal atrophy.

Vigabatrin

Vigabatrin is an anti-epileptic agent used to treat refractory seizures and can lead to irreversible, bilateral, severe visual field constriction. Retinal nerve fibre layer atrophy and nasal optic disc atrophy may occur. Baseline visual field testing should be performed prior to starting treatment, repeated every 6 months for 5 years, and then continued annually.

Tamoxifen

Tamoxifen is a non-steroidal oestrogen antagonist used to treat breast cancer. Retinopathy has been reported in patients receiving >180 mg/day for over 1 year, with a mild reduction in visual acuity and the formation of small white refractile deposits in the perimacular region being characteristic findings. However, the drug is typically used at much lower doses, so retinopathy is rare.

Desferrioxamine

Desferrioxamine is a chelating agent used to remove toxic overloads of metals such as iron in multiple transfusion patients, or aluminium in renal dialysis patients. Symptoms of retinal toxicity include nyctalopia, colour vision problems, central or centrocaecal scotomas, and reduced vision. Macular pigmentary and/or peripheral pigmentary changes may occur.

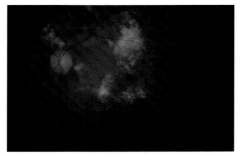

Fig 6.56 Colour photograph showing retinal microaneurysms, telangiectasia, haemorrhage, and exudate in radiation retinopathy

Courtesy of James Leong

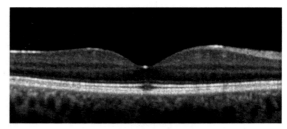

Fig 6.57 Optical coherence tomography showing a defect at the inner segment–outer segment photoreceptor junction in solar retinopathy

Courtesy of Pearse Keane

Chapter 7

Uveitis and medical ophthalmology

Edward Hughes, Miles Stanford, and Dania Qatarneh

Basic sciences

Clinical knowledge

Practical skills

241

7.1 Uveal anatomy

The uvea derives its name from the Latin meaning 'grape', after its appearance when hanging from the optic nerve following dissection from the sclera. It is a highly vascular, pigmented layer of loose connective tissue lying within the corneo-scleral coating of the eye. Macroscopically, the elements of the uvea are black or very dark, owing to the numerous melanin-laden melanocytes within the stroma, and melanosome within the pigmented epithelial layer.

The uvea may be divided into three anatomically and functionally distinct but structurally contiguous parts (see Figure 7.1):

* Iris
* Ciliary body
* Choroid

Iris

The iris is a thin, contractile diaphragm with a central aperture (the pupil). It is an anterior extension of the ciliary body and lies anterior to the lens, with which it makes light contact centrally. The iris is thickest 2 mm from the pupil margin and thinnest at its peripheral extent (ciliary margin). The thickest point is marked by a circular ridge (the collarette), which divides the iris into pupillary and ciliary zones. The iris stroma consists of fibroblasts, melanocytes, blood vessels, and collagen, with both radial and circumferential muscle fibres. The radial fibres (dilator pupillae: myoepithelial processes originating from the pigmented iris epithelium) are sympathetically innervated and located in the ciliary zone, being responsible for pupil dilatation (mydriasis), whereas the circumferential fibres (sphincter pupillae) are arranged around the pupil margin and are under parasympathetic control of pupillary constriction (miosis). The vasculature derives from the anterior ciliary circulation and runs radially apart from at the collarette, where the circumferential minor arterial/venous circle is located. The vascular endothelium under normal conditions contains tight junctions, thus forming part of the blood–ocular barrier. The stroma is bare anteriorly, where crypts may be evident on slit lamp examination (Fuchs crypts). Posteriorly, it is bordered by the bilayered iris epithelium, which is pigmented anteriorly and unpigmented posteriorly.

Ciliary body

The ciliary body, a circumferential structure surrounding the lens and the vitreous base and bordered externally by the sclera, is responsible for aqueous production and accommodation. It may be divided into a corrugated part anteriorly (pars plicata, ciliary processes), which gives rise to the lens zonule, and a flattened part posteriorly (pars plana). The highly vascular and pigmented stroma contains muscle fibres arranged radially (these alter trabecular pore size by inserting into the scleral spur), circumferentially (these relax the zonular fibres to allow accommodation), and longitudinally. The epithelium is bilayered: an innermost unpigmented layer (representing an anterior extension of the neurosensory retina) and a pigmented layer (an anterior continuation of the retinal pigment epithelium (RPE)). The epithelium covering the ciliary processes is thought to be responsible for aqueous production, which flows anteriorly via the posterior chamber, through the pupil, and into the anterior chamber.

Choroid

The choroid is a thin, highly vascular layer lying between the retina internally and the sclera externally. It has a vital role in the functioning of the outer retinal layers by providing vascular supply (via the vascular plexus) and maintaining photoreceptor disc and visual pigment recycling (in the RPE), as well as forming the blood–retinal barrier (tight junctions of the RPE). The stroma contains an outermost vessel layer consisting of large and medium-sized arteries and veins originating from the posterior ciliary arteries and draining via the vortex veins. Internal to this and just beneath Bruchs membrane is the capillary layer: wide-bore capillaries with fenestrated epithelium. Bruchs membrane is a 2–4 µm-thick layer of elastic fibres and collagen and forms the basement membrane layer of the choroidal capillaries externally and the RPE internally. It plays an important role in anatomically separating the choroidal vasculature from the retina and its pigment epithelium. The RPE is the epithelial layer of the choroid: a monolayer of hexagonal cells with microvilli at their apical surface and which surround the photoreceptor outer segments. Junctions between RPE cells are 'tight', thus forming the outer blood–retinal barrier (the inner barrier being formed by retinal vascular endothelium).

Uveal immunology

The human uvea contains small numbers of antigen-presenting cells (dendritic cells and macrophages), and its ability to generate immune responses may differ from those of other tissues. Ocular immune privilege has been proposed by some authors, following observations of anergic responses to novel antigens first delivered to the anterior chamber, and because of the tight blood–ocular barrier. The immune system may indeed be naive to certain antigens within the confines of the blood–ocular barrier, and some of these antigens have been proposed to be the target of autoimmune attack in non-infectious uveitis (putative autoantigens, e.g. interphotoreceptor retinoid-binding protein). However, it is clear that, once inflammation begins, the eye is no longer a 'sanctuary site', as the blood–ocular barrier becomes porous to both proteins and cells (e.g. anterior chamber flare; see Section 7.2).

Background

Uveitis is an umbrella term for a diverse collection of diseases affecting the uveal system. The Standardization of Uveitis Nomenclature group concluded in 2005 that an anatomic classification should be used for subsequent work on diagnostic criteria for specific uveitis syndromes. The classification should be on the basis of location of uveitis, and not the presence of structural complications.

The most common form of uveitis in the developed world is acute anterior uveitis, which fortunately tends to have the best visual prognosis. Uveitis can cause significant visual impairment because of ocular complications, with the most frequent cause of reduced vision being cystoid macular oedema.

Diagnosis and treatment can be complex, with a significant number of patients requiring polypharmacy to control the disease. The paucity of randomized controlled trials makes it difficult to compare immunosuppressive agents, and great care needs to be taken to understand individual needs and disease behaviour in choice of treatment.

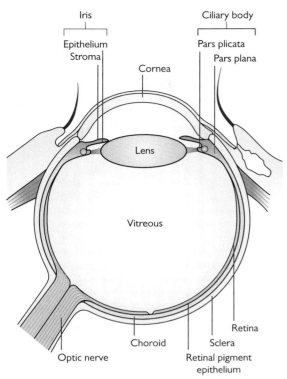

Fig 7.1 Gross uveal anatomy

7.2 Anterior uveitis

Anterior uveitis is an inflammation of the iris and the ciliary body, usually resulting in pain, photophobia, and blurring of vision. The idiopathic form usually affects young adults.

Aetiology

Non-infectious
- Idiopathic (most common)
- Associated with human leucocyte antigen (HLA) B27; relative risk of 26 (seronegative arthritis, inflammatory bowel disease)
- Sarcoidosis; Behcets disease
- Juvenile idiopathic arthritis
- Other: traumatic; Fuchs heterochromic cyclitis; hypermature cataract

Infectious
- Herpes simplex virus (HSV)/ herpes zoster virus (HZV)
- Tuberculosis, syphilis, Lyme disease
- Delayed post-operative endophthalmitis (see Chapter 3, Section 3.6)

Pathophysiology
- Multiple underlying causes, including immune dysregulation and infection
- Common end points; most are predominantly mediated by T-lymphocytes and/or macrophages
- Blood–ocular barrier breakdown leads to the presence of protein (seen as flare) and cells in the aqueous humour.
- Clinical correlations include granulomatous and non-granulomatous types, the presence of which may aid diagnosis.

Clinical evaluation

History
- Pain (aching) and photophobia are typical (NB: occasionally painless; e.g. Fuchs heterochromic cyclitis, and juvenile idiopathic arthritis-associated uveitis)
- Blurred vision
- Epiphora

Examination
- Red eye: often circumcorneal injection
- Cornea: endothelial white-blood cell deposits (keratic precipitates), hazy stroma; look for signs of herpetic keratitis (including sensation). Keratic precipitates may be the large, so-called mutton-fat type (see Figure 7.2), which are seen in granulomatous uveitis (e.g. in tuberculosis, syphilis, Lyme disease, and sarcoidosis uveitis).
- Iris: vascular congestion, nodules in granulomatous disease (Koeppe nodules: pupillary margin; Busacca nodules: ciliary zone; see Figure 7.3), posterior synechiae (irido-lenticular adhesions), fibrin, transillumination (herpetic), heterochromia (Fuchs heterochromic cyclitis). Look for signs of anterior bowing (bombé) when posterior synechiae are extensive.
- Anterior chamber: cells and flare (Grade 0 to 4+; see Table 7.1), fibrin, hypopyon
- Pupil: miosis, irregularity due to posterior synechiae (see Figures 7.3 and 7.4)

Table 7.1 The grading of anterior chamber activity according to the Standardization of Uveitis Nomenclature group

Cells (in 1 mm × 1 mm beam)*	Grade	Flare
<1	0	None
1–5	0.5+	–
6–15	1+	Faint
16–25	2+	Moderate
26–50	3+	Marked (iris details hazy)
>50	4+	Intense (fibrin/plastic aqueous)

*In practice, counting cells would be tedious and an estimate is usually made.
Reprinted from *American Journal of Ophthalmology*, 140, 3,'Standardization of Uveitis Nomenclature for Reporting Clinical Data. Results of the First International Workshop', pp. 509–516. Copyright (2005) with permission from Elsevier.

- Intraocular pressure (IOP): may be low (ciliary body 'shut-down' or failure), normal or high (perform gonioscopy: synechial angle closure/iris bombé)
- Lens assessment: check for capsular abscess (white deposits) in recent pseudophakia.
- Dilated posterior segment examination: it is **mandatory** to exclude signs of posterior segment inflammation (including vitritis), retinal detachment, and other pathology.

Differential diagnosis
- Endophthalmitis
- Pan-uveitis/posterior segment intraocular inflammation
- Keratitis (examine the whole cornea)
- Retinal detachment (may cause anterior chamber reaction)
- Microhyphaema (red blood cells suspended in aqueous)
- Pigment dispersion (iris transillumination, Krukenburg spindle)
- Scleritis

Investigations
- These should be tailored to the clinical history and include a systems review; obtain information about high-risk behaviour (suspicion of HIV, intravenous drug use) and tuberculosis exposure.
- In straightforward cases of non-granulomatous inflammation without systemic symptoms/signs, no laboratory or radiological investigations are indicated.
- If there is clinical suspicion of infectious aetiology or associated systemic disease, consider targeted investigation:
  - Chest X-ray (CXR; for tuberculosis, sarcoidosis)
  - Syphilis serology
  - Serum angiotensin-converting enzyme (ACE), calcium (sarcoidosis)
  - Full blood count (FBC)
  - Inflammatory markers: erythrocyte sedimentation rate (ESR), C-reactive protein (CRP)
  - Mantoux test, Quantiferon test (for tuberculosis)
  - HLA B27
  - Urinalysis

Treatment

Initial treatment
1. **Cycloplegia:** relieves pain, prevents posterior synechiae; e.g. cyclopentolate 1% eye drops three times a day or atropine 1% eye drops; NB: blurs vision

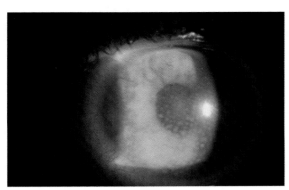

Fig 7.2 Mutton-fat keratic precipitates in a case of granulomatous anterior uveitis

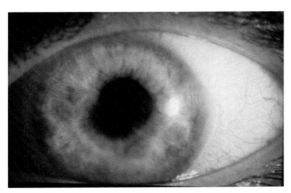

Fig 7.3 Posterior synechiae and iris granulomata (Busacca nodules)

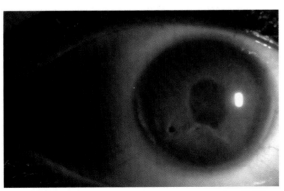

Fig 7.4 Fibrinous anterior uveitis and seclusion pupillae (360° posterior synechiae) treated by laser iridotomy (ideal position for the iridotomy is superiorly in most cases)

2. **Topical corticosteroid treatment:** the great majority of cases will respond to topical corticosteroids (e.g. dexamethasone 0.1% eye drops or prednisolone 1% eye drops) which may have to be given hourly, day and night, in severe cases. Steroid ointment may be used at night to allow sleep when control is achieved. Alternatives include:
   * Subconjunctival delivery (e.g. 1 ml betamethasone 0.1%) for severe cases
   * Periocular steroid (sub-Tenons/orbital floor): very rarely indicated
   * Systemic steroid: very rarely indicated

3. Ocular hypotensive treatment: if necessary
4. Appropriate antimicrobial treatment in infectious cases

Subsequent treatment
* Gradual tapering of topical steroid is necessary to avoid recurrence/rebound of inflammation.
* Should be tailored according to case, but a four-week taper may be suitable in most cases
* Some cases (e.g. sarcoidosis, juvenile idiopathic arthritis) require chronic therapy.

Complications
* Posterior synechiae
  – Adhesions between iris and anterior lens surface
  – If acute, may be broken, with cycloplegia; treat with intensive drops, hot pad, or subconjunctival mydricaine
  – Seclusio pupillae (360° posterior synechiae) may lead to acute angle closure through iris bombé (shallow anterior chamber, iris bowing forward)
* Cataract
* Secondary glaucoma
  – Steroid response
  – Cellular trabecular block
  – Synechial angle closure
  – Acute angle closure 2° iris bombé: dilate pupil; may need surgical iridotomy or intracameral tissue plasminogen activator. Nd:YAG laser iridotomy can trigger more inflammation and does not achieve a large-enough iridotomy to ensure patency with subsequent inflammatory episodes.
* Ocular hypotension (hypotony)
  – Usually resolves with adequate control of inflammation but, if chronic, may lead to maculopathy and phthisis
  – No specific treatment, except eye shield if severe
* Cystoid macular oedema
  – Seen with severe anterior uveitis; especially associated with HLA B27 and juvenile idiopathic arthritis
  – Consider oral acetazolamide or periocular steroid if no resolution with topical treatment.
  – Recent trials have shown intravitreal injections of agents inhibiting vascular endothelial growth factor (VEGF) to be effective in reducing the oedema, with fewer side effects than when intravitreal triamcinolone is used, although this approach seems to be slightly less potent than triamcinolone in reducing the amount of oedema.
* Band keratopathy
  – Commonly seen in chronic anterior uveitis associated with juvenile idiopathic arthritis

Prognosis
Recurrence/relapse
Anterior uveitis is most commonly an acute condition but recurrence is common (66%). The condition may be chronic, requiring long-term topical therapy.

Visual loss
Significant, irreversible visual loss is very uncommon in the acute, relapsing form of anterior uveitis. It is more commonly seen in chronic anterior uveitis (approximately 10% of cases develop severe visual loss in at least one eye). Uveitis associated with juvenile idiopathic arthritis carries a worse prognosis, with up to 25% of cases developing significant visual loss.

7.3 Intermediate uveitis

Intermediate uveitis is a type of posterior segment intraocular inflammation predominantly involving the vitreous body (vitritis), with minimal or no anterior segment and chorioretinal signs (see Table 7.2 *for grading system*). It is most commonly seen in young adults and is usually bilateral but often asymmetric. The combination of vitritis, peripheral retinal vasculitis, and pars plana exudation (previously known as pars planitis) probably represents the severe end of the spectrum of intermediate uveitis.

Aetiology

Intermediate uveitis is usually an idiopathic condition with a presumed immunological basis. Similar features may be found in association with infectious and other aetiologies (see 'Differential diagnosis').

Pathophysiology

Predominantly T-lymphocytic infiltration of the vitreous and pars plana is found on pathological studies performed post mortem or following enucleation.

Clinical evaluation

History
* Symptoms usually subacute/chronic
* Painless
* Blurred vision
* Floaters

Examination
* Typically, a lack of conjunctival injection or severe anterior segment inflammatory signs (i.e. no keratic precipitates, posterior synechiae)
* Cells in the vitreous (differentiate from anterior vitreous spillover in severe anterior uveitis), vitreous haze (see Figure 7.5)
* Pars plana exudation ('snow banking')
* Preretinal inflammatory aggregates inferiorly ('snow balls')
* Peripheral retinal vascular cuffing/sheathing
* Absence of choroidal pathology (e.g. scars/choroiditis)
* Macular oedema: a common complication
* Optic disc swelling: especially with severe inflammation
* Optic disc or retinal neovascularization
* Occasional association with retinoschisis

Differential diagnosis
* Multiple sclerosis
* Sarcoidosis
* Lymphoma
* Fuchs heterochromic cyclitis (usually unilateral with other signs including 'stellate' keratic precipitates, iris stromal atrophy)
* Infectious: syphilis, tuberculosis, Lyme disease, Whipples disease, endophthalmitis, immune recovery uveitis in HIV
* Anterior vitreous cells spillover in severe anterior uveitis
* Vitreous syneresis, haemorrhage, or pigment (retinal tear/detachment, Shafers sign)

Investigations
* Tailor to clinical history. Carry out a systems review but ask specifically for symptoms suggestive of sarcoidosis (dry cough, weight loss, rashes, etc.), multiple sclerosis, and tuberculosis.
* Investigations are not mandatory in intermediate uveitis, and in straightforward cases may not be necessary. If undertaken, they may include (according to clinical suspicion):
  - CXR (tuberculosis, sarcoidosis)
  - Syphilis serology
  - Serum ACE, calcium (sarcoidosis)
  - FBC
  - Inflammatory markers: ESR, CRP
  - Mantoux test, Quantiferon test
  - *Borrelia burgdorferi* serology (Lyme disease)
* Optical coherence tomography (OCT) helps to identify and monitor macular oedema.
* Fundus fluorescein angiography (FFA) identifies macular oedema (see Figure 7.6), capillary non-perfusion, and neovascularization.
* Consider vitreous biopsy for cytology in older patients with new-onset intermediate uveitis or for those not responding to systemic corticosteroid (consider lymphoma).

Treatment

Observation only is recommended for mild or moderate cases with good visual function. Treatment is indicated for cases with reduced vision (usually cystoid macular oedema; see 'Cystoid macular oedema in this section') or severe floaters and is as follows:
* Topical corticosteroids: these rarely provide any benefit but may be worth a brief trial.
* Periocular corticosteroids: sub-Tenons or orbital floor depot steroid injections are particularly useful for unilateral or asymmetric disease
* Intraocular corticosteroids (by injection or slow-release implant/pellet): this approach is being used with increasing frequency, particularly for unilateral or asymmetric disease
* Systemic therapy: bilateral severe/sight-threatening disease may necessitate systemic treatment, initially with corticosteroids. Second-line drugs (see Section 7.15) may be required as steroid-sparing agents or to obtain control of inflammation.

Table 7.2	The binocular indirect ophthalmoscopy score
Bio score	**Fundus details**
0	Clear view
1	Haze, but vessel details visible
2	Vessels visible but no detail
3	Disc, but not vessels, is visible
4	No view (disc or vessels)

Reprinted from *Ophthalmology*, 92, 4, Nussenblatt, R.B. et al., 'Standardizatlon of Vitreal inflammatory Activity in Intermediate and Posterior Uveitis', pp. 467–471. Copyright (1985) with permission from Elsevier.

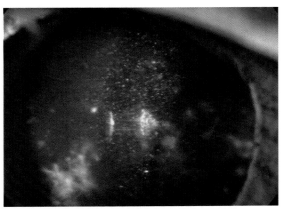

Fig 7.5 Vitreous opacities and cells in intermediate uveitis

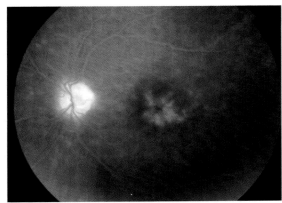

Fig 7.6 Cystoid macular oedema demonstrated by fluorescein angiography

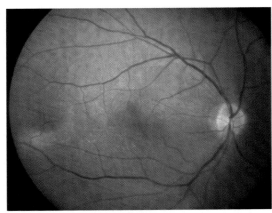

Fig 7.7 Right macular epiretinal membrane causing wrinkling of the retina

- Surgery: vitrectomy may be useful in intermediate uveitis for:
  - Removal of visually significant vitreous opacity not responding to medical treatment
  - Vitreous haemorrhage
  - Epiretinal membrane
  - Improved control of inflammation (controversial)

Complications

- Cystoid macular oedema
  - A major cause of visual loss in intermediate uveitis
  - Detectable clinically and confirmed with OCT or FFA
  - Often rapidly responsive to treatment in acute stages but less so if chronic; therefore treat early (peri-/intraocular or systemic steroids
- Retinal neovascularization/vitreous haemorrhage
  - Neovascularization on the optic disc or peripheral arcades may occur because of inflammation or capillary non-perfusion.
  - Predominantly 'inflammatory' new vessels may regress with adequate control of inflammation alone.
  - Extensive ischaemia may prompt targeted retinal photocoagulation.
  - Vitreous haemorrhage from vitreous traction on new vessels may necessitate vitrectomy if recurrent or dense.
- Cataract
- Secondary glaucoma
  - Steroid response
  - Cellular trabecular block
- Ocular hypotension (hypotony)
- Retinal tear and detachment
- Epiretinal membrane/macular pucker (see Figure 7.7)

Prognosis

Visual prognosis is largely determined by the state of the macula. The condition may remain mild, requiring no treatment, but severe disease is associated with a poor visual outcome (≤6/60) in 20% of cases. Spontaneous remission after several years often occurs. Development of multiple sclerosis occurs in approximately 15% of cases with long-term follow-up.

7.4 Posterior uveitis

The term 'posterior uveitis' encompasses a broad and diverse spectrum of intraocular inflammation primarily affecting the retina and choroid but not infrequently with associated involvement of the vitreous and anterior uvea, when the term 'pan-uveitis' may be used. Inflammatory changes may appear to principally target the tissues themselves (choroiditis, retinitis, papillitis), the vasculature (retinal vasculitis, choroidal vasculitis, optic disc vasculitis), or both. The main distinction to be made clinically is between cases of immune-mediated aetiology and those of an infectious or neoplastic nature, since this distinction will direct appropriate treatment.

Aetiology

Posterior uveitis may be infectious, immunological (non-infectious), or neoplastic ('masquerade'). Infectious cases may be bacterial, viral, or fungal, whereas non-infectious cases may or may not be a manifestation of an underlying systemic disease (see Table 7.3).

Pathophysiology

The concept that the eye harbours uveitogenic proteins or peptides has been supported by animal studies in which subcutaneous vaccination distant from the eye and with proteins such as S antigen (arrestin) or interphotoreceptor retinoid-binding protein induces experimental uveitis. These models have been very useful in the study of non-infectious posterior uveitis and have shown in general that CD4+ T-lymphocytes and monocytes/macrophages are the pre-eminent cellular components in the acute stages. The trigger for immune dysregulation towards uveal/retinal peptides is unknown, although molecular mimicry may play a role. In some instances, a clear genetic predisposition has been demonstrated (e.g. birdshot chorioretinopathy, HLA A29).

Table 7.3 Posterior uveitis: Aetiology

Non-infectious	Infectious
Retinal vasculitis	**Viruses**
Primary retinal vasculitis	**(typically retinitis)**
Sarcoidosis	Cytomegalovirus
Behcets disease	Herpes simplex virus
Multiple sclerosis	Herpes zoster virus
Choroiditis	Epstein–Barr virus
Sarcoidosis	HIV
Multifocal choroiditis	**Fungi**
Birdshot chorioretinopathy	**(typically chorioretinitis)**
Vogt–Koyanagi–Harada syndrome	Candida
Punctate inner choroidopathy	Aspergillus
Acute posterior multifocal placoid	Cryptococcus
pigment epitheliopathy	Histoplasma
Multiple evanescent white dot	**Protozoa/nematodes**
syndrome	**(typically chorioretinitis)**
Sympathetic ophthalmia	Toxoplasma gondii
Serpiginous choroidopathy	Toxocara canis
	Bacterial diseases
	(variable presentation)
	Tuberculosis
	Syphilis
	Lyme disease (Borrelia burgdorferi)
	Endogenous endophthalmitis (endocarditis/sepsis)
	Post-operative (e.g. after cataract surgery)
	Post-traumatic

Clinical evaluation

History

- Symptoms may be acute or chronic
- Usually painless, except when anterior uveitis coexists
- Blurred vision
- Floaters
- Photopsia, nyctalopia; dyschromatopsia in some cases

Examination

- Anterior uveitis may be present and may give a clue to aetiology (e.g. sarcoidosis, Behcets disease, infectious).
- Vitritis (cells and haze)
- Choroiditis (see Figure 7.8): active ('fluffy', white/grey, sometimes raised) or inactive (sharp borders, flat, often with pigment), granuloma (tuberculosis)
- Retinal vascular inflammatory changes: cuffing (see Figure 7.9), attenuation, dilatation, closure, neovascularization; associated haemorrhages and cotton wool spots
- Macular oedema
- Retinitis (e.g. infectious, or Behcets disease): pale/white areas within retina; may be associated with haemorrhage if retinal necrosis (viral, bacterial) is present
- Optic nerve head swelling/infiltration
- Exudative retinal detachment (e.g. VKH syndrome)

Differential diagnosis

The wide differential for posterior uveitis is evident, and identifying infectious or neoplastic aetiologies is key for correct management. A high index of suspicion for infectious aetiology is necessary in patients at risk of HIV/AIDS or on immunosuppression/chemotherapy, those from tuberculosis-endemic areas, and intravenous drug users.

Investigations

A thorough history and examination is mandatory and will enable targeted investigation to discern between likely diagnoses. The only mandatory test is syphilis serology, since syphilis may present in such a wide variety of ways and is easily treatable. Other investigations facilitating diagnosis may include:

- Blood tests:
  - Biochemistry: e.g. serum ACE, renal function, calcium, CRP, liver function test
  - Haematology: e.g. FBC, ESR, T-cell subsets
  - Immunology: e.g. anti-nuclear antibody (ANA), anti-neutrophil cytoplasmic antibody (ANCA), anti-cardiolipin/lupus anticoagulant, Quantiferon test
  - Microbiology: e.g. blood culture, serology for Toxoplasma, syphilis, HIV, Toxocara, herpes viruses, Lyme disease
  - HLA typing: e.g. HLA A29 in birdshot chorioretinopathy
- Imaging studies: may include CXR or chest CT (sarcoidosis, tuberculosis), brain CT or MRI (depending on clinical need), and gallium scanning (sarcoidosis)
- Blood pressure, urinalysis
- Skin testing: Mantoux for tuberculosis
- Cerebrospinal fluid or aqueous/vitreous analysis: viral/bacterial PCR or cytology

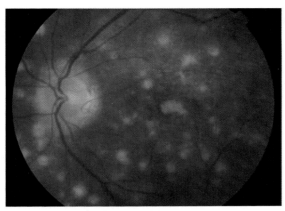

Fig 7.8 Multiple choroidal lesions in a case of multifocal choroiditis involving the fovea

Established/old lesions are discreet, pale, well demarcated, and atrophic in appearance, whereas fresh/active lesions tend to be cream-coloured and have an indistinct margin

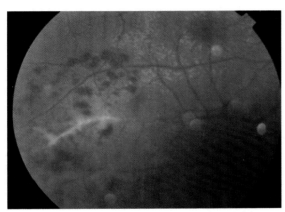

Fig 7.9 Localized venous occlusion due to retinal periphlebitis, as seen by the yellowish venous cuffing

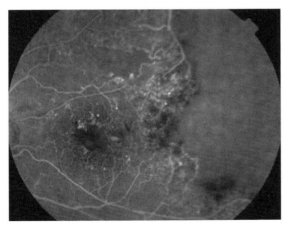

Fig 7.10 Fluorescein angiographic demonstration of capillary closure temporal to the macula in a patient with idiopathic ischaemic retinal vasculitis

* Biopsy: e.g. conjunctiva or lacrimal gland (sarcoidosis), chorioretinal tissue (lymphoproliferative disease), and enlarged lymph node (tuberculosis)
* Ancillary ophthalmic tests for diagnosis and monitoring: OCT, FFA (see Figure 7.10 showing ischaemia), Indocyanine green (ICG) angiography, ultrasound, electrophysiology

Treatment

Observation only is recommended for mild or moderate cases of non-infectious aetiology with good visual function. Assessing risk of bilateral visual loss, presence of systemic disease, and potential reversibility of established visual loss is a fundamental part of treatment planning. Treatments include:

* Appropriate antimicrobial treatment: for infectious aetiologies
* Topical corticosteroids: for anterior uveitis if present
* Periocular, intraocular, and systemic corticosteroids: as for intermediate uveitis (see Section 7.3); dependent upon severity, laterality, and patient factors (e.g. obesity and diabetes mellitus exacerbated by systemic steroids)
* Second-line immunosuppressants/immunomodulatory drugs/biologicals: see Section 7.15

Complications

Posterior uveitis is a sight-threatening condition. Visual loss may be reversible or irreversible, with irreversible loss often resulting from involvement of the macular or optic nerve head.

Potentially reversible visual loss

* Media opacity (corneal oedema, cataract, vitreous inflammation/haemorrhage)
* Macular oedema, submacular fluid
* Some submacular lesions (e.g. choroidal neovascularization (CNV) secondary to choroidal scar, pigment epitheliitis)
* Papillitis
* Transient hypotony
* Retinal detachment (rhegmatogenous, tractional, or exudative)

Irreversible visual loss

* Macular ischaemia/infarction/necrosis
* Submacular fibrosis (following CNV)
* Choroiditis or choroidal infarction involving macular
* Infarction of optic disc
* Secondary glaucoma
* Irreversible hypotony/phthisis

Prognosis

The visual prognosis varies with the diagnosis but, overall, posterior segment intraocular inflammation accounts for over 10% of blind registrations in the United States and is, along with diabetes, a leading cause of blindness in the working-age population, with obvious socio-economic implications. With appropriate treatment, 50% of eyes will retain 6/9 vision in the long term.

Sympathetic ophthalmia

Sympathetic ophthalmia is a rare, bilateral, chronic granulomatous pan-uveitis following previous penetrating trauma or surgery to an eye. The condition may arise many years after the 'exciting' event but 90% will occur within 1 year.

Pathophysiology

Exposure of components of the immune system to intraocular peptides, due to a breakdown of the blood–retinal barrier, breaks tolerance and initiates an autoimmune attack on the uvea of both eyes. Characteristic but not universal pathological findings are the presence of Dalen–Fuchs nodules (containing histiocytes and RPE cells), and lymphocytic infiltration of the choroid.

Clinical evaluation

History

* History of previous penetrating ocular injury or surgery (typically multiple posterior segment procedures)
* Floaters, blurred vision, pain, photophobia

Examination

* Granulomatous anterior uveitis (mutton-fat keratic precipitates)
* Vitritis
* Multifocal choroiditis (lesions may look raised)

Investigations

* Fluorescein angiography may help (multiple punctate lesions block early and stain late).
* ICG shows 'dark spots', which can predate clinical lesions.

Treatment

Treatment is as for non-infectious posterior uveitis. A second-line immunosuppressant (e.g. ciclosporin) is often needed, depending on severity. Sympathetic ophthalmia is often a chronic condition. Prevention by prompt surgical repair of penetrating ocular injuries reduces the risk. Enucleation of the 'exciting' eye after the onset of the condition has been performed in the past without scientific basis, but has no role in current practice.

Vogt–Koyanagi–Harada syndrome

Vogt–Koyanagi–Harada (VKH) syndrome, characterized by intraocular inflammation with cutaneous depigmentation, hearing loss, and meningism, was first described in the early twentieth century. Harada described similar ophthalmic features in the absence of systemic manifestation in 1926 (Haradas disease). It is common in certain racial groups (Japanese, Hispanics) and rare in Northern Europeans. 'Complete' VKH syndrome is diagnosed as the presence of ocular findings with neurological and integumentary changes, the 'incomplete' form has ocular signs together with either neurological or integumentary signs, and 'probable' VKH syndrome is diagnosed when only ocular signs are present.

Pathophysiology

The syndrome is thought by some to involve a specific immune attack on melanocytes. There is an association with HLA DR4.

Clinical evaluation

History

* Bilateral blurred vision, floaters
* Hearing loss, meningism, tinnitus (prodromal), hair/skin depigmentation (late)

Examination

* Poliosis, vitiligo, alopecia, meningism
* Granulomatous anterior uveitis (mutton-fat keratic precipitates, iris nodules)
* Posterior synechiae
* Exudative retinal detachment (the main clue to diagnosis; see Figure 7.11)
* Focal choroiditis
* Retinal and optic disc oedema
* Occasional neovascularization
* 'Sunset glow' fundus: orangey appearance in later stages, due to choroidal and RPE changes

Investigations

* A clinical diagnosis. Patients should have a full neurological examination due to risk of cerebral vasculitis
* Exclude other conditions, e.g. tuberculosis, syphilis, sarcoidosis
* Enquire about risks for sympathetic ophthalmia (penetrating injury/surgery)

Treatment

Systemic treatment is required. VKH is usually responsive to corticosteroids and has a good prognosis (see Section 7.15).

Birdshot chorioretinopathy

Birdshot chorioretinopathy is a painless, bilateral, posterior uveitis syndrome that is more common in women, usually presenting in the third to sixth decades. There are no confirmed systemic features. It is named after the appearance of the choroidal lesions spreading out from the disc, like shot from a shotgun.

Clinical evaluation

History

* Painless, floaters, blurring, nyctalopia

Examination

* Colour vision often defective, even with good visual acuity
* Typically, anterior segments are quiet
* Vitritis, retinal vascular cuffing
* Indistinct, pale (without pigment) choroidal lesions radiating out from the disc (see Figure 7.12)
* Cystoid macular oedema

Investigations

* Clinical diagnosis supported by HLA A29 genotype (strongly associated: over 90%)
* Visual electrophysiology and fields are necessary as a baseline and for monitoring.
* OCT or FFA for macular oedema

Treatment and prognosis

Birdshot chorioretinopathy is a chronic condition with variable response to immunosuppression. Second-line immunosuppression is often required. Visual loss is usually due to cystoid macular oedema, but macular atrophy, choroidal neovascularization, and vitreous haemorrhage also occur. Twenty to thirty per cent of eyes are 6/60 or worse by 5 years.

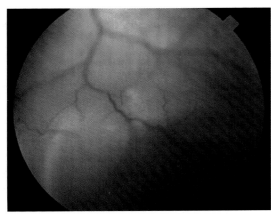

Fig 7.11 Exudative inferior retinal detachment in Vogt–Koyanagi–Harada syndrome

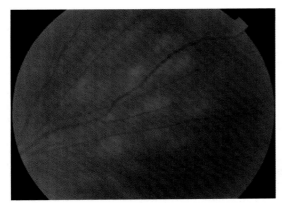

Fig 7.12 Typical indistinct and unpigmented choroidal lesions in birdshot chorioretinopathy
Note the subtle retinal venous cuffing commonly seen with the condition

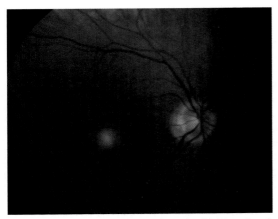

Fig 7.13 Punctate inner choroidopathy with a fresh juxtafoveal lesion in the right eye

White dot syndromes

White dot syndromes comprise a group of posterior segment intraocular inflammatory disorders characterized predominantly by a multifocal choroiditis. Visual loss mainly occurs when the fovea is involved, via either choroiditis or consequent subretinal neovascularization. Certain distinct clinical entities exist, including the following.

Acute posterior multifocal placoid pigment epitheliopathy

Acute posterior multifocal placoid pigment epitheliopathy (APMPPE) presents with an acute onset of blurring and flashes in a young patient, often following a prodromal viral illness. It is usually bilateral, with at most mild anterior segment and vitreous inflammation. Typical lesions are multiple, creamy, flat plaques of varying size, at the level of the RPE. Lesions block fluorescence early on FFA and fluoresce late. Spontaneous resolution after a few weeks is the norm, with good visual outcome. Treatment is not usually required. Recurrence is uncommon.

Multiple evanescent white dot syndrome

Like APMPPE, multiple evanescent white dot syndrome (MEWDS) affects mainly young adults (usually female) but without prodrome. Acute-onset blurring of vision is the main symptom. Examination reveals mild-to-moderate vitritis, occasional retinal vascular cuffing, and typical discreet small white lesions at the posterior pole (at the RPE level) but usually sparing the fovea. The lesions are transient (hence 'evanescent') and usually resolve within 2 months, with return of good vision. Treatment is required only rarely.

Punctate inner choroidopathy

Young myopic women are characteristically affected by punctate inner choroidopathy (PIC), a central choroiditis (see Figure 7.13) causing a central or paracentral scotoma. The creamy yellow lesion often responds to systemic corticosteroids, leaving a scar which is prone to either reactivation or subretinal neovascularization.

Serpiginous choroidopathy

Serpiginous choroidopathy is a poorly understood condition mainly seen in white, middle-aged patients, characterized by choroidal lesions (not dissimilar to those seen in acute posterior multifocal placoid pigment epitheliopathy) of presumed inflammatory origin that progress at the posterior pole in a serpentine fashion (see Figure 7.14). Usually commencing in the peripapillary region, the lesions may cause slight retinal elevation and predispose to subretinal neovascularization. There may be an associated vitritis. The disease is progressive and chronic, with variable response to immunosuppressive treatment.

Retinal vasculitis

Retinal vascular inflammation most commonly affects the venous circulation (phlebitis, periphlebitis). Systemic associations are common and include sarcoidosis, Behcets disease, and multiple sclerosis. Predominantly arterial inflammation (arteritis) is typically seen with infectious uveitis. Some connective tissue diseases and systemic vasculitides, including systemic lupus erythematosus and polyarteritis nodosa, do not manifest with visible retinal arterial inflammation but may cause retinal arterial occlusions. Idiopathic retinal vasculitis may be diagnosed when systemic and infectious disease (e.g. tuberculosis) has been excluded (see Table 7.4).

Clinical evaluation

History

* Painless blurring of vision or scotoma is the norm, sometimes with associated floaters.
* Asymptomatic if the posterior pole is spared

Examination

* Cuffing or sheathing of retinal vessels (usually venules)
* Branch or central vascular occlusion: haemorrhages (venous occlusion)
* Vitritis
* Retinal neovascularization
* Other signs may give clues to diagnosis, e.g. granulomatous anterior uveitis (sarcoidosis, tuberculosis) or retinal infiltrates (Behcets disease).

Investigations

Investigate potential cause with usual blood tests and CXR (see Section 7.4). If arterial disease is present, include ANCA and ANA. Blood pressure and urinalysis are mandatory.

Table 7.4 Conditions associated with retinal vasculitis

Systemic disease	Infectious	Ocular disease
Sarcoidosis	Tuberculosis	Birdshot chorioretinopathy
Behcets disease	Syphilis	Intermediate uveitis
Multiple sclerosis	Toxoplasmosis	Eales disease
Systemic lupus erythematosus	Herpes viruses	
Polyarteritis nodosa	Whipples disease	
Wegeners granulomatosis	Lyme disease	
Crohns disease		

Fluorescein angiography may be useful in demonstrating the extent of involvement and ischaemia, and in identifying early neovascularization. Vessel staining, leakage, and closure are common angiographic features.

Treatment

* Systemic immunosuppression may be necessary for sight-threatening disease or underlying disease once an infectious cause has been excluded.
* Laser treatment has been used to ablate ischaemic retina when vitreous haemorrhage occurs from new vessels.
* Surgery for complications, which include cataract, glaucoma, vitreous haemorrhage, and tractional retinal detachment.

Eales disease

In 1880 Henry Eales described a condition in which recurrent vitreous haemorrhage occurred in young men. Eales disease is now recognized as an obliterative retinal vasculitis, commencing peripherally, usually in the absence of significant vitritis. New vessels will often form, hence the vitreous haemorrhage. An association with tuberculosis has evolved in Eales disease, which is particularly common on the Indian subcontinent. This association is based on the frequency of positive tuberculin tests and the finding of an increased frequency of *Mycobacterium tuberculosis* DNA in vitreous and epiretinal membranes from Eales patients, as indicated by PCR.

Masquerade syndromes

Posterior uveitis presenting in older patients should raise suspicion of a masquerade, most commonly primary intraocular non-Hodgkins lymphoma.

Aetiology

* Non-Hodgkins lymphoma: most commonly primary CNS non-Hodgkins lymphoma presenting within the eye (well patient). Rarely, it is systemic non-Hodgkins lymphoma metastasized to the eye (sick patient).
* Leukaemia
* Metastatic carcinoma
* Hodgkins lymphoma: rarely metastasizes to the eye

Clinical evaluation

Ocular lymphoma usually (but not always) presents in patients >50 years old, with painless floaters and blurred vision. Subretinal infiltrates and vitritis are the most common signs.

Investigations

If suspicion is high, then brain MRI and cerebrospinal fluid sampling may provide the diagnosis; otherwise, vitrectomy and cytological analysis of vitreous cells may be required. Multiple vitreous samples (at different times) may be necessary before a diagnosis is made. Liaise with the oncology service.

Treatment

The type of treatment depends on the stage and grade of the lymphoma. Ocular treatments include intravitreal methotrexate and ocular radiotherapy. Systemic chemotherapy is commonly employed. Rituximab is also used.

Prognosis

An initial response is often good but recurrence is common. CNS non-Hodgkins lymphoma has a 5-year survival rate of 5%.

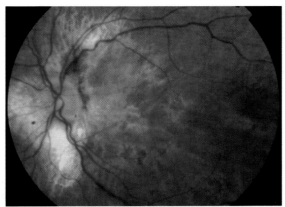

Fig 7.14 Extensive peripapillary atrophy and scarring in the later stages of serpiginous choroidopathy

7.7 Viral infectious uveitis

Intraocular viral infection is most commonly due to the herpes viruses, including HSV1 and 2, varicella-zoster virus (VZV), cytomegalovirus (CMV), and more rarely Epstein–Barr virus (EBV). In the anterior segment, HSV and HZV may manifest as keratitis, uveitis, or keratouveitis. The classical presentation in the posterior segment is retinitis with retinal necrosis.

HSV keratouveitis

HSV keratouveitis is most commonly seen with HSV stromal keratitis, and is rare with just epithelial disease.

Aetiology

HSV keratitis is discussed in Chapter 2, Section 2.18. It is caused by the reactivation of latent infection in the trigeminal ganglion. It is unclear whether uveitis is due to active viral infection of the iris or a reaction to corneal stromal infection.

Clinical evaluation

History

* May have had recurrent corneal disease
* Pain, photophobia, blurred vision

Examination

* Corneal stromal opacity or oedema, with or without keratic precipitates
* Corneal stromal vascularization, reduced sensation
* Aqueous cells and flare
* Regional iris transillumination, posterior synechiae
* Reduced corneal sensation

Differential diagnosis

* HZV
* Bacterial/fungal/*Acanthamoeba* keratitis

Investigations

* Consider corneal scrape to exclude bacterial keratitis

Treatment

* Aciclovir ointment for epithelial disease
* Topical steroid for uveitis (consider delaying until epithelial disease treated)
* The role of oral antiviral drugs is unclear but some practitioners use aciclovir 400 mg twice a day for several weeks/months for chronic disease or recurrence prevention.

Complications

Glaucoma and cataract are common.

Herpes zoster uveitis

Aetiology

Herpes zoster uveitis is usually directly preceded by herpes zoster ophthalmicus (HZO). There may be concurrent or antecedent corneal epithelial and/or stromal VZV disease.

Clinical evaluation

History

* Painful forehead rash in a V_1 distribution
* Pain, photophobia, blurred vision

Examination

* Vesicular unilateral rash in a V_1 distribution

* Ocular signs are similar to HSV keratouveitis, although sector iris atrophy is more prominent and corneal opacity may be absent.

Differential diagnosis

* HSV keratouveitis
* Chronic idiopathic anterior uveitis

Investigations

* Consider investigating for immunocompromise (e.g. HIV) if there is severe disease in a young patient.

Treatment

* HZO should be treated with an oral antiviral agent such as aciclovir 800 mg five times a day or famciclovir 500 mg three times a day for 7 days. If commenced early in the disease (within 3 days of the appearance of the rash) this approach may reduce the risk of complications such as uveitis and postherpetic neuralgia.
* Uveitis is treated in the usual way, with topical corticosteroid and cycloplegia.
* Topical ocular hypotensives are frequently needed and the inflammation may be prolonged, necessitating slow tapering of topical corticosteroid.

Complications

* Dry eye, corneal opacity, neurotrophic cornea
* Glaucoma, cataract

Retinitis

Viral retinitis has been described with somewhat confusing nomenclature, including the pathology-based terms acute retinal necrosis and progressive outer retinal necrosis (PORN), and the aetiology-based term CMV retinitis. Acute retinal necrosis is usually caused by HSV or VZV in immunocompetent individuals, whereas PORN (HSV or VZV) and CMV retinitis are seen in the immunocompromised. CMV and PORN disease are discussed in Section 7.11.

Acute retinal necrosis

Acute retinal necrosis is a necrotizing, herpetic retinopathy usually presenting unilaterally in a well individual but progressing to bilateral disease in one-third of patients within 6 weeks (although second eye involvement may be delayed by many years).

Aetiology

DNA from HSV1 and 2 and VZV has been found in the vitreous of patients with acute retinal necrosis, via PCR, and both electron microscopy and immunohistochemistry have shown herpes virus within retinal biopsies. These viruses appear likely to be the cause of the disease. EBV may be an infrequent cause.

Pathophysiology

* T- and B-lymphocyte infiltration, arteritis with vascular closure, full-thickness retinal necrosis
* Abrupt demarcation with healthy retina

Clinical evaluation

* History
  – Usually well but some have recent history of varicella/shingles/herpes
  – Pain, red eye, floaters, blurred vision

- Examination
  - Anterior uveitis, granulomatous keratic precipitates
  - Vitritis
  - White-yellow retinal lesions (see Figures 7.15 and 7.16), becoming coalescent, often multifocal, usually mid-peripheral; rapid circumferential spread
  - Arteritis; occasionally haemorrhages
  - Disc swelling
- Differential diagnosis
  - CMV retinitis/PORN (immunocompromise)
  - *Toxoplasma* (pigmented scars, choroidal involvement)
  - Syphilis
  - Lymphoma
  - Endogenous bacterial/fungal endophthalmitis
  - Behcets disease (retinal infiltrates)
  - Commotio retinae
- Investigations.
  - Appropriate history and investigation for potential immunocompromise, e.g. HIV
  - Syphilis serology
  - Most perform diagnostic anterior chamber tap or vitreous biopsy with PCR for herpes viruses.

Treatment
- May reduce retinal damage and risk of contralateral eye involvement
- Standard treatment: intravenous acyclovir in three divided doses (10 mg/kg × 3/day) over a period of 10 to 15 days, followed by oral treatment with acyclovir 4 g/day or acyclovir 1 g × 3/day for an additional period of 1–3 months before tapering (NB: watch renal function)
- Alternatively, oral treatment with valacyclovir alone; the standard dose would be 1 g three times a day, although some advocate 2 g three times a day for the first week. Watch renal function and encourage high oral fluid intake.
- Close monitoring of the retina is necessary in order to confirm the efficacy of the antiviral.
- If the patient is resistant to aciclovir or immunocompromised, use ganciclovir (5 mg/kg twice a day for 2 weeks then 5 mg/kg once a day) or foscarnet (180 mg/kg in two or three divided doses).
- Intravitreal foscarnet (2.4 mg in 0.1 ml), given at time of biopsy
- Adjunctive oral prednisolone (0.5–1 mg/kg per day) may be used for the inflammatory component in immunocompetent patients, commencing 48 hours after antiviral treatment and tapering according to clinical signs.
- Laser prophylaxis for retinal detachment remains controversial.

Complications
- Retinal detachment is common.
- Optic neuropathy (poor prognosis)
- Contralateral eye involvement

Prognosis
Retinal detachment (up to 84% of patients) and optic neuropathy are the major causes of sight loss. Contralateral eye involvement is approximately halved (from 75% to 35%) at 2 years by antiviral treatment; 48% of eyes finish with a visual acuity of 6/60 or worse.

Other viral retinitis
CMV retinitis and PORN will be discussed in Section 7.11.

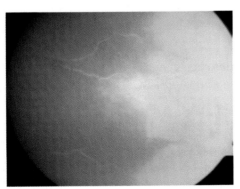

Fig 7.15 A large confluent area of peripheral retinal necrosis due to herpes zoster retinitis in a renal transplant patient on high-dose immunosuppression
Note the associated retinal arterial sheathing

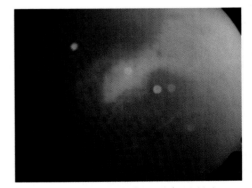

Fig 7.16 Healing retinal necrosis from viral retinitis is seen as a margin of pigment epithelial atrophy at the leading edge. The retinal arterial changes have persisted

Toxoplasma retinochoroiditis

Infection by the protozoan parasite *Toxoplasma gondii* results in disseminated infection which is often asymptomatic in adults but may have profound effects upon the developing foetus in the event of congenital (trans-placental) infection or in the immunosuppressed. The parasite has a predilection for muscle and the CNS and is thought to lie dormant in tissue cysts for many years. Besides the syndrome of congenital toxoplasmosis, human infection-related morbidity is mainly restricted to retinochoroiditis resulting from reactivation in immunocompetent individuals, and CNS manifestations in the presence of immunocompromise.

Aetiology

The definitive host is the cat, in whose intestinal mucosa the parasite undergoes sexual reproduction. Human infection is acquired following ingestion of cysts, initially shed in cat faeces, which may contaminate drinking water or meat from ground-dwelling animals that have ingested cysts. Thorough cooking destroys the cysts.

Pathophysiology

Retinochoroiditis occurs as a result of *Toxoplasma* tachyzoite proliferation, either with primary infection (congenital or acquired) or with delayed (often by many years) infection when bradyzoites within tissue cysts convert into tachyzoites. Intense inflammatory responses, dominated by CD4+ T-lymphocytes, are seen in immunocompetent individuals. Tissue damage (necrosis) is extensive and a full-thickness chorioretinal scar develops after tachyzoites convert back to the encysted bradyzoite stage. Recurrent episodes of reactivation, typically at the margin of a scar, are common, but the cause of reactivation is unknown.

Clinical evaluation

History

* Particularly common in patients from West Africa and South America
* May have had previous uveitis episodes
* Pain, blurred vision, floaters

Examination

* Aqueous cells and flare; large keratic precipitates
* IOP often raised in the acute stage
* Vitritis, vitreoretinal adhesions
* Fluffy yellow/white chorioretinal infiltration (see Figures 7.17 and 7.18), often at the margin of an established chorioretinal scar (typically pigmented).
* Retinal vascular (arterial or venous) cuffing/sheathing.

Differential diagnosis

* Viral, fungal, or bacterial retinitis
* *Toxocara* retinitis.

Investigations

* Usually a clinical diagnosis
* Serology may be useful for suspected primary infection (IgM positive, no pigmented scar) or to exclude *Toxoplasma* (IgG-positive state does not confirm the diagnosis).
* Vitreous biopsy for PCR, with or without IgG, in suspicious cases
* Consider HIV testing if severe/progressive disease

Treatment

* No randomized controlled trials proving benefit of treatment
* Peripheral lesions may be left to spontaneously remit.
* Lesions threatening or involving the macular or optic disc or a major arcade vessel should be treated with one of the following regimens:
  — Clindamycin, with or without sulphadiazine
  — Trimethoprim plus sulphamethoxazole (Septrin)
  — Pyrimethamine plus sulphadiazine and folinic acid (check FBC)
  — Azithromycin, with or without sulphadiazine
* Treatment is usually combined with prednisolone if immunocompetent host (e.g. 0.5 mg/kg), commencing 24 hours after the first dose of antibiotic.
* Treatment should generally continue for 3 weeks at least.
* Prolonged use of low-dose sulphamethoxazole/trimethoprim (Bactrin, Septrin) has been shown to reduce the number of recurrences and should be considered in patients with high risk of visual loss (macular scar).

Complications

* Transiently raised IOP
* Cataract
* Chronic vitreous opacities/floaters
* Macular scar
* Papillitis, retinal vascular occlusion
* Epiretinal membrane
* Retinal tear, vitreous haemorrhage, retinal detachment (due to abnormal vitreoretinal adhesion)

Prognosis

Twenty-four per cent of cases have a visual acuity of less than 6/60 in the affected eye. Bilateral severe visual loss is rare (about 1% of cases).

Toxocariasis

The parasitic nematode *Toxocara canis* infects humans via ingestion of its eggs, which are found in dog faeces (puppies in particular). Larvae invade the intestine and migrate via the bloodstream throughout the body, often causing an acute systemic manifestation, visceral larva migrans.

Pathophysiology

The presence of a *Toxocara* worm in the eye causes an initial intense eosinophilic inflammatory response followed by a granulomatous reaction.

Clinical evaluation

* Typically affects children (mean age 7.5 years) and is a cause of leucocoria
* May be asymptomatic or cause red eye, pain, blurred vision, and strabismus

Examination

* Typically causes raised, white chorioretinal granuloma at posterior pole or periphery; may be large
* Usually accompanied by intense vitritis and anterior uveitis in the active stage; occasionally, hypopyon
* May present with retinitis or optic nerve disease (rare)

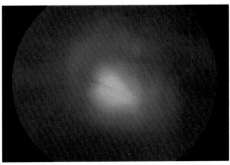

Fig 7.17 'Headlight in the fog': an active *Toxoplasma* retinochoroiditis lesion at the margin of a pigmented scar (seen superior to the fluffy white, full-thickness infiltrate)

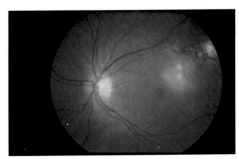

Fig 7.18 Two small foci of active *Toxoplasma* retinochoroiditis adjacent to an old scar. The full extent of the lesion is evident by the size of the resulting scar after resolution of the inflammation

Differential diagnosis
* Retinoblastoma, *Toxoplasma*
* Persistent hyperplastic primary vitreous
* Coats disease
* Retinopathy of prematurity

Investigations
* Serology
* Ultrasound

Treatment
* Consult paediatricians/physicians.
* Use anti-helminthics (e.g. thiabendazole) and topical and systemic corticosteroids for inflammatory response.

Complications
* Tractional retinal detachment
* Epiretinal membranes
* Macular granuloma

Other parasitic causes of uveitis

Onchocerciasis ('river blindness') is a major cause of blindness in endemic areas (mainly central Africa). The causative nematode *Onchocerca volvulus* is transmitted by a bite from the infected *Simulium* black fly. Adult worms then form nodules throughout the body but especially in the skin. Microfilariae are the main cause of the ocular pathology, typically a sclerosing keratitis (the main cause of visual loss), and anterior uveitis. Cataract, glaucoma, vitritis, and choroiditis may develop. Toxocariasis was traditionally diagnosed on 'skin snip' but new methods (serology and antigen dipstick) are now available. It is treated by physicians specializing in infectious diseases.

257

7.9 Fungal infectious uveitis

Endogenous endophthalmitis

Blood-borne spread of fungi from distant sites to the eye is a rare but important cause of endophthalmitis, as fungal infection uveitis benefits from early recognition and treatment. Typical sites of primary infection include indwelling urinary and venous catheters (particularly patients requiring prolonged hospital care) and injection sites of intravenous drug abuse. Immuno-compromised individuals are at particular risk (including those receiving systemic corticosteroids).

Candida

Candida albicans is the most common cause of fungal endoph-thalmitis, usually seen in intravenous drug users and the chroni-cally ill. *Candida* may contaminate lemon juice used as a solvent for diamorphine.

Clinical evaluation

Examination

- Acute or subacute; floaters, blurring of vision, pain
- Susceptible individual
- May be asymptomatic; found on screening of patients in the intensive care unit

Signs

- Anterior uveitis (occasionally hypopyon), vitritis (see Figure 7.19)
- Fluffy white 'puffballs' originating in the choroid and mi-grating through the retina and into the vitreous (see Figure 7.20)
- Occasionally retinal haemorrhages and vascular cuffing.

Differential diagnosis

- *Toxoplasma* (look for pigmented scars, choroidal involvement)
- Bacterial endophthalmitis (tends to progress much faster)
- Viral retinitis
- Syphilis
- Lymphoma
- Sarcoidosis

Investigations

- Serology to exclude differential diagnoses
- Cultures from blood and likely sources of fungaemia
- Other investigations to identify source (e.g. abdominal ultra-sound, echocardiogram)
- Vitrectomy and removal of vitreous infiltrates may be neces-sary to confirm diagnosis (e.g. if cultures are negative from blood and other sites); debulk infection; deliver intravitreal amphoteracin.

Treatment

- Intravitreal 5–10 µg amphoteracin B (at time of vitreous sampling)

- Intravenous/oral fluconazole or intravenous amphoteracin B (watch renal function)
- Flucytosine may be used but resistance is not uncommon.

Complications

- Retinal detachment
- Progressive infection
- Complications of disseminated fungal infection

Aspergillus

Aspergillus species are ubiquitous, filamentous fungi which may cause invasive human disease at any site but in particular the lungs. Immunocompromised hosts are at greatest risk, as are in-travenous drug users.

Clinical evaluation

The clinical features and context will be similar to *Candida* en-dophthalmitis. Unlike allergic bronchopulmonary aspergillosis, serology is of limited value in invasive *Aspergillus* disease.

Treatment

Consult the infectious diseases team. Intravitreal and intrave-nous amphoteracin B has been the gold standard for treatment; however, voriconazole has better in vitro efficacy and is not as toxic. Choice should depend on general condition, renal status, and site of primary infection.

Prognosis

The systemic prognosis with invasive *Aspergillus* is poor, as is the ocular prognosis, particularly if diagnosis and treatment are delayed.

Presumed ocular histoplasmosis

Histoplasma capsulatum, a fungus endemic to the mid-western United States, has been associated with a specific form of pos-terior uveitis found most commonly in that region but rarely elsewhere in the world. Although *Histoplasma* has been recov-ered from eyes in the rare event of endogenous *Histoplasma* endophthalmitis, this has not been the case for the ocular his-toplasmosis syndrome, hence the use of the term 'presumed' in the name for this condition. An association with HLA B7 has supported the concept that the syndrome represents a form of hypersensitivity reaction to *Histoplasma* antigens.

Clinical evaluation

The typical findings are multiple discreet choroiditis lesions which predispose to subretinal neovascularization, macular pigmentary disturbance, peripapillary atrophy, and clear ocular media.

Treatment

Antifungal treatment is of no benefit, and treatment is aimed at controlling the choroiditis with immunosuppression and dealing with the subretinal neovascularization, which is often amenable to surgical membrane removal.

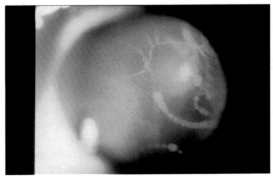

Fig 7.19 'String of pearls' in the vitreous in *Candida* endophthalmitis

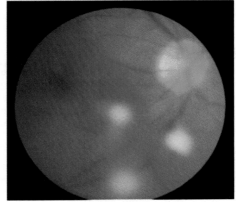

Fig 7.20 Retinal and preretinal 'puffballs' in *Candida* infection

7.10 Bacterial infectious uveitis

Tuberculosis

Mycobacterium tuberculosis infection should be considered in almost any form of ocular and adnexal inflammation. The condition is amenable to definitive (curative) antibiotic treatment, whereas injudicious immunosuppressive treatment has the potential to exacerbate ocular and systemic disease, with potentially fatal consequences.

Pathophysiology

Primary ocular tuberculosis affects the ocular surface and adnexae as a result of direct (exogenous) infection. Secondary ocular tuberculosis occurs following haematogenous dissemination from a distant source of primary infection (commonly the lung) and most typically affects the deep ocular structures and the optic nerve. Tuberculous uveitis may result from active mycobacterial infection of the eye (e.g. choroidal tubercle) or as part of an immunological delayed-type hypersensitivity reaction (e.g. retinal vasculitis, phlyctenular conjunctivitis). Granulomatous inflammation is the hallmark of tuberculous disease.

Clinical evaluation

Patients originating from tuberculosis-endemic areas, and those with known tuberculosis (past or present) or tuberculosis contacts should raise suspicion. There is a wide spectrum of clinical presentation. Systemic symptoms (e.g. fever, weight loss, malaise, lymphadenopathy, cough) may or may not be present.

Ophthalmic presentations

These include:

* Eyelid tubercle
* Phlyctenular conjunctivitis
* Interstitial keratitis
* Scleritis
* Granulomatous anterior uveitis/pan-uveitis
* Retinal periphlebitis (venous inflammation with haemorrhagic veno-occlusion; see Figure 7.21)
* Choroidal granuloma (fluffy, pale, raised subretinal lesion with or without subretinal fluid)
* Serpiginous-like choroiditis
* Optic neuropathy/orbital apex syndrome

Investigations

* CXR, lymph node biopsy
* FBC, CRP, ESR, liver function test, renal profile
* Serum ACE (sarcoidosis) plus syphilis serology (differential diagnoses)
* Tuberculin skin test or new in vitro lymphocyte stimulation tests (e.g. Quantiferon)

Treatment

Consult the infectious diseases/respiratory medicine team. Antituberculous treatment (e.g. rifampicin, pyrizinamide, isoniazid) for 6–12 months, usually combined with systemic corticosteroid to suppress the inflammatory component and a potential Jarisch–Herxheimer reaction (exaggerated inflammatory response due to massive bacterial lysis on commencing antibiotics). Prednisolone dose needs to be doubled when rifampicin is used because of liver enzyme induction.

Syphilis

The classical systemic manifestations of *Treponema pallidum* infection, almost exclusively sexually transmitted, can be subdivided into four phases:

* **Primary syphilis**: the chancre, a painless ulcer, usually on the genitalia, occurring 4 weeks after infection
* **Secondary syphilis**: 4–10 weeks after infection; generalized maculopapular rash, fever, headache, malaise, joint pain, lymphadenopathy, condylomata lata
* **Latent syphilis**: spontaneous remission of symptoms after 6–12 months, with occasional relapse; 30% of cases progress to the tertiary phase
* **Tertiary syphilis**: benign syphilis (gummas), cardiovascular syphilis, and neurosyphilis; neurosyphilis presents in a variety of ways, including aseptic meningitis, encephalitis, tabes dorsalis, cranial nerve palsies, and Argyll Robertson pupils (small, irregular with light-near dissociation)

Clinical evaluation

Ophthalmic manifestations are seen with congenital syphilis (interstitial keratitis, pigmentary retinopathy, glaucoma) and all the phases of acquired disease, although primary disease is limited to chancres of the lids and conjunctiva. Syphilis may cause almost any inflammatory ophthalmic disease, including dacryoadenitis, conjunctivitis, scleritis/episcleritis, keratitis, uveitis, and optic neuropathy. The typical features of syphilitic intraocular inflammation are a granulomatous anterior uveitis (mutton-fat keratic precipitates, iris nodules), vitritis, posterior placoid chorioretinitis (see Figure 7.22), retinal vasculitis, neuroretinitis, and macular oedema.

Investigations

Investigations include dark field microscopy, PCR, and serological tests, for example the Venereal Disease Research Laboratory (VDRL) test, and rapid plasma reagin. Be cautious about false-positive results (e.g. other spirochetal disease, connective tissue disease, pregnancy). Neurosyphilis is confirmed on cerebrospinal fluid sampling. Always check for HIV status, as coinfection is common.

Treatment

Penicillin is the mainstay of treatment, which should be overseen by an infectious diseases specialist. The Jarisch–Herxheimer reaction (see 'Treatment' under the heading 'Tuberculosis') may complicate initial antibiotic therapy.

Prognosis

Syphilis usually responds well to appropriate treatment.

Lyme disease

Lyme disease is caused by the spirochaete *B. burgdorferi*, transmitted by the bite of *Ixodes* ticks, which commonly parasitize deer. Patients may recall a tick bite and will usually have been in parkland or woodland containing deer. The characteristic first symptom is a spreading rash called erythema chronicum migrans. Later features include fever, arthralgia, cardiac involvement, meningitis, and cranial nerve palsies. The eyes may be affected by seventh nerve palsy, conjunctivitis, episcleritis, anterior uveitis, choroiditis, and retinal vasculitis. Diagnosis is made

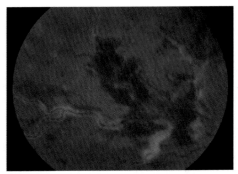

Fig 7.21 Tuberculosis hypersensitivity occlusive retinal periphlebitis with venous cuffing and associated haemorrhagic occlusion

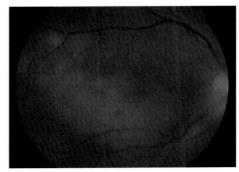

Fig 7.22 A syphilitic choroidal plaque

serologically, and treatment with oral tetracycline or amoxicillin is usually effective. Severe neurological or uveal involvement may necessitate intravenous penicillin/cephalosporin treatment.

Endogenous bacterial endophthalmitis

The clinical presentation of endophthalmitis (severe, painful intraocular inflammation with or without hypopyon) in the absence of an exogenous source (e.g. surgery, penetrating injury, suture abscess) should prompt the diagnosis of endogenous (blood-borne) intraocular infection. The presentation may, however, not be as florid, and subtle signs such as Roth spots (white-centred retinal haemorrhages representing microabscesses) should also raise the same suspicion. Common sources include endocarditis, urinary infection, intravenous lines, intravenous drug use, skin infection, pneumonia, and abdominal abscess.

Clinical evaluation

History

There may be an obvious source of infection or fever. Ask about infective symptoms and intravenous drug use.

Examination

- Varied findings
- Mild to severe intraocular inflammation
- Hypopyon not uncommonly seen
- Typical posterior segment findings are vitritis and areas of white retina (retinitis/retinal necrosis).
- Severe infections may evolve into pan-ophthalmitis (involving ocular adnexae).

Investigations

- Thorough clinical examination for source of sepsis (including the entire skin)

- Cultures of urine, blood, intravenous catheters, etc., with or without vitreous
- Imaging (e.g. echocardiography, CXR, abdominal ultrasound/CT)
- Involve general physicians

Treatment

- Dependent upon clinical scenario
- Intravitreal antibiotics should be given at the time of vitreous sampling (e.g. ceftazidime 2.25 mg and vancomycin 1 mg).
- Broad spectrum intravenous antibiotics should be given until culture and sensitivities available.
- Evisceration may be required in severe cases.
- Topical steroid and cycloplegia

Prognosis

- Very poor in severe cases

Exogenous bacterial endophthalmitis

Exogenous bacterial endophthalmitis is the result of infection introduced locally to the eye, most commonly after surgery (e.g. after cataract surgery) or trauma but also following ocular surface infections such as microbial keratitis or blebitis. Postoperative endophthalmitis is discussed in Chapter 3, Section 3.6. Vitreous sampling and injection of intravitreal antibiotics are important to identify the infecting organism and its sensitivity to antibiotics and to deliver high-dose antibiotic in an attempt to limit the damage caused by the infection are also necessary. Topical antibiotics and topical steroids with cycloplegia may also be used. Some use systemic steroids from 24 to 48 hours after commencing antibiotic.

7.11 HIV-related disease

Much of the contents of this section may be applied to patients without HIV/AIDS but with immunocompromise for other reasons (e.g. lymphoproliferative/bone marrow disease, immunosuppressive drugs).

HIV

HIV1 and 2 are retroviruses which ultimately cause severe immunocompromise, mainly through the infection and subsequent depletion of CD4+ T-cells. Infection is transmitted most commonly through sexual intercourse, although vertical transmission via needle-sharing by intravenous drug users is another common route.

Clinical evaluation

Many individuals will experience an acute viral syndrome within 6 weeks of acquiring the infection. Fever, rash, pharyngitis, myalgia, and headache are common. The disease is then typically asymptomatic for several years before the onset of AIDS, when low CD4+ counts lead to opportunistic infections by organisms such as *Pneumocystis carinii* (pneumonia), *Cryptococcus* (e.g. meningitis), and CMV (e.g. retinitis) or to the development of malignancies such as Kaposi sarcoma and lymphoma. HIV may cause encephalopathy, which sometimes leads to dementia, and a progressive multifocal leucoencephalopathy caused by a papovavirus known as the JC virus may also be seen. HIV has no known therapy other than to improve the immunocompromise.

Treatment

Highly active antiretroviral therapy (HAART) has revolutionized the management and outlook for patients with HIV and AIDS. HAART usually consists of triple (or quadruple) therapy including reverse transcriptase inhibitors with or without protease inhibitors. The decision to commence treatment depends upon the CD4+ count, viral load, and presence of opportunistic infections.

Ophthalmic manifestations of HIV/AIDS

Lids

* Molluscum, Kaposi sarcoma

Conjunctiva/cornea

* Kaposi sarcoma, HSV/HZV infection, microsporidial conjunctivitis/keratitis, dry eye (common)

Posterior segment

* Retinal microvasculopathy (common)
* Opportunistic infections:
  - CMV retinitis (common)
  - PORN (usually HZV)
  - Syphilis, tuberculosis
  - *Toxoplasma* (more severe than in immunocompetency)
  - Cryptococcal or *Pneumocystis* choroidopathy
  - *Candida*
* Intraocular non-Hodgkins lymphoma
* Optic neuropathy:
  - Acute, inflammatory during seroconversion
  - Chronic atrophy (possibly ischaemic) during later stages
  - Infiltrative/infective (cryptococcal, syphilis, tuberculosis)
* Herpetic acute retinal necrosis (may have normal CD4+ count)

Retinal microvasculopathy

Retinal microvasculopathy is the most common ocular manifestation of HIV, occurring in 40%–60% patients, and is commonly seen with low CD4+ counts.

Aetiology

* The exact cause of retinal microvasculopathy is unknown.
* Hypotheses include immunoglobulin deposition and endothelial cell HIV infection.

Clinical evaluation

* Usually asymptomatic, but may cause scotoma or blurring

Signs

* Multiple cotton wool spots and occasionally microaneurysms and haemorrhage (see Figure 7.23)
* No vitreous inflammation

Treatment

* Not indicated

CMV retinitis

* Rare in immunocompetent individuals but common in AIDS (up to 40% before the availability of HAART)
* CD4+ counts are usually fewer than 50 cells/µl.
* Also a recognized complication of organ transplantation with antirejection therapy

Aetiology

* Either haematogenous spread to the retina or reactivation of latent infection, due to immunocompromise

Pathophysiology

* Viral proliferation within the sensory retina, causing retinal necrosis and retinal vasculitis

Clinical evaluation

History

* Subacute presentation with blurring, field loss.
* May be asymptomatic

Examination

* Mild vitritis (unlike acute retinal necrosis in immunocompetent patients)
* May be peripheral or posterior pole, multifocal or unifocal.
* Initially small white retinal infiltrates (similar to cotton wool spots)
* Spreading white areas of retina (necrosis) with associated intraretinal haemorrhage (so-called pizza fundus; see Figure 7.24). Progression is slower than in acute retinal necrosis.
* Retinal vascular cuffing (especially arterial)
* Rarely, frosted branch angiitis (widespread arterial cuffing)
* RPE atrophy/granularity in areas of clearing
* Progression is usually slow.

Differential diagnosis in a known HIV+ patient

* HSV/VZV retinitis, syphilis, *Toxoplasma* (see Figure 7.25)
* Retinal microvasculopathy
* Lymphoma

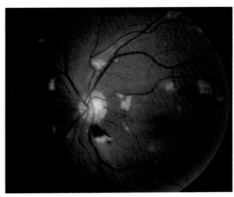

Fig 7.23 Asymptomatic retinopathy in HIV infection (HIV microangiopathy)
Cotton wool spots are typical but haemorrhages may occur also

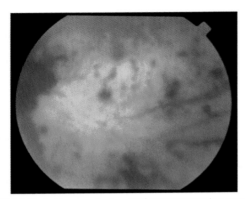

Fig 7.24 Typical haemorrhagic retinal necrosis seen in cytomegalovirus retinitis in AIDS (CD4+ count usually <50 cells/μl)

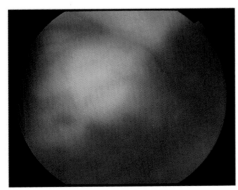

Fig 7.25 Extensive, progressive *Toxoplasma* retinochoroiditis in AIDS

Investigations
* Usually, HIV/low CD4+ count will have already been diagnosed: a clinical diagnosis can usually be made in typical cases.
* HIV test and CD4+ count if not already done
* Liaison with HIV physician
* Vitreous sampling rarely needed unless diagnosis is in doubt.

Treatment
Previously, intravenous ganciclovir or foscarnet and intravitreal ganciclovir implants were the mainstay of treatment.

Contemporary management depends upon the location of the lesion and immediate threat to vision. HAART may be used to control the disease in the absence of anti-CMV treatment with peripheral lesions, but response may take months, so close observation is necessary. For sight-threatening disease, HAART should be combined with ant-CMV treatments, which may include:
* Intravenous ganciclovir (watch for neutropenia; may be combined with granulocyte colony-stimulating factor, or implant.
* Intravitreal foscarnet (2.4 mg in 0.1 ml), given at time of biopsy.
* Foscarnet (watch renal function and electrolytes).
* Cidofovir (watch renal function).
* Valganciclovir (an orally administered ganciclovir prodrug).

Complications
* Macular or optic nerve involvement.
* Retinal detachment.
* Cystoid macular oedema (reversible).

Screening
Since patients with early CMV retinitis may be asymptomatic, some clinicians recommend screening of all patients with CD4+ counts of fewer than 50 cells/μl every 3–4 months.

Immune recovery uveitis
* A non-infectious intraocular inflammation developing in a patient with CMV retinitis (may be inactive) in whom HAART causes a rise in CD4+ count
* Thought to represent an appropriate immune attack upon viral antigens
* Usually manifests with vitritis and anterior uveitis
* May require treatment with topical, periocular, or intraocular steroid (avoid systemic treatment if possible)

Other posterior segment manifestations

PORN
The use of the term 'PORN' may be less useful than simply using the term 'viral retinitis' since these two conditions have overlap and, although most cases of PORN have been shown to be due to VZV, HSV has also been found. PORN represents a manifestation of herpetic retinitis in the immunocompromised, although classical acute retinal necrosis may also be seen.

Clinical evaluation
* History
  — Blurring and floaters
* Examination
  — Deep retinal white patches which spare the inner retina and retinal vessels initially
  — Usually multifocal and at posterior pole
* Treatment
  — Systemic acyclovir or valaciclovir and HAART
  — Variable response to treatment

Toxoplasma retinochoroiditis

- More severe in immunocompromised hosts than in healthy individuals (see Section 7.8), often presenting bilaterally.
- Tends not to spontaneously regress, with progressive disease causing extensive tissue destruction.
- Treatment in immunocompromised individuals differs from that used in the normal situation: antibiotic therapy without corticosteroid for all lesions, often with a good response.

Choroiditis

Choroiditis due to opportunistic infection by either *P. carinii* or *Cryptococcus* is a relatively unusual presentation (*Pneumocystis* choroiditis is more common). It typically presents as a multifocal choroiditis without significant vitritis; patients will usually be severely immunocompromised and may have disseminated infection. *Pneumocystis* may respond to systemic pentamidine or co-trimoxazole, whereas cryptococcal disease requires amphotericin B followed by fluconazole.

Optic neuropathy

- Acute painful retrobulbar optic neuropathy has been described during HIV seroconversion. This condition may respond to corticosteroid therapy.
- Other optic neuropathies in HIV-positive patients, particularly in the immunocompromised, should prompt a search for an infective cause. MRI is helpful to exclude perineuritis, which is often seen with syphilis, tuberculosis, and *Cryptococcus*:
  - Exclude syphilis (serology).
  - Consider CMV (serology, serum DNA quantification).
  - Consider tuberculosis (CXR, Mantoux test, MRI).
  - Consider *Cryptococcus* (MRI with or without cerebrospinal fluid).
- Chronic optic atrophy: may be due to microvasculopathy

Sarcoidosis

Sarcoidosis is a chronic, multisystem, granulomatory disease affecting almost any organ but most typically the lungs, skin, and eyes. It is most common in Afro-Caribbeans.

Aetiology

The cause of sarcoidosis remains unknown, although various hypotheses have developed over the years. The most credible of these include the involvement of an infectious agent, either persisting intracellularly (e.g. mycobacteria, *Propionibacterium acnes*) or causing sensitization after a previous infection. The fact that the disease clusters geographically (e.g. outbreaks on the Isle of Man, UK) and seasonally (most commonly presents in spring/summer) supports the hypothesis that an environmental agent is a possible cause of this condition.

Pathophysiology

Non-caseating granulomata composed of macrophages and T-lymphocytes are seen on histology. Depressed cell-mediated immunity may be seen, potentially causing anergic responses on skin testing with tuberculin.

Clinical evaluation

Non-ocular

- Constitutional: patients with active sarcoidosis may complain of fever, sweats (particularly at night), and weight loss.
- Thoracic (90% patients): bilateral hilar lymphadenopathy is common and the absence of parenchymal lung disease is described as Stage 1 on CXR staging. Parenchymal lung disease (Stage 2 with bilateral hilar lymphadenopathy (see Figure 7.26), Stage 3 without bilateral hilar lymphadenopathy) may progress to pulmonary fibrosis with bullae and bronchiectasis (Stage 4). Symptoms are breathlessness and a persistent dry cough.
- Cutaneous: erythema nodosum (tender, red/dark nodules on the lower leg), cutaneous granulomata, lupus pernio (superficial, blue/purple patches, often on the nose and the cheeks)
- Lymphadenopathy
- Musculoskeletal: arthralgia, dactylitis, lytic bone lesions
- Neurosarcoid: CNS parenchymal and meningeal disease, cranial neuropathies
- Cardiac: conduction block, cardiomyopathy, cor pulmonale
- Gastrointestinal: liver granulomas are common but bowel involvement is rare.
- Renal: stones due to hypercalcaemia, nephritis
- Other: parotid, submandibular, and lacrimal gland involvement

Ocular (25%–75% of patients)

- **Lacrimal gland:** enlargement, dry eye
- **Conjunctiva:** granulomata (see Figure 7.27) ; biopsy of these may confirm diagnosis
- **Uvea:** granulomatous uveitis is the typical finding in ocular sarcoidosis; anterior uveitis may be chronic or acute, painful or painless; iris nodules, posterior synechiae, and mutton-fat keratic precipitates are all common.

Posterior segment findings

Posterior segment findings include:

- **Vitritis:** commonly forms inferior 'snowballs'
- **Retinal vasculitis:** typically a periphlebitis with 'skip' lesions; occasionally, marked perivenous granuloma/exudation, termed 'taches de bougie' or 'candle wax dripping'; may cause retinal ischaemia and neovascularization (see Figure 7.28)
- **Cystoid macular oedema**
- **Retinal granulomata:** these are uncommon; preretinal granulomata (Lander's sign)
- **Choroidal disease:** can be varied; choroidal granulomata, atrophy, subretinal neovascularization
- **Optic disc:** swelling (function usually preserved), infiltration, and papillitis (function affected)
- **Optic nerve:** optic neuropathy from perineural/dural involvement (see Figure 7.29) or parenchymal granuloma

Investigations

Presumptive diagnosis may be based on findings of CXR/high-resolution chest CT, and raised serum ACE but definitive diagnosis requires histological confirmation. Common biopsy sites include transbronchial sites, conjunctival sites, lacrimal glands, lymph nodes, or the skin (in the presence of a rash). The Kveim test (intradermal injection of sarcoid tissue) is no longer used in routine practice. Supportive investigation findings include hypercalcaemia, lymphopaenia, polyclonal hypergammaglobulinaemia, pathological uptake on gallium scanning, and anergy on tuberculin testing.

Treatment

Treatment may be dictated by ocular or systemic morbidity, and patients are usually best managed by working in conjunction with a respiratory physician. Topical, periocular, and systemic corticosteroids are frequently used for ocular disease and are usually effective. Second-line agents may be necessary (methotrexate and anti-tumour necrosis factor (TNF) alpha are highly effective but beware of tuberculosis).

Prognosis

The ocular prognosis is variable and dependent on clinical features. Secondary glaucoma, macular involvement (oedema or choroiditis), and optic neuropathy are common causes of irreversible visual loss. Systemic sarcoidosis spontaneously resolves within 5 years in 60% of cases.

Behcets disease

Behcets disease is a chronic multisystem vasculitis characterized by oro-genital ulceration and is associated most commonly with inflammatory lesions of the eyes, skin, and joints. CNS involvement, gastrointestinal involvement, and thrombo-occlusive events are also seen and can prove fatal. The disease is notable for its geographic variation, with a predilection for inhabitants of the Mediterranean Basin and the Far East; the disease is most prevalent in Turkey (42/10 000 population). The disease is slightly more common and tends to be more severe in males than in females.

Aetiology

The aetiology of Behcets disease remains unclear but environmental factors such as infectious triggers are likely to be involved in conjunction with a background of genetic suscepti-bility. In particular, there has been interest in the role of micro-bial heat-shock proteins, which have sequence homology with human mitochondrial heat-shock proteins. A well-documented association exists between Behcets disease and HLA-B 51.

Pathophysiology

The pathological basis for Behcets disease appears to be a vasculitis, with lymphocytes, macrophages, and neutrophils in-filtrating vessel walls and the perivascular space. Neutrophil hyperreactivity and abnormal T-lymphocyte homeostasis are found.

Clinical evaluation

In 1990, the International Study Group for Behcet Disease proposed a set of classification criteria similar to that shown in Table 7.5 but stipulated the absolute need for recurrent oral ulceration to make the diagnosis. Recurrent oral ulceration (see Figure 7.30) is the hallmark of Behcets disease and may be found on the gums, lips, tongue, palate, or pharynx. Cuta-neous hypersensitivity is a common finding, with patients often describing a pustule forming at sites of skin injury (e.g. needle-entry site), so-called pathergy. Major morbidity and mortality are the result of vascular occlusions (e.g. hepatic portal vein, cerebral venous sinus) and CNS involvement.

Ocular disease

- Anterior uveitis, typically painless; hypopyon common; pain-less hypopyon is almost pathognomonic of Behcets disease (see Figure 7.31)
- Posterior segment signs:
  - Vitritis
  - Occlusive retinal periphlebitis (see Figure 7.32); may mimic branch retinal vein occlusion (BRVO).
  - Retinal infiltrates
  - Papillitis, disc swelling
  - Retinal (with or without anterior segment) neovascularization

Investigations

Behcets disease is a clinical diagnosis. HLA testing (for B51) is rarely contributory because of the low specificity and sensitivity.

Management

Management is best carried out with a multidisciplinary team including rheumatologists and oral physicians. Patients usually need prolonged systemic immunosuppression.

Common medications

- **Colchicine:** particularly used for mucocutaneous disease and Japanese patients

- **Systemic corticosteroid:** may be useful for acute exacer-bations but rarely practical as a single therapy
- **Ciclosporin and azathioprine:** evidence of benefit, often used in conjunction with steroid; tacrolimus (FK506) and mycophenolate may be used in the same way
- **Cyclophosphamide**
- **Interferon alpha:** expensive and with significant side ef-fects, but shown to be particularly efficacious
- **Infliximab:** proven useful in cases refractory to other treat-ments, with good control of both ocular and extraocular manifestations
- **Adalumimab.**

Complications

Ischaemic complications are the main cause of visual loss, in-cluding BRVO or central retinal vein occlusion (CRVO), optic atrophy, and neovascularization causing vitreous haemorrhage, tractional detachment, or glaucoma.

Prognosis

In the past, severe visual loss was seen in over 50% of males but, in an era of greater treatment options, this frequency has been reduced, with only about 25% of cases becoming blind in one or both eyes.

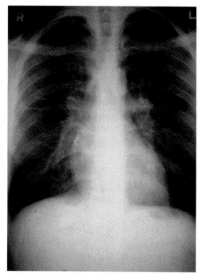

Fig 7.26 Bilateral hilar lymphadenopathy in sarcoidosis

Table 7.5 **Diagnostic criteria for Behcets disease, from the Research Committee of Japan (1987 revision)***	
Major criteria	**Minor criteria**
Recurrent oral ulceration	Arthritis
Skin lesions:	Intestinal involvement
—Erythema nodosum	Vascular occlusion
—Pathergy	Epididymitis
—Folliculitis	Neuropsychiatric symptoms
Genital ulceration	
Ocular inflammation (uveitis)	

*Complete Behcets disease requires all four major criteria. Incomplete Behcets dis-ease needs three major criteria, two major criteria and two minor criteria, or typical ocular disease with either one other major criterion or two minor criteria.
Data from Annual Report of the Behcet's Disease Research Committee of Japan, The Ministry of Health and Welfare of Japan, 1987

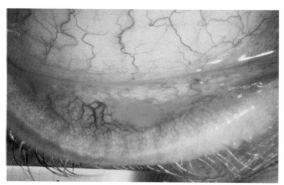

Fig 7.27 Conjunctival granuloma in sarcoidosis

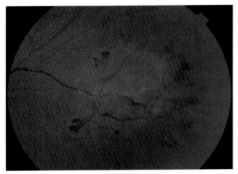

Fig 7.28 Peripheral new vessels in ischaemic retinal vasculitis due to sarcoidosis

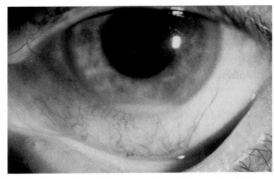

Fig 7.31 Severe, but painless anterior uveitis causing a hypopyon in Behcets disease

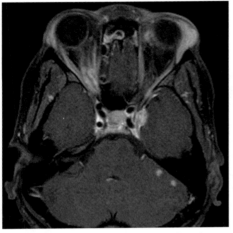

Fig 7.29 Optic nerve sheath disease on the right side in sarcoidosis, shown in a contrast-enhanced T1-weighted MRI

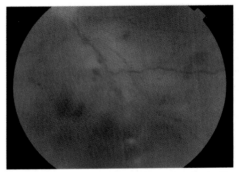

Fig 7.32 Vitritis, occlusive retinal phlebitis and retinal infiltrates (inferiorly) in Behcets disease

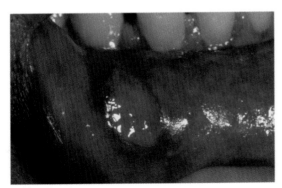

Fig 7.30 Aphthous ulceration of the oral mucosa in Behcets disease

Multiple sclerosis

Multiple sclerosis is a neuroinflammatory disorder characterized by the demyelination of CNS axons. Onset is usually in the third to fifth decades in persons spending their childhood in temperate regions of the northern hemisphere (e.g. northern Europe, North America). The condition is associated with intermediate uveitis (pars planitis) and retinal vasculitis.

Aetiology

The aetiology of multiple sclerosis remains unclear, although environmental and genetic factors are likely to be involved. The fact that the prevalence of the disease increases with increasing distance from the equator is supportive evidence of an environmental trigger; there are also hypotheses that suggest that a persistent viral infection or antecedent infection may cause autoimmunity through molecular mimicry. First-degree relatives of multiple sclerosis patients have an increased risk of the disease.

Pathophysiology

CNS lesions or plaques consist of axonal demyelination with predominantly lymphocytic infiltration. Within the retina, a segmental perivenous lympho-plasmacytic infiltrate is seen.

Ophthalmic features

The foremost ophthalmic manifestation of multiple sclerosis is an acute demyelinating optic neuropathy and ocular motility disturbances which are discussed in detail in Chapter 10, Section 10.10. Retinal periphlebitis is relatively common (approximately 10% of cases) and often asymptomatic, with rare visual morbidity. Intermediate uveitis and anterior uveitis are both seen more commonly in multiple sclerosis patients than in patients without multiple sclerosis. Vitreous haemorrhage may occur in patients with intermediate uveitis and retinal periphlebitis (see Figure 7.33), owing to retinal neovascularization.

Investigations and management

The investigations for multiple sclerosis are discussed further in Chapter 10, Section 10.10. Management of the uveitis does not differ from the management of other cases of non-infectious anterior and intermediate uveitis, although anti-TNF-alpha treatment should be avoided because of reports that it may exacerbate multiple sclerosis.

Seronegative arthritides

This group of conditions, which are negative for rheumatoid factor, is associated with HLA B27 and predisposes to ocular inflammation, which is usually an anterior uveitis. In the United Kingdom, 52% of anterior uveitis patients are positive for HLA B27.

Ankylosing spondylitis

Ankylosing spondylitis is a chronic, painful arthritis, predominantly affecting the spine and sacroiliac joints and often causing eventual fusion (so-called bamboo spine). Males are more commonly affected than females are (3 : 1), with onset usually between 16 and 40 years of age. Other large joints may be affected (e.g. hips, knees). Approximately 90% of cases are positive for HLA B27. Extra-articular manifestations include anterior uveitis, aortitis (leading to aortic regurgitation), and pulmonary fibrosis. The diagnosis is usually made on the basis of a sacroiliac X-ray. Management usually involves physiotherapy and NSAIDs.

Ophthalmic features

Recurrent non-granulomatous anterior uveitis is common, typically acute rather than chronic, unilateral (alternating), and often severe (occasional hypopyon) and painful with a high incidence of posterior synechiae. Cystoid macular oedema is not uncommon.

Reiter syndrome

In 1916, Hans Reiter described an acute febrile illness with arthritis, conjunctivitis, and urethritis following an episode of bloody diarrhoea. The disease classically follows an infection of the bowel (e.g. by *Shigella*, *Campylobacter*, *Salmonella*) or genital tract (*Chlamydia*), which is thought to trigger autoimmunity through molecular mimicry in susceptible individuals. Approximately 60% of cases are positive for HLA B27.

Systemic features

Unlike ankylosing spondylitis, Reiter syndrome has an acute onset, often with associated fever.

Cardinal features

- **Arthritis:** pauciarticular, usually affecting the sacroiliac joints and larger joints of the lower limb
- **Urethritis:** will be sterile unless the trigger was *Chlamydia*; a circinate balanitis (ulceration of the glans penis) may be present
- **Conjunctivitis**: sterile and bilateral
- **Other systemic features:** keratoderma blennorrhagica (a pustular rash usually found on palms and soles), oral ulcers, onycholysis, aortitis

Ophthalmic features

The conjunctivitis is non-cicatrizing, mucopurulent, and usually mild and self-limiting. There may be papillary change. A keratitis has been reported. Acute anterior uveitis with Reiter syndrome behaves similarly to ankylosing spondylitis, with acute, painful non-granulomatous recurrences.

Psoriatic arthritis

Arthritis is seen in 10% of patients with psoriasis, a common (2% prevalence) inflammatory skin condition characterized by scaly plaques. Those patients with nail changes are more predisposed to arthritis, which may be an asymmetric oligoarthritis (similar to other seronegative arthritides) or a symmetric polyarthritis sometimes causing a severe destructive picture (arthritis mutilans). Psoriasis patients with arthritis appear to be more prone to anterior uveitis than arthritis-free psoriasis sufferers are. In comparison with ankylosing spondylitis and Reiter syndrome, the rate of HLA B27 positivity is lower (30%–40%) and the uveitis less frequent (7%) and more likely to be chronic and involve the vitreous.

Inflammatory bowel disease

Some 2% of patients with inflammatory bowel disease (Crohns disease and ulcerative colitis) will develop uveitis. Although this is most commonly a recurrent anterior uveitis similar to that seen in ankylosing spondylitis, these patients may also develop posterior segment inflammation, including vitritis and retinal periphlebitis.

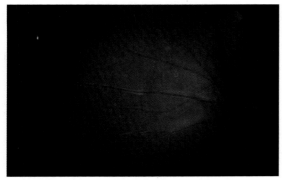

Fig 7.33 Asymptomatic retinal periphlebitis associated with multiple sclerosis

7.14 Scleritis and episcleritis

Episcleritis is an acute, relatively mild, and non-sight-threatening inflammation involving the episclera (loose vascular connective tissue between Tenons capsule and the surface of the sclera). In contrast, scleritis is usually a chronic and frequently severe sight-threatening inflammation of the sclera, often associated with systemic diseases which themselves may carry significant morbidity and mortality. Clinical distinction between the two is important because of the implications for management and prognosis.

Aetiology

Whereas both scleritis and episcleritis may have infectious aetiologies, both conditions are usually immune mediated. Episcleritis is more commonly idiopathic but shares many of the systemic associations of scleritis, which is a manifestation of a systemic disease in 50% cases (see Table 7.6).

Pathophysiology

The strong association between scleritis and systemic vasculitides, connective tissue disorders, and arthritides implies that a primary immunological basis, which may be mediated by both cell and immune complexes, may underlie most cases. Histopathologic studies have shown chronic inflammatory changes with combined lymphocytic and macrophage infiltration of the sclera and, in some aetiologies, granulomata will be present. Severe scleritis additionally involves fibrinoid necrosis with consequent tissue loss seen clinically as scleral thinning (scleromalacia).

Clinical evaluation

The distinction between episcleritis and scleritis is made purely on clinical grounds and is based on both a careful history and an examination. Particular attention should be paid to the severity and character of the pain and to the presence of any systemic symptoms. See Table 7.7 for a classification system.

History

Episcleritis
- Mild or no discomfort; often gritty or at most a mild ache
- Pain may be worse on ocular movement
- Vision unaffected

Scleritis
- Usually severe 'boring'/aching pain (except in the case of scleromalacia perforans)
- Pain often disturbs sleep.

Table 7.6 Aetiologies and associated diseases of episcleritis and scleritis

Non-infectious	Infectious
Rheumatoid arthritis	Syphilis
Granulomatosis with polyangiitis	Herpes zoster virus
Gout	Tuberculosis
Seronegative arthropathy (including Reiter syndrome)	Hepatitis B
Relapsing polychondritis	Lyme disease
Polyarteritis nodosa	
Systemic lupus erythematosus	
Sarcoidosis	
Inflammatory bowel disease	
Surgically induced	

Table 7.7 Classification of scleritis and episcleritis

Episcleritis	Scleritis
Simple	Anterior
Nodular	Diffuse
	Nodular
	Necrotizing:
	— With inflammation
	— Without inflammation (scleromalacia perforans)
	Posterior

- Pain often radiates to the brow.
- Pain may be worse on ocular movement.
- Tender globe, nausea.
- Vision may be affected (especially posterior scleritis).
- Redness may be diffuse, regional, or absent (posterior scleritis, scleromalacia perforans).

Examination

Examining in natural light (via the naked eye) and red-free light (via the slit lamp) is very helpful for distinguishing the blueish-red discolouration and deep vascular involvement seen with scleritis.

Episcleritis
- Vasodilatation of superficial episcleral plexus vessels (usually radially orientated, blanching with topical 10% phenylephrine)
- Episcleral oedema (occasionally nodules; see Figure 7.34)
- Globe usually not tender
- No intraocular signs

Scleritis
- Blueish-red tinge in natural light
- Tender
- Vasodilatation of deep and superficial episcleral plexus vessels (seen in red-free light)
- Scleral oedema, nodules
- Corneal changes (infiltrates, thinning)
- Intraocular inflammation
- Raised IOP
- Chorioretinal folds, exudative retinal detachment, disc swelling, proptosis (posterior scleritis)
- **Look for capillary closure and areas of necrosis/thinning.**
- Scleromalacia perforans: distinct type of painless, necrotizing scleritis without inflammation seen in rheumatoid arthritis

Differential diagnosis

Episcleritis
- Dry eye, blepharitis, conjunctivitis
- Superior limbic keratoconjunctivitis
- Foreign body granuloma (nodular episcleritis)
- Inflamed pingueculum
- Phlyctenulosis
- Lymphoma

Scleritis
* Episcleritis
* Anterior uveitis (more photophobia and anterior chamber reaction)
* Acute glaucoma (based on symptoms)
* Orbital inflammation/cellulitis (posterior scleritis)
* Optic neuritis (posterior scleritis)
* Orbital myositis (posterior scleritis)
* Posterior uveitis, uveal effusion, sympathetic ophthalmia, choroidal tumour (posterior scleritis)
* Lymphoma

Investigations
* Systemic history and examination
* Look for signs of associated systemic diseases, especially rheumatoid arthritis and granulomatosis with polyangiitis (cough, sinus symptoms, nosebleeds).

Episcleritis
Investigations are not necessary in simple episcleritis unless as-yet-undiagnosed systemic disease is suspected.

Scleritis
Scleritis may be the presenting feature of a potentially fatal systemic disease, so all new cases should be investigated, preferably targeted by systemic history and examination:
* Rheumatoid factor, ANA, ANCA, anti-double-stranded DNA
* FBC, urea and electrolytes, ESR, CRP, urate, syphilis serology

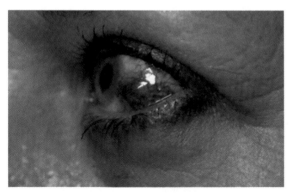

Fig 7.34 Nodular episcleritis, showing injection of the radially orientated superficial episcleral plexus vessels

* Urinalysis (look for casts) and blood pressure
* Ultrasound may be very useful in confirming the presence of posterior scleritis (scleral thickening, fluid in the sub-Tenons space).
* Orbital imaging (MRI/CT) may be necessary to exclude orbital disease.

Management

Episcleritis
For mild or moderate cases, no treatment may be necessary.

Short courses of topical corticosteroid or systemic NSAIDs (e.g. flurbiprofen, indomethacin) will usually prove effective if treatment is required (if not effective, consider revising diagnosis).

Scleritis
Scleritis requires systemic treatment with NSAIDs (flurbiprofen 50–100 mg three times a day, indomethacin), corticosteroids, or other immunosuppressive agents (including azathioprine, ciclosporin, methotrexate, and cyclophosphamide). The treatment should be tailored to the individual patient and will depend upon severity and any associated disease. Surgery is indicated if the diagnosis is in doubt (e.g. biopsy for lymphoma/masquerade) or to repair complications such as perforations and glaucoma.

Complications
* Scleral necrosis, thinning, perforation
* Keratitis/keratolysis
* Uveitis, cataract, secondary glaucoma

Posterior segment
* Exudative retinal detachment
* Macular oedema
* Disc oedema/atrophy

Prognosis
Episcleritis is benign and does not result in long-term complications or visual loss but is often recurrent. Treatment is usually effective but may need to be given long term for chronic or frequently recurrent cases.

The prognosis of scleritis is variable and involves both ocular and systemic morbidity (and mortality). Diffuse anterior scleritis (see Figure 7.35) not associated with systemic disease usually carries a better prognosis than nodular scleritis (see Figure 7.36), whereas necrotizing scleritis has the worst ocular outcome.

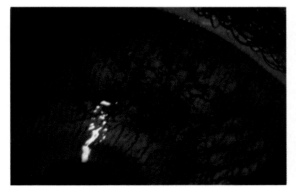

Fig 7.35 Beefy redness in diffuse anterior scleritis

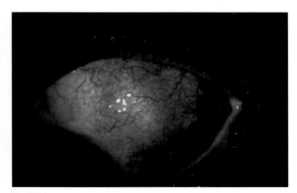

Fig 7.36 Nodular scleritis

7.15 Systemic treatment of ocular inflammatory disorders

Posterior segment intraocular inflammation and scleritis are sight-threatening diseases in which topical corticosteroids are generally ineffective. Since 50% of ocular inflammatory disorders are linked to systemic multisystem diseases, such as sarcoidosis, Behcets disease, or systemic vasculitis, systemic immunosuppression may be necessary both for the eyes and for extraocular disease manifestations. For posterior segment intraocular inflammation without systemic manifestations, periocular and intraocular drug delivery may be an effective option.

Corticosteroids have been the mainstay of systemic therapy for ocular inflammation and are usually very effective but may require high doses. However, supplementary immunosuppression may be required in the following circumstances:

- Disease control is inadequate with corticosteroids alone.
- The patient is on high doses of steroids (>10 mg/day of maintenance therapy).
- Recurrent high-dose steroid rescue for relapsing disease
- Steroid side effects necessitate a steroid-sparing agent.

Under these circumstances, other immunosuppressive agents (e.g. ciclosporin, mycophenolate mofetil (CellCept), azathioprine, tacrolimus) or new 'biological' treatments have a role to play. The use of corticosteroids and immunosuppressants carries with it the risk of serious and sometimes life-threatening side effects and these should be discussed with the patient at the outset and weighed against the perceived benefits. Exclusion of infective causes of ocular inflammation and latent tuberculosis infection is important prior to considering systemic immunosuppression.

The decision to commence immunosuppression and the choice of which drugs to use will depend upon numerous factors which should be discussed with the patient; these factors are as follows:

- General health and state of the patient:
  - Corticosteroids may have particular hazards in the very young and the very old, the obese, diabetics, and those with osteoporosis. Local therapies may be considered.
  - Ciclosporin may be nephrotoxic and so is relatively contraindicated in those with renal disease; in addition, it can cause hirsutism, so may be best to avoid using it in young females.
- Location, nature, and severity of the inflammation:
  - Mild symptoms may not warrant the risks of immunosuppression unless the risk of irreversible visual loss is high (e.g. in Behcets disease).
  - Unilateral disease with good contralateral vision may be considered inappropriate for the risks of heavy immunosuppression.
  - Experience may dictate preference for a choice of drug with proven efficacy in a particular disease.
- Reversibility:
  - Established, irreversible causes of visual loss (e.g. macular ischaemia, optic atrophy) will not benefit from treatment.
  - Vitritis and macular oedema of recent onset are typical causes of reversible visual loss.

- Patient reliability and follow-up potential:
  - Compliance with treatment and regular monitoring is essential for patients taking these potentially dangerous drugs.

General monitoring

Baseline assessment of patients prior to commencement of immunosuppression should include:

- Weight, blood pressure, urinalysis
- Blood tests appropriate to each drug
- Discussion of potential risks and benefits
- Patient information sheets provided where possible
- Other investigations as required, e.g. CXR to exclude tuberculosis
- Contraceptive advice for women of childbearing age
- A check of the varicella-zoster immune status (if patient is uncertain as to whether the disease was contracted, then serology should be checked)
- Vaccination advice: avoid live vaccination unless immunosuppressives are stopped at least 3 months beforehand

Systemic corticosteroids

Indications
Systemic corticosteroids (e.g. prednisolone) comprise the first-line therapy for most patients with sight-threatening or severe ocular inflammation.

Cautions
- Diabetes
- Obesity
- Osteoporosis
- Concurrent infection or previous tuberculosis
- Peptic ulceration

Dosage
- The maximum adult dose is 1–2 mg/kg orally per day or 'pulsed' intravenous methylprednisolone 0.5–1 g over 1 hour, usually given daily for 3 days.
- Taper slowly to a maintenance dose (adult) of less than 10 mg/day, if possible.
- **Abrupt discontinuation can lead to an Addisonian crisis.**

Important side effects
- Weight gain, cushingoid appearance, fluid retention
- Osteoporosis
- Hypertension, hyperglycaemia, hyperlipidaemia
- Peptic ulceration, pancreatitis
- Sleep disturbance, mania, and steroid psychosis
- Acne, skin thinning, and bruising
- Susceptibility to infection

Monitoring
- Blood pressure, weight, urinalysis (especially glycosuria)
- Occasional lipid levels

- Dual-energy X-ray absorptiometry (DEXA) bone scan for anyone on systemic steroids for >3 months. Prophylaxis should be started if patients is >65 years of age or has a T-score of 0 or lower.

Sensible precautions when prescribing steroids

- Provide a steroid card for information.
- Ask about tuberculosis exposure/symptoms and consider obtaining a CXR.
- Ask about chicken pox history: if the history is negative, consider checking VZV IgG levels (VZV-naive patients on prednisolone are at risk of disseminated VZV infection, which can be fatal; they should be warned to seek VZV immunoglobulin if they come into contact with chicken pox or exposed shingles).
- Consider gastric protection in those with a history of dyspepsia (e.g. proton-pump inhibitor/H2 antagonist) and try to avoid NSAIDs, especially if the patient is on warfarin (risk of gastrointestinal bleeding).
- Obtain regular DEXA scans, treat patients for osteoporosis if they are shown to be osteopaenic on DEXA and consider osteoporosis prophylaxis (e.g. alendronate 70 mg/week) in those at risk, e.g.:
  — Patients who have taken more than 7.5 mg prednisolone/day for more than 6 months
  — Patients who are more than 65 years old
  — Patients who are post-menopausal/amenorrhoeal
  — Patients with a history of fractures
  — Patients who are immobile

Ciclosporin and tacrolimus (FK506)

Mechanism of action

The mechanism of action for ciclosporin and tacrolimus is calcineurin inhibition, as they inhibit interleukin 2 (IL-2) production and T-helper cell function. Ciclosporin is a natural product of fungi, and tacrolimus is a macrolide antibiotic produced by *Streptomyces tsubkubaenis*. Tacrolimus (also known as FK506) is better tolerated and has fewer cardiovascular side effects, compared to ciclosporin; these features render it more useful than ciclosporin in the treatment of uveitis.

Contraindications/cautions

Contraindications/cautions include renal impairment, uncontrolled hypertension, pregnancy (advise barrier contraception), breastfeeding, recent live vaccinations, malignancy, and diabetes (in the case of tacrolimus). Ciclosporin and tacrolimus work in a similar way and should not be prescribed together.

Dosage

- **Ciclosporin:** initially 2.5 mg/kg, given in divided doses and increasing to 5 mg/kg depending on clinical need
- **Tacrolimus:** initially 0.03 mg/kg, increasing to 0.08 mg/kg depending on clinical response
- High doses are used in transplantation cases (but accompanied by an increased risk of nephrotoxicity).

Important side effects

- Renal impairment, hypertension
- Infections (e.g. respiratory tract infections)
- Nausea, vomiting, headache
- Tremors, paraesthesiae, cramps

- Hirsutism, gingival hyperplasia (in the case of ciclosporin)
- Hyperlipidaemia, hypomagnesaemia
- Hyperglycaemia (in the case of tacrolimus)
- Cancer (especially lymphoma, skin cancers)
- Tacrolimus interferes with the metabolism of oral contraceptives. Barrier method contraception should be advocated in addition to use of the pill.

Monitoring

- Blood pressure, weight, urinalysis (especially glycosuria)
- FBC, urea and electrolytes, liver function testing; at 2 weeks, 4 weeks, then every 4–8 weeks
- Lipids and serum magnesium every 3–6 months
- Tacrolimus levels

Antimetabolites: Azathioprine and mycophenolate mofetil (CellCept)

Mechanism of action

- Inhibition of T- and B-lymphocyte function by interfering with nucleotide synthesis

Contraindications

- Pregnancy and breastfeeding
- Recent live vaccinations
- Liver impairment
- Malignancy
- Mycophenolate and azathioprine work by similar mechanisms and should not be prescribed together.

Dosage

- **Azathioprine:** depends on thiopurine methyltransferase (TPMT) level, which should be checked prior to starting. There are genetically determined variations in activity, with low levels predisposing to bone marrow suppression. In the presence of normal TPMT levels, the usual dose is 50–100 mg/day for uveitis. A reduced dose is required when the TPMT level is low or when azathioprine is taken with allopurinol.
- **Mycophenolate:** start with 500 mg twice a day, up to a maximum of 3 g/day if tolerated

Important side effects

- Gastrointestinal symptoms (nausea, diarrhoea, vomiting, ulceration, haemorrhage)
- Abnormal liver function test/hepatotoxicity
- Leucopaenia, bone marrow suppression
- Infections, malignancy
- Mycophenolate is teratogenic.

Monitoring

- FBC should be checked at 1, 2, and 4 weeks after commencement, then every 1–2 months.
- Urea and electrolytes, liver function test checked at each clinic visit

Antimetabolites: Methotrexate

- A favoured drug for children and in rheumatoid disease

Mechanism of action

- Methotrexate is a folate analogue; it impairs nucleotide synthesis.

Contraindications

* Pregnancy, breastfeeding
* Recent live vaccinations
* Liver disease (abstain from alcohol)

Dosage

* Weekly dosing, oral or intramuscular. Intravitreal methotrexate has been shown to be successful in treating uveitic cystoid macular oedema.
* Gradually increase from 7.5 mg/week, watching FBC/liver function test.
* The range is 7.5–25 mg/week, usually 15 mg/week.
* Prescribe folic acid 1-5 mg/day.

Important side effects

* Gastrointestinal symptoms (nausea, diarrhoea, vomiting, ulceration, anorexia)
* Abnormal liver function test/hepatotoxicity
* Leucopaenia, bone marrow suppression
* Pneumonitis
* Infections, malignancy

Monitoring

* FBC should be checked at 1, 2, and 4 weeks after commencement, then every 1–2 months.
* Urea and electrolytes, liver function test checked at each clinic visit

Alkylating agents: Cyclophosphamide and chlorambucil

Mechanism of action

* Impairment of DNA synthesis and repair, by cross-linking DNA strands

Indications

Chlorambucil is rarely used in Behcets disease, where it can be effective against mucosal ulceration. Cyclophosphamide is generally reserved for severe inflammatory conditions, particularly those associated with systemic vasculitis (e.g. granulomatosis with polyangiitis or systemic lupus erythematosus), where it may be administered in 'pulsed' intravenous doses every 2 weeks or as an oral daily dose (1–3 mg/kg per day).

Side effects

The major side effects of cyclophosphamide are bone marrow suppression, infertility, and haemorrhagic cystitis. Mesna may be prescribed to reduce cystitis, and cryopreservation of eggs/sperm may be necessary.

7.16 Biological agents, and periocular treatments of ocular inflammatory disorders

Biological agents

There has been a recent explosion of interest and research into the use of so-called biological agents for inflammatory diseases. These agents are highly specific molecules targeting soluble inflammatory mediators (antibodies or antagonists to cytokines or cell surface receptors). Biological agents have been mostly used in conditions such as rheumatoid arthritis and inflammatory bowel disease, where some startling successes have been seen. Evidence that these agents may also be of benefit in treating ocular inflammatory disease has grown over the past few years. Most of the experience in using biological agents to treat ocular inflammatory disease has been with infliximab (in refractory uveitis), interferon alpha (in Behcets disease), and the anti-TNF-alpha agents infliximab and adalimumab (in retinal vasculitis and juvenile idiopathic arthritis (JIA)); all these agents have shown promising results. Like established immunosuppressants, these agents have their drawbacks, which include the risk of opportunistic infection (e.g. tuberculosis reactivation), hypersensitivity reactions, cardiac failure, malignancy, and paradoxical autoimmune disease. Furthermore, these agents are at present very expensive. Nevertheless, in certain situations, particularly when conventional immunosuppression fails because of inadequate effects or intolerable side effects, they may be of great clinical benefit, owing to their high efficacy. Examples of biological strategies currently available, some of which may be useful in ocular inflammation, are as follows.

- Anti-TNF-alpha treatments:
  - Infliximab and adalimumab: monoclonal antibodies which bind to TNF alpha to prevent receptor binding and thus prevent T-cell and macrophage activation. Studies have shown success in controlling Behcets disease, chronic uveitis resistant to other forms of immunosuppression, and JIA-associated uveitis.
  - Etanercept: a fusion protein composed of human immunoglobulin bound to the TNF receptor; binds membrane-bound TNF
  - Reported adverse events include tuberculosis reactivation, increased risk of malignancy, lupus-like reaction, and exacerbation of multiple sclerosis.
- Monoclonal antibodies directed against CD25, the IL-2 alpha receptor (daclizumab and basiliximab), thus preventing IL-2-mediated lymphocyte activation. Daclizumab has been shown to stabilize vision in 67% of patients with non-infectious intermediate uveitis, posterior uveitis, or pan-uveitis; however, it has been withdrawn from the market owing to low market demand.
- Monoclonal antibodies targeting CD52, a T-cell surface antigen (e.g. alemtuzumab (Campath-1H); as such antibodies cause T-cell depletion and therefore a high risk of infection, they are rarely used.
- Interleukin 1 (IL-1) inhibition by anakinra, a recombinant IL-1-receptor antagonist
- B-cell depletion using an anti-CD20 monoclonal antibody (rituximab). It has been shown to be effective in treatment of scleritis associated with Sjögren syndrome and Wegeners granulomatosis, as well as JIA-associated uveitis. Patients need to be screened for hepatitis B and C and given lamivudine prophylaxis if positive. Rituximab must be administered with full resuscitation facilities immediately available, since fatal infusion reactions due to severe cytokine release have been reported.
- Recombinant human interferon alpha 2a: this agent has shown great promise in ocular and systemic Behcets disease and in cystoid macular oedema related to uveitis. It can be administered subcutaneously. Common side effects include a flu-like illness in the first week of treatment; depression has also been reported.

Periocular drug delivery

Periocular depot steroid injection may be particularly useful when avoidance of systemic side effects is desired or when ocular inflammation is unilateral or asymmetric. This approach may even be combined with systemic therapy, for unilateral relapses. A common indication is the development of cystoid macular oedema, for example in intermediate uveitis. However, these approaches do not prevent systemic steroid effects, as some systemic absorption occurs that can, for example, affect glycaemic control in diabetics. Furthermore, periocular steroid use may be complicated by ocular hypertension, glaucoma, orbital fibrosis, and accidental globe perforation.

Various steroid preparations are available, but 40 mg triamcinolone (Kenalog) or methylprednisolone (Depo-Medrone) are commonly used, either as an orbital floor injection or into the sub-Tenons space. Preinjection OCT is helpful if given for macular oedema, for later comparison.

Orbital floor injection

An orbital floor injection is placed infero-temporally within the orbit, extraconally. It may be given transcutaneously or transconjunctivally.

1. Apply topical anaesthetic if a transconjunctival approach is planned. Clean the lower lid skin with, e.g. an alcohol swab for transcutaneous injections.
2. Draw up the steroid injection and ensure adequate mixing to avoid excessive drug deposits being left within the syringe at the end of the injection.
3. Give the patient a fixation point, keeping the eye in a neutral position within the orbit.
4. Remix the suspension and inject using a 25-gauge needle into the extraconal space infero-temporally, posterior to the equator of the globe. Avoid injecting under the periosteum (painful).
5. Carefully withdraw the needle.
6. Patients rarely need a pad or analgesia.

Posterior sub-Tenons injection

Whereas sub-Tenons anaesthesia is usually given by a blunt cannula through a small infero-nasal conjunctival incision, sub-Tenons steroid injections tend to be given by sharp needle supero-temporally (see Figure 7.37). This method is thought to allow depot steroid to settle behind the posterior pole of the

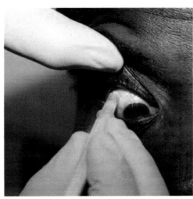

Fig 7.37 Periocular depot steroid injection, showing a posterior sub-Tenons approach

eye and avoids excessive regurgitation of the drug from the conjunctival entry site and unsightly steroid-filled chemosis.

1. Apply topical anaesthetic as drops and then by using an anaesthetic-soaked cotton-tipped applicator placed temporally under the upper lid. The applicator may be left for 5 minutes to ensure adequate anaesthesia.
2. In the meantime, draw up the steroid injection, ensuring adequate mixing (see Step 2 in 'Orbital floor injection').
3. Remove the cotton-tipped applicator.
4. Whilst the patient looks down, elevate the upper lid to expose the supero-temporal bulbar conjunctiva.
5. Insert the 25-gauge needle bevel down under the supero-temporal bulbar conjunctiva posteriorly and advance in the subconjunctival space. Small, gentle horizontal movements of the needle tip whilst advancing ensures that the sclera has not been engaged (ensure the globe does not move with the needle). Inject posterior to the equator.
6. Slowly remove the needle, avoiding excessive regurgitation of the drug.

Follow-up

Patients should be followed up 2–4 weeks after the injection to assess response and check IOP.

7.17 Intraocular treatments of ocular inflammatory disorders

More recently, there has been interest in the delivery of corticosteroids intraocularly, not only for intraocular inflammation but also for post-operative macular oedema (Irvine–Gass syndrome), diabetic macular oedema, and exudative macular degeneration. There have also been recent uncontrolled case series in which anti-VEGF treatments (originally developed for exudative macular degeneration) have been used for uveitic macular oedema.

Intravitreal steroid injection has the advantage of delivering the drug to the site of action, thus maximizing the concentration and reducing the systemic side effects. Rather inevitably, the ocular steroid side effects are maximized, with cataract and glaucoma being particularly prevalent following this approach. Furthermore, each injection carries a small risk of endophthalmitis, retinal detachment, and even lens trauma. The following approaches have been used.

Steroid implant

This approach involves the implantation of a slow-releasing steroid device in the vitreous cavity. Trials of a fluocinolone device (Retisert) implanted through a pars plana incision in non-infectious posterior segment intraocular inflammation showed great promise in terms of efficacy: 87% of implanted eyes showed stable or improved visual acuity during the 34 weeks following implantation, with reduced inflammation recurrence rates and a reduced need for systemic immunosuppression. The implant is thought to work for 2.5–3 years. However, a high incidence of glaucoma and ocular hypertension needing treatment (>50%), trabeculectomy (approximately 30% at 2 years), cataract (nearly 100% at 2 years), and uncertainties about long-term safety have limited their acceptance. The fluocinolone implant can be removed and, on the positive side, those eyes requiring trabeculectomy rarely experienced bleb failure due to the profound suppressive effect of the locally high steroid levels on healing. Ongoing studies will be needed to confirm a favourable risk/benefit profile.

Trials of an injectable, biodegradable dexamethasone pellet (Ozurdex) injected intravitreally for posterior segment intraocular inflammation have been shown to be effective in treating uveitis. The 26-week data also suggested that, despite causing a rise in IOP in 19% of subjects, it did not increase the need for glaucoma surgery, as compared to sham injections. However, a longer follow-up period is required to draw conclusions about increased glaucoma risk.

A large multicentre trial is underway comparing the visual outcomes and disease control achieved with conventional systemic immunosuppressive drugs compared to those achieved with intravitreal steroid implants. The results of this trial will ultimately answer the question of the degree of effectiveness of local therapy in posterior uveitis.

Intravitreal steroid injection

Trans-scleral intravitreal injection of triamcinolone acetonide has become a frequently used (but unlicensed) treatment for a wide variety of posterior segment pathologies resulting in macular oedema including diabetic maculopathy, retinal vein occlusion, subretinal neovascularization, Irvine–Gass syndrome, and posterior segment intraocular inflammation. The effects are not as long-lasting as the fluocinolone implant, with triamcinolone crystals remaining for 3–4 months in the vitreous cavity. As with the fluocinolone implant, glaucoma and cataract are the main complications, with approximately 50% requiring topical antihypertensives. Bacterial endophthalmitis (0.1%), sterile endophthalmitis (0.9%), and pseudohypopyon (crystalline deposits in anterior chamber, 0.8%) may also occur post-operatively. The sterile endophthalmitis may represent a hypersensitivity reaction and usually occurs in the first two post-operative days. Later presentations should raise suspicion of bacterial endophthalmitis, which may present with little pain and redness (presumably because of the immunosuppressive effect of the intraocular steroid).

Intravitreal triamcinolone in uveitis

The main indication is macular oedema, although vitritis may also improve, and the approach has been used in serpiginous choroiditis, Behcets disease, VKH syndrome, and sympathetic ophthalmia. Intravitreal triamcinolone acetonide (2–4 mg) has a beneficial effect on macular oedema (100% resolution in one study of 12 patients) and 75%–83% of patients experience an improvement in visual acuity, although reinjection was necessary to maintain the improvement. Those patients with macular oedema for more than 12 months were less likely to benefit.

Intravitreal injection

Appropriate preinjection counselling of the patient should include the risks of endophthalmitis, glaucoma, cataract, and retinal detachment.

- Apply copious amounts of topical anaesthetic (an anaesthetic-soaked cotton-tipped applicator may be used over the site of injection).
- Prepare the intravitreal injection with e.g. an insulin syringe and ensure adequate mixing of drug suspension.
- Apply povidone iodine to the lids and conjunctival sac and leave for several minutes before sterile draping and then insertion of a speculum.
- Most will inject a small amount of subconjunctival anaesthetic (e.g. 1% lidocaine) over the injection site (usually infero-temporally).
- Using a caliper measure from the limbus: 4 mm for a phakic eye, 3.0–3.5 mm for a pseudophakic eye
- Remix the drug suspension and using an insulin syringe/27-gauge needle enter the conjunctiva a few millimetres away from the sclerotomy so that any vitreous wick is less likely to emerge onto the conjunctival surface.
- Pass the needle perpendicularly through the sclera (see Figure 7.38) into the vitreous, aiming towards the posterior pole and inject (usually 0.1 ml).
- Wait for a few seconds before withdrawing the needle so that the drug dissipates into the vitreous and is not all regurgitated.
- A cotton-tipped applicator may be placed over the sclerostomy when the needle is withdrawn to prevent regurgitation.
- Confirm at least hand-motion vision and check the fundus by indirect ophthalmoscopy. Some clinicians always perform a paracentesis, but most will only do this if the central retinal artery is closed or there is no light perception after injection.
- Prescribe topical antibiotic for 1–2 weeks.
- Some clinicians recommend checking the IOP after half an hour.

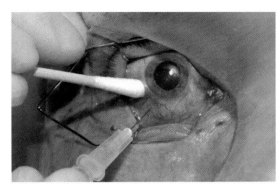

Fig 7.38 Intravitreal injection

A broad spectrum of disease may present to a rheumatologist besides those manifesting with joint disease. So-called connective tissue diseases and vasculitides may also be classed as rheumatological diseases, although they may present to other medical departments as well. Many of these conditions have manifestations within the eye and ocular adnexae.

Systemic lupus erythematosus

Systemic lupus erythematosus (SLE) is a multisystem autoimmune disease typically affecting young women (the female/male ratio is 6 : 1). Afro-Caribbeans and Chinese are particularly affected.

Aetiology

There are various theories concerning the aetiology of SLE, with evidence for both environmental (drug-induced/viruses) and genetic influences. There is 60% concordance of SLE in monozygotic twin studies.

Pathophysiology

Type 3 (immune complex) and possibly Type 2 (antigen-specific antibody-binding) hypersensitivity appear to be involved. Immune complexes are found on glomerular basement membrane in glomerulonephritis. There is widespread small- and medium-vessel vasculitis. Autoantibodies are the hallmark of SLE (e.g. ANA, anti-double-stranded DNA, anti-extractable nuclear antigens, antiphospholipid antibodies).

Clinical evaluation

* Multisystem involvement (lupus is a great imitator of other diseases; see Table 7.8)

Ophthalmic manifestations of SLE

* Lid erythema in malar rash
* Keratoconjunctivitis sicca
* Episcleritis/scleritis
* Uveitis is rare.

* Retinal arterial involvement: occlusive arteritis manifesting usually with cotton wool spot retinopathy but also occasionally as choroidal ischaemia or large retinal arteriolar occlusion

Investigations

Diagnosis is usually made clinically with supportive serological tests:

* ANAs (including anti-double-stranded DNA, anti-extractable nuclear antigens)
* Antiphospholipid antibodies, false-positive VDRL
* Low serum complement

If the diagnosis is suspected (e.g. cotton wool spots in fundus) it is mandatory to check the **blood pressure** and dip the **urine**. Rheumatological input is essential.

Treatment

The treatment usually involves a combination of hydroxychloroquine, corticosteroids, and other immunosuppressants (e.g. azathioprine, cyclophosphamide) depending on the severity of organ involvement.

Antiphospholipid syndrome

A disorder related to SLE in which antiphospholipid antibodies predispose to recurrent abortion, and arterial/venous thromboses which may affect the eye. Other features include thrombocytopaenia and haemolytic anaemia. Diagnosis is made by the detection of anti-cardiolipin antibodies and a coagulation assay called the lupus anticoagulant test.

Rheumatoid arthritis

Rheumatoid arthritis is a common, chronic, inflammatory joint disease characterized by a symmetrical polyarthritis usually affecting the joints of the hand, wrists, knees, and ankles, although any synovial joint can be affected. There are numerous extra-articular manifestations of rheumatoid arthritis (see Table 7.9), including several recognized ocular complications. The condition typically affects females (three times more than men) between 25 and 60 years of age, but it may begin at any age.

Table 7.8 Multisystem involvement in systemic lupus erythematosus

General	**Fever, malaise, weight loss**
Mucocutaneous	Photosensitive, 'butterfly'/malar rash Discoid lupus Alopecia Livedo reticularis Mouth ulcers
Musculoskeletal	Non-erosive arthritis: symmetrical, small joints Proximal myopathy
Renal	Membranous glomerulonephritis Nephrotic syndrome, renal failure
Cardiac	Pericarditis/myocarditis Arrhythmias Hypertension (renal involvement) Libman–Sacks (sterile) endocarditis
Respiratory	Pleurisy, pneumonitis
CNS	Headache, seizures, cranial nerve palsy Chorea, psychiatric disorders
Blood	Leucopaenia, thrombocytopaenia Haemolytic and normochromic anaemia

Table 7.9 Exra-articular manifestations of rheumatoid arthritis

General	**Fever, malaise, weight loss, anaemia, osteoporosis, lymphadenopathy**
Cutaneous	Ulceration, nodules, vasculitis
Renal	Drug-induced nephropathy: NSAIDs, gold, chloroquine; amyloid
Cardiac	Pericarditis, myositis
Respiratory	Pleural effusions, fibrosing alveolitis
Peripheral nervous system	Entrapment neuropathies, mononeuritis multiplex, glove and stocking sensorimotor neuropathy
Gastrointestinal	Splenomegaly, peptic ulceration (NSAIDs); bowel infarction; amyloid; xerostomia (Sjögren syndrome)

Aetiology

Like most autoimmune diseases, there appear to be genetic (HLA DR4/DR1) and environmental (possibly prior exposure to bacteria or viruses) influences.

Pathophysiology

- Synovial attack by T-cells, macrophages, and ultimately fibroblasts, with consequent destruction of cartilage and bone by proteolytic enzymes, resulting in pain, loss of function, and deformity
- Extra-articular involvement may be inflammatory, drug-induced, amyloid-related, or due to immobility (e.g. osteoporosis).

Clinical evaluation

- **Articular:** symmetric polyarthritis (painful joint swelling) most commonly involving hands, wrists, and knees; typical deformities in the hands (e.g. swan neck, boutonniere, ulnar deviation) with muscle wasting and loss of function (see Figure 7.39)

Ophthalmic manifestations of rheumatoid arthritis

- **Dry eye**: may be part of Sjögren syndrome (inflammatory destruction of lacrimal and salivary glands, usually confirmed with anti-SSA(ro) and anti-SSB(la) antibodies). Dry eye in rheumatoid arthritis may be severe and lead to corneal epithelial defects, stromal melting, and perforation. These conditions are discussed further in Chapter 2, Section 2.21.
- **Episcleritis and scleritis (the most common systemic association of scleritis):** scleritis may present painlessly with a white eye and scleromalacia (scleromalacia perforans; see Figure 7.40). Patients with scleromalacia perforans remain asymptomatic until either astigmatism develops or an incidental finding of a blue patch on the eye is made. Contrary to the name, perforation is uncommon in the absence of trauma. No medical treatment is effective or indicated.
- Posterior segment disease is rare in rheumatoid arthritis but retinal arteritis and ischaemic optic neuropathy (presumed vasculitic) may occur.
- Nodular involvement on the superior oblique tendon or inflammation of the trochlea may produce Brown syndrome (see Chapter 9, Section 9.18).

Management

Rheumatoid factor is an antibody directed against the Fc fragment of IgG and is found in 80% patients with rheumatoid arthritis. It may be present in other connective tissue diseases and infection, so it is not 100% specific. X-ray of the hands may show a typical erosive arthritis with soft tissue changes. Systemic treatment has traditionally involved corticosteroids, NSAIDs, hydroxychloroquine, gold, sulphasalazine, penicillamine, and methotrexate. Methotrexate is commonly used for chronic scleritis when associated with rheumatoid arthritis. New biological agents (e.g. infliximab) have been very successful. Dry eye treatment is discussed in Chapter 2, Section 2.6.

Seronegative arthritis

Seronegative arthritides, including ankylosing spondylitis, Reiter syndrome, JIA, and psoriatic arthritis, have an established, strong association with uveitis and are discussed further in Section 7.13

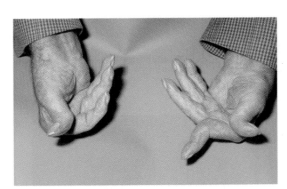

Fig 7.39 Severe joint deformity in rheumatoid arthritis

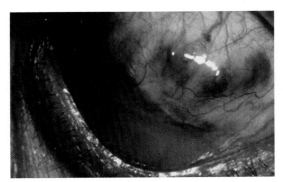

Fig 7.40 Scleromalacia perforans in rheumatoid arthritis
Severe scleral thinning is causing a staphyloma in the absence of overt inflammation. Contrary to the name, perforation is rare

7.19 Vasculitis

Vasculitis comprises a group of presumed autoimmune conditions in which the primary target organ is the vasculature.

Large-/medium-vessel vasculitis

This group includes Takayasus arteritis and giant cell arteritis (GCA; temporal or cranial). Both may result in arterial complications affecting the eye.

Takayasus arteritis (pulseless disease)

Takayasus arteritis is a polyarteritis with a predilection for the aorta and its main branches. It mainly affects young women and children. Manifestations within the eye mainly reflect carotid involvement, typically ocular ischaemic syndrome.

GCA

GCA is found in patients over the age of 55 years, and more commonly affects women than men. It affects medium-sized arteries, particularly branches of the external carotid and is associated with a spectrum of diseases, including polymyalgia rheumatica (proximal muscle pains and weakness, fever). Typical symptoms of GCA are headache (scalp tenderness), jaw pain and claudication, fever, malaise, weight loss and, of course, sudden visual loss due to ischaemic optic neuropathy (see Figure 7.41) or (more rarely) central retinal artery occlusion (CRAO). Diagnosis is made on clinical grounds, with the support of raised ESR and/or CRP and confirmed by typical findings on temporal artery biopsy (chronic intimal inflammation with fragmentation of the elastic lamina). The condition and its ophthalmic manifestations are described in more detail in Chapter 10.

Small-/medium-vessel vasculitis

This group of conditions is uncommon and often severe with life-threatening multisystem involvement. Necrotizing arteritis is a frequent feature.

Granulomatosis with polyangiitis

Previously known as Wegeners granulomatosis, granulomatosis with polyangiitis is a necrotizing, granulomatous arteritis mainly affecting the upper and lower respiratory tract and kidneys. Middle-aged males are most frequently affected.

Common features

- Nasal symptoms are common and may be first feature: rhinitis, nose bleeds, and sinusitis; collapse of the nasal bridge; middle ear involvement may lead to deafness.
- Pulmonary involvement: breathlessness, haemoptysis, pleurisy
- Renal disease: focal and segmental glomerulonephritis, present in 80% of cases, often leading to renal failure
- Multisystem effects: pyrexia, arthritis, purpurae, cutaneous vasculitis, neuropathy

Ophthalmic involvement (up to 58%)

- Adnexae: proptosis, orbital inflammation (may mimic orbital cellulitis), nasolacrimal obstruction
- Conjunctivitis, episcleritis, peripheral keratitis/melts
- Scleritis, particularly the necrotizing variety
- Retinal: rarely, an occlusive retinal arteritis
- Neuro-ophthalmic: optic neuropathy (may be ischaemic), cranial nerve palsies

Investigations

In approximately 16% of cases of granulomatosis with polyangiitis, the presenting feature will be ophthalmic (e.g. scleritis, orbital inflammation). Granulomatosis with polyangiitis is a serious, life-threatening disease with 80% mortality in the first year if left untreated. Maintaining a high index of suspicion is necessary, with appropriate history taking and investigation. ANCAs are present in most cases and are of the cytoplasmic type. Inflammatory markers are usually raised and the CXR may be abnormal. Check the blood pressure and urinalysis.

Treatment

Treatment is usually managed by rheumatologists and nephrologists and usually involves high-dose corticosteroids and cyclophosphamide. Scleritis activity may be gauged clinically and treatment adjusted accordingly. In the event of unilateral visual loss due to optic neuropathy, lengthy immunosuppression is likely to be needed to protect the other eye even in the absence of other symptoms or signs.

Polyarteritis nodosa, microscopic polyarteritis, and Churg–Strauss syndrome

These small-vessel vasculitides may all be associated with the presence of ANCA with a perinuclear staining pattern. Polyarteritis nodosa and microscopic polyarteritis are a spectrum of conditions presenting with fever, weight loss, and renal, cutaneous, and neurological (mononeuritis multiplex) manifestations. Churg–Strauss syndrome primarily affects the pulmonary arteries causing pulmonary eosinophilia. All these conditions may, rarely, cause scleritis, occlusive retinal/choroidal vasculitis, ischaemic optic neuropathy, and cranial nerve palsies.

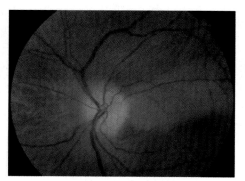

Fig 7.41 Pale disc swelling and associated regional retinal pallor due to arteritic anterior ischaemic optic neuropathy and cilioretinal artery occlusion in giant cell arteritis

7.20 Cardiovascular disease and the eye

Hypertension, atheromatous disease, and embolic phenomena may affect the eye in a variety of ways. Many of these are discussed in Chapter 6.

Systemic hypertension

There are various definitions for systemic hypertension but arterial blood pressure of more than 139/89 mmHg may be considered to be hypertensive and 120–139/80–89 mmHg has been described as pre-hypertension. Prevalence may be as high as 44% in Europe in people over 35 years.

Aetiology

Aetiology may be essential or secondary.

* **Essential:** 30% heritability; multiple environmental factors including salt intake, obesity, exercise, stress, smoking, etc.
* **Secondary:** multiple causes, which should be excluded in suspicious cases (young patients, resistant hypertension); causes include:
  - Renal disease (including renal artery stenosis)
  - Endocrine disease (Cushings/Conns syndromes)
  - Tumours (phaeochromocytoma)
  - Coarctation of the aorta
  - Pregnancy
  - Drugs (e.g. prednisolone, ciclosporin)

Systemic effects

Hypertension is asymptomatic until organ damage occurs.

* Cardiac: left-ventricular hypertrophy, heart failure
* Vascular: contributes to atheromatous diseases
* Stroke (ischaemic and haemorrhagic)
* Nephropathy

Ophthalmic effects

* Hypertensive retinopathy (see Chapter 6. Section 6.8)
* Choroidal infarction (see Figure 7.42)
* Main cause of BRVO
* Contributor to CRVO
* Non-arteritic ischaemic optic neuropathy
* Microvascular cranial nerve palsies

Malignant (accelerated-phase) hypertension

* Severe hypertension causing rapid organ damage in eyes, brain, lungs, and kidneys because of fibrinoid necrosis of vessels
* Blood pressure usually more than 200/140 mmHg
* Effects include:
  - Pulmonary oedema
  - Cardiac ischaemia
  - CNS: headache, vomiting, cerebral infarction, encephalopathy
  - Acute renal failure
  - Papilloedema, optic neuropathy, retinopathy

Management

A wide variety of medications for hypertension is available, including diuretics, beta blockers, calcium channel blockers, ACE inhibitors, angiotensin 2 antagonists, and centrally acting drugs.

Malignant hypertension

Malignant hypertension requires emergency admission under a medical team for cautious control of blood pressure and investigation of cause. It is important not to lower the blood pressure precipitously, since this may exacerbate organ damage (e.g. acute visual loss, stroke) owing to loss of autoregulation.

Atheromatous disease

Atheromatous disease is a major cause of morbidity and mortality in the developed world. Atherosclerosis is the term used to describe arterial changes (including luminal narrowing) due to atheromatous plaque and should be distinguished from arteriosclerosis, which is a loss of elasticity and thickening of the wall due to collagen and hyaline deposition.

Aetiology

Increasing age, male gender, smoking, diabetes mellitus, hypertension, genetic influences, hypercholesterolaemia, obesity, and hypothyroidism are known risk factors.

Pathophysiology

* Initially a sub-intimal fatty streak
* Involvement of macrophages which phagocytose lipid (foam cells); smooth muscle proliferation; ongoing cholesterol deposition; calcification
* Inflammatory component
* Luminal narrowing occurs and occlusion may be gradual, alternatively, it may be sudden if rupture occurs within the atheromatous plaque.

Major effects

* Coronary artery disease (myocardial infarction, angina, ischaemic cardiomyopathy)
* Cerebrovascular disease (cerebrovascular accident, transient ischaemic attacks, multi-infarct dementia)
* Peripheral vascular disease: lower limb ischaemia
* Mesenteric vascular disease: bowel ischaemia and infarction

Ophthalmic presentations

Atherosclerosis may affect the ophthalmic artery, the anterior ciliary artery, the posterior ciliary artery, and the central retinal artery. It may lead to arterial insufficiency and occlusion (e.g. ophthalmic artery occlusion, CRAO, ischaemic optic neuropathy, cilioretinal artery occlusion). In addition, thickening of the arterial wall is thought to cause BRVO and potentially contribute to CRVO, both of which are discussed in Chapter 6. Ischaemic disease may also affect the third, fourth, and sixth cranial nerves (see Chapter 10).

Carotid disease

Carotid disease may manifest in the eye in two ways: as embolic phenomena (CRAO, BRAO, amaurosis fugax) and with vascular insufficiency (ocular ischaemic syndrome). A bruit may or may not be heard (occluded carotid arteries have no flow) in the neck.

Ocular ischaemic syndrome

Ocular ischaemic syndrome may present in a number of ways but common features are:

* **Anterior segment:** uveitis, rubeosis, neovascular glaucoma, cataract

283

- **Posterior segment:** arteriolar narrowing, venous dilatation, mid-peripheral retinal blot haemorrhages, neovascularization of the disc; digital ophthalmodynamometry (gentle pressure on the globe during fundoscopy) may demonstrate an easily collapsible central retinal artery

Carotid ultrasound studies may show stenosis, which is usually severe on at least one side (not necessarily the side of the eye signs). If no stenosis is found and suspicion is high, then angiography may be necessary to further investigate. Ophthalmic artery disease may be a major contributor in these cases.

Management of carotid artery disease affecting the eye

Immediate measures for amaurosis fugax are (1) the exclusion of other causes such as hyperviscosity and GCA, (2) antiplatelet therapy (assuming no contraindication), and (3) addressing risk factors such as hypertension, smoking, diabetes, and cholesterol. Medical treatment of neovascular glaucoma and uveitis in ocular ischaemia may be necessary. The decision to perform carotid endarterectomy is a complex one and, for ophthalmic presentations in the absence of cerebral events, there are conflicting views on the benefits of surgery. Improvements in ocular ischaemia have been seen following endarterectomy. The involvement of a neurologist or stroke physician is recommended.

Other causes of retinal emboli

Emboli appearing in the retinal circulation are most commonly from the internal or common carotid arteries (cholesterol or platelet emboli) but may also originate from the aorta and from the heart because of valvular disease or arrhythmia or from the systemic circulation in the event of an atrial septal defect (paradoxical embolism).

Valvular disease

Degenerative, rheumatic, and congenital valve disease may predispose to embolic phenomena. Degenerative valvular disease may lead to calcific emboli seen in the retinal circulation as white, non-scintillating specks, usually at a branching point. These emboli tend to be larger than platelet or cholesterol emboli. Rheumatic mitral valve disease often leads to atrial fibrillation and left atrial dilatation which predisposes to thrombus formation and subsequent embolism. Opinions are required from specialists in echocardiography and cardiology.

Endocarditis

Infection of the heart valves usually occurs in the presence of pre-existing valvular disease. Common organisms include:

- α-haemolytic streptococci (viridans group): usually following dental work; typically subacute presentation
- Other streptococci: *Streptococcus faecalis, Streptococcus pneumoniae*
- *Staphylococcus aureus*: typically acute presentation, may be on normal valves, usually found in an intravenous drug user or a diabetic
- *Staphylococcus epidermidis*
- *Pseudomonas*

Vegetations on the valve leaflets may dislodge, causing embolic phenomena anywhere in the body, including septic cerebral infarctions.

Common systemic features include heart murmur, fever, weight loss, splinter/nail-bed infarcts (see Figure 7.43), vasculitic skin lesions (Janeway lesions, Oslers nodes), and haematuria.

Ophthalmic manifestations

Retinal artery occlusion is very rare but retinal microabscesses (Roth spots, white-centred haemorrhages; see Figure 7.44) may be seen, as well as areas of retinitis and/or frank endogenous endophthalmitis.

Investigations

Have a high index of suspicion in anyone with a fever and uveitis or retinal haemorrhages. Listen to the heart carefully. Involve cardiologists. Arrange admission if suspicion is high.
Investigations include:

- Blood pressure, urinalysis, FBC, urea and electrolytes, liver function test, CRP, ESR, 3× blood cultures
- Echocardiography: transthoracic, with or without trans-oesophageal

Treatment

Treatment of endocarditis involves prolonged (usually 6 weeks) intravenous antibiotics with or without surgical intervention to repair or replace the affected valve.

NB: bacterial endocarditis has significant mortality and can lead to rapid clinical decline. Do not delay investigations.

Atrial fibrillation

The presence of retinal artery occlusion or a history of amaurosis fugax should always prompt an assessment of the pulse and questions about palpitations. Uncoagulated patients in atrial fibrillation presenting with embolic phenomena should be admitted immediately for formal anticoagulation by the medical team on the assumption of a cardiac source for the embolus. A left atrial thrombus carries the risk of major embolic vessel occlusion.

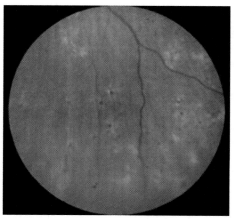

Fig 7.42 Elschnig spots: old choroidal infarcts secondary to severe hypertension

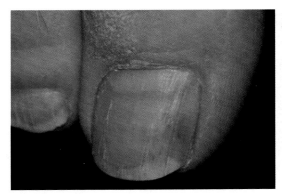

Fig 7.43 Toenail-bed infarction (splinter haemorrhages) in bacterial endocarditis

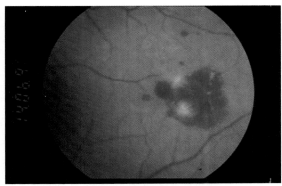

Fig 7.44 A haemorrhagic retinal microabscess (Roth spot, white-centred haemorrhage) due to a septic embolus in bacterial endocarditis

7.21 Endocrine diseases in ophthalmology

Diabetes mellitus (diabetic retinopathy, cataract) and autoimmune thyroid disease (thyroid eye disease, superior limbic keratoconjunctivitis) have well-characterized ophthalmic presentations which are discussed in Chapters 6 and 11, respectively. A brief description of the systemic aspects of diabetes mellitus is given in this section.

Diabetes mellitus

Definition

- Fasting venous blood glucose concentration of more than 6.9 mmol/l, or blood glucose more than 11.0 mmol/l, either on random test or 2 hours following 75 g oral glucose load
- Three main types: type 1 (usually young at onset), type 2 (usually older at onset), and gestational

Aetiology

- **Type 1:** autoimmune destruction of pancreatic islet cells; genetic (HLA DR3/4) and environmental (viral?) influences
- **Type 2:** combination of reduced insulin secretion and insulin resistance (involving the insulin receptor). Genetic influences and obesity are important.

Complications

Acute

- Ketoacidosis (type 1 diabetes) and non-ketotic coma (type 2 diabetes)
- Hypoglycaemia

Chronic

- Microvascular complications including nephropathy, peripheral neuropathy, and retinopathy
- Macrovascular complications relating to contribution of hyperglycaemia to atherosclerosis: ischaemic heart disease, cerebrovascular disease, and peripheral vascular disease

Treatment

The traditional division of diabetes into insulin dependent (type 1) and non-insulin dependent (type 2) has blurred. Whereas all type 1 diabetics require insulin, more and more type 2 diabetics are prescribed insulin in addition to or instead of oral hypoglycaemics to improve glycaemic control.

Reducing the burden of microvascular complications

Glycaemic control

The Diabetes Control and Complications Trial demonstrated the benefit of tight glycaemic control on retinopathy (76% reduction in onset, 56% reduction in need for laser treatment), nephropathy (50% reduction), and peripheral neuropathy (60% reduction) in type 1 diabetics. The UK Prospective Diabetes Study (UKPDS) confirmed the benefit of tight glycaemic control in type 2 diabetics, with a 25% reduction in microvascular complications.

Hypertension

UKPDS demonstrated a relationship in type 2 diabetics between hypertension and diabetic retinopathy and the benefit of tighter control, with a reduction in retinopathy progression and laser of 34% and in worsening visual loss by 47% with blood pressure of less than 150/85 mmHg. This study, in which the mean blood pressure in the tight control group was 144/82 mmHg, also found a 44% reduction in stroke in this group. Blood pressure targets are now lower in diabetics, with many physicians aiming for lower than 130/80 mmHg to prevent long-term complications. ACE inhibitors have an established role in delaying the onset of proteinuria in diabetics.

Lipid profile

The Collaborative Atorvastatin for Diabetes Study showed a non-significant, minor reduction in the need for laser treatment in type 2 diabetics receiving 10 mg atorvastatin, which was for the primary prevention of coronary heart disease and which caused a 26% drop in total cholesterol and a 40% drop in low-density lipoprotein cholesterol. The treatment duration was 4 years. Significant reductions in coronary events and stroke were noted. Further studies of the role of cholesterol lowering on retinopathy are awaited, but there are anecdotal reports of exudate regression in diabetic maculopathy on commencing statins.

Developing strategies

Oral inhibitors of protein kinase C, such as ruboxistaurin, are currently under trial for diabetic microvascular complications. Hyperglycaemia-induced activation of protein kinase C beta appears to be important in the intracellular signalling of VEGF, a principal mediator of retinal neovascularization and permeability in diabetes. Intravitreal anti-VEGF agents are also established therapies for diabetic macular oedema, as discussed in Chapter 6, Section 6.7.

Graves disease

Graves disease is an autoimmune thyroid disease caused by antibodies targeting the thyroid-stimulating hormone receptor. Other antibodies, such as ones to thyroglobulin and the thyroid hormones T_3 and T_4, may also be seen but the primary disease is thought to be an organ-specific (type 2) hypersensitivity reaction. The disease usually affects women (female/male ratio, 7 : 1) in the third to fifth decades. Eye involvement is believed to result from an antigen common to the thyroid gland and the extraocular muscles. The eye disease is discussed in Chapter 11, Section 11.18.

The clinical presentation is usually of hyperthyroidism: weight loss, palpitations, insomnia, irritability, heat intolerance, diarrhoea, and amenorrhoea. Occasionally, eye symptoms are the presenting feature. Pretibial myxoedema and thyroid acropachy (similar to fingernail clubbing) may develop and are specific to Graves disease.

Management (coordinated with an endocrinologist)

- Anti-thyroid drugs, e.g. carbimazole (danger of agranulocytosis), propylthiouracil
- 'Block and replace' strategy: carbimazole and thyroxine
- Beta blockers for symptomatic relief
- Radioiodine
- Thyroid surgery

Eye disease

Eye disease may be exacerbated in Graves disease by smoking, radioiodine (temporarily), and hypothyroidism (raised thyroid-stimulating hormone).

7.22 Respiratory and skin diseases in ophthalmology

Respiratory disease and ocular inflammation

In patients presenting with inflammatory eye disease and respiratory symptoms consider the following unifying diagnoses:

- **Sarcoidosis**: dry cough, breathlessness, weight loss, fever
- **Tuberculosis**: productive cough, haemoptysis, weight loss, lymphadenopathy, travel/from endemic area
- **Wegeners granulomatosis**: nasal/ear symptoms, haemoptysis, breathlessness
- **Churg–Strausssyndrome**: wheeze, cough, weight loss
- **Pneumonia**: acute presentation, fever, cough, breathlessness, pleuritic pain. Consider the possibility of immunocompromise (e.g. *Pneumocystis* in HIV/AIDS/other) or endogenous endophthalmitis (e.g. pneumococcal).

Respiratory disease and papilloedema

Obstructive sleep apnoea

An association exists between obstructive sleep apnoea and intracranial hypertension (discussed in Chapter 10, Section 10.12; see Figure 7.45). Snoring, nocturnal restlessness, morning headache, and excessive daytime somnolence are key features of this condition, which is probably underdiagnosed. Periods of apnoea, with relative upper-airway obstruction via the collapse of soft tissues (e.g. pharynx/palate) occur during sleep. Patients tend to be overweight (e.g. with a large collar size) adults, although children with enlarged adenoids and tonsils and those with reduced tone (e.g. those with Down syndrome) may also be affected. In those with 'idiopathic' intracranial hypertension, formal sleep studies may be indicated if there is a history suggestive of sleep apnoea. Various interventions are available, including continuous positive airway pressure masks for sleep, and surgery for structural airway abnormalities.

Chronic obstructive pulmonary disease

In a patient with severe emphysema or chronic bronchitis, papilloedema may result from hypoxia/hypercapnia in the absence of raised intracranial pressure.

Skin disease and ocular inflammation

Several vesicular/bullous rashes may be associated with ocular inflammation.

Bullous pemphigoid

Usually seen in patients over 60 years old, bullous pemphigoid is a rare, chronic, autoimmune, blistering skin disease. It is caused by IgG autoantibodies specific for hemidesmosomal antigens in the skin basement membrane. Most commonly presents with intact, tense bullae particularly over flexural surfaces. Mucus membrane pemphigoid may develop in association or in isolation: the cicatrizing conjunctivitis is discussed in Chapter 2, Section 2.11. Diagnosis is confirmed by skin or conjunctival biopsy.

Erythema multiforme/Stevens–Johnson syndrome

- An acute blistering skin disease with target lesions (erythema multiforme) and mucus membrane ulceration (Stevens–Johnson syndrome)
- Most common in the second to fourth decades
- Immune-complex-mediated hypersensitivity reaction to drugs (e.g. penicillin, sulphur-containing drugs), infection (e.g. HSV, *Mycoplasma*, tuberculosis, streptococci) and malignancy

- There is significant mortality—up to 30% in the most severe cases—and significant ocular morbidity, with chronic dry eye and keratinization resulting from severe conjunctival disease (discussed in Chapter 2, Section 2.11).
- Urgent in-patient medical care is needed for many cases, involving fluid resuscitation and immunosuppression/intravenous immunoglobulin.

Epidermolysis bullosa acquisita

Unlike other inherited forms of epidermolysis bullosa, epidermolysis bullosa acquisita is acquired and commences in adult life. Blistering skin lesions may be associated with cicatrizing conjunctival inflammation.

Herpes simplex and zoster

Herpetic vesicular rashes around the eye are usually easily recognized. Herpes simplex of the lids may be associated with conjunctivitis, as may chicken pox and HZO (ophthalmic shingles). Anterior uveitis is a rare feature of chicken pox and will usually respond well to topical steroid. Chronic anterior uveitis is a common complication of HZO.

Erythema nodosum

The associations between erythema nodosum and tuberculosis, sarcoidosis, and Behcets disease warrant a brief description. Erythema nodosum is an inflammation of the subcutaneous fat (panniculitis). It causes tender, red nodules (see Figure 7.46) that are usually seen on both shins. It is an immunological response to a variety of different causes. As well as the diseases listed above, causes include drugs (sulphonamides, penicillin), inflammatory bowel disease, pregnancy, and infections, including those caused by streptococci and *Mycoplasma*.

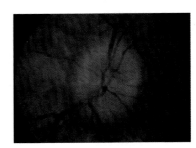

Fig 7.45 Chronic papilloedema in idiopathic intracranial hypertension, which may be associated with obstructive sleep apnoea

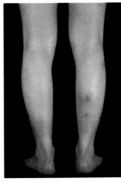

Fig 7.46 Erythema nodosum: raised, tender erythematous lesions on the right lower leg

Chapter 8

Glaucoma

Andrew Tatham and Peng Tee Khaw

The optic nerve head, or optic disc, is the region where retinal ganglion cell (RGC) axons exit the eye through the scleral canal. The optic nerve head represents a weak spot in the corneoscleral envelope and it is therefore subject to intraocular pressure (IOP)-induced stress and strain. The optic nerve head is believed to be the major site of RGC axon damage in glaucoma.

The mean optic disc area is **2.2 ± 0.5 mm²** (measured from Elschnigs rim at the margin of the scleral canal); however, disc size varies considerably between individuals. Hypermetropic eyes, with shorter axial lengths, tend to have small 'crowded' discs, whereas myopic eyes tend to have larger discs. The optic disc also tends to be larger in black populations. Optic disc size should be measured if glaucoma is suspected, as it can influence interpretation of measures such as cup/disc ratio (see Section 8.4).

Zones of the optic nerve head

The OHN represents the intraocular portion of the optic nerve. It consists of **four zones** determined by the relationship of the nerve and lamina cribrosa (see Figure 8.1):

Zone 1: Retinal nerve fibre layer

The retinal nerve fibre layer (RNFL) consists of approximately 1.2 million unmyelinated RGC axons. This point is important, as unmyelinated axons have a much higher energy requirement than do myelinated axons, a fact which may be highly relevant in the pathogenesis of glaucomatous neuroaxonal damage. The axons follow a precise pattern as they course towards the scleral canal. Fibres arising from between the disc and fovea pass directly to the optic nerve head as the papillomacular bundle. Fibres from the nasal, superior, and inferior retina also take a direct route to the optic nerve head. Fibres from the areas temporal to the fovea follow arcuate paths around the papillomacular bundle to enter the optic nerve head at its upper and lower margins.

Zone 2: Prelaminar zone

In the prelaminar zone, RGC axons turn from the retinal plane by 90° to form the optic nerve. Spatial order continues with axons from RGCs in the central retina located near the centre of the nerve, and axons from RGCs in the peripheral retina located in the periphery of the optic nerve. The major supporting cell of the optic nerve head is the astrocyte glial cell. Astrocytes processes are widespread and are in close proximity to the nerve fibres, separating bundles of the fibres. The astrocytes have giant mitochondria, an observation that suggests they supply large amounts of energy to the axons and also provide 'waste disposal' functions.

Zone 3: Lamina zone

The lamina cribrosa is a continuation of the inner sclera. It consists of approximately ten perforated connective tissue beams. Together, the beams form a mesh-like structure spanning the scleral canal. The lamina provides structural and functional support for axons passing through the scleral canal, and a passageway for retinal blood vessels. The lamina is a site of biomechanical weakness in the eye and therefore a location of stress and strain. The lamina is considered the principal site of nerve fibre damage in glaucoma. The dura mater of the optic nerve also begins in this zone as a continuation of the outer sclera.

Zone 4: Post (or retro) lamina zone

This portion of the optic nerve head marks the beginning of myelination of the RGC axons.

Using the slit lamp, it is possible to assess the RNFL, the prelaminar zone, and the anterior lamina cribrosa.

Zones of the optic nerve head on slit lamp examination

Neuroretinal rim

The optic disc can be divided into the neuroretinal rim and the cup. The neuroretinal rim is the tissue between the outer edge of the cup and disc margin. It is composed of neuroglia, astrocytes, and RGC axons that will eventually pass through the lamina cribrosa. A plentiful blood supply and the presence of axoplasm give the healthy rim an orange-red appearance. The neuroretinal rim has a characteristic configuration obeying the **ISNT rule**: the **i**nferior rim is thickest, followed by the **s**uperior rim, the **n**asal rim, and then the **t**emporal rim. If this rule is not obeyed, a pathological condition such as glaucoma is a possibility.

Optic cup

The optic cup is a three-dimensional depression, either round or ovoid, in the centre of the optic disc. The cup represents an absence of axons and partial exposure of the lamina; it therefore appears slightly pale. Pallor of the cup should not be confused with pallor of the neuroretinal rim, as the latter indicates a non-glaucomatous process. The limit of the cup can be determined as the first discernible change in surface contour as the nerve fibres course posteriorly. Within a population, the number of axons in the optic nerve head is relatively constant but the scleral canal (and therefore the size of the disc) varies in size depending on factors such as the size of the globe. As the RGC axons occupy a similar volume, the size of a normal optic cup can vary considerably.

Retinal blood vessels

The central retinal artery, a branch of the ophthalmic artery, tends to be nasal to the central retinal vein. Both vessels enter/exit the optic disc centrally then course nasally, following the edge of the cup. Cilioretinal arteries occur in about 25% of the population, most arising from the temporal rim.

Blood supply

The main arterial supply of the optic nerve head is via the posterior ciliary arteries derived from the ophthalmic artery. Fifteen to twenty short posterior ciliary arteries pierce the sclera close to the optic nerve, forming an incomplete anastomosis within the sclera around the optic nerve (the circle of Zinn–Haller). One or two long posterior ciliary arteries pierce the sclera further away. Small end arterial branches leave the circle of Zinn–Haller to feed the optic nerve head via capillaries within the lamina cribrosa beams. There is no direct blood supply to RGC axons in the laminar region; instead, nutrients arrive by diffusion from laminar capillaries. Venous drainage is via the central retinal vein and also by drainage into the peripapillary choroid.

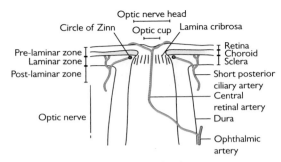

Fig 8.1 Anatomy of the optic nerve head

8.2 Aqueous fluid dynamics

Aqueous humour is a transparent, colourless fluid continually produced by the ciliary body. Aqueous is similar to plasma but has lower levels of glucose and protein (assuming an intact blood–aqueous barrier) and higher levels of ascorbate and lactate than plasma does. Aqueous humour provides structural and nutritional support to the avascular cornea and lens and also removes metabolic waste products. Production and outflow of aqueous humour must be balanced to maintain a steady-state IOP. **Aqueous humour dynamics** describe the balance of aqueous humour production and outflow through the trabecular meshwork (TM) and uveoscleral pathways.

Aqueous production

Aqueous humour is produced by the ciliary body, a triangularly shaped structure attached to the sclera at the scleral spur. Approximately 70 ciliary processes are located on the inner, anterior surface of the ciliary body at the pars plicata. The epithelium of each process has two neuroepithelial layers:

1. An inner, **non-pigmented epithelium** in contact with the posterior chamber (this layer represents a continuation of the retina)
2. An outer, **pigmented epithelium** in contact with the stroma of the ciliary process (this layer represents a continuation of the retinal pigment epithelium)

Tight junctions between the non-pigmented cells form the blood–aqueous barrier. Each process has a central arteriole ending in a rich, highly fenestrated capillary network.

Aqueous humour is formed via a combination of active secretion (70%–80%), ultrafiltration (20%), and diffusion (10%) as follows:

1. Plasma from the fenestrated capillaries in the ciliary processes moves down a hydrostatic pressure gradient into the ciliary process stroma **(ultrafiltration)**.
2. Plasma-derived ions are taken up across the basolateral surface of the outer pigmented epithelium and move to the non-pigmented cells via gap junctions. They are then transported into the intercellular clefts between the non-pigmented cells **(active secretion)**. Carbonic anhydrase mediates the transport of bicarbonate, which in turn affects sodium ions.
3. Active transport produces an osmotic gradient across the ciliary epithelium. Water follows ions into the intercellular spaces, allowing diffusion into the posterior chamber **(diffusion)**. Aquaporin water channels aid the transport of fluid.

After secretion into the posterior chamber, aqueous passes around the lens equator and flows through the pupil into the anterior chamber, where it circulates because of convection currents derived from the temperature difference between the cornea and iris (see Figure 8.2). Some of the aqueous flows directly towards the cornea and then flows downwards in the anterior chamber. In pigmentary dispersion, the pigment granules therefore deposit on the central and inferior cornea.

Ultrafiltration and diffusion are passive processes and depend on capillary hydrostatic pressure, oncotic pressure, and IOP. Active secretion does not depend on IOP but instead relies on enzyme systems including the Na+/K+-ATPase pump, ion transport by symports and antiports, calcium- and voltage-gated channels, and carbonic anhydrase. Active secretion is reduced by inhibitors of metabolism, e.g. hypoxia and hypothermia.

Rate of aqueous flow

Aqueous flow has a circadian rhythm, being higher during the morning than at night. Daytime aqueous humour turnover is estimated to be 1.0% to 1.5% of the anterior chamber volume per minute (approximately 2.9 μl/min in a healthy young adult). The anterior chamber has an average volume of 0.25 ml. Turnover declines by about 2.4% every 10 years.

Aqueous outflow

Conventional (trabecular) route

This passive, pressure-sensitive route represents the primary means of outflow. Aqueous passes first through the TM and then into Schlemms canal. The TM is a sieve-like structure at the anterior chamber angle made up of three anatomically distinct portions: the uveal meshwork (innermost), the corneo-scleral meshwork, and the juxtacanalicular or endothelial meshwork (outermost). Transport into Schlemms canal is by transcellular channels in the form of 'giant vacuoles' of fluid crossing the inner wall. The outer wall of the canal contains the openings of collector channels, which leave at oblique angles to connect either directly or indirectly with episcleral veins. The TM accounts for 75% of resistance to outflow, with 25% occurring beyond Schlemms canal. The major site of resistance within the TM is believed to be the juxtacanalicular TM.

Alternative (uveoscleral) route

The remaining aqueous outflow occurs across the iris root and the face of the ciliary body, passing between the muscle fibres into the supraciliary and suprachoroidal spaces, where it is drained by the choroidal circulation. This route is not pressure dependent and in young individuals can account for 40% to 50% of outflow. The proportion of aqueous outflow via each route differs by age and disease. Patients with primary open-angle glaucoma have increased resistance to flow through the TM.

IOP

The relationships between IOP, aqueous production (flow), and aqueous outflow is described by the modified Goldmann equation:

$$F = C(P_o - P_e) + U,$$

where **F** is the rate of aqueous flow (in healthy young eyes, approximately 2.9 μl/min, decreasing by 2.4% per decade, lower during sleep than during waking hours), **C** is facility of outflow (in healthy eyes, between 0.1 and 0.4 μl/min/mmHg); **P$_o$** is IOP, **P$_e$** is the episcleral venous pressure (in healthy eyes, between 8 and 10 mmHg) and **U** is uveoscleral outflow. Episcleral venous pressure is subject to circadian variation and also varies with posture (higher when supine than when standing up).

Aqueous fluid dynamics

Conventional and alternative routes

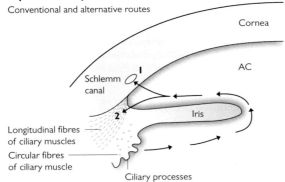

1 Conventional (trabecular) pathway – 90% outflow
2 Alternative (uveoscleral) pathway – 10% outflow

Fig 8.2 Diagram of aqueous fluid dynamics showing normal flow from the ciliary body through from the posterior chamber to the anterior chamber and then the angle

8.3 Glaucoma pathogenesis

Glaucoma is defined as 'a disease of the optic nerve with characteristic changes in the optic nerve head, and typical defects in the visual field, with or without raised intraocular pressure' (UK National Institute of Clinical Excellence (NICE) guidelines). In other words, glaucoma is an optic neuropathy. Patients are not required to have raised IOP to be diagnosed with glaucoma; however, IOP is usually the only modifiable risk factor. Glaucoma may be primary or secondary and associated with an open or closed angle.

The pathogenesis of glaucomatous optic neuropathy is complex and not fully understood but glaucoma is likely to be due to damage to RGC axons at the level of the lamina cribrosa. Integrity of the RGC axon is essential for survival of the cell. If the axon is damaged, disruption of retrograde transport of neurotrophins from the lateral geniculate nucleus and superior colliculus to the cell body, and anterograde transfer of cellular organelles may lead to RGC apoptosis.

A **direct mechanical** theory and a **vascular or ischaemic** theory have been proposed as potential causes for axon damage. A recent energy theory proposes astrocyte axon dissociation as the primary mechanism of axon damage. A combination of factors is likely to be responsible.

IOP-related stress and strain

Mechanical displacement of the lamina cribrosa due to pathological levels of IOP may directly damage RGC axons passing through its mesh-like pores. Indirect damage may also occur because of the effects of IOP on glial support cells, including disassociation from axons, and RGC blood and nutrient supply.

Normal IOP may be defined by range within a population; however, whether an IOP is normal for a particular patient is another matter. Two eyes exposed to the same IOP may respond in different ways; that is, some optic nerves are sensitive to relatively low pressures whereas others are resilient to relatively high pressures.

Corneal thickness, hysteresis, hydration, and curvature can affect IOP measurements. IOP is also affected by breath holding, eyelid squeezing, strenuous wind instrument playing, and wearing a tight necktie (all lead to an increase in IOP).

Impaired blood flow and nutrient diffusion

An insufficient blood supply may contribute to glaucomatous retinal ganglion cell damage by reducing oxygen and nutrient delivery to the RGCs, supporting cells, and optic nerve head connective tissues. Impaired blood flow may also increase the susceptibility of the RGC axons to mechanical damage and explain why glaucomatous damage occurs in some eyes at relatively low levels of IOP.

Ocular perfusion pressure

* The Barbados Eye Study showed a link between glaucoma and low ocular perfusion pressure (OPP).
* A mean OPP <40 mmHg was associated with a 2.6 relative risk of glaucoma.
* Low OPP can be due to high IOP or low systemic BP, where mean $BP = diastolic\ BP + 1/3(systolic\ BP - diastolic\ BP)$L

$$OPP = 2/3(mean\ BP) - IOP.$$

Low systemic BP

* Low systemic BP has been associated with an increased risk of glaucoma progression.
* Progression of primary open-angle glaucoma and normal tension glaucoma has also been associated with nocturnal BP dipping.
* Dipping is classified as a 10%–20% reduction in mean BP between waking and sleeping; extreme dipping occurs if there is a >20% reduction.
* Glaucoma has also been associated with systemic vascular disorders such as hypertension and cardiovascular disease.

Vasospasm

* Vasospastic conditions such as migraine and Raynauds syndrome are associated with glaucoma, possibly because of impaired autoregulation of the blood supply.
* The Collaborative Normal Tension Glaucoma Study found a significant association between the rate of glaucoma progression and migraines in normal tension glaucoma.

Autoimmune and inflammatory factors

* Cytokines released by injured RGCs or glial cells may contribute to the death of adjacent cells.

8.4 Optic nerve head assessment in glaucoma

Glaucoma is a specific form of optic neuropathy, and recognition of optic nerve head changes typical of glaucoma is key to diagnosing glaucoma. Raised IOP is of importance but primarily for stratifying risk and does not need to be present to diagnose glaucoma.

Optic nerve and/or RNFL changes are often the first signs of glaucoma. Abnormalities can be difficult to detect but are best seen stereoscopically; therefore, the pupil should be dilated. Use the slit lamp and indirect fundus lenses (e.g. 78 dioptres (D)). Detailed disc drawings should be taken and, at baseline, optic disc imaging is essential. Further images should be taken if any change is noted. Increasingly, optic nerve and RNFL imaging techniques are also used to provide quantitative measurements.

Scheme for optic nerve head examination

It is important to have a system for optic nerve head examination, to ensure signs are not missed. Specifically search for each feature.

Size
Measure the size of the optic disc as the vertical diameter from scleral rim to scleral rim. The normal disc is vertically oval.

Optic discs vary in size, with an average vertical diameter of 1.8 mm. Discs can be categorized as:

- Small: <1.5 mm
- Medium: 1.5–2.0 mm
- Large: >2.0 mm

The size of the normal optic cup depends on the size of the optic disc. Small cups can be glaucomatous in eyes with small discs. The disc diameter can be measured by projecting a narrow, bright beam from the slit lamp, and the height of the beam can adjusted to measure the vertical dimension of the disc as the slit overlies it. A correction factor must be applied depending on the power of the fundus lens used:

- A **60 D** lens has a correction factor of **1.0×**
- A **78 D** lens has a correction factor of **1.1×**
- A **90 D** lens has a correction factor of **1.3×**

Neuroretinal rim
The edge of the neuroretinal rim can be detected as the first contour change at the surface of the optic disc. This contour change corresponds to the first bend in the retinal vessels as they dip into the cup, not to the extent of pallor. Glaucoma is characterized by progressive loss of the neuroretinal rim; this loss is generally greater at the inferior and superior poles than elsewhere. Loss may be diffuse (see Figure 8.3) or localized (see Figure 8.4).

The Werner–Jones **ISNT** rule determines the normal rim configuration (see Section 8.1). If this rule is not followed, the disc is likely to be glaucomatous, unless there are other abnormal features of the disc that would explain deviation (e.g. tilting).

Tilting of the optic disc produces a gently sloping rim in one sector, and a narrow, sharply defined rim in the opposite sector (see Figure 8.5). A normal optic nerve has a 15° tilt of the inferior pole towards the fovea. If the nerve is very tilted, it may be difficult to assess the neuroretinal rim accurately. Assess the colour of the rim, as pallor increases the likelihood of a non-glaucomatous process.

RNFL
Loss of nerve fibres may initially be detectable as defects in the RNFL. Like rim loss, RNFL loss may be diffuse or localized (see Figure 8.6). The healthy RNFL glistens and has fine striations visible. Localized defects appear as slits or wedge-shaped defects in the usual uniformly reflective sheen of the RNFL. The defects follow the pattern of retinal striations (i.e. they are arcuate) and are best seen at the transition point between normal and abnormal areas within two disc diameters of the disc, under red-free (green) illumination.

Diffuse defects can be harder to visualize but may be appreciated owing to a difference in the brightness of the RNFL on comparing the two eyes, or on comparing superior and inferior peripapillary RNFLs in the same eye. Vessels running within the RNFL will also become more visible with diffuse thinning.

Peripapillary atrophy
Chorioretinal atrophy surrounding the optic nerve head consists of two zones: an inner beta zone (i.e. beside the optic disc), and an outer alpha zone (i.e. away from optic disc). Alpha-zone atrophy is due to variable irregular hyper- and hypopigmentation of the retinal pigment epithelium (RPE) and is common in normal eyes. Beta-zone atrophy is more important and is correlated with neuroretinal rim loss; it enlarges as glaucoma progresses. In beta atrophy, there is visibility of the sclera and choroidal vessels because of atrophy occurring in the RPE and the choriocapillaris (see Figure 8.7).

RNFL haemorrhages
Optic disc or RNFL haemorrhages are found in **4%–7%** of glaucomatous eyes, most frequently in areas of focal neuroretinal rim loss. They are common in normal tension glaucoma. Haemorrhages can be located either on the optic disc itself, where they appear blot-like, as small splinter haemorrhages, or in the immediate peripapillary area, with a flame-shaped configuration due to their location within the RNFL (see Figure 8.8).

Haemorrhages may be difficult to see and are best detected after dilatation. Under red-free light, the haemorrhage appears dark. Haemorrhages are most common in the infero- or supero-temporal regions and take 6 weeks to 9 months to clear.

The presence of an optic disc haemorrhage indicates likely glaucoma progression. The site of a haemorrhage should be documented, as it can represent a marker for future focal disc damage and visual field loss.

Other features

Vertical cup/disc ratio
Enlargement of the vertical cup/disc ratio (CDR) is secondary to the loss of RGCs leading to a thinning of the neuroretinal rim. A problem with CDR is that it is highly variable, with a normal range of 0 to 0.85; however, a CDR >0.65 is found in less than 5% of the normal Caucasian population. Whether a CDR is normal depends on the size of the optic disc. Asymmetry between the CDR of fellow eyes usually does not exceed 0.2 (assuming equal refractive status).

Notching
An increase in cup size may occur by concentric enlargement or focal loss of the neuroretinal rim. Focal loss can cause a notch. Notching occurs most frequently inferiorly. A notch may indicate an area of the disc in which circulation has been compromised.

Saucerization

Saucerization is a gentle concavity extending over most of the disc diameter, resulting in indiscernible cup edges.

Pallor

Pallor should be not be confused with cupping. Pallor within the cup and of the rim may indicate a non-glaucomatous cause for the optic neuropathy.

Laminar dot sign

Loss of neuroretinal tissue may expose the underlying pores of the lamina cribrosa.

Nasalization

The central retinal vessels emerge in the centre of the optic disc and initially course nasally. If the nasal rim becomes eroded, the vessels will follow the erosion and become displaced nasally (nasalization).

Bayoneting

In a healthy disc, vessels pass over the sloping rim of the cup to reach the retina. This creates a mild kink or change in direction of the vessel. With loss of the neuroretinal rim, a vessel may pass into a recess below the rim before climbing on to its surface. This creates a double angulation (a z-shaped bend) which looks like a bayonet.

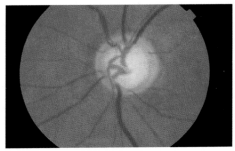

Fig 8.3 Colour fundus photograph showing diffuse thinning of the neuroretinal rim and significant glaucomatous cupping

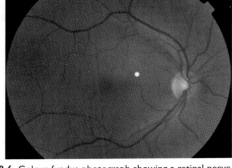

Fig 8.6 Colour fundus photograph showing a retinal nerve fibre layer defect as a dark band extending from the optic disc supero-temporally

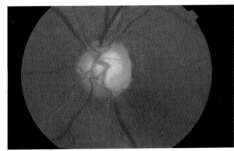

Fig 8.4 Colour fundus photograph showing a focal notch of the inferior neuroretinal rim

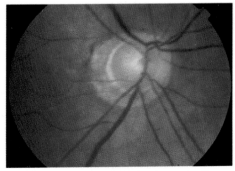

Fig 8.7 Colour fundus photograph showing peripapillary atrophy around a glaucomatous optic disc

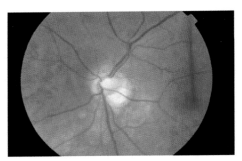

Fig 8.5 Colour fundus photograph showing a tilted optic nerve head

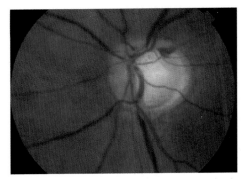

Fig 8.8 Colour fundus photograph showing an optic disc haemorrhage at the superior pole of the disc

8.5 Glaucoma imaging devices

Optic nerve imaging is useful for the diagnosis of glaucoma and detection of progression.

Optic disc stereophotographs

Stereoscopic photography provides high-resolution images of the optic disc and peripapillary retina, creating a permanent record for comparative purposes. A dilated pupil and clear media are required for quality photographs. The evaluation of glaucomatous progression will be subjective, with both inter- and intra-observer variability, even when the images are viewed by highly trained glaucoma experts. RNFL defects are sometimes more easily detected on photographs than by fundus examination.

Confocal scanning laser ophthalmoscopy

The Heidelberg retinal tomograph (HRT; developed by Heidelberg Engineering) provides quantitative data regarding the topography of the optic nerve head and the peripapillary retina. HRT uses a **diode laser** with a **670 nm** light source to scan the optic nerve head and peripapillary retina. Following the scan, the operator is required to manually draw an outline around the disc. A reference plane is then created 50 μm deep with respect to the temporal edge of the disc. Everything within the disc outline and deeper than the reference plane is considered to be the cup. Everything above the reference plane is considered to be neuroretinal rim. Distances of structures from the reference plane are analysed by computer software to produce three-dimensional reconstructions of the disc and retina.

Moorfield's regression analysis

HRT provides information regarding neuroretinal rim area, disc area, and cup size. An assessment is made as to whether sectors of the disc are abnormal, and a probability map is generated. The Moorfields regression analysis (MRA) compares the global and sectorial rim areas, adjusted for age and disc size, to a database of normal eyes. Sectors are then classified as normal, borderline, or abnormal (see Figure 8.9).

Glaucoma probability score

The glaucoma probability score (GPS) is another automated algorithm that generates a probability score of having glaucoma. The GPS uses information regarding horizontal and vertical RNFL curvature, cup size and depth, and neuroretinal rim steepness. An advantage of the GPS is that it does not need the manually drawn disc margin contour line. The values in the MRA and GPS results are displayed as red crosses when outside normal limits, yellow exclamation points when borderline, and green ticks when within normal limits.

Loss of neuroretinal rim area on HRT has been associated with glaucoma progression. HRT 2, Version 3, includes software that allows longitudinal analysis (topographic change analysis). This version also includes an enlarged race-specific normative database.

Disadvantages

Variation occurs because of the need to manually draw the reference outline around the optic disc. Thickness measurements depend on the position of the reference plane along the z-axis.

Scanning laser polarimetry

The **GDx** (developed by Carl Zeiss Meditec, Inc.) is a **confocal scanning laser polarimeter** used to assess the thickness of the peripapillary RNFL. It uses a polarized infrared (**780 nm**) light source.

RGC axons have birefringent properties because of their arrangement in parallel bundles. When a birefringent tissue reflects polarized light, the light undergoes a phase shift corresponding to the thickness of tissue through which it has passed. The GDx quantifies RNFL thickness by measuring the phase shift (or retardation) of reflected light and then using that value to estimate RNFL thickness. Compensation for other birefringent ocular structures such as the cornea and lens is made. The **GDxVCC** (for **v**ariable **c**orneal **c**ompensation) takes account of corneal birefringence. **GDxECC** (for **e**nhanced **c**orneal **c**ompensation) is more advanced than the other two polarimeters and eliminates other artefacts.

The data provided include a TSNIT (thickness in **t**emporal, **s**uperior, **n**asal, **i**nferior, and **t**emporal quadrants) graph, which in normal eyes has a double hump (greater thickness in superior and inferior sectors). The RNFL thickness is classified as being within normal limits, borderline, or outside normal limits. A **guided progression analysis** is available for comparing serial GDx images. GDxVCC is repeatable to within 4 μm.

Disadvantages

Data from different generations of GDx are not interchangeable. Opacities in the media can create abnormal retardation patterns.

Optical coherence tomography

Optical coherence tomography (OCT) uses low-coherence (near-infrared) interferometry to measure light backscattered from the retinal layers. Light scattered from different layers has different frequencies. The principle is similar to ultrasonography except that light is used rather than sound. Many single A-scans are acquired to provide a cross-sectional image of the retina, from which tissue thickness layers can be measured. The RNFL has particularly high reflectance because of its parallel nerve fibre bundles.

The original form of OCT was time domain OCT (TD-OCT). TD-OCT detects the echo time delay between the sample and a moving reference arm. A new version of OCT, spectral domain OCT (SD-OCT) has a stationary reference arm and collects backscattered light of different frequencies (due to different layers) simultaneously. This method reduces the acquisition time, which leads to fewer movement artefacts and allows resampling, to ensure precise placement of the scan. SD-OCT provides more A-scans and has a better axial resolution (3–6 μm) than TD-OCT does.

Peripapillary RNFL thickness is assessed using a single circular scan that is centred on the optic nerve head and has a diameter of approximately 3.4 mm. The circle scan is unwound and a linear result presented. The optic nerve head itself can be assessed using multiple radial linear scans to provide data on cupping and neuroretinal rim. SD-OCT is able to generate a RNFL thickness map, and thickness values can be averaged for different sectors or globally (see Figure 8.10). Global measurements are more reproducible.

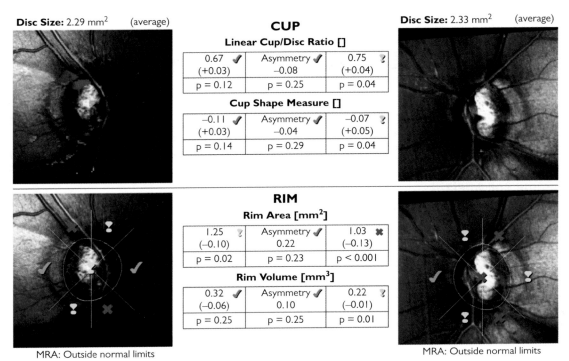

Disc Size: 2.29 mm² (average)   **Disc Size:** 2.33 mm² (average)

CUP
Linear Cup/Disc Ratio []

0.67 ✓ (+0.03)	Asymmetry ✓ −0.08	0.75 ? (+0.04)
p = 0.12	p = 0.25	p = 0.04

Cup Shape Measure []

−0.11 ✓ (+0.03)	Asymmetry ✓ −0.04	−0.07 ? (+0.05)
p = 0.14	p = 0.29	p = 0.04

RIM
Rim Area [mm²]

1.25 ? (−0.10)	Asymmetry ✓ 0.22	1.03 ✗ (−0.13)
p = 0.02	p = 0.23	p < 0.001

Rim Volume [mm³]

0.32 ✓ (−0.06)	Asymmetry ✓ 0.10	0.22 ? (−0.01)
p = 0.25	p = 0.25	p = 0.01

MRA: Outside normal limits   MRA: Outside normal limits

Fig 8.9 Heidelberg retinal tomograph report for both eyes of a subject with glaucoma
The Moorfields regression analysis results are outside normal limits

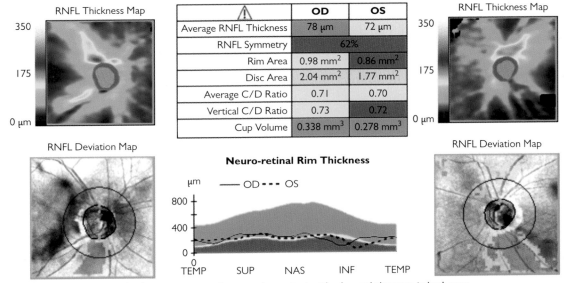

RNFL Thickness Map   RNFL Thickness Map

⚠	OD	OS
Average RNFL Thickness	78 μm	72 μm
RNFL Symmetry	62%	
Rim Area	0.98 mm²	0.86 mm²
Disc Area	2.04 mm²	1.77 mm²
Average C/D Ratio	0.71	0.70
Vertical C/D Ratio	0.73	0.72
Cup Volume	0.338 mm³	0.278 mm³

RNFL Deviation Map   RNFL Deviation Map

Neuro-retinal Rim Thickness
μm — OD - - - OS
800
400
0
0 TEMP   SUP   NAS   INF   TEMP

Fig 8.10 Example of an optical coherence tomography report in a patient with advanced glaucoma in both eyes

The higher resolution of SD-OCT also allows imaging of the ganglion cell complex (GCC) in the inner retina in the macular region. RGC loss is a key pathological feature of glaucoma, so imaging of the GCC is of great interest for the future. Other recent developments include enhanced depth imaging OCT, which allows examination of deeper structures in the optic nerve head, such as the lamina cribrosa.

Disadvantages

One disadvantages of OCT is that it may be less able to detect change in patients with advanced glaucoma, compared to functional tests. Also, OCT is not able to detect disc haemorrhages, so it should not replace clinical examination.

Imaging the angle

Imaging of the anterior chamber drainage angle can be useful in assessing patients with suspected angle closure. It is particularly useful for determining the mechanism of angle closure. At present, the role of imaging is to supplement, not replace, gonioscopy. The drainage angle may be imaged using anterior segment OCT or ultrasound biomicroscopy (UBM).

Anterior segment OCT

Anterior segment OCT uses the scleral spur as the reference point (see Figure 8.11). Look for apposition anterior to the scleral spur to diagnose angle closure. This method has good sensitivity but poor specificity for detecting angle closure, as compared to gonioscopy.

Advantages

- Non-contact procedure (can be done immediately after surgery)
- Can be done in darkness, avoiding light-induced pupil constriction
- Can use quantitative tools to assess the angle

Disadvantages

- Cross-sectional rather than 360° view
- Not able to assess pigmentation or angle vessels
- Poor view of structures behind the iris, such as the ciliary body

UBM

UBM is similar to conventional ultrasound imaging. An eyecup holding a coupling medium is used and the patient must be in a supine position.

Advantages

- Good view of structures behind the iris, such as the ciliary body
- Not limited to optically transparent tissues (can be done in eyes with opaque corneas)

Disadvantages

- Direct contact procedure

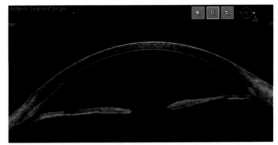

Fig 8.11 Example of anterior segment optical coherence tomography in an eye with an open angle

8.6 Tonometry and pachymetry

Tonometry

Tonometry is the clinical measurement of IOP. Tonometers measure IOP indirectly through the cornea and rely on the principle that, the higher the pressure in a sphere, the greater the force required to indent it. Tonometry may be by contact or non-contact (using a jet of air).

Goldmann applanation tonometry

Goldmann applanation tonometry (GAT) is the current gold standard of tonometry, although its accuracy is affected by corneal properties.

Imbert–Fick principle

GAT is based on the Imbert–Fick principle, which states that the pressure of a sphere equals the force of flattening (F) divided by the surface area of flattening (A), or $P = F/A$.

The Imbert–Fick principle assumes that the sphere has a constant radius of curvature, is dry, infinitely thin, and that aqueous humour does not move during testing. These assumptions are untrue of the globe. Goldmann took into account tear-film capillary action, which draws the tonometer towards the cornea, and the elastic repulsive force of the cornea. He calculated that, when applanation occurred over a circular area with a diameter of **3.06 mm**, these two forces would cancel each other.

GAT consists of a prismatic doubling device in the centre of a cone-shaped, 3.06 mm plastic head (the biprism head). The head is mounted on a metal rod attached to a coiled spring. The spring may be adjusted to change the forwards force of the head. The tonometer is mounted on a slit lamp and aligned so the examiner looks down the barrel of the tip using **one eye**. Oblique illumination with a cobalt-blue light is used. Fluorescein and topical anaesthesia are instilled. When the biprism head comes into contact with the cornea, two yellow-green semicircles are seen in the image of the tear-film meniscus. The dial, and thus the forwards force in the head, is adjusted until the inner margins of the semicircles just touch, so that the applanation area becomes 3.06 mm in diameter. The semicircles oscillate with each ocular pulse, so the reading is taken when the inner borders meet at the midpoint of the movement. The grams of force applied (as read from the dial) are multiplied by ten to give a reading in millimetres of mercury.

Compensation for corneal astigmatism of more than 3 D is achieved by placing the flattest corneal meridian at 45° to the axis of the biprism head (align the red mark on the prism holder with axis of the minus cylinder). In high or irregular astigmatism, take the average of two measurements: one when the biprism is horizontal, and another with it vertical.

Sources of error with GAT

- Overestimates of true IOP:
  - Examiner pressing on globe whilst holding lids
  - Wide meniscus (excessive fluorescein or tears)
  - Unequal semicircles due to misalignment
  - Against-the-rule astigmatism
  - Thick or rigid cornea (including corneal scar)
  - Patient squeezing (apprehension or blepharospasm)
  - Valsalva manoeuvre (breath holding)
  - Restrictive clothing around neck (tie, shirt collar)
  - Eccentric gaze (accentuated in restrictive orbital disease)

- Underestimates of true IOP:
  - Thin meniscus (too little fluorescein or poor tear film)
  - Thin cornea (including previous corneal refractive surgery)
  - Corneal oedema (easier to indent)
  - Ocular 'massage' (gonioscopy or repeated measurements)
  - With-the-rule astigmatism
  - Poor or infrequent calibration of instrument
  - Inter-observer variability

Other problems with GAT

- Infection risk: need strict adherence to hygiene and sterilization protocols
- Use disposable prisms in known infection (particularly prion protein diseases).
- Corneal abrasion: possible with inappropriate or repeated measures

Non-contact tonometry

Non-contact tonometry uses the same principles as GAT, but a puff of air is used to flatten the cornea. The force of airflow required to flatten is proportional to IOP. There is no requirement for topical anaesthesia. This technique is less accurate with high IOPs than with low or normal IOPs.

Perkins tonometry

Perkins tonometry is similar to GAT but uses a handheld battery-powered device. The technique is more difficult than GAT is and therefore less accurate; however, it can be used in a vertical or a supine position, so is useful for bed-bound patients and those unable to position on the slit lamp; 59% of readings are within 2 mmHg of GAT. Tonometer heads of different weight (e.g. disposable heads) may be inaccurate.

The Tono-Pen

The Tono-Pen is a battery-powered device held like a pen. A microprocessor within the device is connected to a strain-gauge transducer that measures the force of the central plate, which is 1.02 mm in diameter, as the plate applanates the corneal surface. The tip is covered with a disposable latex sleeve to prevent infection. Several measurements are taken and averaged to provide a digital readout. The Tono-Pen is useful for eyes with distorted or oedematous corneas but tends to overestimate at low IOPs and underestimate at high IOPs; 48% of readings are within 2 mmHg of GAT.

The iCare rebound tonometer

The iCare tonometer is a handheld device with a trigger and a thin, disposable, stainless steel probe with a length of 50 mm. The device is held 4 to 8 mm from the cornea; the probe, repelled by a magnet, bounces off the cornea. The deceleration of the probe is used to calculate the IOP. A series of measurements can be taken rapidly. This tonometer does not require anaesthesia and is particularly useful when GAT may not be possible, such as in young children and in patients who cannot hold their eyelids open for Goldmann tonometry, including some patients with dementia. It is also useful in eyes with an irregular corneal surface; 52% of measurements are within 2 mmHg of GAT.

Factors such as corneal hysteresis (a measurement of the dynamic properties of the cornea) play a role in IOP measurement accuracy. New devices such as dynamic contour tonometry and the ocular response analyser are thought to offer more accurate measures of IOP, independent of corneal thickness.

Dynamic contour tonometry

Dynamic contour tonometry uses a slit-lamp-mounted contact tonometer designed to compensate for the effects of the cornea on tonometry (see Figure 8.12): The effects of the cornea are reduced, as the tonometer head is contour matched to the cornea. IOP is recorded using a miniature pressure sensor; 100 IOP readings are taken every second over a 5–8-second period. The ocular pulse amplitude is also measured; 49% of measurements are within 2 mmHg of GAT. DCT tends to give higher readings than GAT does at low IOPs.

Ocular response analyser

The ocular response analyser is a non-contact air impulse tonometer. It provides two applanation pressures with each measurement. An air impulse causes the cornea to move in until applanation. The cornea then becomes slightly concave, before moving outward, where there is a second applanation. The difference between the inward and outward applanation pressure depends on the viscoelastic properties of the cornea (corneal hysteresis). A corneal compensated IOP measurement is thus provided which is thought to be less influenced by corneal properties than ones provided by GAT; 46% of measurements are repeatable within 2 mmHg of GAT.

Pachymetry

Pachymetry is used to measure central corneal thickness (CCT). 'The measurement of CCT aids in the interpretation of IOP measurement results and the stratification of patient risk for glaucoma' (American Academy of Ophthalmologists' Glaucoma Guidelines, 2005). The mean CCT is 550 μm, whereas the peripheral cornea can be up to 1 mm thick.

The Ocular Hypertension Treatment Study showed CCT to be a powerful predictor for the development of glaucoma (eyes with CCT <555 μm were at three times greater risk of developing glaucoma than those with a CCT >588 μm). Part of this finding is attributed to the inaccuracies induced in IOP measurement because of varying CCT. IOP tends to be underestimated in eyes with thin corneas because of increased deformability, whereas IOP is overestimated in eyes with thick corneas. In addition, a thin cornea may reflect a thin eye and weak optic nerve head tissues.

Pachymetry can be performed using ultrasonic or optical techniques. Although there are slight differences between the two methods of measurement, for the purposes of clinical practice, they are equally efficacious.

The most user-friendly and thus most commonly used method is that of ultrasound. This method has a range of 280–1000 μm, and a clinical accuracy of ±5 μm. Ultrasound energy is emitted from the probe tip, and some of the energy is reflected back towards the probe in the form of an echo at the first tissue interface it reaches (i.e. endothelium to aqueous humour). Measurement data are then calculated on the time it takes for the echo to travel back to the probe.

Method

* The eye is anaesthetized with drop of local anaesthetic.
* The patient is asked to look straight ahead.
* The probe is touched lightly against the central cornea, ensuring perpendicular alignment throughout testing (see Figure 8.13).

Several measurements are taken to provide an average. The accuracy of ultrasonic pachymetry is dependent upon the perpendicularity of the probe to the cornea, whilst the reproducibility relies on probe placement at the exact corneal centre.

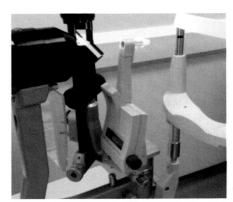

Fig 8.12 The dynamic contour tonometer, mounted to the slit lamp

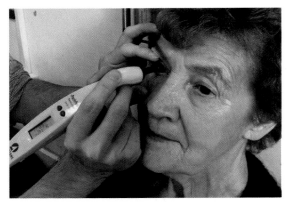

Fig 8.13 Use of a pachymeter
The eye is anaesthetized and the probe placed onto the central cornea

Examination of the anterior chamber or the iridocorneal angle is essential in all patients with suspected glaucoma. It allows one to differentiate between open- and closed-angle glaucomas and to identify pathological changes. The drainage angle cannot be visualized directly because of the internal reflection of light by the peripheral cornea. Gonioscopy is a technique that allows visualization of the angle by replacing the tear-film–air interface with a tear-film–goniolens interface.

Limbal chamber depth

Before gonioscopy, assess limbal chamber depth (LCD), as follows:

* Using the slit lamp, offset the illumination column from the axis of the microscope by 60°.
* Direct the brightest, narrowest beam of vertical light at the limbal cornea, at the most peripheral part that permits a clear view of the peripheral iris.
* The resulting slit image of the cornea is used as a reference for the anterior chamber depth (represented by the optically empty gap between the posterior corneal surface and the iris).
* LCD is expressed as a percentage or fraction of the thickness of the cornea (Van Hericks grade).

Van Hericks grades

* **Grade 1:** LCD < ¼ corneal thickness
* **Grade 2:** LCD = ¼ corneal thickness (see Figure 8.14)
* **Grade 3:** LCD = ¼ to ½ corneal thickness
* **Grade 4:** LCD ≥ the full thickness of the peripheral cornea (see Figure 8.15)

There is good correlation between LCD and angle grading by gonioscopy; however, LCD is not a substitute for gonioscopy. LCD ≤ 25% has a sensitivity of >95% and a specificity of 66% for detecting gonioscopically occludable angles.

Direct gonioscopy

Direct goniolenses or gonioprisms are used to allow direct visualization of the angle. There are several types (e.g. Koeppe (360°), Barkan (120°), and Swan–Jacob lenses) and their main use is in the direct visualization of the angle in the operating room for surgical procedures (e.g. goniotomy, or synechiolysis). The technique requires high magnification with illuminated loupes, a portable slit lamp or operating microscope, and the patient to be lying supine. A four-mirror direct gonioscope (Khaw) can also be used for standard slit lamp examination and for laser treatment of the angle.

Indirect gonioscopy

Indirect goniolenses or goniomirrors are used to provide a mirror image of the opposite angle and are used in conjunction with a slit lamp. There are two main types: Goldmann lenses and Zeiss lenses (see Figure 8.16).

Goldmann lenses

* Single- or double-mirror lens with a contact-surface diameter of 12 mm (greater than the surface area of the cornea)
* The concave surface of the lens is steeper than that of the cornea, so a coupling agent is required to bridge the gap (this agent may cause temporary blurring of vision afterwards).

* Provides excellent view of angle structures and stabilizes the globe
* If an iris convexity obscures the view, one can still see 'over the hill' if the patient looks in the direction of the mirror. Take care not to indent the cornea, as this will result in iatrogenic opening of the angle.

Method

* Instil topical anaesthetic (e.g. benoxinate).
* Ensure lens is disinfected with appropriate solution.
* Instil coupling agent (e.g. Viscotears or methylcellulose) in lens concavity.
* Needs to be performed in a **dark room,** as light causes pupillary constriction and may lead to a falsely open angle. Also avoid shining the slit lamp beam across the pupil.
* Hold down lower lid and ask patient to look up.
* Insert lens, with the mirror at the 12 o'clock position and ask the patient to look straight ahead.
* Use a 2 mm slit beam, with the axis perpendicular to the mirror.
* Rotate lens clockwise until all quadrants are viewed.

Zeiss lenses

* Four-mirror lens on a handle, with a contact-surface diameter of 9 mm (less than the corneal diameter)
* The curvature of the lens is flatter than the cornea is, so no coupling agent is required.
* Can be used for indentation gonioscopy; axial pressure on the central cornea by lens will cause flattening of the anterior chamber and force aqueous humour into the angle, thus opening it if possible (allowing distinction between appositional and synaechial closure and identification of plateau)
* Entire circumference of angle visualized with minimal rotation

Method

* As for 'Zeiss lenses', but tear film is adequate as a coupling agent, and the lens is placed directly on the centre of the cornea (see Figure 8.17)
* Minimal or no rotation is required.
* It is important not to press too firmly until indentation is desired, as pressing too firmly will artificially open the angle. The aim is to hold the lens in gentle apposition with the cornea so that the contact meniscus is occasionally lost. If corneal tension lines are seen, too much force is being applied. Indentation is achieved by anterior–posterior force.

Identification of angle structures

The key to gonioscopy is the **corneal wedge** (see Figure 8.18). The wedge is an image created by a thin slit lamp beam, offset at 15°–45°, and viewed through the goniolens. The beam creates two reflections forming a wedge shape. The apex of the corneal wedge is used to locate Schwalbes line as the location where the two reflections meet. Identification of the corneal wedge helps avoid mistaking secondary pigmented lines for the TM. There are four main structures to examine, which can be remembered via the mnemonic **'S-T-S-C'**:

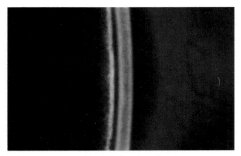

Fig 8.14 Assessment of limbal chamber depth
The clear gap behind the cornea is approximately one-quarter the width of the cornea (Van Hericks Grade 2), indicating a potentially occludable angle

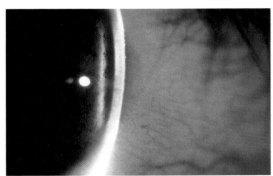

Fig 8.15 Assessment of limbal chamber depth
The clear gap behind the cornea is almost the width of the clear cornea (Van Hericks Grade 4)

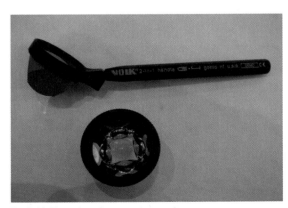

Fig 8.16 Examples of two gonioscopy lenses

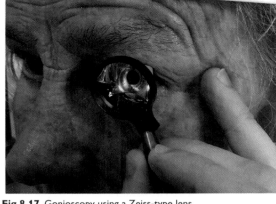

Fig 8.17 Gonioscopy using a Zeiss-type lens

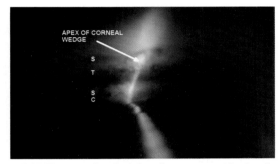

APEX OF CORNEAL WEDGE

S
T
S
C

Fig 8.18 The corneal wedge light reflex in an eye with a heavily pigmented angle

S: Schwalbes line

- Schwalbes line is the most anterior angle structure and represents the peripheral termination of Descemets membrane and the anterior limit of the TM.
- Circumferential whitish, glistening ridge, occasionally pigmented

T: Trabecular Meshwork

- Extends from Schwalbes line to the scleral spur with a 'ground glass' appearance. The anterior portion of the TM is non-pigmented.
- The pigmented posterior functional portion adjacent to scleral spur is grey-blue. Pigmentation increases with age and is most marked inferiorly.
- Increased pigmentation may be evident in pigment dispersion syndrome or pseudoexfoliation.

S: Scleral spur

- Narrow whitish band posterior to the trabeculum
- Represents the most anterior projection of the sclera and is the site of attachment of the ciliary body longitudinal muscle

C: Ciliary body

- Brown-grey circumferential band
- The root of the iris inserts into the anterior portion of the ciliary body.
- The width of the ciliary body varies depending on iris insertion: it is narrow in hyperopes and wide in myopes.

Other structures

Schlemms canal

- Occasionally seen as a slightly darker line deep with respect to the posterior trabeculum
- Blood seen in canal, with raised episcleral venous pressure (compression by Goldmann goniolens or pathological process)

Iris processes

- Small extensions of the iris inserting at level of the scleral spur
- Present in one-third of normal eyes; does not draw the iris up in the way that peripheral anterior synechiae (PAS) do

Blood vessels

- Form a radial pattern at the base of the angle recess and, as a general rule, do not cross the scleral spur
- Pathological vessels follow a random pattern, beginning as fine lacy fronds, and are later accompanied by a fibrous 'scaffold'.

Angle grading

Spaeth grading system

In this system, three features are assessed:

- Iris insertion: the system for grading iris insertion can be remembered via the mnemonic 'ABCDE' (an insertion anterior to a C grade is pathological):
  — A: **A**nterior to Schwalbes line
  — B: **B**ehind Schwalbes line
  — C: s**C**leral spur visible
  — D: **D**eep; ciliary body visible
  — E: **E**xtremely deep (>1 mm of the ciliary body visible)
- Anterior chamber angle
  — Estimate the angle width in degrees between two tangents; one drawn from the pigmented TM along the posterior surface of cornea, and another from the pigmented TM along the peripheral iris.
  — If the pigmented TM is not visible, the angle is 0°.
- Curvature of the iris; assessed as follows:
  — **b**: Bowing anteriorly
  — **p**: Plateau configuration (sudden steep rise after insertion before the iris flattens)
  — **f**: Flat
  — **c**: Concave posterior bowing
  — The features can be combined and abbreviated, e.g. D30p for a deep, 30° angle with a plateau configuration.

Shaffer grading system

The angle is graded 0–4 according to the most posterior angle structure visualized (see Table 8.1). The amount of trabecular pigmentation should also be noted. An **occludable angle** is defined as an angle in which there are **two or more quadrants (≥180°) of iridotrabecular contact (ITC)**. Indentation gonioscopy should be used to determine whether angle closure is due to apposition or PAS.

Table 8.1 The Shaffer grading system			
Grade	Angle size	Angle structure seen	Angle description
4	35–45°	Ciliary body	Wide open
3	20–35°	Scleral spur	Open
2	20°	Posterior pigmented TM	Moderately narrow
1	10°	Schwalbe's line	Very narrow
0	0°	No structures visible	Closed

TM, trabecular meshwork.
Reprinted from *American Journal of Ophthalmology*, 68, 4, Van Herick et al., 'Estimation of Width of Angle of Anterior Chamber Incidence and Significance of the Narrow Angle', pp. 626–629. Copyright (1969) with permission from Elsevier

Perimetry is a psychophysical test to evaluate a patient's visual field. This test is an essential part of glaucoma management, as loss of visual function reduces quality of life. Glaucomatous RGC damage leads to specific patterns of field loss. Visual field defects may occur before detectable structural defects or vice versa. Serial field tests should be used to assess for progression. Perimetry is also valuable in the identification and monitoring of certain neurological diseases.

The visual field is described as 'an island of vision surrounded by a sea of darkness'. This island is depicted as a hill with maximum height at fixation, owing to the high density of photoreceptors at the fovea. Visual acuity decreases towards the periphery in a steep fashion nasally and more gradually temporally. There is a 'blind spot' 10°–20° temporal to fixation; this spot corresponds to the optic nerve head. The normal visual field extends 60° superiorly, 60° nasally, 80° inferiorly, and 90° temporally.

An overall reduction in field sensitivity (e.g. cataract) will flatten the hill. A localized defect is known as a scotoma, which can be 'absolute' (total loss of vision) or 'relative' (area of partial visual loss with reduced sensitivity).

Kinetic perimetry

Kinetic perimetry can be performed by simple confrontation, a tangent (Bjerrum) screen, Lister perimeter, or Goldmann perimeter. It provides a two-dimensional measure of the boundary of the hill of vision. A stimulus of fixed size and intensity is steadily moved from a non-seeing to a seeing area of the field along set meridians at 15° intervals. The points at which the stimulus is perceived are plotted on a chart and joined by a line to form isoptres. Using stimuli of different intensities will provide a contour map of the visual field.

Goldmann perimeter

The Goldmann perimeter is the most commonly used kinetic perimeter. It is useful for patients unable to perform reliable automated perimetry, for low visual acuity, and if a neurological defect is suspected. The patient sits one side of the bowl and presses a button when a stimulus is seen; the examiner sits at the other side to present targets and record responses.

- Roman numerals 0–V represent increasing target size.
- Arabic numerals 1–4 represent increasing light intensity.
- Lowercase letters represent the use of filters (a = darkest; e = brightest).

Advantages

The test can be carried out at any speed. The examiner can assess patient responses and adapt to them.

Disadvantages

Small scotomas may be missed between isoptres. Results depend on the skill of the examiner. No statistical analysis is made. This test is not suitable for the detection of early glaucomatous defects.

Static perimetry

Automated static perimetry uses a machine with preset programs, for example Henson, Octopus, and Humphrey perimeters. It provides a three-dimensional measure of the vertical boundaries of the visual field. The size and location of the target are constant but a varying luminance of the target is used to determine 'threshold' retinal sensitivity at different locations of the field.

Standard automated perimetry (SAP) is static computerized threshold perimetry with a white-on-white stimulus. The Humphrey perimeter is the most frequently used analyser in the United Kingdom. It consists of a hemispherical bowl onto which the target is projected. The patient presses a button when the target is seen. A background luminance of 31.5 apostilb (asb) is used. The examiner can choose testing strategies, including suprathreshold and full-threshold tests.

Suprathreshold testing

Suprathreshold testing is mainly used for screening. Points of light at luminance levels 2–6 dB above the expected normal threshold values are presented at various locations in the visual field. Missed targets will reflect areas of decreased sensitivity that can be further analysed if required. The Humphrey analyser can be used to perform 120-point screening, in which a positive test is defined by a total of 17 missed points, or 8 missed points in any one quadrant.

Threshold testing

Threshold testing is used for more detailed assessment. Threshold luminance values are plotted and compared with age-matched normal values. The Humphrey analyser increases the intensity of its stimulus in 4 dB steps until a threshold is crossed. The threshold is then rechecked by decreasing the intensity by 2 dB steps. Testing may be of the central 10°, 24°, or 30°.

Full-threshold 30–2

- Tests 76 points (6° apart) in the central 30° of the field
- Long and laborious test

Full-threshold 24–2

- Tests 54 points (6° apart) in the central 24° of the field
- Cuts test time by one-fifth
- Gold standard for monitoring glaucoma

Full-threshold 10–2

- Tests 68 points (2° apart) in the central 10° of the field
- Used in advanced glaucoma where fixation is threatened

The Swedish Interactive Thresholding Algorithm (SITA) Standard or the SITA Fast programs have generally replaced full-threshold testing.

SITA Standard

- Uses computerized algorithms based upon a normative database
- Utilizes threshold values of adjacent points to determine starting points, thus saving time by asking fewer 'questions'

SITA Fast

- Same method as the SITA Standard but less scrutiny at each point
- Faster but less reliable than the standard test

All automated test procedures have a significant learning curve that should be taken into account. Often three to four consecutive tests are required before reliable fields are obtained.

Esterman visual field testing

An Esterman chart/program using static perimetry is part of the UK's DVLA visual standards for driving. The Group 1 (ordinary licence) standard specifies a field of at least 120° on the horizontal; the field is measured using a white target equivalent to the Goldmann III4e setting. In addition, there should be no significant defect in the binocular field which encroaches within 20° of fixation above or below the meridian. Acceptable central loss includes scattered single missed points or a single cluster of up to three contiguous points. Those who have been driving with static defects and non-progressive eye conditions for many years can be considered on an individual basis. The Group 2 (vocational licence) standard requires a 'normal binocular visual field' with no provision for exceptional cases.

Humphrey analyser displays

Numerical

- Gives a threshold (in decibels) for each point
- Figures in parentheses for the same point are checked a second time.

Greyscale

- Decreasing sensitivity represented by darker tones
- Useful for examining the gross shape of the field defect

Total deviation

- Represents the deviation of a patient's result from age-matched controls
- Upper numerical and lower greyscale displays

Pattern deviation

- Total deviation adjusted for generalized depression in the overall field
- Can correct for diffuse loss such as that induced by the presence of cataract
- Upper numerical and lower greyscale displays

Probability values

- Probability values (represented as *p*) indicate the significance of defects.
- Refers to the probability that the sensitivity is normal
- Shown as <5%, <2%, <1%, and <0.5%

Humphrey analyser reliability indices

Fixation losses

- Stimuli are presented within the blind spot.
- If the losses are seen by the patient, he/she is clearly not fixating correctly.
- If losses exceed 20%–30%, reliability should be questioned.

False positives

- 'Trigger-happy' patients who press the button with no stimulus present
- Greyscale printout is abnormally pale
- Should be <10% for a reliable test

False negatives

- Test points of known sensitivity are rechecked with a brighter stimulus.
- If not seen by patient, may be due to inattention or fatigue
- A greyscale printout with a high number of false negatives has a cloverleaf pattern.
- Should be <20% for a reliable test

Global indices

Mean deviation

- Mean elevation or depression of the field compared with age-corrected normal
- May be due to overall defect or localized loss

Visual field index

- Similar to the mean deviation but expressed as a percentage and centrally weighted
- The visual field index (VFI) takes into account cataract.

Glaucoma hemifield test

- Assesses asymmetry between the top and bottom halves of the field (one hemifield tends to be damaged first in glaucoma)
- The results are graded as being outside normal limits, borderline, or within normal limits.

Other indices include the pattern standard deviation, which is a measure of focal loss or variability within the field compared to an age-corrected normal, and short-term fluctuation, which is a test of intra-test consistency where ten preselected points are tested twice.

Sources of error in perimetry

Poor reliability or performance by patient

- Check reliability indices.

Incorrect date of birth

- Threshold testing takes patient age into account.

Miosis

- Apparent loss of peripheral field: dilate if <3 mm

Media opacities

- Overall depression of whole field: corrected by pattern standard deviation plot

Uncorrected refractive error

- Overall depression, particularly central sensitivity
- Error greater than 1 D cylinder uncorrected may cause peripheral scotoma.
- Testing should be performed with near-vision correction after the age of 40 or in aphakes/pseudophakes.

Spectacles

- Can cause rim artefacts (concentric scotoma)

Ptosis/blepharochalasis

- Superior field defects (tape lids up during test)

Facial anatomy

- A large nose or protruding supraorbital margins may cause pseudodefects.

Visual field practicalities

- Watch for a 'learning effect'.
- A visual field defect should only be considered real after repeat testing.
- Disc features should match the visual field defects.
- Other causes of visual field defects should be ruled out, e.g. chorioretinal lesions and tilted discs.

Other perimetry devices

Short-wavelength automated perimetry

Short-wavelength automated perimetry (SWAP) was developed with the hope that field defects might be detected earlier than with SAP (e.g. the Humphrey visual field test), but this expectation has not been confirmed. SWAP uses static threshold testing with a large blue stimulus against a bright yellow background. The theory is that the blue visual pathways are preferentially damaged in glaucoma. Blue pathways also have less redundancy than other pathways and thus any glaucomatous loss of blue-pathway nerve fibres manifests as a visual field defect early in the condition. SWAP is sensitive but is less specific than SAP. SWAP has greater short-term and long-term fluctuation than SAP does, making detection of progression difficult. SWAP also takes longer and is affected more significantly by media opacities, compared to SAP.

Frequency-doubling perimetry

Frequency-doubling technology measures the function of the magnocellular pathway, which includes a subset of RGCs (parasol RGCs, which have large dendritic trees and cell bodies) that detect motion and which are lost early in glaucoma. Testing is performed by rapid reversal of a grating of low spatial frequency (narrow black and white bars) at a high temporal frequency (25 flickers per second) to create a doubling-frequency illusion. The contrast of the stimulus is varied during the test, and the patient presses a button when the flickering stimulus is detected. The perimeter is a compact and portable unit, screening takes less than 1 minute per eye, and the technique has good sensitivity and specificity.

Glaucoma field defects

Diagnostic criteria for glaucomatous visual field defects (European Glaucoma Society Guidelines)

In the absence of retinal or neurological disease affecting the visual field, visual field loss is considered significant when:

1. An abnormal glaucoma hemifield test is confirmed on two consecutive tests.
2. Three abnormal points are confirmed on two consecutive tests, with p <5% probability of being normal, with point one having p <1%, and all being not contiguous with the blind spot.
3. Corrected pattern standard deviation is less than 5% if the visual field is otherwise normal, as confirmed on two consecutive tests.

Any defect or suspected defect must be confirmed by repeated testing.

Typical glaucomatous field defects

Arcuate defect

Axons from ganglion cells temporal to the optic nerve follow an arcuate course. Damage to these axons results in an arcuate field defect (see Figure 8.19). Axons in the superior and inferior retina are separated by the horizontal raphe, a line intersecting the fovea and optic nerve. Ganglion cells superior to the raphe arc superiorly and those inferior to it arc inferiorly.

Nasal step

A nasal step is a nasal defect due to a peripheral temporal lesion that respects the horizontal midline, again because of the horizontal raphe (see Figure 8.20). Nasal step may be superior or inferior.

Temporal wedge defect

Axons from ganglion cells in the nasal fundus travel directly to the optic. Damage to this axon group produces a wedge-type visual field defect.

Paracentral defect

Although paracentral defects may appear small, they are serious and vision-threatening due to their proximity to fixation (see Figure 8.21). Most commonly found supero-nasally, they tend to respect the horizontal raphe. Superior and inferior defects may thus not be aligned. Paracentral defects can coalesce to form arcuate defects.

As glaucoma progresses, multiple defects can present which enlarge and deepen with time. End-stage defects are characterized by a small remaining island of central vision with an accompanying isolated patch of temporal field. Typically central vision is preserved until late (see Figure 8.22); however, paracentral defects can develop early in disease, particularly in normal tension glaucoma.

Glaucoma severity staging

Visual fields are often used to stage glaucoma. A classification based on that of Hodapp is:

- **Early glaucoma:** mean deviation <−6 dB and no points in the central 5°, with <15 dB sensitivity
- **Moderate glaucoma:** mean deviation < −12 dB, with no point in the central 5° with 0 dB sensitivity and only one hemifield with a sensitivity <15 dB within the central 5°
- **Severe glaucoma:** mean deviation worse than that for moderate glaucoma

Detecting progression

Progression can be examined via **event-based** analysis (determines whether a specific visual field has changed from a previous visual field by an amount greater than that expected owing to test–test variability) or a **trend-based** analysis (determines the rate of change).

A simple global trend analysis might consist of plotting the mean deviation or VFI value of an eye over time. This analysis can help predict whether progression is likely to lead to loss of vision during a patient's life (see Figure 8.23).

The **Glaucoma Progression Analysis** program compares pattern deviation values to determine if progression has occurred (see Figure 8.23). At least three SAP tests are needed. In the graphical output, a square means the point has not worsened, an open triangle indicates the point has worsened on one visit, a half-filled triangle indicates that the point has worsened on two consecutive visits, and a filled triangle indicates that the point has worsened on three consecutive visits.

The **Progressor** program performs a trend-based analysis using linear regression of the threshold values from each test point. Results are presented for each test location by a series of bars representing different SAP test dates (see Figure 8.24). A short bar indicates a near-normal sensitivity, and a long bar indicates an abnormally low sensitivity. The significance of change is colour coded, with hot colours (white, red) indicating significant change, and grey meaning no change.

CENTRAL 24-2 THRESHOLD TEST

FIXATION MONITOR: BLINOSPOT

FIXATION TARGET: CENTRAL

FIXATION LOSSES: 0/17

FALSE POS ERRORS: 3 %

FALSE NEG ERRORS: 3 %

TEST DURATION: 07:24

FOVEA: 38 DB

STIMULUS: III, WHITE

BACKGROUND: 31.5 ASB

STRATEGY: SITA-STANDARD

PUPIL DIAMETER:

VISUAL ACUITY:

RX: +4.25 DS   DC X

DATE: 01-11-2004

TIME: 16:36

AGE: 73

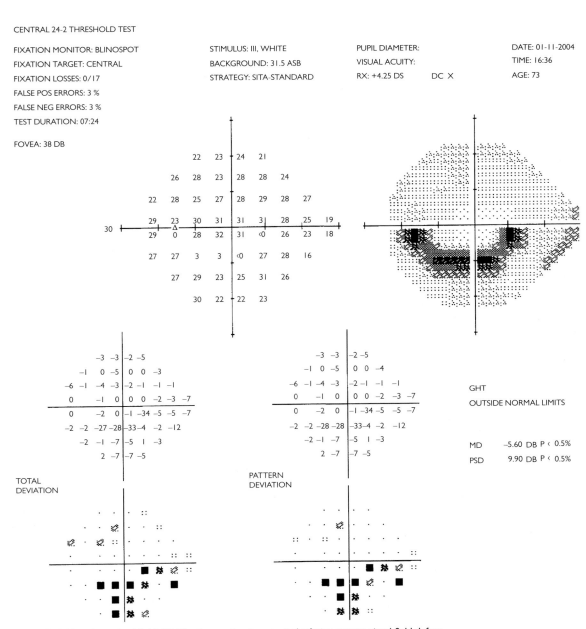

GHT

OUTSIDE NORMAL LIMITS

MD   −5.60 DB P < 0.5%

PSD   9.90 DB P < 0.5%

TOTAL DEVIATION

PATTERN DEVIATION

Fig 8.19 A Humphrey visual field (24–2) printout showing a typical inferior arcuate visual field defect

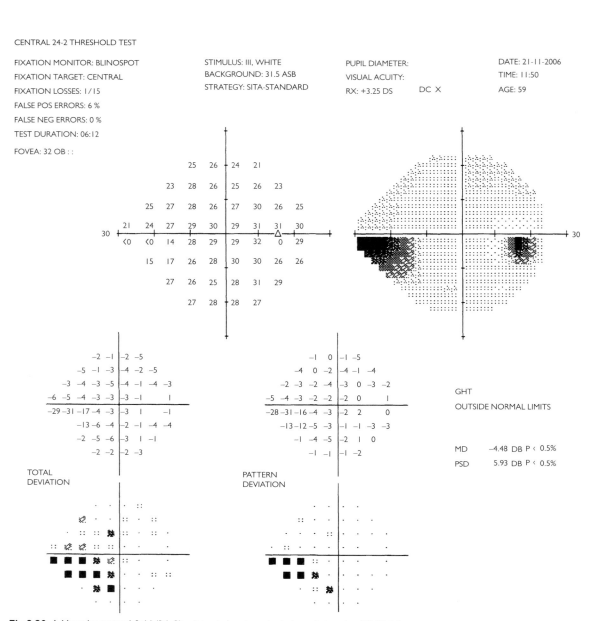

CENTRAL 24-2 THRESHOLD TEST

FIXATION MONITOR: BLINOSPOT
FIXATION TARGET: CENTRAL
FIXATION LOSSES: 1/15
FALSE POS ERRORS: 6 %
FALSE NEG ERRORS: 0 %
TEST DURATION: 06:12

FOVEA: 32 OB : :

STIMULUS: III, WHITE
BACKGROUND: 31.5 ASB
STRATEGY: SITA-STANDARD

PUPIL DIAMETER:
VISUAL ACUITY:
RX: +3.25 DS   DC X

DATE: 21-11-2006
TIME: 11:50
AGE: 59

```
              25  26 | 24  21
          23  28  26 | 25  26  23
      25  27  28  26 | 27  30  26  25
  21  24  27  29  30 | 29  31  31  30
30 <0  <0  14  28  29 | 29  32  △  29
      15  17  26  28 | 30  30  26  26
          27  26  25 | 28  31  29
              27  28 | 28  27
```

```
           -2  -1 | -2  -5                          -1   0 | -1  -5
       -5  -1  -3 | -4  -2  -5                   -4   0  -2 | -4  -1  -4
   -3  -4  -3  -5 | -4  -1  -4  -3            -2  -3  -2  -4 | -3   0  -3  -2
-6 -5  -4  -3  -3 | -3  -1       1         -5  -4  -3  -2  -2 | -2   0       1
-29 -31 -17 -4 -3 | -3   1      -1        -28 -31 -16 -4 -3 | -2   2       0
   -13 -6  -4 | -2  -1  -4  -4             -13 -12 -5 -3 | -1  -1  -3  -3
    -2  -5  -6 | -3   1  -1                    -1  -4  -5 | -2   1   0
        -2  -2 | -2  -3                            -1  -1 | -1  -2
```

TOTAL
DEVIATION

PATTERN
DEVIATION

GHT
OUTSIDE NORMAL LIMITS

MD   −4.48 DB P < 0.5%
PSD   5.93 DB P < 0.5%

Fig 8.20 A Humphrey visual field (24–2) printout showing a typical nasal step visual field defect

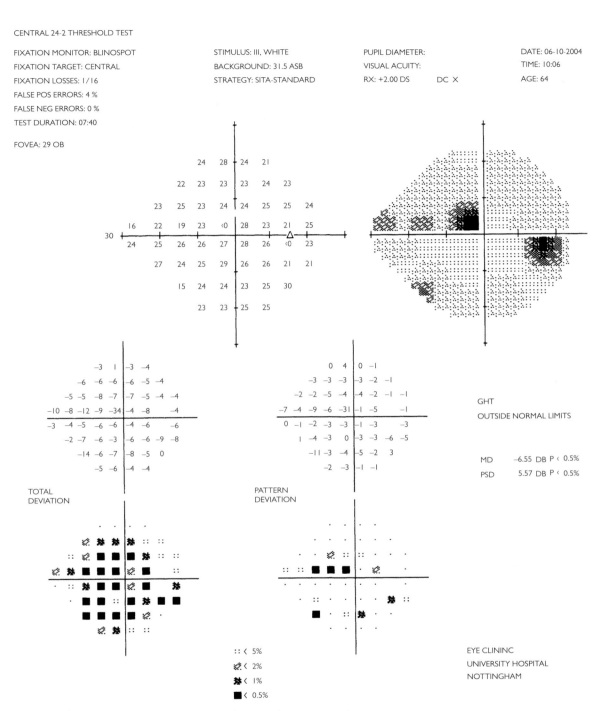

CENTRAL 24-2 THRESHOLD TEST

FIXATION MONITOR: BLINOSPOT
FIXATION TARGET: CENTRAL
FIXATION LOSSES: 1/16
FALSE POS ERRORS: 4 %
FALSE NEG ERRORS: 0 %
TEST DURATION: 07:40

FOVEA: 29 OB

STIMULUS: III, WHITE
BACKGROUND: 31.5 ASB
STRATEGY: SITA-STANDARD

PUPIL DIAMETER:
VISUAL ACUITY:
RX: +2.00 DS   DC X

DATE: 06-10-2004
TIME: 10:06
AGE: 64

```
              24  28   24  21
          22  23  23   23  24  23
      23  25  23  24   24  25  25  24
  16  22  19  23  ‹0   28  23  21  25
30                    △‹0
  24  25  26  26  27   28  26  ‹0  23
      27  24  25  29   26  26  21  21
          15  24  24   23  25  30
              23  23   25  25
```

TOTAL
DEVIATION

```
              -3   1   -3  -4
          -6  -6  -6   -6  -5  -4
      -5  -5  -8  -7   -7  -5  -4  -4
  -10  -8 -12  -9 -34  -4  -8      -4
  -3  -4  -5  -6  -6   -4  -6
      -2  -7  -6  -3   -6  -6  -9  -8
         -14  -6  -7   -8  -5   0
              -5  -6   -4  -4
```

PATTERN
DEVIATION

```
               0   4   0  -1
          -3  -3  -3   -3  -2  -1
      -2  -2  -5  -4   -4  -2  -1  -1
  -7  -4  -9  -6 -31  -1  -5      -1
   0  -1  -2  -3  -3  -1  -3      -3
       1  -4  -3   0  -3  -3  -6  -5
         -11  -3  -4  -5  -2   3
              -2  -3  -1  -1
```

GHT
OUTSIDE NORMAL LIMITS

MD   -6.55 DB P ‹ 0.5%
PSD   5.57 DB P ‹ 0.5%

:: ‹ 5%
⍩ ‹ 2%
⧳ ‹ 1%
■ ‹ 0.5%

EYE CLININC
UNIVERSITY HOSPITAL
NOTTINGHAM

Fig 8.21 A Humphrey visual field (24–2) printout showing a dense paracentral scotoma

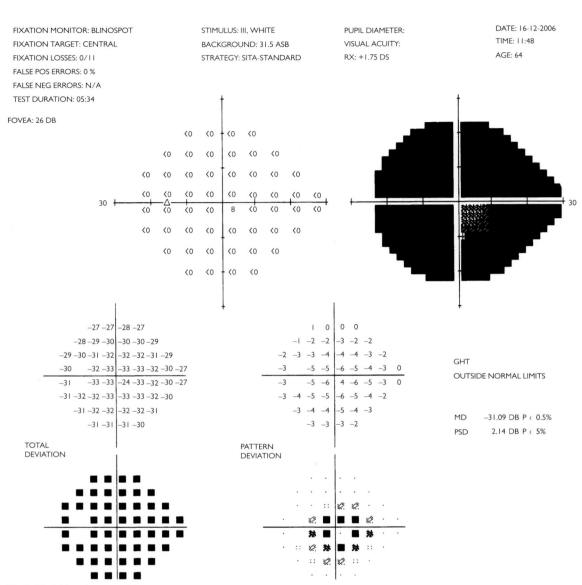

Fig 8.22 A Humphrey visual field (24–2) printout showing end-stage glaucoma
Such patients should be assessed using a 10–2 program

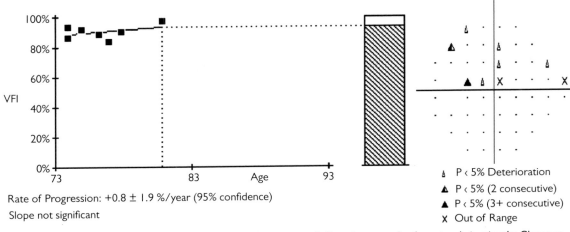

P ‹ 5% Deterioration

P ‹ 5% (2 consecutive)

P ‹ 5% (3+ consecutive)

X Out of Range

Rate of Progression: +0.8 ± 1.9 %/year (95% confidence)

Slope not significant

Fig 8.23 An example of trend analysis of the visual field index over time (left), and an example of event analysis using the Glaucoma Progression Analysis program (right)

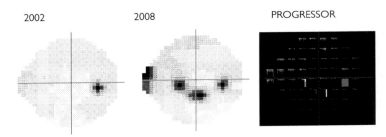

2002   2008   PROGRESSOR

Fig 8.24 Example of progression in a right eye

The Progressor software shows hot colours in the progressing points

8.10 Ocular hypertension

Ocular hypertension (OHT) is a condition characterized by consistently raised IOP and with anatomically open angles in which the optic nerve and visual field show no signs of glaucomatous damage.

Prevalence

Population studies show that IOP has a normal distribution with the curve skewed to the right, as there are more normal people with an IOP above the mean pressure of 16 mmHg than there are with an IOP below it. The statistical definition of the upper limit for 'normal' IOP is 21 mmHg, which is two standard deviations above the mean value. An IOP >21 mmHg is used as the cut-off for the definition of OHT: 4%–10% of the population over 40 years of age will have an IOP >21 mmHg but no detectable signs of glaucoma.

Risk factors

* Increased age
* Female
* Ethnic origin: those of black African or Afro-Caribbean origin are more at risk than those of other ethnic origins are
* Systemic hypertension
* Corticosteroid use: oral or inhaled
* Diabetes mellitus
* Positive family history of glaucoma

Clinical evaluation

History

* Asymptomatic
* Family history of glaucoma

Examination

* Applanation tonometry
* Gonioscopy
* Pachymetry
* Stereoscopic slit lamp optic disc evaluation
* Visual field assessment
* Baseline optic disc imaging

Management

OHT treatment is indicated only in those individuals recognized to be at increased risk of conversion to open-angle glaucoma. The Ocular Hypertension Treatment Study trial from 2002 provides useful information regarding risk. This study was a multicentre randomized controlled trial in which patients with OHT were assigned to either observation or topical medications (IOP needed to be lowered 20% from baseline). The probability of developing glaucoma over 5 years was halved by treatment, from 9.5% in the observed group to 4.4% in the treated group. The conclusion was that treatment should be considered for individuals with OHT who are at moderate-to-high risk.

The challenge is to assess the risk of glaucomatous damage for a particular individual, at a particular IOP, and in a particular eye.

Risk factors for conversion to glaucoma

Ocular risk factors

* High presenting IOP
* Large vertical CDR

* CDR asymmetry >0.2
* Disc haemorrhage
* RNFL defect
* Thin central corneal thickness: in the Ocular Hypertension Treatment Study, those with a CCT <555 µm were three times more likely to develop glaucoma than those with thicker corneas

Systemic risk factors

* Age
* Family history
* Black African or Afro-Caribbean origin

The UK NICE guidance on OHT recommends:

* Start treatment when IOP is >32 mmHg, no matter the CCT.
* If the CCT is >590 µm, treat only if the IOP is >32 mmHg.
* If the CCT is 555–90 µm, treat if the IOP is >25 mmHg, but only until the age of 60.
* If the CCT is <555 µm, there should be a low threshold for treatment in patients younger than 60; for patients over 60, the threshold should be slightly higher than that for patients under 60.

Ultimately the decision to treat is an individual one for the clinician and patient, and the above is only a guide. The decision to treat must take into account the risk/benefit ratio of treatment and weigh the side effects of medication and the individual's life expectancy with the probability of functional visual loss. An IOP of >32 mmHg may be treated in an effort to reduce the risk of central retinal vein occlusion, especially in a patient with other cardiovascular risk factors predisposing to central retinal vein occlusion (CRVO) or in whom CRVO has already occurred in the fellow eye.

Treatment is usually with topical ocular hypertensives such as prostaglandin analogues or beta blockers. The aim is to lower the IOP to a safe level for the individual patient; one would expect at least a 20% reduction.

Follow-up

After the initial visit, if medication has been commenced, a 1–4 month review is recommended to assess the response to treatment. Depending on the risk factors present, follow-up is then normally performed every 6–12 months. After several visits, a patient with mild OHT but with no signs of conversion to glaucoma may be able to be discharged to the community for optometric follow-up on a 1–2 yearly basis. Increasingly, low-risk patients are managed in shared care with optometrists, either in hospital or in the community.

Prognosis

Although the Ocular Hypertension Treatment Study found that 9.5% of untreated individuals with OHT and an IOP of 24 mmHg or more convert to glaucoma over a 5-year period, the individual risk of conversion depends on the presence or absence of the risk factors (see 'Risk factors for conversion to glaucoma').

Primary open-angle glaucoma is a progressive, chronic optic neuropathy with characteristic structural changes to the optic nerve head and RNFL. Patients develop reproducible visual field defects, which are often, but not always, consistent with the extent of RNFL damage. Typical visual field defects include a nasal step or an arcuate or paracentral defect. Gonioscopy shows a macroscopically normal and open drainage angle and there is no identifiable secondary cause.

Elevated IOP is not included in the definition of primary open-angle glaucoma as the disease may occur when the IOP is within the normal population-based range (see Section 8.14). The susceptibility of the optic nerve to damage varies among patients and at different stages of disease.

Eyes may be labelled **'glaucoma suspect'** if they have optic disc appearances suspicious of glaucoma but without evidence of progressive changes, and normal visual fields.

Prevalence

Primary open-angle glaucoma is the most prevalent of all the glaucomas and is the third leading cause of blindness worldwide. It occurs in approximately **2%** of the population **over the age of 40**, increasing with age to over **4%** of those **over 80**. The incidence is similar in males and females.

Clinical evaluation

History

- Asymptomatic until there is significant loss of the visual field, especially as early visual field loss tends to involve the nasal field, which overlaps with the fellow eye
- Damage results in negative scotomas.
- The patient may have difficulty in moving from bright to dark rooms and in judging steps and kerbs. Inability to deal with contrast, particularly rapidly changing contrast, may become a major issue.

Risk factors for the development of primary open-angle glaucoma

- Factors increasing risk of conversion of OHT to glaucoma (see Section 8.10)
- Positive family history in a first-degree relative: risk is doubled for a parent but quadrupled for a sibling
- Myopia
- Diabetes mellitus
- Risk rises continuously with increasing IOP
- Also enquire about other risk factors such as systemic hypotension, anaemia, and vasospastic disorders (migraine, Raynauds syndrome).

The inheritance of primary open-angle glaucoma is multifactorial. Relatives of patients with primary open-angle glaucoma have a 22% risk of developing glaucoma, compared to 2%–3% of controls. The myocillin gene on Chromosome 1q was the first gene associated with glaucoma. Myocillin, which is also known as the TM-inducible glucocorticoid response (TIGR) protein, is found in the TM but its role is unknown. The presence of mutated myocillin may increase the vulnerability of the TM to cellular insults. The discovered genes predisposing to glaucoma only account for about 5% of cases of primary open-angle glaucoma.

Risk factors for blindness in primary open-angle glaucoma

- Advanced disease at presentation
- Suboptimal IOP control
- Black African or Afro-Caribbean race
- Low socio-economic status

Examination

- Visual acuity
- GAT: reveals a raised IOP, usually in the region of 24–32 mmHg. There may be fluctuations in IOP (90% of patients have diurnal variations up to 5 mmHg).
- CCT
- Gonioscopy: open angle with normal appearance is a key feature in making the diagnosis
- Blood pressure
- Stereoscopic dilated optic disc examination
- SAP

Screening

Screening should be routinely performed for patients over the age of 40 who have first-degree relatives with primary open-angle glaucoma. Free eye tests on the UK National Health Service are available for this group and for all individuals over 60. If IOP is normal, screening should occur every 2 years until age 50, then annually thereafter. Screening should begin earlier if a family member developed glaucoma at a young age.

Management

The aim of treatment in primary open-angle glaucoma is to preserve visual function. This aim is achieved by controlling the IOP whilst minimizing any adverse effects of treatment. It is important to realize that primary open-angle glaucoma cannot be cured but that control of IOP can slow progression. Large randomized control trials have shown the benefit of lowering IOP; some of these are summarized in Section 8.27.

In most cases, medical treatment is used as the first resort and will often involve a prostaglandin analogue. Additional medications may be added if needed. Surgery may be considered as a first-line treatment if advanced damage is present at presentation. Laser treatment (e.g. selective laser trabeculoplasty (SLT)) may also be considered as a first-line option, particularly in those with early disease, ocular surface disease, or in those who find instilling eye drops difficult. Specific pharmacological and surgical management options are discussed in later chapters.

Target IOP

It is useful to set a target pressure when initiating treatment. The target IOP should be individualized and based on factors such as the IOP at presentation and the IOP at which documented damage has occurred. Patients with a low baseline IOP are likely to need a low target IOP; however, the target depends on the risk of sight loss. Factors such as age, family history, the severity of glaucoma, the rate of progression, and the status of the fellow eye are important when deciding a target IOP. Ensure the patient is at the centre of decisions regarding treatment. The target IOP level should be re-evaluated at each visit in light of the visual field and optic disc.

Follow-up

After a decision to treat, reassessment of IOP should be performed within 6 weeks and any side effects evaluated. If IOP reduction is satisfactory, this interval may be extended to 3 to 6 months, depending on disease severity.

8.12 Primary angle closure

The defining feature of angle closure is contact between the iris and posterior pigmented TM, or **ITC**. ITC causes damage to the TM, resulting in PAS and increased IOP with resultant damage to RGCs and glaucoma. ITC may be due to the **iris being pushed forwards**, as in cases of pupil block, or being **pulled back** towards the TM, for example by inflammatory PAS. Secondary causes of angle closure are discussed in Section 8.13.

Pathophysiology

A physiological situation of **relative pupillary block** occurs in all eyes, owing to contact between the posterior iris at the pupil margin and the anterior lens surface (see Figure 8.25). The result is resistance to aqueous flow from the posterior chamber to the anterior chamber. The pressure differential causes the peripheral iris to bow forwards (**iris bombé**). If the angle is predisposed, ITC may occur and aqueous outflow become blocked.

Some eyes are anatomically predisposed to angle closure because of (i) the relative anterior location of the iris lens diaphragm, (ii) a shallow anterior chamber, and (iii) a narrow chamber angle. Irido-lenticular contact is at its maximum with a mid-dilated pupil; therefore, dim lighting and mydriatics may provoke angle closure.

PAC may also occur without pupil block because of angle crowding and the occlusion of the drainage angle by thick iris folds, or as a manifestation of the **plateau iris configuration**. In plateau iris configuration, the central anterior chamber depth is normal and the iris plane is flat, until a steep insertion into the ciliary body at the periphery.

Classification of PAC

Previous nomenclature regarding angle closure has been confusing. The following staging is now used:

1. Primary angle closure suspect (PACS)
   * PACS is defined as the presence of two or more quadrants of ITC (≥180°).
   * The IOP is normal and there is no evidence of PAS or glaucomatous optic neuropathy.
   * Eyes with PACS are at risk of primary angle-closure glaucoma (PACG) or an acute attack of angle closure.
   * About one in four eyes with PACS develop either an elevation in IOP or PAS within 5 years.
2. Primary angle closure (PAC)
   * In primary angle closure, ITC is present but there are also features indicating that obstruction of the TM by the peripheral iris has occurred, namely, PAS and/or raised IOP.
   * There is no evidence of glaucomatous optic neuropathy.
   * An eye with primary angle closure has a 1 in 3 chance of progressing to PACG within 5 years.
3. PACG
   * PACG is defined as the presence of both ITC and glaucomatous optic neuropathy.

In these definitions, ITC should not be secondary to other ocular pathologies causing PAS, for example uveitis, trauma, or neovascularization.

Prevalence

The prevalence of primary open-angle glaucoma in European populations has recently been estimated as 0.4%. Three-quarters of those affected are female. There is a much higher prevalence of primary open-angle glaucoma in Inuit and Chinese populations than in other populations. The worldwide prevalence of primary open-angle glaucoma is estimated at 0.7% in those aged over 40 years. Primary open-angle glaucoma is a more blinding disease than primary open-angle glaucoma is.

Clinical evaluation

History

Symptoms associated with PAC and raised IOP, for example pain, redness, blurring, and haloes, may be present; however, these symptoms have poor sensitivity and specificity, and most patients with PAC are asymptomatic.

Assess the following risk factors:

* Increased age
* Female gender
* Inuit and/or Far-Eastern descent: PAC is rare in black populations
* Positive family history
* Use of topical or systemic medications associated with angle closure, e.g. nebulized bronchodilators, muscle relaxants, and other sympathomimetic or anticholinergic drugs

Examination

* Visual acuity
* Assess refractive status: hypermetropia is a risk factor
* GAT
* CCT
* Gonioscopy
* Shallow anterior chamber: assess LCD and central anterior chamber depth
* Narrow drainage angle: perform gonioscopy of both eyes
* Short axial length: nanophthalmic eyes are at particular risk; therefore, if the axial length is less than 21 mm, also assess scleral thickness
* A dilated exam is not advisable in eyes with PAC until treatment has been performed.

Differential diagnosis

* Neovascular glaucoma
* Inflammatory glaucoma
* Lens-induced angle closure
* Uveal effusion, e.g. with systemic medication (topiramate, sulphonamides), scleritis, pan-retinal photocoagulation (PRP)
* Aqueous misdirection
* Secondary causes of pupil block, e.g. silicone oil, anterior chamber intraocular lens (AC-IOL)
* Axenfeld–Reiger syndrome (see Section 8.22)
* Iridocorneal endothelial syndrome

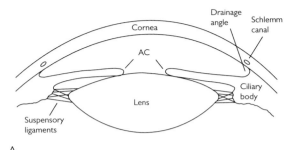

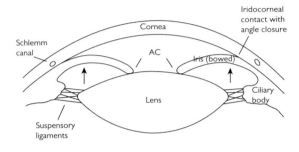

A

B

Fig 8.25 Diagram of the mechanism of pupil block

Management

It is recommended that PACS should be treated, usually with laser peripheral iridotomy (Laser PI). A Laser PI allows aqueous humour to bypass the pupil block, thus reducing iris bombé and contact between the iris and the TM. Patients with primary angle closure or PACG can also be treated initially by Laser PI; however, lens extraction may also be a good option.

If ITC is still present following Laser PI, options include long-term pilocarpine (although this is not well tolerated and should only be continued if it successfully opens the angle), argon Laser PI (ALPI), or lens extraction. If IOP remains high, glaucoma surgery such as trabeculectomy may be needed. Glaucoma surgery should be avoided in eyes with very small axial lengths because of the high risk of complications, particularly aqueous misdirection. Laser treatment for primary angle closure is discussed in Section 8.25.

Acute angle closure

Acute angle closure (see Figure 8.26) is one of the few ophthalmic emergencies, because, if left untreated, it can result in irreversible visual loss.

Clinical evaluation

History

- Consider the risk factors listed under primary angle closure.
- May be asymptomatic but often patients have ocular pain, red eye, and tearing
- Haloes around lights
- Reduced vision
- Nausea and vomiting
- Headache
- Previous intermittent episodes of blurred vision and ocular pain

Examination

- Ciliary injection
- Corneal oedema (fine ground glass) and epithelial bullae
- Shallow anterior chamber: assess LCD
- Aqueous flare with and without cells
- Stromal iris atrophy with a spiral-like configuration
- Fixed/sluggish mid-dilated pupil; vertically oval
- IOP greater than 40 mmHg; can be up to 100 mmHg
- Closed angle on gonioscopy
- Glaucomflecken: small grey-white anterior subcapsular opacities; indicate previous episodes of markedly raised IOP
- Optic disc oedema and hyperaemia
- Gonioscopic examination of the fellow eye is essential to look for an occludable angle.

Differential diagnosis

- Primary open-angle glaucoma with unusually high IOP
- Uveitic glaucoma
- Neovascular glaucoma
- Malignant glaucoma
- Pigment dispersion syndrome/glaucoma
- Anterior chamber angle tumour or mass
- Other causes of ocular pain (migraine, cluster headache)

Management

Initial

The aims of treatment are to break the pupil block, lower IOP, and control inflammation. It is usually possible to lower IOP via medications. Aqueous suppressants, including acetazolamide, topical beta blockers, and topical alpha agonists, should be given immediately.

- Acetazolamide 500 mg intravenously
- Timolol eye drops, 0.25% or 0.5%
- Iopidine eye drops, 1%
- Dexamethasone eye drops, 1%
- Pilocarpine eye drops, 2% or 4%, to both eyes; may not be effective in high IOP because of iris ischaemia; avoid intensive pilocarpine
- Have the patient lie in a supine position.
- Analgesics and anti-emetics, if needed

After 1 hour

- Recheck IOP; if IOP has fallen and corneal clarity permits, perform Laser PI.

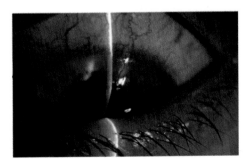

Fig 8.26 Colour anterior segment photograph showing the eye of a patient in acute angle-closure glaucoma
There is ciliary injection, the pupil is mid-dilated, and the cornea is slightly oedematous

If IOP still high, consider:
- Corneal indentation
- ALPI: can be performed more easily through an oedematous cornea than Laser PI
- Mannitol 20% (1–2 g/kg) intravenously over 45 minutes
- Oral glycerol 50% (1.0–1.5 g/kg) in lemon juice
- Be cautious if using mannitol/glycerol in elderly patients with cardiovascular and/or renal disease.

After a further 1 hour
If IOP is not reduced by the above measures, options might include surgical iridectomy or use of a cyclodiode laser with the eventual aim being to remove the crystalline lens. If there is an adequate corneal view, consider Laser PI. Glycerine can be used to clear the cornea. Laser PI is indicated in the fellow eye, as more than 50% of patients will develop symptoms in the second eye if it is left untreated.

Follow-up

Patients should not be discharged following acute angle closure until they have a patent Laser PI. Following laser iridotomy to both eyes, if the IOP is controlled, then patients can be discharged but should continue to use pilocarpine eye drops, 2% (or 4% if the iris is dark), four times a day and topical steroid such as dexamethasone eye drops, 0.1%, every two hours to the affected eye and four times a day to the fellow eye. Once patency of the Laser PI is confirmed, the pilocarpine can be stopped and gonioscopy repeated to ensure the angle remains open.

Persistent angle closure may be due to PAS, a plateau iris configuration, or a phacomorphic component. In such cases, glaucoma drainage surgery, ALPI, or cataract extraction may be considered. The urgency of the procedure will depend on whether the IOP can be controlled medically. If the pressure is controlled medically, it is better to defer surgery until inflammation has resolved.

Prognosis

Prognosis depends on the duration and severity of the attack. Prompt IOP lowering is essential to prevent irreversible optic nerve damage. There may also be permanent TM damage because of inflammation, appositional angle closure, and PAS causing the IOP to increase over time. Occasionally, the IOP will spike because of the recovery of temporary ciliary body shutdown, which resulted from ischaemia induced by the high IOP.

8.13 Secondary angle closure

The management of eyes with secondary angle closure is often different to those with primary angle closure. A warning sign that there may be a secondary cause is a difference in anterior chamber depth between eyes.

Angle closure can be due to **four mechanisms,** although there is often a combination involved:

1. Pupil block (80%)
   - Discussed in Section 8.12; however, in secondary angle closure, it may be due to secondary causes such as anterior lens dislocation, posterior synechiae, vitreous, silicone oil, or an AC-IOL
2. Obstruction at the level of the iris or ciliary body (10%)
   - This condition may occur because of a thick iris, an anterior iris insertion, or an anteriorly located ciliary body; an example is plateau iris.
3. Obstruction at the level of the lens (8%)
   - The lens plays a role in most types of angle closure; however, angle closure can be primarily 'phacomorphic'. In these cases, the lens is usually hypermature or may be subluxed.
4. Posterior pushing mechanism (2%)
   - Due to forwards movement of the iris lens diaphragm, secondary to an abnormality behind the lens
   - Causes include cilio-choroidal effusion and aqueous misdirection. Posterior pushing mechanisms usually cause shallowing of the central as well as the peripheral anterior chamber (i.e. there is not iris bombé).

This section discusses Mechanisms 2–4.

Obstruction at the level of the iris or ciliary body

Angle closure at the level of the iris may be secondary to the proliferation of abnormal tissue in the angle, for example due to neovascularization or iridocorneal endothelial syndrome. These are anterior pulling mechanisms. Angle closure at the level of the iris may also occur due to an abnormal iris configuration.

Plateau iris configuration

- Defined as a narrow or closed angle on gonioscopy, with a flat iris plane and a **deep central anterior chamber**

- Indentation gonioscopy shows the **double hump sign**: the peripheral hump is due to an anteriorly positioned ciliary body, which keeps the peripheral iris close to the TM, and the central hump is due to the iris resting on the lens surface.
- Other features are a thick iris, anterior iris insertion, and prominent last iris roll.
- Another possible cause is the presence of iridociliary cysts, which may be seen on UBM.

Plateau iris syndrome

- Diagnosed when an Laser PI has failed to reverse appositional angle closure in an eye with a plateau iris configuration
- More common in women than in men and tends to present at a younger age than primary angle closure does
- Accounts for 50% of patients who have angle closure with a patent Laser PI
- Recurrent or prolonged apposition leads to PAS and irreversible angle closure.

Eyes with plateau iris configuration should be treated with Laser PI, as there may be an element of pupil block. If plateau iris syndrome follows, treatment may be with ALPI or long-term pilocarpine.

Obstruction at the level of the lens

Increased lens thickness and anterior positioning of the lens contribute to primary angle closure; however, secondary angle closure, in which the lens is the primary cause, is usually due to factors such as lens subluxation (e.g. Marfan syndrome, trauma) or a very large (and usually white) cataract.

Posterior pushing mechanism

Causes include:

1. Aqueous misdirection
2. Choroidal effusion
   - A choroidal effusion is due to an accumulation of fluid in the suprachoroidal space.
   - May be due to inflammation (scleritis, uveitis), increased choroidal venous pressure (nanophthalmos, scleral buckling, PRP), tumours, or drugs (topiramate)

8.14 Normal tension glaucoma

Normal tension glaucoma is a form of open-angle glaucoma characterized by a peak IOP that is consistently within the statistically normal range, that is, there is glaucomatous optic neuropathy with an IOP of less than 21 mmHg, in the absence of a secondary cause. Normal tension glaucoma should be considered a diagnosis of exclusion.

Pathogenesis

Although IOP remains a significant factor, non-pressure-dependent processes are likely to be important. For example, there is evidence that systemic vascular dysregulation and localized vasospasm are risk factors. Such evidence suggests that impaired blood flow to the optic nerve may contribute to glaucomatous damage.

Prevalence

Although once thought to be uncommon, up to one-third of patients with open-angle glaucoma can be classified as having normal tension glaucoma (Beaver Dam Study). It is more common in the elderly than in other age groups, but up to 30% of patients are under 50 years. The overall prevalence of normal tension glaucoma in the general population is estimated at 0.15%; however, NTG accounts for 90% of glaucoma in the Japanese population.

General risk factors for normal tension glaucoma

* IOP: the optic nerve is susceptible to damage at relatively low levels of IOP
* Thin CCT
* Increased age
* Female gender (2 : 1)
* Race: Japanese
* Positive family history
* Diabetes mellitus
* Myopia

Risk factors for reduced blood flow to the optic nerve head

* Vasospasm: history of migraine or Raynauds phenomenon
* Hypercoagulability
* Nocturnal hypotension
* Autoimmune disorders
* Sleep apnoea

Clinical evaluation

History

* Need to specifically enquire about risk factors for reduced blood flow

Examination

* As for OHT/ primary open-angle glaucoma
* Phasing (diurnal IOP curve) to elucidate any IOP spikes. Office-hour phasing may still miss a nocturnal peak in IOP.

Specific clinical features for normal tension glaucoma

* Visual field defects are often more localized, deeper, steeper, and closer to fixation than those in primary open-angle glaucoma.
* The amount of visual field loss may be greater than expected on optic disc appearance.
* Localized (slit or wedge) defects of RNFL
* Increased propensity for optic disc haemorrhages
* Acquired optic disc pits
* Peripapillary atrophy more common

Further investigations (as appropriate)

* Blood pressure, blood glucose level, serum autoantibodies, erythrocyte sedimentation rate, C-reactive protein test
* 24-hour BP monitoring
* OPP
* Laboratory testing for infectious or inflammatory conditions

Neuroimaging if compressive disease suspected because of the following features:

* Age less than 50 years
* Poor visual acuity
* Pallor of neuroretinal rim
* Discrepancy between disc cupping and visual field loss
* Visual field loss that respects the vertical midline

Differential diagnosis

* Primary open-angle glaucoma with diurnal fluctuations
* Intermittent angle closure
* Hereditary optic neuropathy
* Compressive lesions of anterior visual pathway
* Acquired optic neuropathies (ischaemic, toxic, drug-induced, or nutritional optic neuropathy)
* Systemic disorders (syphilis, tuberculosis, sarcoidosis, and multiple sclerosis)
* Hypoperfusion (including history of large-volume blood loss)
* Optic disc anomalies (drusen, large pits, colobomas)

Management

Despite the IOP being statistically within the normal range, reduction of IOP reduces the risk of progression. The Collaborative Normal Tension Glaucoma Study showed that lowering IOP by 30% significantly reduced the rate of progression (12% of treated vs 34% of untreated progressed at 7 years). Although many untreated eyes showed no progression, there was a significant minority that had rapid loss of vision.

Medical

- Prostaglandin analogues (greater IOP-lowering effect at night)
- Alpha 2 agonists (may have additional neuroprotective effects)
- Carbonic anhydrase inhibitors (may increase ocular blood flow)
- Beta blockers (if needed, consider once a day morning use only, because of possible adverse effects on BP and on optic nerve head perfusion)
- Trial of supramaximal medical therapy and effect on progression of field loss may help to establish optimal management.

Improve optic nerve head blood flow

There may be some specific circumstances where a 'blood flow risk factor' can be addressed in collaboration with the patients GP or physician. First, treat any underlying medical conditions.

- Prevent nocturnal hypotension: Patients with normal tension glaucoma may have a low night-time BP. In patients who show progression despite a low IOP, consider 24-hour ambulatory BP monitoring to look for a nocturnal dip (>20% decreased from baseline is considered to be a large dip). Nocturnal dipping may have a reversible cause (e.g. use of an oral hypotensive drug, particularly at night).
- If the patient has migraines or peripheral vasospasm (Raynauds disease), consider calcium channel blockers (may decrease vasospasm and increase capillary dilatation).
- Consider gingko biloba (but not if patient has a bleeding tendency or is on clopidogrel or warfarin). Should be stopped before surgery.

Surgical

- Laser trabeculoplasty (less likely to achieve a low enough IOP in normal tension glaucoma than in primary open-angle glaucoma)
- Trabeculectomy, probably combined with antimetabolite and adjustable releasable sutures to achieve low range pressures (there may be a very small 'target pressure' window)

Follow-up

- As for primary open-angle glaucoma

8.15 Steroid-induced glaucoma

Raised IOP and eventually glaucoma may occur following corticosteroid administration in so-called steroid responders. Steroid-induced glaucoma is most common with the use of topical steroids such as dexamethasone or prednisolone but can also occur with oral, intravenous, or inhaled steroids and with the use of over-the-counter steroid creams for conditions such as eczema (especially if used on the face). Ask every patient with suspected glaucoma about current and past steroid use.

With the increasing use of periocular and intravitreal steroids, steroid-induced glaucoma will probably increase. A DRCR.net study of intravitreal triamcinolone for diabetic macular oedema found that 20% of eyes treated with **1 mg triamcinolone** had significant elevation of IOP, and **6%** of eyes needed **IOP-lowering medication at 2 years**.

Pathophysiology

The condition is not completely understood, but steroids are known to have several effects on the TM, all of which contribute to an increased outflow resistance and hence increased IOP. Changes to the TM include an increase in glycosaminoglycans, decreased membrane permeability, reduced breakdown of extracellular and intracellular structural proteins, and reduced local phagocytic activity by cells that filter and clean debris from the aqueous humour. These effects usually take about 2–4 weeks to manifest, but sometimes the IOP rise is acute.

Several genes are responsible for TM changes; however, the most extensively studied is *MYOC*, which encodes the protein **myocillin** (also known as TIGR). This protein is induced in human cultured TM cells after they have been exposed to dexamethasone for 2–3 weeks, a timescale which appears to fit with that for steroid-induced IOP elevation.

Risk factors

* Past or current steroid use of any type: e.g. for asthma, skin disorders, allergies, autoimmune disease, uveitis
* Endogenous elevation of steroid (Cushings syndrome)
* Primary open-angle glaucoma or pigmentary glaucoma
* Family history of glaucoma
* Age over 40
* Diabetes mellitus
* High myopia
* Connective tissue disease

Prevalence of steroid response

Armaly et al. examined the IOP response to a 4-week course of topical dexamethasone. They reported **three groups** with steroid-induced raised IOP:

* **Five per cent** of the population showed a **high response**, with an IOP increase >15 mmHg.

* **One-third** of the population showed a **moderate response**, with an IOP increase of 6 to 15 mmHg.
* **Two-thirds** of the population are **non-responders**.

A response was more likely in primary open-angle glaucoma patients, with more than 90% showing a moderate or high response.

Clinical evaluation

History

* Use of topical, intraocular, periocular, inhaled, nasal, oral, intravenous, or dermatological steroid
* Presence of known risk factors

Examination

* Usually unremarkable; chronicity tends to prevent corneal oedema
* Stopping steroids may confirm the diagnosis

Management

* A baseline measurement of IOP should be taken prior to starting steroid therapy.
* Discontinue steroids if IOP rises.
* Use ocular steroids that are weaker or less pressure-inducing than the one(s) currently used by the patient, e.g. fluorometholone (FML™), rimexolone (Vexol™), or loteprednol (Lotemax™).
* IOP-lowering therapy as for primary open-angle glaucoma
* If induced by a depot steroid, surgical removal may be indicated.

Follow-up

* Careful monitoring of patients at risk is required because of the insidious nature of this condition.
* Topical therapy: measure IOP a few weeks after start of therapy then at regular intervals
* Intravitreal injections: patients must be monitored for up to a year after injection
* Patients on long-term systemic steroids should visit their own optometrist for regular IOP checks.

Prognosis

IOP usually returns to normal within 1 to 4 weeks of cessation of treatment; however, in about 3% of cases, IOP remains elevated.

8.16 Traumatic glaucoma

Blunt ocular trauma results in ocular indentation and a sudden expansion of tissues in the opposite plane. As the vitreous offers some resistance, most of the transmitted force is directed laterally along the iris towards the TM, the ciliary body, and the zonules. This force can tear these tissues in addition to tearing the associated blood vessels and thus causing a hyphaema.

Penetrating trauma may lead to direct damage to any of the ocular structures. Secondary open- or closed-angle glaucoma may occur via a variety of mechanisms and may develop years after the injury.

Pathophysiology

Early-onset traumatic raised IOP

One-third of eyes with hyphaema develop raised IOP. The presence of a hyphaema and low IOP should alert to the presence of a ruptured globe. IOP may be raised because of:

* TM obstruction with fresh red blood cells and fibrin
* Pupillary block due to blood clot
* Haemolytic glaucoma (due to breakdown products)
* Steroid-induced glaucoma due to treatment

Late traumatic glaucoma

* Ghost cell glaucoma: Ghost cells are rigid, haemolysed erythrocytes that may block the TM; typically results in elevation of IOP 1 to 3 months after a vitreous haemorrhage. Ghost cells are khaki or tan coloured.
* Haemolytic glaucoma: occurs when red blood cells and macrophages block the TM
* Haemosiderotic glaucoma: very rare glaucoma due to intraocular haemorrhage with iron deposition in the TM; may occur years after the injury
* PAS formation
* Posterior synechiae formation with iris bombé
* Angle recession: a tear in the ciliary body between longitudinal and circular muscle layers; an indicator of direct TM damage, not the direct cause of the raised IOP

Prevalence of raised IOP following trauma

The larger the hyphaema, the more likely the IOP to be raised; however, there are exceptions, and patients with sickle cell may have a small hyphaema but high IOP. Rebleeding increases the risk. Coles et al. found raised IOP in the following groups:

* **In 13.5%** of those with a hyphaema that was **up to half** the size of the anterior chamber
* **In 27%** of those with a hyphaema that was **greater than half** of the size of the anterior chamber
* **In 52%** of those with **total** hyphaema

Risk factors for raised IOP following trauma

* Young age
* Male gender (3 : 1)
* Black populations and Hispanics (related to the presence of sickle cell disease or trait):
  - Rigid cells more easily trapped in TM
  - Vascular occlusion and optic nerve damage at lower IOP
* Predisposition to primary open-angle glaucoma
* Antiplatelet or anticoagulant drugs (including alcohol)
* Large initial hyphaema

* Eight-ball hyphaema: total black hyphaema clot; black colour related to the ischaemic environment in the anterior chamber
* Delayed presentation
* Rebleed

Clinical evaluation

History

* Details of injury (exact time, type of injury)
* Family history of a bleeding disorder or sickle cell disease
* Drug history (aspirin, NSAIDs, anticoagulants, alcohol)
* Previous history of trauma (chronic glaucoma)
* May be asymptomatic or have decreased vision, photophobia, pain, nausea, or vomiting

Examination

* Subconjunctival haemorrhage
* Hyphaema (or microhyphaema)
* Anterior chamber may be deeper than that in the fellow eye
* Iris sphincter tear or iridodialysis
* Gonioscopy:
  - Angle recession (see 'Management of angle-recession glaucoma')
  - Cyclodialysis cleft (see 'Management of cyclodialysis cleft')
  - PAS
* Lens subluxation, cataract, or phacodonesis
* Vitreous haemorrhage
* Choroidal rupture
* Retinal dialysis or detachment; commotio retinae

Investigations

* B-scan ultrasonography (if no view of posterior pole)
* CT scan (if suspect orbital fracture or intraorbital foreign body)
* Haemoglobin electrophoresis (if suspected sickle cell disease)

Management of traumatic hyphaema

Complications of hyphaema include PAS and corneal blooding staining. Risk factors for corneal bloodstaining are high IOP, a large hyphaema, prolonged clot duration, rebleeding, and corneal endothelial cell dysfunction. An early sign is a straw-yellow discolouration of the corneal stroma. Patients with sickle cell disease or trait have a higher incidence of rebleeding and raised IOP. Sickled erythrocytes are less able to pass through the TM. Avoid drugs that promote acidosis and sickling (acetazolamide, mannitol), and consider surgical evacuation at an early stage.

General

* Protective eye shield
* Bed rest
* Elevation of head
* Anti-emetics
* Systemic BP control
* Avoid antiplatelet and anticoagulant drugs

325

Medical

* Topical cycloplegic and corticosteroid
* The use of cycloplegic agents is controversial; movement of the iris may theoretically predispose to dislodgement of the clot and a rebleed.
* Consider using an antifibrinolytic drug in high-risk patients.
* Topical aqueous suppressants
* Systemic carbonic anhydrase inhibitors and hyperosmotics (contraindicated in sickle cell)
* Avoid miotics.

Surgical

* Anterior chamber washout may be required if IOP is uncontrolled.
* Anterior vitrectomy
* Trabeculectomy with antimetabolites
* Surgery indicated with healthy optic nerve if:
  - IOP **>60 mmHg** for **2 days** (to prevent optic atrophy)
  - IOP **>35 mmHg** for **5 days** (to prevent corneal blood staining)
  - **Sickle cell** patients if IOP **>24 mmHg** for **24 hours**
  - Hyphaema fails to resolve to **<50% of the anterior chamber by Day 8** (to prevent PAS)

The aim of surgery is to reduce the risk of irreversible corneal bloodstaining. Earlier intervention is advised if the optic nerve is compromised or there is endothelial dysfunction.

Follow-up

* Daily monitoring is necessary until the hyphaema clears (rebleed risk highest at 2–5 days after injury).
* Perform gonioscopy 4–6 weeks after injury to look for angle recession.
* Glaucoma may develop weeks to years after the event; therefore, inform patients of glaucoma risk and ensure annual IOP checks with a local optometrist. If there is a large degree of angle recession, close follow-up may be appropriate.

Prognosis

* The prognosis is highly dependent upon the degree of initial damage and the amount of disruption to the TM.
* Rebleeds tend to result in more IOP-related problems than the initial bleed does.
* In high-risk patients with markedly uncontrolled IOP, the visual prognosis may be guarded.

Management of angle-recession glaucoma

Angle recession occurs when a cleft forms **between the circular and longitudinal muscles** of the ciliary body. It is visible as an irregular widening of the ciliary body band on gonioscopy (see Section 8.7; compare the two eyes).

Angle recession is common after a hyphaema; however, only **6% to 7%** of eyes with angle recession eventually develop glaucoma. The greater the circumference recessed, the greater the risk of glaucoma. Eyes with less than 180° of recession are unlikely to develop glaucoma. Patients that develop angle-recession glaucoma have a high incidence of primary open-angle glaucoma in the contralateral eye.

Treatment

* Aqueous suppressants
* Hyperosmotics
* Trabeculectomy (increased rate of failure compared to primary open-angle glaucoma)
* Argon laser trabeculoplasty (ALT) has limited success and may exacerbate angle damage.

Management of cyclodialysis cleft

A cyclodialysis cleft is a **focal detachment of the ciliary body from its insertion at the scleral spur**. The cleft creates an abnormal pathway for aqueous humour to drain into the suprachoroidal space, thus resulting in low IOP. A cyclodialysis cleft appears as a deep angle recess with a gap between the sclera and ciliary body but, because of very low IOP, it may be difficult to detect on gonioscopy. Anterior segment OCT or UBM may be useful.

Treatment

* Initially, conservative treatment should be tried.
* Atropine 1% three times a day (allows the ciliary muscle to relax and come into contact with the sclera)
* Avoiding topical steroids may facilitate this process.
* Closure may take 6 to 8 weeks.
* Cryotherapy (often successful in small clefts that have not closed with atropine)
* Surgical closure (direct cyclopexy (surgical fixation) may be needed for moderate to large clefts).

Follow-up

* Following successful closure, there may be a very high spike in IOP, requiring treatment with aqueous suppressants and hyperosmotics.

8.17 Inflammatory glaucomas

Inflammation within the anterior segment and which is caused by uveitic conditions can result in raised IOP (secondary OHT). If raised IOP causes glaucomatous optic nerve damage or visual field defects, it is known as inflammatory or uveitic glaucoma.

Pathophysiology

Ocular inflammation causes breakdown of the blood–aqueous barrier, resulting in the liberation of protein and inflammatory cells into the aqueous. Inflammatory glaucoma may occur with an open or closed angle and be secondary to a systemic or ocular uveitic condition. Patients may also develop glaucoma secondary to steroid use for treating ocular inflammation.

Secondary open-angle glaucoma

May be caused by:

- Obstruction of the TM by cellular debris, protein, or macrophages
- Trabeculitis: inflammation and oedema of the TM, leading to a reduction in intertrabecular pores, or the formation of precipitates which reduce aqueous outflow
- Prostaglandins: released in the inflammatory process; may contribute to raised IOP by compromising the blood–aqueous barrier)

Secondary angle-closure glaucoma

With pupil block

- Anterior segment inflammation may result in the formation of 360° posterior synechiae causing iris bombé.
- Pupil block may lead to shallowing of the anterior chamber, to appositional angle closure, and to the development of permanent PAS.

Without pupil block

- In chronic anterior uveitis, contraction of inflammatory debris within the angle can pull peripheral iris over the trabeculum, causing gradual but progressive angle closure.
- Angle neovascularization from ischaemic processes may also result in the formation of PAS.
- Ciliary body swelling due to intraocular inflammation may result in the forwards rotation of the ciliary body, also causing angle closure.

Prevalence

Ten per cent of uveitics have chronically elevated IOP with many having wide and episodic fluctuations. There may be long periods where the pressure is normal and therefore patients may progress with apparently normal IOP.

Risk factors

- Pre-existing primary open-angle glaucoma
- Being post surgery
- Being post trauma
- Drugs (1% of patients on prostaglandin analogues develop uveitis)

- Rigid AC- IOL (uveitis-glaucoma-hyphaema syndrome)
- Presence of uveitic conditions associated with secondary glaucoma:
  - Juvenile rheumatoid arthritis
  - Ankylosing spondylitis
  - Reiters syndrome
  - Psoriatic arthritis
  - Herpetic uveitis: herpes simplex virus (HSV), varicella-zoster virus, rubella, mumps
  - Lens-induced uveitis: phacoanaphylactic, phacolytic, lens particle
  - Sarcoidosis
  - Vogt–Koyanagi–Harada syndrome
  - Behçets disease
  - Sympathetic ophthalmia
  - Syphilis
  - Tuberculosis

Clinical evaluation

History

- Symptoms of acute uveitis
- Previous history of uveitic episodes
- Systemic history of associated disorder

Examination

- Signs of acute or chronic uveitis or of a previous uveitic episode
- The signs present will depend on the primary cause of the uveitis.
- Gonioscopy is most important, as it will elucidate the primary mechanism and thus the treatment.

Investigations

- Basic uveitic screen, including bloods and chest X-ray
- Additional tests as appropriate for the suspected uveitic process

Management

For all mechanisms, find and treat any cause for the uveitis.

Control intraocular inflammation

- Topical, periocular, or sub-Tenons corticosteroid
- Oral corticosteroid: up to 1 mg/kg per day, depending on severity
- Steroid-sparing agents: ciclosporin, methotrexate, azathioprine, mycophenolate
- Prevent and break synechiae, and relieve ciliary and iris sphincter spasm (regular cycloplegics).

Reduction of IOP

- Aqueous suppressants: beta blockers, alpha agonists, topical carbonic anhydrase inhibitors
- Systemic carbonic anhydrase inhibitors: acetazolamide
- Hyperosmotic agents: mannitol, glycerol
- Avoid prostaglandins because of the risk of inducing cystoid macular oedema.

For secondary angle closure with pupil block

* Laser iridotomy is less likely to be effective in uveitis than in other conditions, because of the presence of inflammatory membrane behind the pupil; thus surgical iridectomy may be a better option.

For secondary angle closure without pupil block

* Trabeculectomy (with adjunctive antimetabolites)
* Glaucoma drainage devices
* Avoid cyclodestructive procedures.

Follow-up

It is extremely important to monitor patients closely as there may be permanent compromise of aqueous outflow. IOP may increase after inflammation has resolved, owing to the recovery of ciliary body shutdown.

Prognosis

The prognosis depends on the extent of permanent damage to the drainage mechanism and the recurrent nature of the uveitic condition. The prognosis is worse than for primary open-angle glaucoma (higher pressures, more likely to need surgery than in primary open-angle glaucoma).

Specific inflammatory glaucoma syndromes

Posner–Schlossman syndrome

Also known as glaucomatocyclitic crisis, Posner–Schlossman syndrome is a condition in which there are recurrent episodes of unilateral mild anterior uveitis associated with marked elevation of IOP (40–80 mmHg) thought to be due to a trabeculitis. Patients tend to be asymptomatic. There is only mild inflammation visible in the anterior chamber.

Fuchs heterochromic iridocyclitis

Also known as Fuchs uveitis syndrome, Fuchs heterochromic iridocyclitis is a low-grade, chronic, anterior uveitis associated with secondary cataract and glaucoma. It is almost always unilateral. The classic presentation is of stellate keratic precipitates scattered throughout the endothelium. The iris may be hypochromic (see Figure 8.27). Posterior synechiae are not a feature. Initially, the rise in IOP is intermittent before becoming chronic. Approximately 30% of cases develop glaucoma. The condition may have an infective cause (rubella, cytomegalovirus).

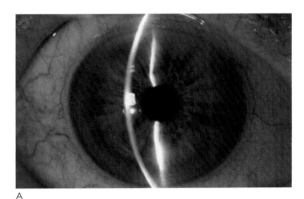

A

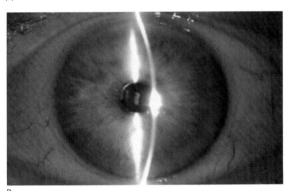

B

Fig 8.27 Colour anterior segment photographs of both eyes of the same patient, showing marked heterochromia

8.18 Pseudoexfoliative glaucoma

Pseudoexfoliation syndrome (PXF) is a systemic condition thought to be a generalized **basement membrane disorder**, which results in white powdery deposits within the anterior segment of the eye, with weakness of the zonules. PXF material impairs aqueous outflow, resulting in raised IOP and secondary open-angle glaucoma.

Pathophysiology

PXF material is composed of filamentous proteoglycosaminoglycans, which aggregate to form granular, electron-dense grey/white fibrillar deposits. It is thought to occur because of abnormal extracellular matrix material metabolism. PXF is associated with mutations in the **LOXL1 gene**, which encodes a protein involved in elastin cross-linking.

PXF material is believed to be produced by the lens epithelium, iris pigmented epithelium, and non-pigmented epithelium of the ciliary body. It is visible on the iris, the lens, the ciliary body, the TM, the anterior vitreous face, the corneal endothelium, and the conjunctiva and has been found in the endothelial cells of blood vessels within the eye and orbit. PXF material has also been identified in the skin, the myocardium, the lung, the liver, the gall bladder, the kidney, and the cerebral meninges; this observation suggests that PXF is an ocular manifestation of a systemic disorder.

Increased IOP is due to 'clogging' of the TM both by PXF material and by pigment released from the iris as a result of pathological friction against the rough deposits on the anterior lens capsule. In addition, trabecular endothelial dysfunction occurs, increasing outflow resistance in the TM and raising IOP. PXF differs from **true exfoliation syndrome**, which is often observed in glass-blowers and where **schisis of the anterior lens capsule** occurs.

Prevalence

* The prevalence of PXF varies by country. It is typically thought of as having a Scandinavian genetic origin (Iceland and Norway have 20%–25% prevalence), but it also occurs in populations as diverse as Japanese and Aboriginal Australians.
* Prevalence increases with age.
* The Framingham Eye Study found that:
  - The prevalence of PXF was **0.6%** of people aged **52–64 years**.
  - The prevalence of PXF was **5%** of people aged **75–85 years**.
* The risk of glaucoma is **five times greater** in PXF patients than in the normal population (Blue Mountains Eye Study).
* Overall, approximately 25% of open-angle glaucoma worldwide is pseudoexfoliation related.

Risk factors

* Age
* Female gender (3 : 2) for PXF (males = females for pseudoexfoliative glaucoma)
* Race (Scandinavian)

Clinical evaluation

History

* Rarely symptomatic
* May have foreign body sensation (possibly because of subclinical involvement of conjunctiva)
* History of complicated cataract surgery

Examination

* Signs may be unilateral or bilateral with asymmetry.
* Deposition of pseudoexfoliation flakes or of pigment within the anterior segment
* IOP spikes may occur following pharmacological mydriasis.
* Patchy increase in trabecular pigmentation
* Sampaolesi's line may be present (see Figure 8.18).
* Peripupillary iris transillumination defects
* Depigmented (moth-eaten) pupillary ruff (see Figure 8.28)
* Classic concentric (bullseye) deposition on anterior lens capsule (see Figure 8.29): (i) a central translucent zone, (ii) a clear zone (pseudoexfoliation rubbed off by pupil movement), and (iii) a peripheral granular zone
* Nuclear sclerotic cataract, lens subluxation, phacodonesis

Management

Medical therapy is as for primary open-angle glaucoma, although pseudoexfoliative glaucoma is more resistant than primary open-angle glaucoma. Laser trabeculoplasty may be more effective in pseudoexfoliative glaucoma than in primary open-angle glaucoma because of the presence of trabecular hyperpigmentation, which results in an increased uptake of laser energy. Trabeculectomy in pseudoexfoliative glaucoma has the same success rate as in primary open-angle glaucoma. However, PXF causes challenges for cataract surgery, including small pupils, zonular instability, an increased risk of vitreous loss, and post-operative IOP elevation.

Follow-up

Pseudoexfoliative glaucoma tends to progress more rapidly than primary open-angle glaucoma does, so needs watching closely. Patients with PXF but not glaucoma should have at least annual glaucoma screening.

Prognosis

Pseudoexfoliative glaucoma has a poorer prognosis than primary open-angle glaucoma does because of the high IOP present at the time of diagnosis, significant diurnal IOP fluctuation, and often a rapid progression of glaucomatous damage.

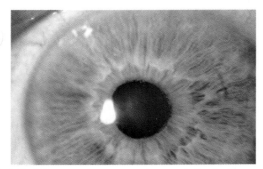

Fig 8.28 Colour anterior segment photograph showing fine pseudoexfoliative material at the pupil margin

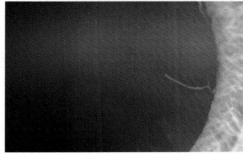

Fig 8.29 Colour anterior segment photograph showing the pseudoexfoliative material on the anterior surface of the lens

8.19 Pigmentary glaucoma

Pigment dispersion syndrome (PDS) is a bilateral condition characterized by dislodgement of pigment from the posterior iris pigment epithelium, resulting in mid-peripheral transillumination defects. The pigment particles are carried by aqueous convection currents and deposited on structures throughout the anterior segment. Obstruction of the TM by pigment can result in increased IOP (pigmentary OHT) and a secondary open-angle glaucoma known as pigmentary glaucoma.

Pathophysiology

PDS may be inherited as an autosomal dominant trait with variable penetrance. The anterior chamber is deep, and the iris appears to bow posteriorly in a concave configuration. **Posterior bowing** is due to **reverse pupil block** caused by a relative increase in pressure in the anterior chamber. There is friction between the posterior pigment layer of the iris and the underlying lens zonules. The friction causes pigment release into the anterior chamber; the released pigment leads to obstruction of the intertrabecular spaces, reduced aqueous outflow facility, and permanent damage to the TM via damage to phagocytic trabeculocytes though pigment overload, denudation, collapse, and sclerosis. Exercise, mydriasis, and accommodation can increase posterior iris concavity, leading to additional irido-zonular contact and pigment dispersion. In some patients, strenuous exercise leads to a 'pigment storm' and high IOP spikes.

Prevalence

Prevalence of PDS is approximately 2.5%. Estimates for conversion to pigmentary glaucoma are **5.0%–10.0%** at **5 years, 15.0%** at **15 years,** and **35.0%** at **35 years**. Pigmentary glaucoma accounts for 1.0%–1.5% of all glaucoma. Risk factors for conversion include male gender, myopia, the presence of a Krukenberg spindle, and, most importantly, a high initial IOP.

Risk factors

* Age 20–45 years; later in females
* Male gender: PDS affects men and women equally but men are more likely to develop pigmentary glaucoma
* Race: Caucasian
* Myopia

Clinical evaluation

History

* Usually asymptomatic
* May have blurred vision, haloes, or headache during 'pigment storm', e.g. after exercise

Examination

* Krukenberg spindle: vertical deposition of pigment on and within the corneal endothelial cells
* Endotheliopathy: endothelial cells in PDS show pleomorphism and polymegathism
* Deep anterior chamber
* Pigment showers: small pigment specks floating within the anterior chamber
* Iris transillumination defects: mid-peripheral radial spokes, present in 86% of cases, retroilluminate (see Figure 8.30)

* Pigment on anterior surface of iris (preferentially within furrows), possibly causing heterochromia
* Pigment on anterior and posterior lens surfaces
* Glaucomatous optic atrophy
* Lattice degeneration: present in up to one-third of cases; also higher incidence of retinal detachment than in the general population.

Gonioscopy

* Wide-open angle
* Concavity of iris near insertion; backwards bowing of the iris
* Diffuse trabecular hyperpigmentation; the degree of pigmentation correlates with severity
* A pigmented Schwalbes line creates a dark line that is similar to Sampaolesi's line in PXF.

Differential diagnosis

* Primary open-angle glaucoma with hyperpigmented trabeculum
* Pseudoexfoliative glaucoma
* Pseudophakic pigmentary glaucoma: rubbing of haptics/optics against the posterior iris
* Uveitis
* Melanoma
* Iris and ciliary body cysts
* Trauma

Management

* Medical therapy as for primary open-angle glaucoma
* Pilocarpine should be considered, as it can increase aqueous outflow, reverse posterior iris bowing, and prevent pupil dilation; however, it is poorly tolerated.
* Trabeculectomy: success rate similar to primary open-angle glaucoma
* Prophylactic Laser PI can theoretically be used to relieve reverse pupil block in PDS but the long-term benefits in the prevention of glaucoma are not proven and the treatment is controversial. Laser PI is only likely to succeed in the active stages of the disease and in the presence of observable posterior iris bowing. Laser treatment also carries the risk of further TM damage due to pigment release.

Follow-up

Patients with PDS and a normal IOP with no signs of glaucoma need regular IOP checks only, which can be done by their own optometrist; otherwise, follow-up is as for primary open-angle glaucoma.

Prognosis

Long-term prognosis is good. Pigment dispersion tends to decrease with age because of miosis and gradual lens enlargement, which increases relative pupil block, thus lifting the peripheral iris away from the zonules.

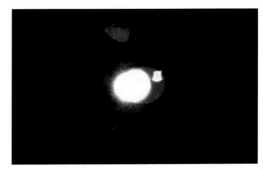

Fig 8.30 Colour anterior segment photograph showing typical slit-like iris transillumination defects
The patient has also had a trabeculectomy and has a superior peripheral iridectomy

8.20 Neovascular glaucoma

Neovascularization of the iris (NVI, or rubeosis iridis) can be initiated by any process causing widespread posterior segment hypoxia with subsequent raised levels of vascular endothelial growth factor (VEGF). If neovascularization of the angle occurs and treatment is not initiated in the early stages, synechial angle closure and glaucoma will result.

Pathophysiology

In an attempt to revascularize, the ischaemic retina produces vasoproliferative factors (e.g. VEGF), which diffuse throughout the eye, including into the anterior segment. Vasoproliferative factors stimulate angiogenesis. Neovascularization usually starts with endothelial budding from capillaries at the pupil margin (although it can also start within the angle). The new vessels then grow in an irregular pattern over the surface of the iris towards the angle (see Figure 8.31).

Neovascular tissue invading the angle (see Figure 8.32) arborizes with proliferating connective tissue from myofibroblasts to form a fibrovascular membrane. This membrane may block the TM, thus causing a rise in IOP. The condition is reversible initially; however, if untreated, the myofibroblasts, which have smooth muscle characteristics, will contract and pull peripheral iris over the TM in a zip-like manner, resulting in PAS.

Prevalence

* Ischaemic CRVO: 16%–60% of patients develop neovascular glaucoma (depending on the extent of capillary non-perfusion).
* Proliferative diabetic retinopathy: approximately 20% of type 1 diabetes mellitus patients with proliferative diabetic retinopathy eventually develop neovascular glaucoma.
* CRAO: approximately 18%

Risk factors

* Ischaemic CRVO (most common cause of unilateral neovascular glaucoma):
  — Age
  — Systemic hypertension
  — OHT/ primary open-angle glaucoma
  — Hypercoagulable state
  — Vasculitis
  — Drugs: diuretics
  — Retrobulbar external compression: e.g. from thyroid eye disease, orbital tumour
* Diabetes mellitus: the most common cause of bilateral neovascular glaucoma
* Ocular ischaemic syndrome; e.g. from carotid artery disease
* BRVO
* CRAO/BRAO
* Chronic retinal detachment
* Sickle cell retinopathy
* Ocular neoplasm
* Chronic uveitis
* Endophthalmitis
* Sympathetic ophthalmia
* Radiation retinopathy

Clinical evaluation

History
* Asymptomatic in early stages
* Ocular pain or photophobia
* Red eye
* Reduced vision

Examination
* Congestion of globe
* Corneal oedema
* Raised IOP
* Aqueous flare
* Possible hyphaema
* Rubeosis iridis: check the angle gonioscopically prior to dilation
* Synechial angle closure
* Distorted pupil with ectropion uveae

Differential diagnosis
* Angle-closure glaucoma
* Post-vitrectomy inflammation
* Uveitis: radial engorged vessels
* Intraocular tumours

Management

* Prevention is the best treatment.
* PRP: should be done as soon as neovascularization is detected, not deferred to a routine laser list
* Intravitreal anti-VEGF agents: in conjunction with PRP may prevent glaucoma occurring in eyes with NVI; not effective alone at controlling IOP once PAS and neovascular glaucoma are established; also show promise as an adjunct to glaucoma surgery because of their effects on wound healing
* Aqueous suppressants
* Atropine eye drops, 1%, twice a day: increases uveoscleral outflow
* Topical corticosteroid: controls congestion and inflammation
* Trabeculectomy: with antimetabolites combined with an intravitreal anti-VEGF drug; guarded prognosis
* Glaucoma drainage device
* Cyclodestructive procedure: cyclodiode laser
* Enucleation

Follow-up

* Close follow-up is crucial, as neovascular glaucoma can be reversible in early stages.
* Fill-in PRP is applied as required.
* An ischaemic CRVO can cause neovascular glaucoma within 3 months (so-called 90-day glaucoma) or up to 2 years later.

Prognosis

* Excellent if condition is fully treated in early stages
* Extremely poor once synechial angle closure has occurred

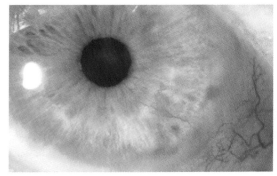

Fig 8.31 Neovascularization of the iris

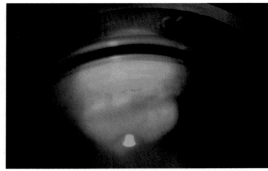

Fig 8.32 Gonioscopic view of new vessels within the angle

8.21 Aqueous misdirection

Aqueous misdirection (malignant glaucoma), also known as ciliary block glaucoma, is a type of secondary angle-closure glaucoma. Aqueous misdirection usually follows penetrating surgery in eyes that are anatomically predisposed, particularly eyes with a short axial length.

Pathophysiology

Ocular surgery causes a not fully understood initiating event (postulated to be sudden anterior chamber decompression) that changes the direction of aqueous humour flow. UBM has shown the ciliary body to be anteriorly rotated so that it causes the ciliary processes and lens equator to come into contact (see Figure 8.33). The anterior vitreous face may also contact the iris and ciliary processes. There may be an underlying shallow peripheral ciliochoroidal effusion.

These changes may prevent the aqueous humour from flowing forwards through the pupil into the anterior chamber. Instead, the aqueous humour may flow into the vitreous, leading to an increase in vitreous volume, increased posterior segment pressure, forwards displacement of the lens–iris diaphragm, and shallowing of the anterior chamber. In contrast to the case with pupil block, there is **shallowing both centrally and peripherally**.

Aqueous misdirection may present days, months, or years after surgery. IOP may be normal or high and may be associated with secondary angle closure. Aqueous misdirection has been reported after trabeculectomy, cataract surgery, laser iridotomy, laser suture lysis, scleral buckling, and anterior segment laser procedures; it has also been reported to occur spontaneously.

Differential diagnosis

* Choroidal effusions: B-scan ultrasonography should be performed
* Suprachoroidal haemorrhage: may be associated with sudden pain
* Pupil block: anterior chamber remains deep centrally
* Overfiltration and wound leak : anterior chamber may be shallow but the IOP will be low

Risk factors

* Choroidal effusions
* Filtration surgery: particularly for PACG
* Cataract surgery
* Nd:YAG capsulotomy or laser iridotomy
* Nanophthalmos: small globe with normal lens size
* Increased age or cataract: increased lens size
* Trauma or pseudoexfoliation: decreased anterior–posterior lens position due to weak or ruptured zonules

* Inflammation or vascular engorgement: swelling of the ciliary body
* Chronic miotic use

Clinical evaluation

History
* Recent eye surgery: can be up to months post-operatively
* Blurred vision
* Usually no pain

Examination
* Shallow anterior chamber: central and peripheral
* No iris bombé
* High IOP, or relative increase after glaucoma surgery
* Corneal oedema, if the IOP is high or there is lens–endothelial contact

Investigations
* UBM

Management

Medical (50% respond)
* Topical cycloplegics/mydriatics (atropine 1% four times a day): paralyses the ciliary muscles, tightens the zonules, and helps pull the lens posteriorly
* Topical aqueous suppressants: reduce the amount of aqueous humour entering the vitreous
* Oral or systemic hyperosmotic agents
* Topical corticosteroids
* Discontinue miotics

Surgical
* Cyclodiode laser: 10–15 shots at 1500 mW for 1500 milliseconds in 1 quadrant
* Decompartmentalize the eye: aim to create communication between the anterior and posterior segments to allow the free movement of aqueous humour
* Pseudophakic eye:
  – Nd:YAG laser to the peripheral anterior hyaloid face through a pre-existing peripheral iridectomy
  – Surgical decompartmentalization with pars plana vitrectomy and removal of anterior hyaloid as far peripherally as possible
* Phakic eye:
  – Surgical decompartmentalization with a lens extraction–posterior capsulectomy–vitrectomy procedure

1 Normal direction of aqueous flow

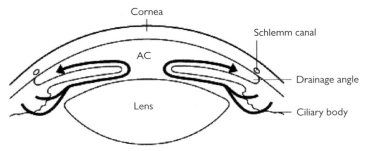

2 Aqueous misdirection

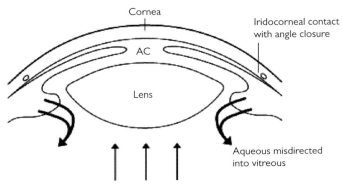

Increased posterior segment pressure causes
anterior movement of the lens/iris diaphragm

Key features:

Shallow AC (central and peripheral)
No iris bombé
High IOP

Fig 8.33 Diagram showing the proposed mechanism of malignant glaucoma

8.22 Iridocorneal endothelial syndrome and iridocorneal dysgenesis

Iridocorneal endothelial syndrome

Iridocorneal endothelial syndrome is an acquired condition consisting of three separate entities with overlapping features:

1. Essential iris atrophy
2. Chandlers syndrome
3. Cogan–Reese syndrome

These entities have in common an abnormal corneal endothelial cell layer, which forms a membrane over the angle structures and iris, initially causing secondary open-angle glaucoma but eventually leading to angle closure because of iridocorneal adhesions and contraction of the membrane.

Pathophysiology

Endothelial cells in iridocorneal endothelial syndrome have been found to be morphologically similar to epithelial cells; this observation suggests that the cells are derived from an embryological ectopia or a metaplastic process. HSV has been implicated in the aetiology of this condition, as HSV DNA has been found in a large number of iridocorneal endothelial syndrome corneal specimens by PCR; however, a definite link has not been proven. The pathological membrane complex migrates over the drainage angle, causing obstruction and secondary angle closure with formation of PAS. Tractional forces may cause distortion of the iris in opposing quadrants. Corneal opacity/oedema is also a feature because of increased IOP and reduced endothelial cell count.

Prevalence

* Rare, but exact incidence is not known
* Approximately **50%** of iridocorneal endothelial syndrome patients **develop glaucoma**.
* Patients with the Cogan–Reece variant are at greatest risk of developing raised IOP.

Risk factors

* Age: 20–50 years
* Sex: female
* History of HSV
* Race: Caucasian

Clinical evaluation

History

* Asymptomatic in early stages; often an incidental finding
* Later on:
  - Decreased vision
  - Ocular pain
  - Red eye
  - Iris abnormalities

Examination

The three entities are based on signs present in early stages of the disease. During the later stages, they can be indistinguishable. Signs are **always unilateral**. There are no non-ocular features. Corneal specular microscopy is useful and shows pleomorphic endothelial cells with intracellular dark spots.

* Common signs:
  - Asymptomatic in early stages; often an incidental finding
  - Corectopia: distortion of pupil (see Figure 8.34)
  - Pseudopolycoria: 'extra' pupils
  - Iris atrophy: moth-eaten iris; of varying severity
  - 'Hammered silver' appearance to endothelium
  - Broad-based PAS

Chandlers syndrome (most common)

* Characterized by severe corneal changes, blurred vision, and haloes
* Normal or mild iris changes; no iris holes

Progressive iris atrophy

* Characterized by severe iris changes, corectopia, pseudopolycoria, atrophy, and ectropion uveae

Cogan–Reese (iris naevus) syndrome

* Characterized by the presence of pigmented nodules in the iris stroma
* A sheet of membrane-like material covers the iris; naevi form where the iris tissue protrudes through.
* The iris has a flattened appearance.

Management

* Topical therapy is often ineffective
* Hypertonic saline for corneal oedema
* Trabeculectomy plus antimetabolites: the filtration site should be in an area free of membrane; there is a high failure rate, owing to membrane growing over the sclerostomy, and high post-operative inflammation
* Glaucoma drainage devices (also high failure rate)
* Cyclodestructive therapy
* Penetrating keratoplasty for corneal changes
* Laser trabeculoplasty is not recommended, as it increases the formation of PAS.

Follow-up

* To assess corneal clarity and development of glaucoma

Prognosis

* Poor, owing to resistance to therapy

Axenfeld–Riegers syndrome

Pathophysiology

* Represents a spectrum of anterior segment maldevelopment with or without iris and systemic abnormalities
* Unlike iridocorneal endothelial syndrome, Axenfeld–Riegers syndrome is present at birth (see also Section 9.26).
* **Axenfeld anomaly:** a prominent anteriorly displaced Schwalbes line (posterior embryotoxon) is present with associated iridocorneal adhesions. The posterior embryotoxon appears as a white line in the peripheral cornea (partial or 360°) visible on slit lamp examination in most, or by gonioscopy. NB: Posterior embryotoxon is seen in 15% of normal eyes and is not associated with glaucoma if present in isolation.
* **Reiger anomaly:** Axenfeld anomaly plus iris changes (see *Chapter 9*, Figure 9.36)

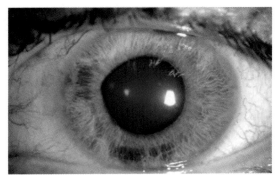

Fig 8.34 Mild corectopia in iridocorneal endothelial syndrome

- **Reiger syndrome:** Reiger anomaly with non-ocular features
- **Genetics:** typically autosomal dominant, with associated mutations described in the *PITX2* gene (Chromosome 4q25), the *FOXC1* gene (Chromosome 6p25), and on Chromosome 13q

Clinical features

Corneal
- The hallmark is a posterior embryotoxon.
- The central cornea is typically normal.

Angle abnormalities
- Iris processes/bands/sheets extend across the angle to the TM or even up to the posterior embryotoxon.
- High insertion of the iris can obscure the scleral spur.

Iris abnormalities
- May be absent
- Include iris hypoplasia with easily visible iris sphincter, corectopia (displaced pupil), and polycoria (iris holes)

Glaucoma
- There is a **50% risk of raised IOP**; glaucoma usually develops in the second or third decade (very rarely in infancy).
- Patients with high iris insertion are more prone to developing glaucoma.

Non-ocular features
- **Facial:** maxillary hypoplasia, broad nasal bridge, telecanthus, prominent lower lip, micro/hypodontia
- **CNS:** mental retardation, empty sella syndrome
- **Genital:** hypospadias
- **Endocrine:** growth hormone deficiency

Treatment

- Consider physician referral.
- Angle surgery in children can be considered.
- Treat glaucoma as in primary open-angle glaucoma: medically initially then surgery (trabeculectomy/glaucoma drainage devices).
- Laser trabeculoplasty is not possible/is contraindicated, owing to angle abnormalities.

8.23 Ocular hypotensive agents I

Ocular hypotensive agents lower IOP by increasing aqueous humour outflow (e.g. prostaglandin analogues) and/or suppressing aqueous humour production (e.g. carbonic anhydrase inhibitors).

Prostaglandin analogues

Mechanism of action
Agonists of prostaglandin F2 alpha increase outflow mainly through the uveoscleral pathway. This effect is thought to be due to the activation of matrix metalloproteinases and consequent increase in the turnover of the extracellular matrix. IOP reduction in an excess of 30% is often achieved.

Side effects
Local

* Stinging
* Tearing
* Hyperaemia
* Darkening of the iris
* Thicker and longer lashes
* Cystoid macular oedema
* Anterior uveitis

Systemic

* Upper respiratory tract infection
* Backache
* Chest pain
* Myalgia
* Exacerbation of angina, and new shortness of breath

Contraindications

* Pregnancy
* Inflammatory conditions, including post-surgical (aphakic and pseudophakic with posterior capsule breaks at greatest risk)

Preparations

* Latanoprost (Xalatan): available as 0.005%
* Travoprost (Travatan): available as 0.004%
* Bimatoprost (Lumigan): available as 0.03% and 0.01%
* Tafluprost (Saflutan): available as 0.0015% (preservative free)
* Generally used as a first-line therapy, owing to proven efficacy and tolerability
* All have a duration of action of 24 hours.
* All have once-daily night-time dosing.

Beta blockers

Mechanism of action
Beta adrenergic antagonists block the beta receptors of the ciliary body, thus decreasing aqueous humour production. They can be non-selective, acting on both beta 1 receptors and beta 2 receptors, or cardioselective and thus more potent at beta 1 receptors. Beta blockers are less effective at reducing the nocturnal diurnal IOP peak than other agents are.

Side effects

* Most occur within the first week.

Local

* Stinging
* Dry eye
* Hyperaemia

Systemic

* Bradycardia or heart block
* Bronchospasm
* Fatigue
* Mood change
* Impotence

Contraindications

* Asthma, chronic obstructive pulmonary disease, bradycardia (resting heart rate of less than 60 bpm), heart block, congestive cardiac failure
* Patients already on systemic beta blockade or calcium channel blockers should be monitored for potential additive toxicity.

Preparations
Timolol maleate (Timoptol)

* Non-selective
* The majority of patients achieve 20% IOP reduction but 10% of the population are unresponsive.
* Effectiveness can diminish in the first 2 weeks (short-term escape).
* Further diminishing efficacy may occur within 3 months (long-term drift).
* Onset of action within 30 minutes; peak at 2 hours.
* Available as 0.25% and 0.5% (similar efficacy; therefore, 0.25% should be first choice)
* Twice-daily dosing

Timolol LA (0.25% or 0.5%)

* Long-acting variant
* Changes from liquid to gel-like state when instilled
* Once-daily dosing
* Transient blurring for up to 5 minutes often occurs

Levobunolol (Betagan; 0.25% or 0.5%)

* Non-selective
* Onset of action within 1 hour; peak at 2–6 hours

Betaxolol (Betoptic; 0.5%)

* Selective beta 1 blocker
* Use with great care in patients with respiratory conditions.
* Cardiac patients still contraindicated.
* Onset of action within 30 minutes; peak at 2 hours; duration up to 12 hours
* Twice-daily dosing

Alpha agonists

Mechanism of action
Alpha 2 adrenergic agonists act on alpha receptors in the ciliary body to inhibit aqueous secretion.

Side effects

Local

- Irritation
- Allergy
- Dry eye

Systemic

- Dry mouth
- Hypotension
- Sedation

Contraindications

- Monoamine oxidase inhibitor use
- Brimonidine is contraindicated in children less than 7, as it crosses the blood–brain barrier and causes respiratory depression.

Preparations

Brimonidine (Alphagan; 0.2%)

- Also increases uveoscleral outflow
- Animal studies suggest that there may be neuroprotective properties.
- Peak effect at 2 hours; duration of action, 12 hours
- Twice-daily dosing
- Allergy occurs frequently with long-term therapy, presenting sometimes months later.

Apraclonidine (Iopidine)

- Onset of action within 1 hour; duration of at least 2 hours
- Available as 0.5% (27% IOP reduction) or 1% (37% IOP reduction)
- Causes allergic conjunctivitis in 9% within 3 months and in 50% after long-term treatment
- Exhibits tachyphylaxis (decreased therapeutic response following initial doses)
- Its main use is for the prevention of IOP spikes in the short term, e.g. after anterior segment laser and in angle-closure glaucoma patients.
- Also plays a role in those already on maximal medical therapy who are unsuitable for surgery

Cholinergic agents

Mechanism of action

Cholinergics act on muscarinic receptors of the ciliary muscle, causing the ciliary muscle to contract and move anteriorly. The anterior tendons of the ciliary muscle insert into the TM; therefore, contraction causes the TM to spread, Schlemms canal to dilate, and outflow resistance to decrease.

Side effects

Local

- Brow ache
- Accommodative spasm
- Variable myopia
- Retinal tear/detachment
- Decreased peripheral and night vision

Systemic

- Gastrointestinal upset
- Abdominal cramping

- Salivation
- Potential heart block

Contraindications

- Peripheral retinal pathology
- Central media opacity
- Young age: increased myopic effect
- Uveitic patients
- Less effective in patients with damaged TMs
- Chronic use can result in permanent miosis: problems with dilated fundoscopy.

Preparations

Pilocarpine

- Onset of action within 20 minutes; peak at 2 hours; duration up to 6 hours
- Available as 0.5%, 1%, 2%, 3%, and 4%
- Administered four times a day; short duration of action
- Dosage increased in stepwise increments
- Maximum concentrations usually 2% for light irises, 4% for brown/dark irises

Topical carbonic anhydrase inhibitors

Mechanism of action

- Inhibition of the enzyme carbonic anhydrase decreases aqueous humour production in the ciliary body.
- Achieves a 20% reduction in IOP

Side effects

Local

- Mild hyperaemia
- Stinging
- Bitter taste

Systemic

- Diuresis
- Fatigue
- Gastrointestinal upset
- Stevens–Johnson syndrome
- Aplastic anaemia

Contraindications

- Sulphonamide sensitivity
- Use with caution in corneal decompensation (carbonic anhydrase is an important enzyme in the corneal endothelial pump).

Preparations

Dorzolamide (Trusopt)

- Available as 2%
- Dose three times a day alone, or twice a day with concurrent beta blocker use.

Brinzolamide (Azopt)

- Available as 1%
- Twice-daily dosing
- The suspension form allows the drug to be buffered at physiological pH (so that it is therefore more comfortable and with fewer allergic reactions, compared to other preparations).

341

Systemic carbonic anhydrase inhibitors

Mechanism of action

* As for topical treatment
* Oral or intravenous administration will also cause dehydration of the vitreous.

Side effects

* As for topical carbonic anhydrase inhibitors
* Additional systemic concerns: hypokalaemia, renal stones, paraesthesia (tingling of hands and feet), nausea, cramps, malaise, depression, impotence

Contraindications

* Sulphonamide sensitivity
* Hyponatraemia
* Hypokalaemia
* Renal stones
* Use of thiazide diuretics or digitalis
* Pregnancy

Preparations

Acetazolamide (Diamox)

* IOP reduction up to 35%
* Available as 125 mg or 250 mg tablets or 250 mg slow-release capsules orally, or as 500 mg vials for use intravenously
* Dosing four times a day for tablets, twice a day for slow-release capsules, or stat dosing as required for intravenous use
* Maximum dosage: 1000 mg in 24 hours

Hyperosmotic agents

Mechanism of action

* Dehydrates the vitreous and reduces intraocular volume by increasing plasma osmolality, thereby drawing fluid into the intravascular space

Side effects

* Diuresis, cardiac failure, urinary retention (in men), backache, headache, myocardial infarction, confusion
* Also vomiting, when glycerine is used

Contraindications

* Congestive cardiac failure, pre-existing dehydration
* Also watch for diabetic ketoacidosis with glycerine (broken down to glucose).
* Caution in elderly patients and those with renal disease
* Only used when rapid reduction is required when IOP is dangerously high

Preparations

Glycerine

* Oral agent in 50% solution
* Needs rapid ingestion to maximally change osmolality
* Serve mixed with orange juice or over ice to reduce vomiting

Mannitol

* Drug of choice, as no penetration into vitreous cavity
* Dosage 1–2 g/kg of 20% solution given intravenously over 45 minutes

Fixed dose combinations

The fact that only two drops of the fixed dose combinations need to be used decreases the preservative load and may improve compliance. A disadvantage is that all the fixed dose combinations include beta blockers, which may be contraindicated; also, the fixed dose combinations contain the highest available concentration of the drugs (e.g. timolol 0.5%). These agents should not be used as first-line therapy and should only be utilized when the efficacy and tolerability of the individual components have been established.

Preparations

Cosopt

* A combination of 0.5% timolol and 2% dorzolamide
* Twice-daily dosing

Combigan

* A combination of 0.5% timolol and 0.2% brimonidine
* Twice-daily dosing

Xalacom/DuoTrav/GanFort

* A combination of 0.5% timolol and Xalatan/Travatan/Lumigan, respectively
* Once-daily dosing

Use of ocular hypotensive agents during pregnancy and lactation

Discuss plans for management of glaucoma during pregnancy in all women of childbearing age. The risks of medication to the foetus must be balanced against the risk of visual loss to the mother. Ideally, all glaucoma medications should be avoided, particularly prior to conception and during the first trimester. IOP tends to decrease during pregnancy.

The FDA categorizes medication safety during pregnancy into Categories A to D:

* **Category A:** Safety established using human studies
  - No glaucoma medications are in this category
* **Category B:** Presumed safe based on animal studies
  - Brimonidine (although it does cross the placenta and may cause respiratory depression; contraindicated in children <7 years old)
* **Category C:** Uncertain safety. No human studies but animal studies show adverse effect.
  - Beta blockers: fetal bradycardia
  - Carbonic anhydrase inhibitors: reports of forelimb deformities with oral use in animals
  - Prostaglandin analogues: risk of premature labour
* **Category D:** Unsafe

If medications cannot be stopped, beta blockers are probably the best option in early pregnancy but consider stopping prior to birth. Advice should be given on punctal occlusion and consider using the once-daily gel form. Prostaglandin analogues should be avoided at all stages.

Beta blockers are not recommended during lactation, but topical carbonic anhydrase inhibitors and prostaglandin analogues are reasonable options.

Consult the latest safety information before prescribing in pregnancy.

8.25 Laser therapy for glaucoma

Argon Laser Trabeculoplasty (ALT)

ALT involves the application of discrete laser burns to the TM (see Figure 8.35). The Glaucoma Laser Trial (1990) found ALT to be as effective as timolol for the initial treatment of glaucoma; however, as patients in that trial had used ALT in one eye and timolol in the other, a drug crossover effect could have biased results. The effectiveness of ALT also decreases with time. In eyes with initial success (at least a 20% reduction in IOP), approximately 19% fail after 1 year and an additional 10% fail each year thereafter, reaching a **65% failure rate at 5 years**. With the introduction of better medications, ALT is not a first-line treatment.

Mode of action

There are two main theories concerning the mode of action of ALT:

1. **Mechanical theory:** coagulative damage to the TM causes collagen shrinkage and scarring, thus exerting traction on the adjacent TM and opening intertrabecular spaces.
2. **Cellular theory:** migration of macrophages into the TM occurs in response to coagulative damage. Macrophages phagocytose any debris present, thus improving aqueous outflow.

Indications

* Primary open-angle glaucoma, pigmentary glaucoma, and pseudoexfoliative glaucoma
* Ineffective in paediatric glaucoma and secondary glaucoma
* Not suitable if angle abnormalities are present

Laser settings

* Use a 50 μm spot with a 0.1-second duration at 300–850 mW.
* Start with low power setting and increase if reaction is inadequate; less power is required if the pigment is heavy than if otherwise.

Method

* Follow laser safety protocols.
* Gain patient consent (including advising on failure and complications).
* Instil topical anaesthetic and apraclonidine 1% (to prevent IOP spike).
* Insert Latina goniolens at the 12 o'clock position (as the inferior angle is easiest to visualize).
* Identify the anterior border of the pigmented TM as the site to treat.
* Focus the aiming beam perpendicular to the TM (round spot with a clear edge).
* Look for blanching or small bubbles whilst treating.
* Place 50 equally spaced shots over 180° (or entire circumference with 100 burns).
* Instil additional apraclonidine 1%.

Post-procedure guidelines

* Check for IOP spike after 1 hour.
* Prescribe topical steroid four times a day for 1 week and continue usual glaucoma medication.
* Arrange follow-up in 4–6 weeks.

* If IOP reduction is inadequate after 180° treatment, consider ALT for the remaining superior 180°.
* Do not treat the same area twice.

Complications

* PAS: if burns applied too posteriorly or energy too high
* Bleeding: if blood vessels inadvertently treated (apply pressure with goniolens)
* IOP spike
* Anterior uveitis

Selective Laser Trabeculoplasty (SLT)

SLT is a newer procedure, which is employed in a similar manner as ALT but uses a Q-switched, frequency-doubled Nd:YAG laser with a frequency of 532 nm (see Figure 8.36). Pulse duration of 3 nanoseconds is used (ALT is 0.1 seconds). The energy used in SLT is several thousand times lower than that used in ALT.

In theory, SLT selectively targets pigmented TM cells and spares adjacent tissue from collateral thermal damage. The exact mechanism of action is unknown but it appears to be cellular rather than mechanical.

Indications

* Indications are similar to those for ALT.

Laser settings

* Fixed spot size, 3-nanosecond duration; start at 0.4 mJ (high pigment) to 0.8 mJ (low pigment)
* Adjust according to response.

Method

* Follow laser safety protocols.
* Gain patient consent (including advising on failure and complications).
* Instil topical anaesthetic and apraclonidine 1% (to prevent IOP spike).
* Insert Latina goniolens (or equivalent with zero magnification).
* Start with low power setting and increase if reaction is inadequate.
* Look for fine champagne bubbles; reduce energy level to 0.1 mJ below bubble formation threshold.
* Treat 180° or 360° with 50 or 100 shots, respectively.
* Instil additional apraclonidine 1%.

Post-procedure guidelines

* Topical NSAIDs (not steroids) four times a day for 4 days post-treatment
* Arrange follow-up in 2–6 weeks.
  Success is more likely with 360° of treatment (approximately 80% of cases achieve a 20% reduction in IOP, and 60% achieve a 30% reduction in IOP when SLT is used as the initial treatment). A response may take 4 to 6 weeks to be maximal. As with ALT, the effects of SLT wear off over time; however, unlike ALT, SLT can be repeated. If there has been no IOP-lowering effect with the first treatment, retreatment is not recommended.

Complications

* Rare; but anterior chamber inflammation and IOP spike may occur

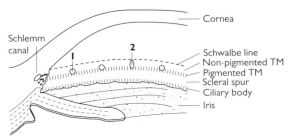

Fig 8.35 Technique of ALT

The laser is aimed at the junction of pigmented and non-pigmented TM. (1) The appearance of evenly spaced, round spots of blanching with clear edges with or without a small bubble is the ideal reaction. (2) Production of an oval spot means the aiming beam is not perpendicular to the TM and thus requires refocusing

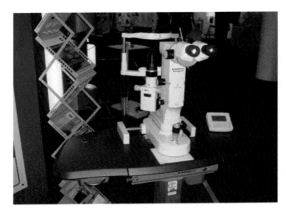

Fig 8.36 Selective laser trabeculoplasty machine

Cyclodiode laser

Cyclodestructive procedures lower IOP by destroying part of the ciliary body, thus reducing aqueous inflow. The most common method at present employs a trans-scleral diode laser (a cyclodiode laser). Endoscopic cyclophotocoagulation is also available in some centres.

The success rate of cyclodiode laser treatment depends on the type of glaucoma treated. Often the procedure needs to be repeated.

Indications

- Uncontrolled end-stage secondary glaucoma, e.g. for pain relief
- Patients with multiple previous failed glaucoma procedures
- Primary procedure in certain eyes where surgery is inappropriate
- To reduce IOP; as a temporizing measure before undertaking surgery

Laser settings

- Typical settings for the laser are 1500 milliseconds at 1500 mW.
- If popping occurs, reduce the power with or without increasing the duration.
- The number of burns given can be varied depending on the eye but 30 are typical.

Method

- Follow laser safety protocols.
- Gain patient consent (including advising on failure/retreatment and complications).
- Administer sub-Tenons or peribulbar anaesthetic (diode laser treatment is painful).
- Patient lies flat and an eyelid speculum is inserted.
- Use transillumination to confirm the location of the ciliary body.
- The ciliary body appears as a dark area 0.5–2.0 mm from the limbus.
- Eyes that have undergone multiple previous surgeries may have abnormally placed ciliary bodies or even areas where the ciliary body is absent.
- Place the diode probe against the globe with the heel at the anterior margin of the ciliary body (see Figure 8.37).
- Apply burns circumferentially, avoiding 3 and 9 o'clock (positions of posterior ciliary nerves), areas of subconjunctival haemorrhage (will reduce laser penetration), and areas of scleral thinning (risk of perforation).
- Treat 270°, sparing one quadrant.

Post-procedure guidelines

- Prescribe topical steroid (e.g. dexamethasone 0.1%) 6–8 times per day for 1 week.
- Continue all usual glaucoma medication; arrange follow-up in 1–2 weeks.

Complications

- Conjunctival burns
- Iris burns (if too anterior)
- Localized scleral thinning
- Corneal decompensation
- Anterior uveitis
- Bleeding (hyphaema or vitreous haemorrhage)
- Hypotony (including phthisis bulbi)
- Aqueous misdirection/malignant glaucoma
- Cataract
- Retinal or choroidal detachment
- Sympathetic ophthalmitis

Peripheral iridotomy (PI)

Laser PI involves creating a conduit for the flow of aqueous humour via a laser-induced puncture through the peripheral iris (see Figure 8.38). This procedure allows for the free passage of aqueous humour between the posterior and anterior chambers.

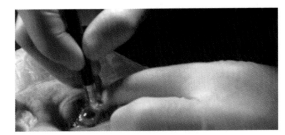

Fig 8.37 The technique of cyclodiode laser

The probe is placed vertically on the anaesthetized eye with the base of the probe against the limbus

The position of the iridotomy should be within the superior iris, covered by the upper lid to minimize risk of monocular diplopia and glare, and as peripheral as possible to prevent damage to the lens. Three-quarters of cases of appositional angle closure are reversed following Laser PI.

Indications

* PACS, primary angle closure, primary angle glaucoma
* Secondary angle closure where pupil block is a component

Laser settings

* Use the lowest energy possible to achieve a patent Laser PI.
* Typically use single 0.8 to 1.5 mJ shots and expect to use a total energy of up to 50 mJ.
* Thin blue irises need a lower power setting than thick brown irises do; the latter should have argon laser pretreatment.

Method

* Follow laser safety protocols.
* Gain patient consent (including advising on risks).
* Gonioscopy should have been performed before the procedure, and the findings documented.
* If the patient is taking warfarin, check recent international normalized ratio.
* Instil pilocarpine 2% at least 30 minutes before treatment (miosis will 'unfold' peripheral iris).
* Instil apraclonidine (iopidine) 1% (to prevent IOP spike).
* Instil topical anaesthetic.
* Insert contact lens, such as an Abraham iridotomy lens.
* Position the Laser PI between 11 and 1 o'clock but never at the level of the lid margin.
* Look for iris crypts or thin areas that will be easier to penetrate.
* A 'pigment gush' indicates successful penetration.
* If there is bleeding (occurs in 50% of cases), gentle pressure on the iridotomy lens should stop it.
* Instil additional apraclonidine 1% at the end of the procedure.

Post-procedure guidelines

* Prescribe topical steroid (e.g. dexamethasone 0.1%) hourly for 24 hours (day only) and then four times a day for 1 week. The aim is to limit any inflammatory response, which could increase PAS if the angle remains narrow.
* Check IOP after 1 hour.
* Arrange follow-up for 1 week to check IOP and assess patency of peripheral iridotomy.
* Gonioscopy should be repeated to detect any deepening in the angle and to exclude residual narrowing due to phacomorphic or plateau iris components.

Complications

* One in four risk of a short-term change in vision; vision change usually will resolve by 6 weeks.
* Glare: most likely if Laser PI positioned at the level of the lid margin, owing to the prismatic effect of the marginal tear strip
* Bright horizontal line (marginal tear strip) or dark vertical lines (lashes)
* Transient pressure rise: tends to occur within 1 hour; more common if high pretreatment IOP or PAS

* Anterior chamber inflammation
* Corneal burns: increased risk with shallow anterior chamber
* Lens opacities: can occur at treatment site but tend to be localized and non-progressive; lens rupture has been reported
* Macular damage: theoretical risk if beam is aimed perpendicularly
* Visual loss (1 in 7000)

Argon laser pretreatment

* Use the Wise or Abraham contact lens and treat in two phases:
  1. Low power: 80–130 mW, 0.05 seconds, 50 μm; make a rosette pattern of soft pitting in the iris using 15–20 shots
  2. High power: 700–750 mW, 0.1 second, 50 μm; apply 10–20 shots until the radial muscle fibres are visible
* Complete the iridotomy using the Nd:YAG laser as for PI.

Argon laser peripheral iridoplasty (ALPI)

In ALPI, the argon laser is used to shrink the peripheral iris and draw it away from the TM. ALPI is useful for the treatment of plateau iris syndrome and primary angle closure (acute or chronic). It is successful in about 50% of cases. ALPI is not appropriate for most patients with PAS and may worsen them.

* Prepare the patient using the same steps as for iridotomy.
* Use a 500 μm spot, 0.5–0.7 seconds; start with low power (100 mW) and increase (up to 180–300 mW).
* Apply 15–20 shots around the peripheral circumference of the iris.
* Avoid the cornea.
* Look for a gentle contraction of the iris stroma.
* Post-operative treatment is the same as for Laser PI but continue pilocarpine for at least 1 week to prevent PAS developing. ALPI can be used in the acute setting for primary angle closure but must be followed by Laser PI.

Complications

* Transient pressure rise
* Ache
* Reduced vision
* Dilated pupil, unresponsive to light causing glare; can be avoided with appropriate spacing of the burns
* Corneal burns

Argon laser suture lysis

Following trabeculectomy, an argon laser may be used to lyse fixed nylon sutures in the scleral flap. Laser treatment can be performed through the tip of a glass rod or by using a Blumenthal laser lens. When a suture is lysed, there is likely to be increased flow under the scleral flap into the subconjunctival space and the sub-Tenons space (the bleb). Whether or not laser suture lysis is necessary depends on the surgical technique and wound healing. Sutures may be obscured by subconjunctival haemorrhage or a thick Tenons capsule.

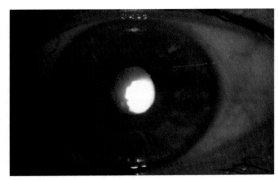

Fig 8.38 Iris transillumination defects seen after laser peripheral iridotomies

Only one Laser PI is necessary and, if placed under the upper lid, it should be as peripheral and as close to 12 o'clock as possible. Laser PIs are now also done at 3 o'clock and at 9 o'clock to avoid a meniscus effect diverting light to the 12 o'clock peripheral iridotomy and thus causing visual disturbance; one randomized trial has suggested that the incidence of visual disturbance is reduced with fully interpalpebral iridotomies

8.26 Glaucoma surgery

Glaucoma surgery may be indicated when IOP is not satisfactorily controlled with medication, when medication is contraindicated, or when compliance is poor. Surgery may also be offered as initial treatment in patients who present with advanced disease.

The main surgical options are trabeculectomy, or insertion of a glaucoma drainage device (tube). There are also a growing number of alternative procedures, including non-penetrating surgery. The type of surgery selected should be tailored to suit the individual, as each has its own specific risk–benefit profile. This section focuses on adult glaucoma surgery.

Trabeculectomy

The aim of trabeculectomy is to create a fistula that is guarded by a superficial scleral flap. The fistula allows aqueous humour to flow from the anterior chamber to the sub-Tenons space, forming a 'bleb' of fluid that is then absorbed into the episcleral vessels (see Figure 8.39). A challenge of trabeculectomy is managing wound healing. Fibrosis and scarring can lead to closure of the fistula and surgical failure; therefore, intra- and post-operative anti-fibrotics such as mitomycin C and 5-fluorouracil can be used to prevent fibrosis and are increasingly used in all patients; however, they are associated with complications, including corneal epithelial defects, post-operative wound leaks, and cystic thin-walled blebs that predispose to chronic hypotony, late-onset bleb leak, and endophthalmitis.

The problems associated with anti-fibrotics can be largely avoided by adopting a meticulous surgical technique. Using modern techniques such as 'The Moorfields Safer Surgery System' trabeculectomy with adjunctive anti-fibrotics can achieve success rates of 80%–90% in primary open-angle glaucoma.

Method

1. Place a 7–0 silk traction suture into the superior cornea.
2. Create a fornix-based conjunctival flap.
3. Clear episcleral tissue and wet-field cauterize the proposed flap area.
4. Create a rectangular scleral flap that is two-thirds of the scleral thickness. Ensure the flap is wider than it is long to encourage posterior drainage (see Figure 8.40).
5. Dissect the scleral flap forwards until clear cornea is reached.
6. Pre-place at least two 10–0 nylon sutures in the scleral flap (to enable quick closure).
7. Perform a temporal paracentesis. Consider placement of an anterior chamber maintainer.
8. Make an incision into the anterior chamber.
9. Complete the sclerostomy posteriorly using a punch (Kelly or Khaw punch).
10. Perform peripheral iridectomy (see Figure 8.41).
11. Ensure adequate flow.
12. Tie the scleral flap sutures (fixed, releasable, or adjustable sutures; see Figure 8.42).
13. Aim for no flow after sutures are secured (see Figure 8.43).
14. Close the conjunctiva so that it is 'watertight', with 10–0 nylon.
15. Inject steroid/antibiotic subconjunctivally.

Augmented trabeculectomy

Treatment with mitomycin C or 5-fluorouracil can take place before or after creation of the scleral flap but must occur before the anterior chamber is entered. A typical treatment is mitomycin C 0.2 mg/ml for 3 minutes, applied using polyvinyl alcohol sponges placed under the conjunctival/Tenons flap (with or without a scleral flap; see Figure 8.44). We use 3 minutes, as tissue absorption plateaus after this time. Great care should be taken to avoid contact with the cornea or with the conjunctival wound edge. The area is then thoroughly irrigated with balanced salt solution before completion of the trabeculectomy.

- Note that 5-fluorouracil (50 mg/ml) inhibits DNA synthesis.
- Mitomycin C (0.2–0.5 mg/ml) alkylates DNA.
- Anti-fibrotic use can be titrated to the risk of scarring.

Risk factors for scarring

- Neovascular glaucoma
- Previous failed trabeculectomy
- Secondary glaucoma (e.g. inflammatory, post-traumatic, or iridocorneal endothelial syndrome)
- Prolonged use of antiglaucoma medication (particularly adrenergic drugs)
- Previous conjunctival or cataract surgery
- African ancestry
- Age less than 40 years

Post-operative care

- Topical steroid every 2 hours for 2–4 weeks, then four times a day for a further 2 months
- Topical antibiotic four times a day for 1 month
- Follow-up at 1 day and then weekly for the first month

Frequent follow-up is needed to allow manipulation of the bleb. For example, if the IOP is too high, the eye may be massaged and sutures loosened, removed, or lysed with a laser. 5-Fluorouracil and steroids can be injected adjacent to the bleb to modify the healing response. A sudden drop in IOP during surgery should be avoided; it is preferable to have a high IOP in the first days after surgery and then to gradually lower the pressure through bleb manipulation.

Early post-operative complications

Shallow anterior chamber

- Causes
  - Wound leak: low IOP, Seidel positive, peripheral iridectomy patent, bleb poor/flat
  - Ciliary body shutdown: low IOP, Seidel negative, peripheral iridectomy patent, bleb poor/flat
  - Overfiltration: low IOP, Seidel negative, peripheral iridectomy patent, bleb good/large
  - Pupil block: high IOP, Seidel negative, peripheral iridectomy non-patent, bleb flat, iris bombé
  - Aqueous misdirection: high IOP, Seidel negative, peripheral iridectomy patent, bleb flat, shallow central anterior chamber
  - Suprachoroidal haemorrhage: variable IOP, Seidel negative, peripheral iridotomy patent, bleb variable, pain

Specific treatment depends on cause but if the anterior chamber is flat, there is a risk of corneal decompensation due

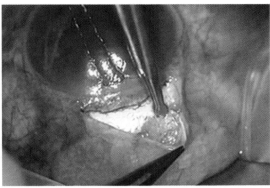

Fig 8.39 Example of trabeculectomy with mitomycin C
Placement of mitomycin C polyvinyl alcohol sponges under the
Tenons capsule

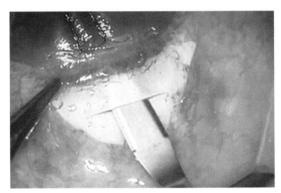

Fig 8.40 Creation of a scleral flap

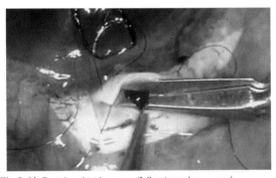

Fig 8.41 Peripheral iridectomy (following sclerostomy)

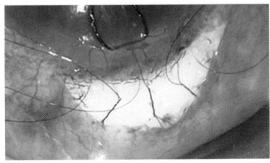

Fig 8.42 Three releasable sutures

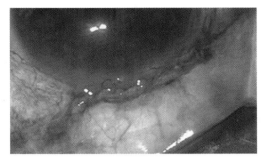

Fig 8.43 End of surgery with releasable sutures visible through
conjunctiva

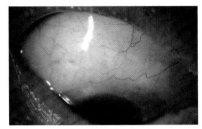

Fig 8.44 Slit lamp examination of trabeculectomy bleb

to lenticulo-corneal touch. In such cases, the anterior chamber
needs to be reformed urgently using balanced salt solution, a
viscoelastic, or gas.

Low IOP (hypotony)

* Causes:
  — Wound leak
  — Ciliary body shutdown
  — Overfiltration
* Consequences:
  — Shallowing of the anterior chamber
  — Choroidal detachment
  — Hypotonous maculopathy
  — Corneal oedema
  — Suprachoroidal haemorrhage
* Management:
  — Taper or stop topical steroids.
  — Cycloplegics to reduce shallowing of anterior chamber
  — May need reformation of the anterior chamber or
    revision of the trabeculectomy
  — Large choroidal effusions (especially if 'kissing') may need
    drainage.

Wound leak

* Consider bandage contact lens.
* Taper or stop steroids.
* May require suturing

Overfiltration

* Topical atropine to prevent shallowing of anterior chamber
* Aqueous suppressants to assist spontaneous healing of fis-
  tula by temporarily reducing aqueous flow through it.
* Autologous blood injection into bleb
* Bleb revision, with resuturing of the sclera flap

Suprachoroidal haemorrhage

- Very rare with the precautions of 'safer surgery'
- Increased risk if poorly controlled BP, anticoagulant use
- Drainage may be necessary.

Filtration failure

- The bleb may be flat, e.g. because of obstruction of the sclerostomy or scleral flap, or because of subconjunctival fibrosis.
- A specific cause of failure is an encapsulated bleb (Tenons cyst), which is a firm, dome-shaped cavity made of hypertrophied Tenons capsule with engorged surface vessels. It tends to develop 2–8 weeks post-operatively and may or may not result in raised IOP.
- Management.
  - Bleb manipulation: removal of releasable sutures, loosening of adjustable sutures, or laser suture lysis of fixed sutures
  - Needling, with or without 5-fluorouracil and steroids. Local anaesthetic injected beforehand will reduce intra- and post-procedure pain and may also reduce scarring

Visual loss

- May be due to 'wipe-out' of visual field, suprachoroidal haemorrhage, or hypotonous maculopathy

Late post-operative complications

Filtration failure

- Rate of failure is 10% in 1 year, and 25% in 5 years.
- May be treated with needling and 5-fluorouracil, e.g. if subconjunctival fibrosis ('ring of steel')
- Repeat surgery in the form of mitomycin C trabeculectomy or placement of a glaucoma drainage device may be required.

Blebitis

In contrast to bleb-related endophthalmitis, blebitis is an isolated bleb infection. It may be due to direct spread through a leaking bleb or transconjunctival migration of bacteria. Streptococcal species are the most common pathogens found in this condition.

- Causes
  - Thin-walled, avascular, cystic blebs
  - Inferior bleb location
  - Bleb leak
  - Blepharitis
  - Contact lens use
  - Ocular trauma
  - Advanced age
  - Immunosuppression
- Symptoms
  - Red, uncomfortable eye
  - Discharge
  - Tends to have a prodrome of a few days
- Signs
  - 'Milky' bleb; if the anterior chamber has more than 1+ anterior chamber cells, treat as endophthalmitis
- Management
  - Admit.
  - Conjunctival swab

- Topical ofloxacin/cefuroxime hourly day and night
- Oral moxifloxacin 400 mg in the morning for 10 days; Augmentin 625 mg three times a day
- Review within 4 hours to check progression.
- Start Pred Forte 1% four times a day 24–48 hours later if improving.

Bleb-related endophthalmitis

- Risk factors:
  - As for blebitis
- Symptoms:
  - Red, painful eye with reduced vision; usually sudden onset
- Signs:
  - 'Milky' bleb
  - Anterior uveitis
  - May have hypopyon, vitritis
- Management:
  - As for blebitis but also requires urgent vitreous tap and intravitreal vancomycin 2 mg and amikacin 0.4 mg (or ceftazidime 2 mg)
  - Intravitreal dexamethasone 0.4 mg is also given.
  - Any risk factors for infection can be treated later.

Leaking bleb

- A key concern is the development of endophthalmitis.
- Bleb revision may be required (e.g. conjunctival advancement, free patch autograft, or sclera allograft patching).

Visual loss

- Often due to surgically induced cataract; cataract surgery increases the risk of bleb failure
- If cataract surgery is performed, use topical steroids every 2 hours and consider subconjunctival 5-fluorouracil post-operatively.

Bleb dysesthesia

- Ten per cent risk; may require bleb revision

Glaucoma drainage devices

Glaucoma drainage devices (GDDs) consist of a silicone tube attached to an endplate secured to the equatorial episclera. The tube is inserted into the anterior chamber to create a direct communication between the chamber and the sub-Tenons space (see Figure 8.45). The endplate acts as a surface for bleb formation. IOP reduction is by passive, pressure-dependent

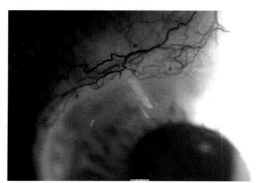

Fig 8.45 The tip of a Baerveldt tube visible in anterior chamber with a Supramid suture visible inside

outflow of aqueous humour. Some devices also have regulatory valves. GDDs include Molteno tubes, Baerveldt tubes, and Ahmed valves. GDDs are increasingly used once medication or trabeculectomy has failed. The Tube versus Trabeculectomy Study also suggested that GDDs be used more frequently in patients who have had previous conjunctival surgery, including cataract surgery.

GDDs can be classified into those with resistance (Ahmed valves) and those without resistance (Molteno tubes and Baerveldt tubes). Surgery using tubes with no resistance will result in hypotony in the early post-operative period unless the tube is ligated (with nylon or Vicryl) or blocked with an internal stenting suture (using Supramid). The aim of tube ligation is to prevent excess flow until healing offers some resistance to flow at the endplate. The ligature may dissolve or be removed, depending on the material used.

The Ahmed valve is a unidirectional, pressure-sensitive valve designed to open when the IOP is 8 mmHg; however, there is a wide variation in the true opening pressure.

A reduction in IOP can generally be obtained through the use of endplates with a large surface area. The Baerveldt tube has a surface area of 250 mm^2 or 350 mm^2, the Molteno tube has a surface area of 135 mm^2, and the Ahmed valve has a surface area of 185 mm^2.

Indications
* Uncontrolled glaucoma despite previous surgery
* Secondary glaucoma where trabeculectomy is likely to fail, e.g. neovascular and post-traumatic, iridocorneal endothelial syndrome
* Presence of conjunctival scarring
* Contact lens wearer who needs glaucoma surgery

Complications
* Over-drainage
* Malposition: endothelial or lenticular touch
* Erosion/exposure of tube: occurs in 2% of cases
* Failure of drainage: blocked tube or encapsulation of bleb over footplate
* Diplopia: occurs in 5% of cases

Non-penetrating surgery

Non-penetrating surgery is a term used to describe a group of surgeries in which the rate of aqueous drainage is controlled by the TM and Descemets membrane rather than tension in the scleral flap. It is more technically challenging than penetrating surgery. Non-penetrating surgery minimizes the risks associated with penetration into the eye, but the reduction in IOP is less.

Non-penetrating surgery is not appropriate in some glaucoma types (e.g. neovascular glaucoma). A narrow drainage angle is a relative contraindication. It may be a good option in eyes that do not need a low target pressure or in patients with mild glaucoma.

Deep sclerectomy
* Two scleral flaps are fashioned and the deep flap excised to leave a thin membrane consisting of TM/Descemets membrane (Descemets window).
* The window allows the diffusion of aqueous humour from the anterior chamber into the subconjunctival space and can result in a shallow filtration bleb.
* Inadvertent perforation of Descemets window requires conversion to a trabeculectomy.
* Goniopuncture using an Nd:YAG laser can be used to convert a deep sclerectomy to a penetrating procedure (needed in 50% of cases).

Viscocanalostomy
* As for a deep sclerectomy but, in addition, Schlemms canal is dilated with high-density viscoelastic, and the superficial scleral flap is sutured tightly to minimize bleb formation.
* Canaloplasty is a similar procedure but involves 360°Cannulation of Schlemms canal with a microcatheter. A suture can be threaded into Schlemms canal to permanently distend that structure.

Other surgical procedures for glaucoma

Peripheral iridectomy
* To relieve pupil block, when Laser PI is not possible

Goniotomy
* Indicated for primary congenital glaucoma, to open the abnormal angle (see Chapter 9, Section 9.26)

Trabeculotomy
* Indicated for congenital glaucoma, to open Schlemms canal directly to the anterior chamber (see Chapter 9, Section 9.26)

Other devices
* Several new surgical devices for glaucoma have been launched recently, including those working by increasing meshwork, such as via Schlemm canal flow (iStent, Hydrus, Trabectome), micro shunts draining to the subconjunctival space (Ex-PRESS, Xen, and Inn Focus microtube implants) and suprachoroidal space implants (Cypass, Istent supra). Further studies are currently underway to determine their long-term efficacy.

8.27 Glaucoma clinical trials

Treatment versus no treatment

Collaborative Normal Tension Glaucoma Study

- Compared treatment vs no treatment in normal tension glaucoma
- The treatment goal was a 30% reduction in IOP through the use of medications, ALT, or trabeculectomy.
- Showed that 12% of treated versus 35% of controls progressed (optic disc or visual field) after 5 years
- Surgically treated eyes were more likely than eyes that were not surgically treated to develop cataracts.
- Showed that, as a group, patients with normal tension glaucoma benefit from IOP reduction
- The effect of CCT was not examined.

Early Manifest Glaucoma Treatment Study

- Compared treatment vs no treatment in early to moderate glaucoma
- Recruitment through population screening
- Treatment with ALT and betaxolol
- Showed that a 25% reduction in IOP reduced risk of progression by 50%
- Risk of progression decreased 10% for each 1 mmHg reduction in IOP.

Ocular Hypertension Treatment Study

- Compared treatment vs no treatment in OHT
- Patients had IOPs between 21 and 32 mmHg.
- Treatment to lower IOP by at least 20% was associated with a 50% reduction in risk of glaucoma (4.4% of treated vs 9% of controls at 60 months).
- Both the optic disc and the visual field need to be monitored, as conversion occurred almost equally frequently by visual field defect alone or disc changes alone.
- Not every patient with OHT needs treatment; patients with OHT should be risk stratified.
- Thin CCT, increased age, high IOP, and a large vertical cup : disc ratio were risk factors for conversion.

Comparison of treatments

Collaborative Initial Glaucoma Treatment Study

- Compared medical treatment and trabeculectomy in newly diagnosed glaucoma
- Surgery reduced IOP more than medications did (40% vs 31%, respectively).
- There was no difference in progression between the groups.

Advanced Glaucoma Intervention Study

- Compared two treatment protocols involving ALT and trabeculectomy in uncontrolled glaucoma
- Showed that low IOP and low IOP fluctuation are associated with reduced progression, with a likely dose–response relationship
- Eyes with an average IOP >17.5 mmHg progressed more than eyes with an average IOP <14 mmHg did.

Fluorouracil Filtering Surgery Study

- Compared trabeculectomy alone to trabeculectomy with 5-fluorouracil, in eyes with previous cataract surgery or failed filtering surgery
- 5-Fluorouracil was given via post-operative injections (twice a day for 1 week, then once a day for 1 week).
- The 1-year failure rates were 28% with 5-fluorouracil vs 50% without (the difference was sustained at 5 years).

Tube versus Trabeculectomy Study

- Compared mitomycin C trabeculectomy to GDD surgery (350 mm^2 Baerveldt tube)
- Included eyes with previous cataract extraction with or without unsuccessful trabeculectomy
- At 5 years, there was equally good IOP reduction in each group (64% in both groups had an IOP of 14 mmHg or less).
- Neither glaucoma operation was superior to the other; the results support the use of tube surgery in eyes other than just those with refractory glaucoma.

Ahmed Baerveldt Comparison Study

- Compared Ahmed valves and Baerveldt tubes in patients with inadequately controlled glaucoma on maximal medial therapy
- Included primary glaucomas with previous intraocular surgery, and secondary glaucomas known to have a high failure rate with trabeculectomy
- One-year results showed that IOP reduction was greater with the Baerveldt tube than with the Ahmed valve.
- Both GDDs had a similar safety profile but the Baerveldt group needed more post-operative interventions.

The Effectiveness of Early Lens Extraction for the Treatment of PACG Study

- Ongoing study comparing early lens extraction to laser iridotomy for the treatment of PACG.

Chapter 9

Paediatric ophthalmology and strabismus

Lucy Barker, Kelly MacKenzie, Joanne Hancox, Wanda Kozlowska, and Andrew Tatham

353

The bony orbit is pyramidal in shape, with the medial wall lying parallel to the sagittal plane and with the medial and the lateral walls forming a 45° angle at their apex. The central orbital axis forms an angle of 22.5° with the medial walls and the lateral walls, and with the visual axis in primary position. The eyes make yaw, pitch, and roll movements, which can be considered as rotations around the *axes of Fick* (see Figure 9.1):

*   Horizontal movements take place around the z-axis
*   Vertical movements take place around the x-axis, which is horizontal
*   Torsional movements take place around the y-axis, which extends from anterior to posterior

The extraocular muscles act in consort to produce eye movements, and the action of the individual muscles depend on the position of the eye at the start of muscle contraction. The four recti originate from a ring of condensed orbital fascia at the orbital apex called the *annulus of Zinn*. The superior oblique originates from the back of the roof of the orbit, above and medial to the optic foramen. It passes through the trochlea anteriorly at the junction of the roof and medial wall of the orbit; this route alters the muscle's direction of action. The inferior oblique muscle originates from a tubercle on the anterior orbital floor just lateral to the lacrimal fossa.

Insertions, and the spiral of Tillaux

The extraocular muscles insert partially into a fibromuscular pulley system formed by the fascia of the orbit, and partially into sclera. The insertions of the rectus muscles into the sclera form an anticlockwise spiral known as the *spiral of Tillaux* (see Figure 9.2), with the medial rectus insertion closest to the limbus (5.5 mm behind the limbus), followed by the inferior (6.5 mm), lateral (6.9 mm), and superior (7.7 mm) recti. The obliques insert behind the equator in much more variable positions than the recti do. The superior oblique inserts in the posterior upper temporal quadrant of the globe, whilst the inferior oblique inserts in the lower posterior quadrant close to the macular.

Nerve supply

The six extraocular muscles are innervated by the third, fourth, and sixth cranial nerves:

*   The trochlear (fourth) cranial nerve supplies the superior oblique
*   The abducens (sixth) cranial nerve supplies the lateral rectus
*   The oculomotor (third) cranial nerve supplies all the other extraocular muscles and is subdivided into:
    *   The superior division, which innervates the superior rectus and the levator palpebrae superioris.
    *   The inferior division, which innervates the inferior rectus, the medial rectus, the inferior oblique, and both intraocular muscles (the sphincter pupillae and the ciliary muscle).

The course of each cranial nerve is discussed in Chapter 10.

Blood supply

The extraocular muscles all receive their blood supply from the ophthalmic artery. In turn, the blood supply of the anterior segment arises from that of the four recti via the anterior ciliary arteries. The lateral rectus provides one anterior ciliary artery, and the other recti have two each. Hence, surgery on two or more recti, particularly the vertical recti, can lead to anterior segment ischaemia.

Actions of the extraocular muscles

Individual extraocular muscle actions are given in Table 9.1. The superior muscles are incycloductors; the inferior muscles, excycloductors. The vertical rectus muscles are adductors; the oblique muscles, abductors.

To achieve a wide range of coordinated eye movements, each extraocular muscle interacts with the other muscles in the same eye and the fellow eye in a number of ways:

*   When a muscle's contraction causes a specific movement to occur, the muscle is termed the agonist
*   When a muscle's contraction opposes that particular movement, it is termed the antagonist
*   Agonist–antagonist pairs are pairs of muscles that have opposing actions; e.g. for adduction of the right eye, the right medial rectus is the agonist, and the right lateral rectus is the antagonist
*   Synergists are muscles that work together to generate a particular movement; e.g. the left inferior rectus and the left superior oblique act as synergists for depression of the left eye
*   Yoke muscles (contralateral synergists) are paired muscles that are located in opposite eyes and which move the two eyes in the same direction; e.g. the right superior rectus is the yoke muscle of the left inferior oblique, with both muscles acting in dextroelevation

Laws that govern eye movements

Herings law

Herings law states that, during conjugate eye movements (both eyes moving in the same direction), when one muscle contracts, its partner, or yoke muscle, receives equal and simultaneous innervation so that the eyes move the same amount; for example, when the eye is looking to the right, a contraction of the right lateral rectus is accompanied by an equal contraction of the contralateral left medial rectus.

Table 9.1 Actions of the extraocular muscles			
Muscle	**Primary action**	**Secondary action**	**Tertiary action**
Medial rectus	Adduction	—	—
Lateral rectus	Abduction	—	—
Superior rectus	Elevation max. in abduction	Intorsion max. in adduction	Adduction
Inferior rectus	Depression max. in abduction	Extorsion max. in adduction	Adduction
Superior oblique	Intorsion max. in abduction	Depression max. in adduction	Abduction
Inferior oblique	Extorsion max. in abduction	Elevation max. in adduction	Abduction

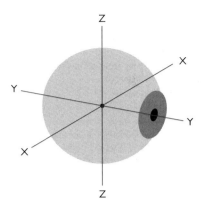

Fig 9.1 Axes of Fick

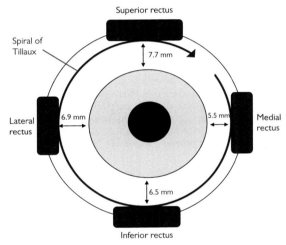

Fig 9.2 The spiral of Tillaux

However, if one muscle is weak, the extra drive required to make the muscle contract sufficiently is also applied to the yoke muscle, which will tend to overact; for example, a right sixth nerve palsy causing right lateral rectus weakness also tends to cause left medial rectus overaction.

Sherringtons law of reciprocal innervation

Sherringtons law of reciprocal innervation states that, when one muscle contracts, its opposite or antagonist muscle relaxes to an equal extent, allowing smooth movement to take place; for example, contraction of medial rectus is accompanied by simultaneous relaxation of the ipsilateral lateral rectus.

During the course of a paresis or paralysis, the actions of the extraocular muscles change because of these laws. The extent and time over which muscle sequelae develop varies greatly between patients. There are three stages in the development of the sequelae:

1. Overaction of the contralateral synergist, due to Herings law
2. Overaction of the ipsilateral antagonist, due to Sherringtons law
3. Secondary underaction of the contralateral antagonist

For example, in right sixth nerve palsy, the sequelae are:

• Primary underaction in the right lateral rectus
• Overaction in the contralateral synergist, i.e. the left medial rectus
• Overaction of the ipsilateral antagonist, i.e. the right medial rectus
• Secondary underaction of the contralateral antagonist, i.e., the left lateral rectus

Types of eye movements

Versions

Versions are rotary movements of both eyes from the primary position in the same direction and are driven by yoke muscles. Versions bring the eyes into six cardinal positions:

• Dextroversion: right gaze (driven by the right lateral rectus and the left medial rectus)
• Laevoversion: left gaze (driven by the left lateral rectus and the right medial rectus)
• Dextroelevation: gaze to the right and upwards (driven by the right superior rectus and the left inferior oblique)
• Dextrodepression: gaze to the right and downwards (driven by the right inferior rectus and the left superior oblique)
• Laevoelevation: gaze to the left and upwards (driven by the left superior rectus and the right inferior oblique)
• Laevodepression: gaze to the left and downwards (driven by the left inferior rectus and the right superior oblique)

Ductions

Ductions are rotary movements of one eye from the primary position and can be examined to elicit any limitation:

• Horizontal excursions: adduction (inwards movement) and abduction (outwards movement)
• Vertical excursions: supraduction (elevation/upwards movement) and infraduction (depression/downwards movement).
• Rotation excursions: excycloduction (rotating the upper part of the cornea temporally) and incycloduction (rotating the upper part of the cornea nasally)

Vergences

Vergences are disconjugate bilateral eye movements; that is, the eyes move in opposite directions:

• Convergence: eyes turn inwards
• Divergence: eyes turn outwards

Eye movement systems

There are five systems that govern eye movements, explained in more detail in Chapter 10:

• Smooth pursuit: eye movements slower than 40°/second
• Saccadic: fast eye movements (400–700°/second)
• Vestibular: slow eye movements in response to head movements
• Optokinetic: eye movements in response to image movement
• Vergence: eye movements to maintain fixation of an object as its distance changes

9.2 Embryology

Development of the eye begins early in the first trimester and continues postnatally. A summary of the embryological derivative tissues is given in Table 9.2; the major events in embryological development are summarized in this section.

Development of the globe

Day 22
Optic peduncles develop from bilateral invaginations of the neuroectoderm of the forebrain (the prosencephalon).

Day 27
The peduncles proliferate laterally to become primary optic vesicles connected to the third ventricle of the brain via the optic stalks. On reaching the overlying surface ectoderm, the optic vesicles induce formation of the lens placode. The vesicle then begins to invaginate to form a double-layered optic cup (see Figure 9.3).

Day 29
A groove appears on the inferior surface of the optic stalk and vesicle; this groove later becomes the optic or choroidal fissure (see Figure 9.3).

Day 33
Vascular mesenchyme grows inside the optic fissure, taking with it the hyaloid vessels which will later become the central retinal artery and vein.

Week 5
The lens placode separates from the surface ectoderm to become the lens vesicle and lies within the mouth of the optic cup. The overlying surface ectoderm begins differentiation into a bilayer corneal epithelium. Neural crest cells migrate in waves in the space between the surface ectoderm and lens vesicle to form the corneal endothelium, the trabecular meshwork, and corneal stromal keratocytes. Failure of this process results in **Peters anomaly**.

Week 6
The outer and inner layers of the optic cup begin differentiation into the pigmented and neural layers of the retina, respectively. The surrounding neural crest cells differentiate into the choroid and sclera.

Week 7
The optic fissure fully closes, encasing the hyaloid vessels and mesenchyme, which become the central retinal artery and vein and primary vitreous body. Failure of complete closure results in formation of a **coloboma** (see Figures 9.4 and 9.5). The anterior double layer of the optic cup differentiates into the pigmented (outer) and non-pigmented (inner) layers of the iris. Primary lens fibres develop and fill the optic vesicle, forming the lens nucleus.

Week 9
The ciliary bodies develop from neural crest cells on the inner surface of the developing iris and begin to secrete aqueous humour.

Development of other ocular structures

Extraocular muscles
The extraocular muscles develop from mesenchyme between the fourth and the tenth week of gestation. Differentiation occurs at the muscle insertion first.

Eyelids
The eyelids appear during the sixth week of gestation, as folds of ectoderm encasing a mesenchymal core. They grow towards each other and fuse in the ninth week. They remain fused until the fifth month, when they start to divide, a process which is completed in the seventh month.

The nasolacrimal system
The nasolacrimal system arises from a cord of neural crest cells; this cord is met by proliferating cords of cells from both the developing lids and nasal fossa. Cannulation of the cord begins at 4 months but epithelial membranes cover both the puncta and the nasolacrimal outlet (the membrane of Hasner). The punctal membranes open at term, and the membrane of Hasner shortly after; however, the distal membrane can remain imperforate for a prolonged postnatal period, causing **congenital nasolacrimal duct obstruction.**

The vitreous
The primary (vascular) vitreous body starts to form in the fifth week as the optic fissure begins to close, encasing the hyaloid vessels and the surrounding mesenchymal tissue. The hyaloid artery reaches the developing lens by the sixth week and forms the tunica vascular lentis. The secondary (avascular) vitreous is formed as hyalocytes begin secreting hyaluronic acid. The junction between primary and secondary vitreous becomes the walls of Cloquets canal. The hyaloid vessels regress by the seventh month, leaving the vitreous as an acellular jelly. Failure of complete regression results in **Mittendorfs dot** (an anastomosis between the hyaloid artery and the tunica vascular lentis on the posterior lens surface), **Bergmeisters papillae** (a remnant of the posterior portion of the hyaloid artery) or **persistent hyperplastic primary vitreous** (PHPV; see Figure 9.6).

The retina
All retinal layers are derived from the neuroectodermal optic cup, and differentiation occurs first at the posterior pole before spreading anteriorly. The photoreceptors are formed from the inner layer of the optic cup. Cones develop first, during the fourth, fifth, and sixth months, and rods from the seventh month onwards. Retinal vasculature arises from the hyaloid vessels and spreads anteriorly from the posterior pole. It is not fully developed until the ninth month of gestation, and disruption of this process, as occurs in premature birth, can result in retinopathy of prematurity.

Table 9.2 Summary of embryological derivative tissues	
Neuroectoderm	• Iris epithelium
	• Iris sphincter and dilator
	• Ciliary body epithelium
	• Neurosensory retina
	• Retinal pigment epithelium
	• Optic nerve
Neural crest cells	• Corneal stroma and endothelium
	• Trabecular meshwork
	• Ciliary muscles
	• Sclera
	• Choroidal stroma
Surface ectoderm	• Skin and eyelids
	• Conjunctival epithelium
	• Corneal epithelium
	• Lacrimal gland
	• Nasolacrimal system
	• Lens
Mesoderm	• Extraocular muscles
	• Ocular vasculature

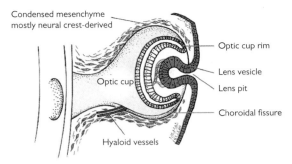

Fig 9.3 Formation of the optic cup and lens vesicle

Reproduced from Snell, R.S and Lemp, M.A, *Clinical Anatomy of the Eye*, 2nd Edition. Copyright (1998) with permission from John Wiley and Sons

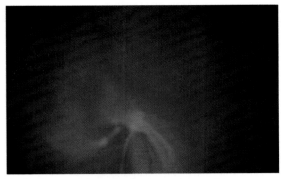

Fig 9.6 Persistent hyperplastic primary vitreous right eye

Courtesy of Prof A T Moore

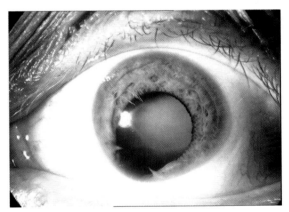

Fig 9.4 Left iris coloboma

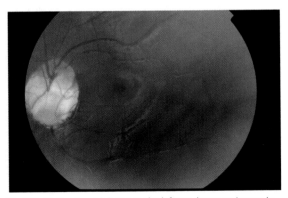

Fig 9.5 Optic disc coloboma in the left eye (same patient as in Figure 9.4)

9.3 Patient assessment I: History and general examination

History

A careful history is crucial for appropriate diagnosis and management of strabismus in paediatric and adult patients. In particular, enquire about the following aspects:

Strabismus

- Duration/age of onset: this can give an indication of the nature of the strabismus, whether gradual, sudden, or intermittent; the earlier the onset, the poorer the prognosis for binocular single vision.
- Variability: intermittent deviations suggest some degree of binocularity; variation with near and distance fixation suggests an accommodative element or convergence disorder.
- Laterality: a constant squint with one eye indicates a high risk of amblyopia in a child; alternating fixation suggests equal visual acuities.

Symptoms

- Asthenopia: what are the precipitating factors for headaches, blurred vision and/or eye strain?
- Diplopia:
  - Constant or intermittent?
  - Monocular or binocular?
  - Horizontal, vertical, torsional, or a combination?
  - Exacerbated by particular positions of gaze?
- Confusion (rare).

Previous treatment

- Spectacles
- Patching
- Orthoptic exercises
- Botulinum toxin therapy
- Surgery

Family history

- Strabismus
- Refractive error
- Ocular defects

Medical history

- Any possible precipitating or attributed causes, such as past or present systemic diseases

Birth history

- There is an increased risk of strabismus and refractive error in children who are premature, have cerebral palsy, or are developmentally delayed

Social history

- In adults, occupation, hobbies, and driving history may all have a bearing on decisions regarding strabismus management

General examination

A number of general examinations should be made to supplement the more specific strabismus examinations:

- Observation: for abnormal head posture, nystagmus, facial and orbital abnormalities, epicanthus, etc
- Visual acuity
- Pupil check
- Refraction: to identify any accommodative or ametropic strabismic drive. All children below the age of 8 should undergo full cycloplegic refraction with repeated refraction on a yearly basis, or sooner if vision fails to improve
- Fundoscopy: mandatory to identify any underlying pathology, e.g. macular scars, optic nerve hypoplasia, retinoblastoma

9.4 Assessment of visual acuity

Measurement of visual acuity is a key part of the assessment of patients with strabismus and amblyopia. For testing to be meaningful, the test chosen must be appropriate to the patient's age and level of literacy.

Definition

Visual acuity is a measure of spatial discrimination; that is, the ability to distinguish two visual stimuli separated in space. However, it is only one aspect of visual function. To fully assess visual function, other factors, such as contrast sensitivity, colour vision, and visual fields, must be considered.

The principles of visual acuity measurement are as follows:

* Acuity is determined by the smallest retinal image whose form can be appreciated.
* This image is usually quantified by the minimum angle of separation (subtended at the nodal point).
* The normal minimum angle of separation is 1 minute of arc or less, corresponding to a Snellen acuity of 6/6, but under optimal conditions a healthy eye may discriminate 0.5 minutes of arc.

Visual acuity testing in infants

Quantifying visual acuity in preverbal children (usually 0–2 years old) may be difficult. In children with strabismus, it is important to assess whether the acuity is equal in both eyes or whether amblyopia is present. A number of techniques can be used, as follows.

Occlusion

If a child objects strongly to occlusion of one eye, observation that is poorer in the uncovered eye than in the covered eye.

Fixing and following

Fixation behaviour can be examined using a small toy or light as a fixation target. Searching, slow, unsteady movements, nystagmus, or inability to follow a moving target may be due to poor vision. Any fixation preference for one eye should be noted; an observation of alternating fixation in infants with strabismus suggests equal vision in the two eyes.

The 10-dioptre base-down prism fixation test

In this test, a 10-dioptre (D) prism is held base down front of one eye as a patient fixes on a target, thereby inducing vertical diplopia. If the vision between the two eyes is equal, both eyes will be seen to alternately fixate. If visual acuity is reduced in one eye, then that eye will be seen to deviate vertically as the better-seeing eye continues to fixate.

Hundreds and thousands

The ability to locate hundreds and thousands at 0.3 m, with an attempt to pick them up, indicates a visual acuity of approximately 6/24. The sweets need to be presented on a plain-coloured background and not on one's hand. The infant needs to be able to use a pincer grasp that develops by 9 months of age.

Optokinetic nystagmus

A series of moving targets across the visual field will produce a slow following eye movement of a target, followed by a re-fixation movement in the opposite direction as the new target enters the visual field; this phenomenon is termed optokinetic nystagmus (OKN). One way to assess it is to use a device known as an OKN drum, which is held 50 cm from the patient and rotated at a constant speed whilst the observer notes the fix and follow of the patient's eye movements. This method is only used for gross assessment of visual function, owing to an inability to quantify the response. Modern approaches use either electrooculography (EOG) or video eye movement recording techniques to measure OKN.

Forced-choice preferential looking

An infant's attention is attracted more by patterned than plain surfaces, provided the pattern is above the visual acuity threshold. Test cards such as Teller acuity cards, Keeler acuity cards, and Cardiff acuity cards have been designed with gratings or pictures of varying spatial frequencies with equal contrast to the background. The grating or picture is on one-half of the card, whilst the other half of the card is plain. The cards are held 50–100 cm from the infant, and the observer watches the child's eyes and head for fixation movements indicating that the grating or picture has been detected.

Visual acuity testing in verbal children and adults

A single-picture or optotype tests may overestimate visual acuity because of the **crowding phenomenon**, whereby symbols of a given size become more difficult to recognize when they are surrounded by similar symbols, such as full rows of letters on a LogMAR chart. This phenomenon is thought to happen because the receptive fields of neurons in the amblyopic visual system are abnormally large. In view of this fact, it is essential to test children on a linear or crowded chart as early as possible, in order to establish if there is any amblyopia that might otherwise be missed.

Picture and optotype matching

As a guide, from the age of 2 years, most children can undertake picture-naming or picture-matching tests such as **Kays pictures**, the Keeler LogMAR, or the Sonksen–Silver test. Crowded versions of these tests are available. The normative value for a child of 3 with Kays pictures is 0.100 (3/3.8).

Snellen chart

The Snellen chart is a widely used eye chart in which letters of diminishing sizes are used to test minimum resolvable acuity.

When viewed at the appropriate distance, each Snellen letter subtends an angle of 5′ of arc at the retina, and the gaps between the letters subtend 1′ of arc; for a person with normal acuity, the largest optotype subtends 5′ when viewed at a distance of 60.0 m, and the smaller ones when viewed at 36.0 m, 24.0 m, 18.0 m, 12.0 m, 9.0 m, 6.0 m, 5.0 m, and 4.5 m, respectively. The acuity is expressed as a Snellen fraction: the distance at which the chart is read/distance at which the smallest optotype read subtends a 5′ arc; for example, 6/60 if only the top line is read. The normal eye has a Snellen acuity of 6/6 or better.

LogMAR chart

The LogMAR chart is designed to record the logarithm of the mean angle of resolution (LogMAR = **log**arithm of the **m**ean **a**ngle of **r**esolution). The original Bailey–Lovie chart is not widely seen in clinical practice; instead, the Early Treatment Diabetic Retinopathy Study (ETDRS) version is most commonly used. The LogMAR chart has a number of advantages over the Snellen chart:

- Every line has five letters proportionally spaced to minimize crowding.
- All the letters are equally legible.
- There is a logical progression in size of letters in each successive line.

The space between each letter is equal to the width of one letter, and the spacing between two rows is equal to the height of one letter in the smaller row. The chart is usually read at 4.0 m. Each correct line (worth 0.10 units) or each correct letter (worth 0.02 units) is subtracted from 1.00 to give the LogMAR acuity; an acuity of 0.00 approximates 6/6 Snellen.

Acuity tests for illiterate adults

Optotype matching can test patients who are illiterate or unable to read the chart because of a language barrier. Tests have also been devised based on Snellen or LogMAR charts with E's (the Illiterate E test) or C's (the Landholt C test) in varying orientations. In these tests, the patient indicates the direction of the prongs of the E's or of the gaps in the C's, respectively.

Near acuity tests

A number of tests exist for near vision. They are read at 0.3 m, and acuity is recorded as an N value plus print point size (tests range from N48 to N5) or recorded as a LogMAR score. The MNRead acuity card is not widely used in clinical practice but assesses reading speed with progressively smaller test sizes. The chart is held at 0.3 m, and the time taken to read the paragraph recorded. A reading speed is then calculated. The MNRead acuity card represents a more accurate test of near reading ability than other near acuity tests do.

9.5 The child who can't see

Investigation of the child who can't see, be it the infant with poor visual behaviour or the older child with visual loss, is often difficult and challenging for the ophthalmologist and the family alike. It is important to involve the paediatrician from the outset, as his/her input is invaluable.

Evaluation of the baby with poor vision from birth

History
A thorough evaluation by both the paediatrician and the ophthalmologist should occur. Birth history requires particular attention, including birth weight, prematurity, and adverse perinatal events. Family history, in particular consanguinity, would guide towards an investigation of potential autosomal recessive traits.

Examination
Even in small infants, the presence of fixation may be established with a large target such as the human face. Problems with fixing and following may become more evident from 2 months onwards. If visual behaviour is abnormal, it is important to examine the patient carefully for nystagmus. Following anterior segment evaluation, a cycloplegic refraction and dilated fundus examination should be carried out. In the majority of cases, the cause of visual impairment will be seen on examination.

Table 9.3 summarizes potential causes of visual impairment in the child with bilaterally poor vision from birth.

Table 9.3 Differential diagnosis of a baby with poor vision	
Abnormal external eye examination	Microphthalmia, coloboma Corneal opacities, anterior segment dysgenesis, aniridia Glaucoma Congenital cataract Albinism Congenital idiopathic nystagmus
Normal external eye examination	High refractive error
Abnormal vitreous	Non-accidental injury Retrolenticular fibroplasia Persistent hyperplastic vitreous Hyaloid abnormalities Retinal dysplasia Retinoblastoma
Abnormal retina	Albinism Coloboma Chorioretinitis (toxoplasma, toxocara, tuberculosis) Haemorrhages Maculopathy Metabolic (cherry-red spot) Retinal dystrophy Retinoblastoma
Abnormal optic disc	Coloboma Optic nerve hypoplasia/anomalous disc Optic atrophy Optic disc swelling (papilloedema, infiltration)

Evaluation of the child with visual loss

It is important to ascertain a good history. Congenital causes of visual loss may only manifest later in life when visual demands increase. It is therefore important to take a birth history. Family history and parental consanguinity should be enquired about.

Examination
Observe the child's behaviour: is it consistent with the amount of visual loss? An accurate assessment of visual acuity as appropriate for age should be carried out by an orthoptist in all cases. A normal examination does not exclude a serious underlying cause. Table 9.4 summarizes potential causes of visual impairment in an older child.

Investigations
Investigation will help elucidate the underlying disorder and should be directed by the history and examination findings. The following should be considered:
* Refraction in all cases
* Tonometry, topography, keratometry
* Electrodiagnostic tests: electroretinogram (ERG)/visual evoked potential (VEP)/EOG
* Neuroimaging: MRI/CT
* Ultrasound
* Metabolic/systemic/uveitis workup
* Genetic testing
* Paediatric referral
* Lumbar puncture

Investigating the child with poor vision and normal fundal findings

It can be difficult in situations where the child demonstrates poor visual behaviour but ocular examination does not reveal an obvious cause (see Table 9.5). It is important to instigate

Table 9.4 Differential diagnosis of a child with poor vision	
Normal external eye examination	Functional Refractive error Retinal dystrophy, e.g. Stargardts disease Cerebral visual impairment Meningitis/encephalitis Hydrocephalus
Abnormal anterior segment examination	Keratoconus Corneal scar/opacity Cataract Ectopia lentis
Glaucoma	
Abnormal retinal/vitreous examination	Trauma Uveitis Tumour Retinal dystrophy Retinal detachment
Abnormal optic disc	Papillitis Chronic papilloedema Optic atrophy Infiltration

Table 9.5 Causes of poor vision in a baby with a normal examination

Delayed visual maturation	Clinical findings and investigations normal; vision develops over time with observation
Cerebral visual impairment	Flash VEP, pattern VEP, MRI, and neuropaediatric examination usually abnormal
Congenital idiopathic nystagmus	Nystagmus with possible head posture; investigations normal except for pattern VEP
Leber congenital amaurosis	Roving eyes, eye poking, photophobia, high hypermetropia, absent flash ERG, and pattern VEP
Achromatopsia/cone dystrophy	Nystagmus, day blindness, colour blindness, photophobia, absent cone response on flash ERG, and abnormal pattern VEP
Retinal dystrophy	Nystagmus, night blindness, abnormal flash ERG, and pattern VEP
Optic nerve hypoplasia	Poor vision, roving eye movements, abnormal flash VEP, and abnormal pattern VEP; MRI may or may not be abnormal; patient may have associated endocrine abnormalities

ERG, electroretinogram; VEP, visual evoked potential.

investigations as soon as possible in order to provide a diagnosis and counsel the parents as appropriate. Electrodiagnostic testing can be diagnostic but neuroimaging with MRI should also be considered in these cases.

Non-organic/functional visual loss in children

Children may present with visual loss symptoms that do not conform to known diseases; alternatively, children may describe symptoms that are difficult to understand. This fact does not necessarily mean that the symptoms are fabricated, and it is important to exclude any possibility of an organic disorder before coming to a diagnosis of functional visual loss. The paediatrician should again be involved early on in the management of these patients.

Background

The child will commonly be aged between 6 and 16 years old. Symptoms usually come on gradually but may worsen over time. Uniocular/binocular or varying degrees of visual loss may be described.

It is important to do a full workup and enquire about home and family circumstances as well as schooling.

Examination

Thorough ocular examination is required, including:

- Visual acuity (appropriate for age)
- Ishihara
- Visual fields
- Orthoptic assessment
- Refraction
- Anterior segment evaluation
- Assessment of pupils, relative afferent pupillary defect
- Dilated fundus examination

Useful tests in ruling out an organic cause

It is important in all cases of suspected non-organic visual loss to gain as much information as possible about visual function. This process can help avoid having to carry out more invasive investigations on the child. The following tests can be particularly helpful in diagnosis:

- **OKN testing:** a normal OKN response rules out severe visual impairment, although it is possible for the patient to look through the drum.
- **The 20 D prism test:** a prism placed base out in front of a seeing eye will usually induce an involuntary fusional movement; this effect will not be seen with severe visual loss.
- **Refraction:** during refraction, the patient may be tricked by inadvertently fogging the good eye and reading with the bad.
- **Stereoacuity:** the Frisby test can be used, as the patient will not be aware they are using both eyes to perform this test; a good stereoacuity means the patient must be using both eyes.

Investigations

Further investigation may be required if there is any doubt. Such investigation would include electrodiagnostic tests such as ERG, pattern ERG, VEP, and EOG, and imaging tests such as MRI/CT.

It is important to remember that some diseases such as Batten disease and Stargardts disease can be difficult to detect initially on clinical examination. Appropriately targeted electrodiagnostics can aid the diagnosis in these cases and may avoid the need for imaging.

Management

It is important to reassure both parent and child that no underlying pathology has been found. The condition should be discussed in full with language appropriate to both. It is useful to mention that these situations can occur in children as part of a reaction to stress and that they usually settle. It is also important to work with the school if that is the source of the child's stress. Most cases can usually be managed by the ophthalmologist and the paediatrician, with close monitoring to ensure symptoms and signs do not progress and to provide support. In difficult cases, it may be necessary to involve a psychologist or a psychiatrist.

The prognosis is usually good, especially in young children, with strong reassurance and an appreciation, on the part of the family, of the underlying psychological nature of the condition.

9.6 Binocular vision and stereopsis

Binocular single vision is the ability to use both eyes simultaneously so that each eye contributes to a common single perception.

Development of binocular single vision in infancy requires:

* Similar image clarity in both eyes
* Overlapping visual fields
* Correct neuromuscular development so that both visual axes can be aligned with the object to allow motor fusion
* Correct central development capable of image interpretation to allow sensory fusion
* Corresponding retinal areas, e.g. normal foveal position in both eyes

Such features permit **normal retinal correspondence**, whereby viewing an object will produce an image at anatomically corresponding points on each retina.

Levels of binocular single vision

Binocular single vision can be graded according to the following levels.

Simultaneous perception

In simultaneous perception, an image is perceived simultaneously on each retina.

Fusion

Fusion has two components:

* **Sensory fusion:** the ability to perceive two images, one on each retina, and interpret them as one
* **Motor fusion:** the ability to maintain sensory fusion through a range of vergences which may be horizontal, vertical, or torsional, e.g. by convergence movements when fixing on a target moving towards the viewer

Sensory fusion is of little value on its own; motor fusion must be present so that sensory fusion can be maintained as the eyes move.

If we consider the field of vision at a given fixation distance as a plane, the plane composed of all object points that are present in the visual space and which are imaged on corresponding retinal elements at that fixation distance is termed the **horopter**, or horizon of vision. Fusional processes allow objects on the plane of the horopter to be seen as a single visual perception.

Stereopsis (depth perception)

Objects viewed at a distance produce images with a slight horizontal disparity between the two eyes, owing to the horizontal separation of the eyes in the skull. Fusion of these slightly disparate images and processing of the disparity gives a three-dimensional perception of depth. Fusion is not limited solely to objects confined to the horopter. There exists a narrow region just in front of and behind the horopter in which, despite disparity, points will be seen as single. This region is called **Panums fusional area**. Objects falling within this area are seen singly and stereoscopically. Objects falling outside Panums area produce physiological diplopia.

Abnormalities of binocular single vision

Diplopia

The stimulation of non-corresponding retinal points by the same image produces diplopia, or double vision, whereby the same object is perceived twice.

Confusion

Confusion occurs when corresponding retinal points are stimulated by two different stimuli and fusion cannot occur. The two images may appear to be on top of one another and projected to the same point in space.

Adaptations to abnormalities of binocular single vision

Abnormal binocular single vision arises before the age of 6–8 years; however, plasticity of the developing visual system may produce adaptations to prevent perception of confusion and diplopia. Such adaptation may be done via suppression or through abnormal retinal correspondence.

Suppression

Suppression is the mental inhibition of visual sensations of one eye in favour of those of the other eye when both eyes are open. Physiological suppression occurs normally in binocular single vision to allow concentration on a viewed object and suppress physiological diplopia from perception of surrounding objects behind or in front of Panums area.

Abnormal retinal correspondence

If the fovea of one eye is paired with a non-foveal area of retina in a deviating fellow eye, some binocular vision with limited fusion may occur by abnormal retinal correspondence despite a manifest deviation. In abnormal retinal correspondence, stimulation of non-corresponding retinal points with a stable relationship leads to stimulation of functionally corresponding cortical points to produce a single percept. This condition is most common in constant small-angle esotropias and microtropia.

Abnormal head posture

Abnormal head posture consists of one or more components:

* Chin elevation or depression
* Face turn to the right or left
* Head tilt to the right or left shoulder
  It can occur to:
* Enable development of binocular single vision
* Maintain binocular single vision in cases of acquired strabismus
* Overcome symptoms, e.g. to avoid painful eye movements
* Improve vision in cases of nystagmus and bilateral ptosis
* Increase separation of diplopia, so that the second image can be ignored

Horizontal deviations produce face turns horizontally, vertical deviations result in elevation or depression of the chin, and torsional deviations cause a head tilt to one or the other shoulder.

Fusion

The presence or absence of fusion (sensory and motor) plays an important part in the prognosis and management of strabismus. Conservative and surgical management are generally aimed at eliciting a functional result. If fusion is absent, binocular single vision cannot be restored. Fusional amplitudes may be affected by:

- **Compensation for deviations:** as a tendency to deviate develops, a patient may show a compensatory increased fusional amplitude for that deviation, e.g. congenital vertical deviations frequently lead to an increased vertical fusion range.
- **State of alertness:** tiredness, illness, etc. may decrease fusional reserves, e.g. converting a heterophoria to a heterotropia and thereby giving rise to asthenopic symptoms.

Fusional amplitudes can be measured using a prism bar, a synoptophore, or a 20 D base-out prism.

Prism fusion range

To determine the prism fusion range, the patient fixates on a target, wearing any refractive correction, and the prism bar strength is gradually increased from 1 D until diplopia occurs or a corrective eye movement is no longer made, both of which indicate that the prism can no longer be overcome by motor fusion.

Normal horizontal fusion range:

- **Near:** 40 D base-out to 14 D base-in
- **Distance:** 14 D base-out to 7 D base-in
  Normal vertical fusion range:
- **Near and distance:** 3 D supra- or infravergence, giving a total of 6 D

Base-out prism test

The base-out prism test is a relatively quick and easy method for detecting binocular single vision in children who are too young or cannot perform the fusion test.

A 20 D base-out prism is placed in front of one eye, displacing the image and causing diplopia. If the prism is placed in front of the right eye, the following movements should be observed:

- A shift of the right eye to the left, to establish foveal fixation
- Herings law causes a matching shift of the left eye to the left (conjugate movement)
- The left eye will then make a convergent movement to re-fixate (disjugate movement)

A child with good binocular single vision should have enough fusion to overcome a 20 D base-out prism. This procedure is then repeated with the prism in front of the other eye. If the child is unable to overcome a 20 D prism, then reduce the prism strength to 15 D or 10 D.

Stereopsis

Stereopsis is the perception of the relative depth of objects on the basis of binocular disparity. Stereoacuity is the angular measurement of minimal resolvable binocular disparity at which stereopsis is appreciated. It is measured in seconds of arc ($1° = 60'$ of arc; $1' = 60$ seconds ($60''$) of arc). The normal value for those with normal visual acuity is $60''$. A number of tests are in widespread use to assess stereopsis.

Lang test

The Lang test is based on two principles: random dots, and cylinder gratings. Images are seen disparately by each eye through intrinsic cylindrical lens elements in the test plates. Two strips of an image are located beneath each vertical cylinder such that one is seen by the right eye and the other by the left. The test plate is held parallel to the plane of the patient's face at 40 cm. The patient is then asked to name or point to a simple shape on the card.

This test is useful in assessing very young children and babies, as they will instinctively reach out and touch the pictures. The degree of disparity ranges from $1,200''$ to $550''$.

Titmus test

The Titmus test uses the principle of linear polarization and consists of three-dimensional polaroid vectographs, which are made up of two plates assembled in the form of a booklet and viewed through polaroid spectacles. It is performed at a distance of 40 cm and has three components, as follows:

Wirt fly

The Wirt fly component tests gross stereopsis ($3000''$ of arc). This test is very useful in children; if stereopsis is present, the fly will appear solid, and the child can be asked to pick up one of its wings. In the absence of gross stereopsis, the fly will appear flat (see Figure 9.7).

Animal

The animal component of the test consists of three rows of animals, one of which should appear to stand out from the page and can be pinpointed by patients with stereopsis. The degree of disparity tested ranges from $400''$ to $100''$.

Circles

The most finely discriminating part of the test consists of nine sets of four circles. One of the circles in each set has a degree of disparity and should be seen as standing out from the page. The degree of disparity tested ranges from $800''$ to $40''$. False positives are possible, as the test contains some monocular clues.

TNO test

The TNO test consists of seven plates of red and green dots. Spectacles are worn with a red filter over one eye, and a green filter over the other. The plates contain various shapes (squares, circles, etc.) created by random dots in complimentary colours. Some shapes can be seen without the spectacles, whereas others are 'hidden' and only become visible to someone with stereopsis who is wearing the red/green glasses (see Figure 9.8).

The first three plates establish the presence of stereopsis, and subsequent plates quantify it; the degree of disparity tested ranges from $480''$ to $15''$. This test is also useful because there are no monocular clues to produce false positives and it can be used in children as young as 3.

Frisby test

The Frisby test consists of three transparent plastic plates of 6.0 mm, 3.0 mm, and 1.0 mm thickness. On the surface of each plate are printed four squares of small random shapes. One of the plates contains a hidden circle, in which the random shapes are printed on the reverse of the plate. The patient is asked to identify the hidden circle. The test does not require special spectacles as the disparity is created by the thickness of the plate. The degree of disparity ranges from $600''$ to $15''$ of arc. Monocular clues are possible if the plate is held incorrectly.

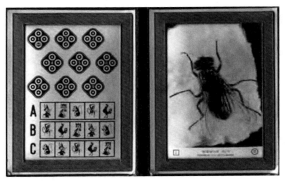

Fig 9.7 The Wirt Fly test

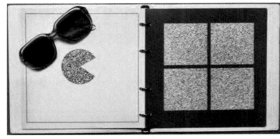

Fig 9.8 The TNO test

9.8 Assessment of retinal correspondence and suppression

The tests described in this section are used to investigate retinal correspondence, are often dissociative, and are usually subjective.

Bagolini glasses test

The Bagolini glasses test is a diplopia-based test of retinal correspondence. Glasses are worn in which the lens have fine parallel striations at 45° in one eye and at 135° in the other. The patient views a spotlight through the glasses, and the glasses convert the spot of light into lines perpendicular to the striations. The patient is then asked to describe the appearance of the lines and lights seen. Patients may see the following patterns:

* One light with two lines crossing in the middle of the light: this pattern indicates that retinal correspondence is present (but could be normal or abnormal).
* One light with two lines crossing in the middle, with a gap in one of the lines around the light: this pattern indicates the presence of a suppression scotoma.
* Two lights and two separate lines: this pattern indicates a manifest deviation with diplopia; a pattern in which the lights become one, and the lines form a cross when the deviation is corrected with prisms suggests that normal retinal correspondence is present.
* One light with only one line: this pattern indicates suppression of one eye.

Worths four-dot test

Worths four-dot test is another test of visual alignment, suppression, dominance, and diplopia. The patient wears glasses with a red filter over one eye, and a green filter over the other. The patient is then asked to view a target consisting of four lights: an uppermost red light, two green lights, and a lowermost white light. If the other eye is occluded, the eye with the green filter can potentially see three lights (the two green lights plus the white light, which is perceived as green by that eye). The eye with the red filter will see two lights (the red light plus the white light, which is perceived as red through the filter) if the other is covered.

The patient is asked how many lights they can see, and of which colours. If the right eye looks through the red filter, and the left through the green, the results are interpreted as follows:

* If there is orthophoria with bifoveal fixation, four lights are seen: the red at the top, two green, and then the white light, which may be perceived as red (if the right eye is dominant), as green (if the left eye is dominant), alternate between the two, or appear mixed.
* If the left eye is suppressing, two red lights are seen.
* If the right eye is suppressing, three green lights are seen.
* If five lights are seen, there is either double vision or rapidly alternating suppression. If the images are crossed (red lights on the left), there is an exo deviation; if the images are uncrossed (red lights on the right), there is an eso deviation.

Area and depth of suppression

The area of suppression can be measured either by using prisms or on the synoptophore.

The depth or density of suppression is measured using a **Sbiza bar** (or Bagolini filter bar), which contains a series of red filters of increasing densities. The bar is held in front of the fixing eye, and a white light is viewed through increasingly dense red filters. The red filter will eventually reduce the illumination to the fixing eye enough to switch fixation to the deviating eye, hence causing diplopia. The filter strength is increased until the patient sees two lights: one red and one white. The filter strength at this point gives a measure of density of suppression. This test is used mainly to assess whether occlusion therapy should be continue in children aged 7 and above, although the filter strength at which occlusion therapy should be stopped remains debatable. If the level of suppression falls below Filter 7, there is a risk of intractable diplopia.

Post-operative diplopia test

This test is undertaken to assess the risk of inducing diplopia post-operatively if cosmetic alignment is successful. It is generally performed on any patient aged 7 or over.

The patient fixates a target at 0.3 m; next, prisms are introduced at the lowest strength and then gradually increased, first to correct the angle of deviation and then to overcorrect it. At each prism strength, the patient is asked to state whether they see diplopia. This test is then repeated, with the patient fixating at distance. If there is concern regarding the outcome of this test, then the diagnostic use of botulinum toxin may be indicated prior to considering surgery.

9.9 Measurement of ocular deviation

Assessment of the size of a manifest deviation is vital when determining management, for example, when planning surgery. There are various ways to measure the deviation and these can be divided into objective, that is, based on neutralization of the movement of the deviating eye as it takes up fixation, and subjective, that is, based on the patient's awareness of images projected from each eye.

Objective

- Hirschberg test
- Prism reflection test
- Krimsky test
- Prism cover test
- Synoptophore

Subjective

- Maddox rod
- Maddox wing
- Synoptophore

To neutralize a deviation, the apex of any prism should point in the direction of the deviation:

- For eso (convergent) deviations, the prisms are held base out
- For exo (divergent) deviations, they are held base in
- For hyper deviations, they are held base down
- For hypo deviations, they are held base up

Hirschberg test (corneal light reflexes)

The Hirschberg test is an objective test used in small infants, uncooperative children with poor fixation, and adults with poor vision who are unable to take up fixation; it allows an estimate of the angle of a heterotropia (manifest squint) to be made by viewing the corneal reflex when a light is shone at the eyes. If both reflexes are centred and symmetrical, no deviation is present. In a manifest deviation, the distance of the light reflex from the centre of the pupil of the deviating eye gives an idea of the size of the strabismus, with each millimetre of deviation equivalent to 15 D in adults and to 20–22 D in children.

As a rough guide, if the corneal reflex falls at the pupil margin, the deviation is 20–30 D; if it falls at the limbus the deviation is about 90 D (see Figures 9.9–9.12).

Prism reflection test

The prism reflection test is used in small children and in patients with poor vision and who do not have foveal fixation. The prisms are placed over the deviating eye until the corneal reflexes appear straight, giving an approximate magnitude of the manifest squint at 0.3 m. The examiner observes the corneal reflections and increases the prism strength until the corneal reflections appear symmetrical.

Krimsky test

The Krimsky test is similar to the prism reflection test, but the prisms are placed over the fixing eye, and the eye actually moves to take up fixation. When the appropriate prism neutralizes the deviation, the corneal light reflexes appear symmetrical and there is no fixation movement.

Prism cover test

The prism cover test is used to measure the total angle of deviation (manifest or latent deviation) and is usually performed with fixation at 3 cm, at 6 m, and occasionally at far distance. This test is the most commonly used method to assess the size of the deviation. The patient needs to be able to see the fixation target with each eye. The alternate cover test is performed and prisms of increasing power placed in front of one eye until the deviation is neutralized. Both horizontal and vertical angles can be measured simultaneously. The end point occurs when there is no further movement to take up fixation.

Maddox rod

The Maddox rod is a subjective dissimilar image test used to measure the angle of a heterophoria (latent deviation), provided normal retinal correspondence is present. The test should be performed at 0.3 m and 6 m, with each eye fixating. It consists of a series of fused cylindrical red glass rods, mounted in a trial lens or a handheld frame. When placed over one eye, it converts the appearance of a white spot of light into a red streak. The streak is at 90° to the long axis of the rods; that is, when the rods are held horizontally, the streak will be vertical. The Maddox rod effectively dissociates the eyes, since dissimilar images are presented to the eyes, removing the stimulus to fuse.

Assessing horizontal heterophoria

The rod is placed horizontally in front of the right eye. The patient is asked to fixate on a distant spot of white light. He/she should see a red line and a white spot. If there is no heterophoria, the line will pass straight through the spot. If the line is to the left of the spot (crossed), there is an exophoria; if the line is to the right of the spot (uncrossed), there is an esophoria. The heterophoria is then quantified by finding the prism required to neutralize it.

Assessing vertical heterophoria

The rod is rotated vertically and the procedure repeated to identify any vertical heterophoria. If the line appears below the spot, there is a hyperphoria; if the line appears above the spot, there is a hypophoria. As with horizontal heterophoria, the vertical heterophoria is quantified by neutralizing with prisms.

Maddox wing

The Maddox wing is another dissimilar image method of measuring heterophorias in the presence of normal retinal correspondence. The device dissociates the eyes for near fixation (0.3 m). The patient (wearing their reading correction) looks through the apertures, and a septum dissociates the eyes so that the left sees a vertical numerical scale and a horizontal numerical scale, and the right sees a white vertical arrow and a red horizontal arrow. Horizontal deviation is measured by asking the patient to which number the white arrow points; an even number indicates an exotropia, and an odd number indicates an esotropia. Similarly, the number indicated by the red arrow indicates a vertical deviation.

Cyclophoria can also be assessed with the Maddox wing. The patient is asked whether the red arrow is parallel to the white line of numbers. If it is not, it can be moved until parallel, and the amount of torsion in degrees is then read from a scale.

The synoptophore

The synoptophore is a haploscopic device via which the two eyes are dissociated so that each eye views a picture on a different slide on a plane mirror. The eyepieces contain +6.5 D lenses to mimic distance viewing. There are various slides to test aspects of simultaneous perception, fusion, and stereopsis.

A full discussion of the synoptophore is outside the scope of this text, but its uses include:

• Measurement of the angle of deviation in the primary position (objectively and subjectively)
• Measurement of angle of deviation in up to eight positions of gaze, for incomitant deviations, including vertical, horizontal, and torsional deviations
• Assessment of retinal correspondence: fusion, stereoacuity, and simultaneous perception
• Assessment of aniseikonia
• Measurement of angle kappa (the angle between the pupillary and optical axes)

Accommodative convergence/ accommodation ratio

Determining the accommodative convergence/accommodation (AC/A) ratio may be valuable when determining management plans in patients with either a convergence excess esotropia or intermittent distance exotropia, to differentiate between true and simulated. This ratio is a measure of the amount of convergence induced (in prism dioptres) by 1 D of accommodation. This ratio remains fixed for a given individual throughout their life, unless altered by treatment such as surgery. A normal range is 3 : 1 to 4 : 1.

The AC/A ratio may be calculated via a number of methods; however, the ones most commonly used in clinical practice are as follows:

• **Gradient method:** This method can be performed with either near (in exo deviations) or distance (in eso deviations) fixation. With near fixation, a prism cover test is performed and then repeated with +3 lenses over both eyes to reduce accommodation. For distance, a prism cover test (PCT) is performed with and without −3 lenses to induce accommodation. The AC/A is then calculated by using the following formula, where *amount of accommodation exerted* = 3 D:

$$AC/A = IPD + (near\ PCT - distance\ PCT) / amount\ of\ accommodation\ exerted$$

• **Heterophoric method:** in this method, a PCT is performed with both near and distance fixation. The interpupillary diameter (IPD; in cm) must be known. The AC/A can then be calculated with the following formula, using a positive sign for eso deviations, and a negative sign for exo deviations, where *amount of accommodation exerted* is in dioptres:

$$AC/A = IPD + ((near\ PCT - distance\ PCT) / amount\ of\ accommodation\ exerted).$$

9.10 Assessment of ocular deviation

Examination for ocular deviation: cover tests

Cover tests are objective dissociative tests to elicit the presence of a manifest or latent deviation. They rely on the observation of the behaviour of the eyes whilst fixation is maintained and when each eye is covered in turn. They should be performed:

- At near fixation (0.3 m) with a:
  - Pen torch to observe corneal reflections (non-accommodative target)
  - Small picture or letter to stimulate accommodation (accommodative target)
- At distance fixation (6 m)
- At far distance fixation (>6 m if necessary)
- With and without any spectacle correction
- With and without abnormal head posture if present

Cover–uncover test

The cover–uncover test has two elements:

Cover test

The cover test looks for **manifest** deviations (heterotropia). One eye is covered with an opaque occluder, and the behaviour of the other eye is observed. If the uncovered eye moves to take up fixation, a manifest deviation is present.

Uncover test

The uncover test looks for **latent** deviations (heterophoria). One eye is covered, and then the same eye is observed as the cover is removed for any corrective movement.

Examination routine

1. Sit facing the patient so you are at eye level.
2. Observe the corneal reflections with a pen torch to see if there is any obvious deviation. If there is a manifest deviation, the corneal reflection from the pen torch will not been symmetrical in both eyes (see Figures 9.9–9.11).
3. Cover one eye with the occluder whilst the patient fixates the near target (pen torch, then accommodative target).
4. If there is no movement of the uncovered eye, then this eye has been fixing on the target and is therefore not deviating.
5. Cover the other eye and again watch the movement of the uncovered eye.
6. If the uncovered eye moves to take up fixation, a manifest deviation is present in that eye. The deviation is present in the opposite direction to the take up of fixation:
   - Temporal movement indicates an esotropia (convergent deviation; see Figure 9.9).
   - Nasal movement indicates an exotropia (divergent deviation; see Figure 9.10).
   - Downwards movement indicates a hypertropia (hyper deviation).

- Upwards movement indicates a hypotropia (hypo deviation; see Figure 9.11).
7. If no movement occurs with either eye, either there is no manifest deviation or there is eccentric fixation. Eccentric fixation may be noted whilst observing the patient's corneal reflections in response to a light; if fixation is eccentric, the reflections will be asymmetric.
8. If there is no manifest deviation in either eye, move on to the uncover test.
9. Again, cover one eye with the occluder whilst the patient fixates the near target.
10. Then observe the eye that is occluded as the cover is removed, for any corrective movement:
    - Temporal movement indicates an esophoria (see Figure 9.12).
    - Nasal movement indicates an exophoria.
    - Downwards movement indicates a hyperphoria.
    - Upwards deviation indicates a hypophoria.
    - When no movement occurs, orthophoria is indicated.
11. The test is then repeated for the other eye.
12. The cover–uncover test is then repeated whilst the patient fixates a distance target, e.g. a Snellen chart.

Information gained from cover testing

For a manifest deviation:
- Type and size of deviation for both near and distance fixation
- Speed for the eye to take up fixation; this measure is a good indication of the level of vision
- Effect of accommodation
- Nystagmus
- Incomitance
- Diplopia or suppression

For a latent deviation:
- Type and size of deviation for both near and distance fixation
- Rate of recovery to achieve binocular single vision and therefore fusion

Alternate cover test

The alternate cover test dissociates the eye to reveal the full deviation (phoria plus tropia). The cover is placed over each eye in turn at about 2-second intervals, and movement of the eye being uncovered is noted as the cover moves to the other eye. Patients with heterophoria may break down to a manifest deviation after dissociation during this test. Dissociated vertical deviation (DVD) and manifest latent nystagmus may also become apparent during cover testing. Orthoptists are expert in identifying and measuring ocular deviations, but ophthalmology trainees should learn to perform and interpret cover tests.

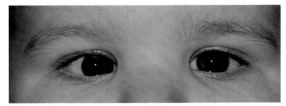

Fig 9.9 Esotropia, right eye

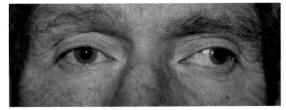

Fig 9.10 Exotropia, left eye

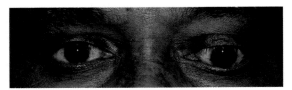

Fig 9.11 Hypotropia left eye

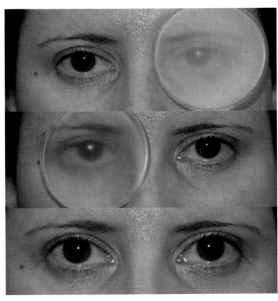

Fig 9.12 Cover/uncover test
No manifest deviation. The eye behind the occluder looks
convergent; therefore, as the cover is removed, the eye makes a
temporal movement (esophoria) to fixate

The aim of ocular movement/motility testing is to observe:
- The extent of movement of each eye in each direction of gaze
- The quality of the movement
- Signs and symptoms associated with defective eye movement

Examination of ocular movements

1. The patient is seated with the head upright. A child may need his/her head gently held by one of his/her parents. Any glasses are removed.
2. Sit in front of the patient at eye level.
3. Hold a pen torch 50 cm from the patient, at eye level.
4. Note the position of corneal reflections; a cover–uncover test is then performed in primary position.
5. The patient is asked to follow the light as it directs the patient's eyes into the six cardinal positions of gaze, up-gaze, and down-gaze, ensuring the light is still within the patient's field of vision (see Figure 9.13).
6. Observe any changes in position of corneal reflections and perform the cover–uncover test in each position of gaze to compare any deviation with that found in the primary position; in addition, observe the duction movements of each eye.

Features to be recorded

- Underaction/overaction: underaction is an insufficient version; the movement is full once the unaffected eye is covered (full ductions). Overaction usually occurs when the patient is fixing with the underacting eye.
- Up-drifts/down-drifts: one eye elevates/depresses on lateral versions; alternatively, or eye overacts/underacts in oblique positions
- Limitation/restriction: an insufficient or incomplete duction movement
- Quality of eye movement: note whether it is consistently smooth or becomes jerky or unstable
- Whether there is a gradual or sudden cessation in movement.
- The ability to sustain movement at limitation of gaze; is there any discomfort on movement or fatigue?
- Presence of end-point nystagmus
- Presence of pathological nystagmus
- Any lid or globe changes
- Presence of torsion; best seen by watching for movement of a conjunctival blood vessel or an iris landmark

Grading of ocular movements

Ocular movements can be recorded diagrammatically or with a written description; the record must include a method of grading the degree of underaction, either by classifying it as slight, moderate, or marked, or by using a numerical grade (see Figure 9.14); for example:

- Grade <−4: the eye does not reach the midline
- Grade = −4: there is no movement of the eye beyond the midline
- Grade = −3: there is only 25% of the normal range of movement into the position of gaze

- Grade = −2: there is only 50% of the normal range of movement into the position of gaze
- Grade = −1: 75% of the normal range of movement into the position of gaze
- Grade = 0: full ocular movements

The guidelines for recording overactions are less specific, and in general an overaction will be recorded as equal to the underaction of the contralateral synergist.

For the oblique muscles, there are some more specific guidelines:

- Grade = +1: vertical deviation present only in the field of action of the oblique
- Grade = +2: small vertical deviation on side gaze; the deviation increases in the field of action of the oblique
- Grade = +3: large vertical deviation on side gaze; the deviation increases in the field of action of the oblique but remains purely vertical
- Grade = +4: large vertical deviation on side gaze

Additional features recorded on diagrammatical ocular movements include:

- Limitations: indicated by a hashed line and then graded from −1 to −4
- Alphabet patterns: indicated by dashed lines in the vertical plane
- Down-drifts and up-drifts: indicated by sweeping arrows in the direction of gaze
- Downshoots and upshoots: indicated by right-angled arrows in the direction of gaze

Alphabet patterns

Alphabet patterns are horizontal deviations that vary in magnitude according to the vertical position of the ocular movement. The horizontal angle changes from up-gaze and down-gaze via the tertiary actions of the vertically acting muscles: the recti adduct and the oblique abduct (see Section 9.1). A and V patterns are primarily classified by the horizontal deviation in primary position.

Alphabet patterns are caused by a variety of aetiologies, such as abnormal muscle insertions, craniofacial abnormalities, vertical muscle dysfunction, and horizontal muscle dysfunction.

Measurements of alphabet patterns can be done with the PCT for distance, with the patient moving his/her head up and down 30° from the primary position; alternatively, the patterns can be measured with the use of a synoptophore.

Surgical management is indicated for symptomatic cases, for patients with abnormal head postures, or for cosmesis, depending on the underlying aetiology.

V pattern

In a V pattern, there is a relative divergence on up-gaze compared to down-gaze. A slight physiological V pattern is normal, so it is only considered clinically significant if divergence increases by 15 D or more in up-gaze.

- V eso pattern: a relative convergence on down-gaze compared to up-gaze; most commonly caused by unilateral or bilateral superior oblique underactions. The inferior oblique will overact, resulting in more abduction on elevation.

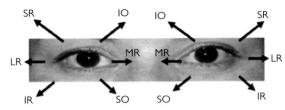

Fig 9.13 Extraocular muscles: positions of main action
IO, inferior oblique; IR, inferior rectus; LR, lateral rectus; MR, medial rectus; SO, superior oblique; SR, superior rectus

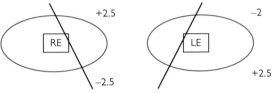

Fig 9.14 Right superior oblique palsy
Right superior oblique underaction (−2.5), right inferior oblique overaction (+2.5), left inferior rectus overaction (+2.5), and left superior rectus underaction (−2) with a V pattern; LE, left eye; RE, right eye

- V exo pattern: a relative divergence on up-gaze compared to down-gaze; is usually due to underaction of one or both superior rectus muscles, with corresponding inferior oblique overaction. It may also be associated with craniofacial abnormalities with shallow orbits.

A pattern

An A pattern is a horizontal deviation in which there is relative convergence on up-gaze and relative divergence on down-gaze, with a minimum of 10 D difference between the two.

- An A eso pattern is commonly due to underaction of one or both inferior oblique muscles.
- An A exo pattern is caused by underaction of one or both inferior rectus muscles and may lead to a chin-down head posture.
- Overaction of one or both superior oblique muscles is frequently seen.

Atypical variants

Other 'alphabet patterns' have been described but are less commonly of clinical significance:

- X pattern: relative divergence in up-gaze and down-gaze but straight in the primary position
- Y pattern: relative divergence on up-gaze but no difference between the primary position and down-gaze
- Lambda pattern: relative divergence on down-gaze with no significant difference between the primary position and up-gaze

373

Convergence

The near point of convergence can be examined and acts as an indicator of the strength of a patient's binocular single vision. A fixation target is placed about 33 cm in front of the patient. The patient is instructed to keep looking at the target as it is moved slowly towards them and to indicate when it becomes blurred, jumps, or appears double. The examiner looks for when convergence breaks and one of the eyes diverges again. The normal near point of convergence is around 6 cm. The RAF rule can be used for accurate measurement of the near point of convergence and accommodation.

9.12 Hess charts and field of binocular single vision

Principles

Hess charts are used in the investigation and monitoring of paretic deviations and are based on:

- Dissociation, either through a mirror or a different coloured image
- Foveal projection; therefore normal retinal correspondence must be present
- Herings and Sherringtons laws of innervation

If the two eyes are dissociated, it is possible to indicate the position of the non-fixing eye when the other eye is fixing in specific positions of gaze. A field is plotted separately with each eye fixing. Each point on the inner field represents fixation at 15° from the primary position, whereas the outer field represents 30° from the primary position. The Hess chart may not pick up defects present more than 30° from primary.

Hess charts can be a valuable diagnostic tool, but results must be interpreted alongside the assessment of ocular movements and the patient's binocular status. The charts are particularly useful for documenting changes over time and responses to any treatment.

Patients must have normal retinal correspondence and central fixation in order for interpretation to be accurate.

Methods

Hess charts can be plotted by dissociating the eyes in one of two ways:

Hess screen

A Hess screen consists of a screen displaying a tangent pattern on a dark grey background. Each small square subtends an angle of 5° at the 50 cm working distance. The patient should be seated squarely 50 cm from the screen, with his/her head centred on the central fixation spot. Dissociation is achieved by means of complimentary colours; the patient wears glasses with a red filter in front of the fixing eye and a green filter in front of the other eye.

The examiner projects a vertical slit of red light onto the screen from a red laser pointer. The red light can only be seen by the fixing eye (red filter). The patient holds a green laser pointer and is asked to superimpose their horizontal slit of green light (visible only to the non-fixing eye) onto the red light. The examiner plots a chart of the indicated positions for the non-fixing eye. In orthophoria, the two lights are more or less superimposed in all nine positions of gaze.

Lees screen

A Lees screen consists of two opalescent white screens placed at 90° apart, with a two-sided plane mirror at 45° between the two to dissociate the eyes (see Figure 9.15). The screens can each display a tangent grid as for the Hess screen. The examiner projects the grid on the screen for the fixing eye and indicates a point on the grid. The patient must use a pointer to indicate where on the other screen they perceive the point to be. The examiner marks the perceived point on the Hess chart to enable comparison between it and the expected point, which is noted as standard.

Interpretation of Hess charts

There are a number of basic rules for interpreting a Hess plot.

1. Compare the right and left field with each other.
   - The smaller of the two represents the eye with the defect.

- If one field is considerably smaller than the other, there may be recent-onset paresis. The size difference may lessen as sequelae take effect.
- Sloping sides to fields indicate an A or a V pattern.

2. Compare each field with the normal field represented by the grid.
   - Small field: the displacement in the primary position is the primary deviation.
   - Large field: the greatest negative or inward displacement represents the muscle with the primary underaction.
   - A positive or outwards displacement indicates an overacting muscle.

Hess chart characteristics of neurogenic defects

- Muscle sequelae are seen to a greater or lesser extent, depending on the duration of the condition; the size difference between the fields may lessen with time.
- The largest underaction is normally in the direction of action of the paretic muscle, and the largest overaction usually represents the contralateral synergist (see Figure 9.16).
- There is proportional spacing between the inner and outer fields.

Hess chart characteristics of mechanical defects

- The affected eye shows a compressed field (compressed vertically or horizontally; see Figure 9.17).
- Muscle sequelae are usually limited to marked overaction of the contralateral synergist.
- There may be no deviation in primary position; the deviation in primary does not represent the extent of the defect.

Possible problems that may be encountered

- Suppression; therefore unable to plot one field.
- Occasionally, the deviation remains controlled despite dissociation using the mirror.
- Gross limitations may prevent the patient from fixing on the points.
- Variable angle
- If both eyes have symmetrical ocular motility deviations, e.g. as in thyroid eye disease, the chart will only indicate the defect of the most deviated eye.

Field of binocular single vision

The field of binocular single vision is plotted on a perimeter to depict the areas of binocular field in which binocular single vision is

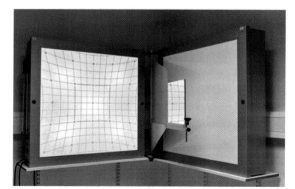

Fig 9.15 Lees screen

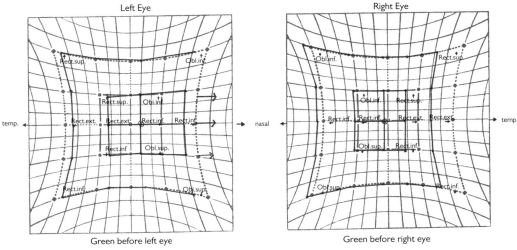

Fig 9.16 Hess chart for recent-onset right sixth nerve palsy
Obl. inf., inferior oblique; Obl. sup., superior oblique; Rect. ext., external rectus (lateral rectus); Rect. inf., inferior rectus; Rect. int., internal rectus (medial rectus); Rect. sup., superior rectus; temp., temporal

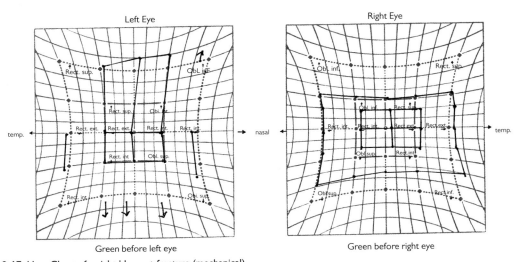

Fig 9.17 Hess Chart of a right blowout fracture (mechanical)
Obl. inf., inferior oblique; Obl. sup., superior oblique; Rect. ext., external rectus (lateral rectus); Rect. inf., inferior rectus; Rect. int., internal rectus (medial rectus); Rect. sup., superior rectus; temp., temporal

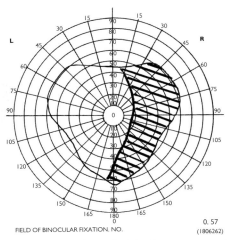

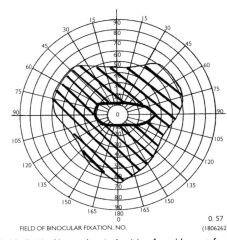

Fig 9.18 Field of binocular single vision for a recent-onset right sixth nerve palsy (hashed area = diplopia)

Fig 9.19 Field of binocular single vision for a blowout fracture (hashed area = diplopia)

maintained, and areas of diplopia. It is indicated for use in patients with diplopia but who are able to fuse the images in some part of the binocular field. It measures the field of binocular single vision in degrees and provides a permanent and repeatable record.

Method

The patient sits at the perimeter, at eye level, looking at a white target that subtends 2°. The area of binocular single vision is then plotted by moving the target from an area of single vision to an area of diplopia. Generally, diplopia is hashed; however, this is not the case in all centres.

Interpretation of the field of binocular single vision

1. Position of field: the field will be displaced away from the direction of maximum limitation of movement, e.g. the field of binocular single vision will be to the left for a right lateral rectus palsy (see Figure 9.18).

2. Size: the greater the limitation of ocular movement, the smaller the field of binocular single vision; field size may be influenced by a patient's amplitude of fusion. The better the fusional amplitude, the larger is the field of binocular single vision.

3. Shape: a narrow field of binocular single vision suggests a mechanical problem; e.g. a blowout fracture of the orbital floor, characteristically placed centrally (see Figure 9.19).

9.13 Amblyopia

Amblyopia is defined as defective visual acuity that persists after correction of the refractive error and removal of any pathological obstacle to vision. Amblyopia has an estimated prevalence of 1.2%–4.4% in childhood, depending on the defining criteria used. Prevention and treatment of amblyopia forms the majority of the workload of most children's eye services.

Aetiology and classification

Normal development of the visual system and central visual processing requires bilateral focused foveal images with retinal correspondence during a critical period lasting until around 8 years of age. Any interruption to such stimulation, for example deprivation of form vision or abnormal binocular interaction, can lead to amblyopia. The degree of amblyopia varies depending on the child's age and the severity of the interruption, with severe reductions in stimulation before the age of 2 years producing the most profound amblyopia. Amblyopia is usually unilateral, but bilateral degradation of visual stimuli may lead to bilateral amblyopia. Amblyopia can be classified as follows, and more than one type may be present in the same patient:

Strabismic
* Strabismic amblyopia is a consequence of abnormal binocular interaction in cases of constant or near constant strabismus and is always unilateral.

Anisometropic
* Anisometropic amblyopia occurs when there is a difference in refractive error between the two eyes such that one eye sees better for all distances. It is frequently associated with microstrabismus and can coexist with strabismic amblyopia.

Ametropic
* Bilateral amblyopia is the result of high uncorrected refractive errors which are typically more than +5.00 D or −10.00 D. This condition is due to visual deprivation and is more common in hypermetropia, as myopes receive some focused retinal images from near stimulation.

Meridional (astigmatism)
* Result of uncorrected astigmatism, where one or both eyes are predominantly astigmatic

Stimulus deprivation (vision deprivation)
* Occurs when no image or a degraded image forms at the fovea, e.g. because of congenital cataract or ptosis

Clinical diagnosis

Visual acuity
* Is reduced with no other detectable organic cause and despite full refractive correction
* The crowding phenomenon may be exaggerated: visual acuity is better with single optotype letters than with charts where letters are in rows or otherwise crowded.

Neutral density filters
* May help to differentiate amblyopia from organic causes of reduced visual acuity. Visual acuity is measured with and without the filter placed over the eye. Acuity is not reduced significantly with a given filter in the amblyopic eye when compared to the normal eye. In cases of organic amblyopia, the affected eye will have further reduction in visual acuity under poor illumination.

Management

Full correction of refractive error if present, with sufficient glasses adaptation time (up to 24 weeks) should be undertaken, as this approach may be sufficient to fully treat the amblyopia in some cases. Occlusion of the non-amblyopic eye, with either a patch or use of atropine penalization, to encourage use of the amblyopic eye is the mainstay of treatment. Ideally, amblyopia should be treated before the end of the sensitive period of visual development (around the age of 8). If picked up later than this point, it is still worth considering, as some children older than 8 and with no prior treatment have shown improvement. Patching should be instigated with caution in children older than 8 because of the risk of the development of diplopia. Not all children will respond equally to treatment, and some will not regain normal visual acuity following treatment. The aim of amblyopia therapy is to ensure the maximum visual acuity, because this condition can carry an increased lifetime risk of serious visual loss in the fellow eye through trauma or ocular pathology.

Prevention
Some countries now have screening programmes to identify reduced vision and strabismus in preschool children.

Correct remediable underlying causes
Amblyogenic stimuli, such as cataracts or ptosis, should be treated as soon as possible. Any refractive error should be corrected with full-time spectacle wear and adequate spectacle adaptation time allowed to occur in children with refractive and strabismic amblyopia. If the vision fails to improve during this time, occlusion or atropine should then be commenced.

Occlusion
Full-time patching is not usually required, and most parents cannot manage more than 3–4 hours a day. The amount of occlusion needed varies with:
* Age at onset of amblyopia
* Aetiology
* Age at presentation
* Severity of the acuity deficit
* Initial response to treatment
* Recurrence of amblyopia
* Compliance with prescribed treatment; at times may be challenging

Careful monitoring is essential, as excessive patching may induce amblyopia in the non-amblyopic eye in very young children (usually under 2 years of age) or dissociate poorly controlled latent deviations.

Atropine
Atropine 1% drops or ointment can be given topically to blur the vision in the better eye, thereby giving the amblyopic eye more stimulus. Atropine is prescribed for twice weekly use and is often used as a reserve treatment for children who do not comply with occlusion.

Atropine has been shown to be as effective as occlusion for patients with moderate and severe amblyopia. Advantages of atropine include the fact that patient cannot cheat, as cheating is possible with patches, and the fact that use of the drops is socially less obvious than use of a patch is.

Amblyopia therapy should be continued until:

- Optimum visual acuity is achieved; indicated by a lack of improvement in vision over two consecutive visits despite good compliance.
- Equal vision is achieved (does not commonly occur).
- Complaints of diplopia, or significantly reducing suppression, as measured by the Sbiza bar in children aged 7 and above. Occlusion must be monitored carefully to prevent intractable diplopia in this group.

The term **concomitant strabismus** describes cases in which the angle of deviation of the eyes remains constant in all positions of gaze. Such cases can be classified as heterophorias or heterotropias.

- Heterophorias are latent deviations that can be controlled by fusion when both eyes are open. Heterophorias may decompensate and become manifest in situations where fusion cannot be maintained or from the effort to maintain fusion; e.g. tiredness, illness, certain visual tasks, incorrect refractive error, medications affecting accommodation, alcohol use, or when the eyes are dissociated.
- Heterotropias are manifest deviations present even with both eyes open. The patient may have a variable degree of control over the deviation.

It should be noted that these conditions are not absolute; individuals may exhibit a heterophoria in one situation (e.g. distance fixation) and a heterotropia in another (e.g. near fixation). Heterophorias and heterotropias can be demonstrated during the cover test (see Section 9.10)

Heterophoria

Esophoria

Esophoria is a latent convergent squint. It is controlled by adequate negative fusional vergence (motor ability to diverge) so binocular single vision is achieved.

Esophoria may:

- Be larger for near vision than for distance vision (convergence excess), so symptoms are more likely to develop during close work than during distance activities
- Be larger for distance vision than for near vision (divergence weakness), so symptoms are more likely during distance activities such as watching TV or driving than during near activities.
- Not vary significantly between near and distance vision (non-specific)

The aetiology of esophoria includes:

- Accommodative and/or refractive errors.
- A high AC/A ratio
- Weak negative fusional reserves, demonstrated by a reduced ability to overcome base-in prisms
- Anatomical features such as a narrow interpalpebral distance, orbital abnormalities, and extraocular muscle abnormalities

Exophoria

Exophoria is a latent divergent squint. It is controlled by adequate positive fusional vergence (the motor ability to converge) so binocular single vision is achieved. As for esophoria,

it may be larger for near fixation than for distance fixation, or vice versa, and is demonstrated by the alternate cover test. Exophoria may:

- Be greater for near fixation than for distance fixation (convergence weakness)
- Be greater for distance fixation than for near fixation (divergence excess)
- Not vary significantly between near and distance fixation (non-specific)

The aetiology of exophoria includes:

- Accommodative errors and/or refractive errors, including myopia and anisometropia
- Divergence excess
- Relatively weak positive fusional reserves, demonstrated by a reduced ability to overcome base-out prisms
- Increasing age
- Anatomical features such as wide interpalpebral distance, orbital abnormalities, and extraocular muscle abnormalities

Hyperphoria/hypophoria

Hyperphoria/hypophoria is a vertical deviation which is demonstrable on alternate cover tests in which one eye rotates upwards and the other eye rotates downwards, depending on fixation.

Management of heterophorias

Heterophorias are asymptomatic in most cases, and binocular single vision is maintained by adequate fusional vergence. Hence, no treatment is required in the majority of cases.

Decompensation of heterophorias may be precipitated by an increase in visual demands, illness, or a change in refractive status or spectacle correction. Exophoria is more common with increasing age, and correction of presbyopia may sometimes precipitate the development of symptoms. Indications for treatment include asthenopic symptoms such as eye strain, blurred vision, headaches, and diplopia.

Management of heterophorias may include the following options:

- Correction of refractive error, particularly full hypermetropic correction in esophorias
- Orthoptic exercises to improve fusional amplitude, and convergence exercises in convergence insufficiency exotropias
- Prisms for small deviations (base in for exophoria and base out for esophoria)
- Botulinum toxin injections to horizontal recti muscles in cases of large deviations (the lateral rectus for exo deviations, and the medial rectus for eso deviations)
- Surgery to horizontal recti muscles for large deviations with persistent symptoms

9.15 Concomitant strabismus II: Esotropia

Esotropia is also known as manifest convergent strabismus.

Pseudo-esotropia

Some children presenting with suspected convergent squints do not have true strabismus but in fact have anatomical variations that mimic esotropias. Pseudo-esotropia may be due to:

- Prominent epicanthic folds
- Large negative angle kappa (the angle between the pupillary and optical axes)
- Narrow interpupillary distance
- Facial or lid asymmetry
- Globe or orbit abnormalities
- Enophthalmos
- Pupil abnormalities, e.g. corectopia

A pseudo-esotropia would show no movement of either eye on the cover–uncover test, and binocular functions would be present.

Classification of esotropia

- **Primary esotropia**: esotropia constitutes the initial defect; it may be intermittent or constant and may be non-specific or related to:
  - Accommodative effort
  - Fixation distance
  - Time (cyclic)
- **Secondary or sensory esotropia:** following loss or impairment of vision
- **Consecutive esotropia:** surgical overcorrection of a divergent strabismus

Primary constant non-accommodative esotropias

Infantile esotropia

Infantile esotropia is an esotropia presenting before 6 months of age. It may represent a neurodevelopmental anomaly, though association with other CNS abnormalities is relatively unusual. Clinical features include:

- No or low and usually hypermetropic refractive error
- Constant esotropia unaffected by accommodation
- Large alternating deviation present at all distances (although amblyopia is uncommon)
- Manifest latent nystagmus may be present later (a horizontal conjugate jerk nystagmus worsened by occluding the fixing eye).
- DVD may be present later on (DVD, an alternating upwards deviation of either eye on occlusion, can be asymmetric).
- No or slight limitation of abduction (bilateral congenital sixth nerve palsy is a differential diagnosis)
- Cross-fixation (where the right eye is used to fix in the left field of gaze, and the left eye is used to fix in the right field of gaze; can be seen on ocular movement testing)
- Asymmetry of optokinetic nystagmus (absent or defective nasal to temporal response)
- Inferior oblique overaction may be present

- A or V patterns may be present.
- No binocular function.

Treatment is surgical and in most cases should be performed under 12–18 months of age. Any amblyopia and refractive error should also be addressed.

Bilateral recession of the medial recti is the standard procedure for infantile esotropia. If DVD is present, inferior oblique or superior rectus weakening may be needed. Amblyopia treatment often needs to continue after surgery, as loss of alternating fixation may actually promote amblyopia.

Timing of surgery in infantile esotropia is controversial. Some experts favour early surgery before 6 months to encourage the development of binocularity, whilst others believe that long-term results improve when surgery is performed at around 4 years of age. Thirty to fifty per cent of children who undergo surgery under 1 year of age develop weak binocular single vision.

Management of infantile esotropia via botulinum toxin injections to both medial recti is also used in a number of cases. This procedure aligns the eyes and may allow sufficient development of fusion to maintain alignment in the long term. Evidence would suggest that botulinum toxin is most useful in patients whose angle is around 30 D.

Sudden-onset constant esotropia

A sudden-onset constant esotropia usually presents in patients over the age of 4 years. Diplopia may be the presenting symptom. The esotropia may be precipitated by febrile illness, a minor head injury, or a temporary occlusion with reduced vision in one eye. In these cases, neurological investigation may be required and optic discs must be examined. If neurological signs are normal, prompt surgical treatment or a botulinum toxin injection may restore alignment permanently.

Nystagmus block esotropia

Nystagmus block esotropia develops in children within the first 6 months of life. The esotropia develops as the patient adducts the fixing eye to dampen congenital nystagmus. Amblyopia is common.

Microtropia (or monofixation syndrome)

Microtropia is a unilateral squint of very small angle (10 D or less) in which some form of binocular single vision occurs. Anisometropia is thought to be the most common aetiological factor. It may not be detectable with cover testing. Microtropia with identity have a small heterophoria, whereas microtropia without identity have a small heterotropia. It is quite common (around 1% of the population). Clinical features are:

- Anisometropia
- Amblyopia in the affected eye (anisometropic and strabismic)
- Good or near-normal fusional amplitudes
- Abnormal retinal correspondence
- Reduced stereopsis
- Central suppression scotoma within the deviating eye prevents diplopia; may be detected with Bagolini striated glasses, with which a cross is seen with a gap at the point of intersection, or with a 4 D base-out prism test, as follows. A 4 D prism placed in front of a normal eye displaces the image to a point just temporal to the fovea, eliciting a refixation movement. In a micro-esotropic eye, the 4 D prism will displace the image into the parafoveal suppression scotoma, and no movement will be seen.

Management consists of correcting the refractive error and performing occlusion therapy to optimize vision in the affected eye.

Primary constant esotropia with accommodative element

Primary constant esotropia with accommodative element is a constant esotropia that improves but is not abolished when full hypermetropic correction is prescribed. It is also known as partial accommodative esotropia. Clinical features are:

* Onset 1–3 years of age.
* Moderate degree of hypermetropia with or without anisometropia
* Amblyopia
* Constant esotropia (usually unilateral) that persists with full hypermetropic correction.
* Binocular single vision that is poor or absent for both near and distance vision (depending on age of onset, size of deviation and retinal correspondence)
* Inferior oblique overaction
* Familial tendency

Initial treatment is with glasses prescribed to the full cycloplegic refraction, and treatment of amblyopia. There are three potential outcomes after glasses have been prescribed:

* Small-angle esotropia with abnormal retinal correspondence: no surgical treatment necessary
* Esotropia with suppression: if cosmesis is an issue, aim to surgically under-correct esotropia to reduce the risk of consecutive exotropia later in life
* Esotropia with potential for binocular single vision: aim for surgical alignment

Intermittent accommodative esotropias

Intermittent accommodative esotropias are the most common group of esotropias. Convergent strabismus is secondary to high accommodative drive, owing to one or both of the following:

* Uncorrected hypermetropia
* High AC/A ratio

Presentation is between 1 and 5 years of age. The esotropia is usually first noticed when the child views near objects. It becomes more apparent with tiredness or illness and may eventually become constant (see Figure 9.20).

Fully accommodative esotropia

Fully accommodative esotropia is an esotropia in which normal binocular single vision is present for all distances when hypermetropia is corrected. Clinical features are:

* Hypermetropia (>+2.00 D).
* Normal AC/A ratio
* Accommodation to overcome uncorrected hypermetropia stimulates convergence, thus resulting in esotropia.
* No esotropia when full hypermetropic correction is worn.
* Normal binocular single vision development if child wears appropriate spectacles
* Amblyopia is unusual unless anisometropic.
* Positive family history

Treatment is with full hypermetropic spectacle correction, and treatment of any amblyopia. Surgery is not needed; this approach must be carefully explained to parents, who may find it difficult to understand why surgical correction is not desirable.

Convergence excess esotropia

Convergence excess esotropia is a condition in which there is normal binocular single vision for distance fixation but esotropia on accommodation for near fixation because of a high AC/A ratio. Clinical features are:

* Low hypermetropia or anisometropia
* High AC/A ratio (higher than 5 : 1)
* Esotropia for near when accommodating
* Esophoria for near when fixating a non-accommodative target
* Esophoria for distance
* Amblyopia is rare
* Binocular single vision is reduced for near but normal for distance

There are two treatment options: bifocals or surgery. **Executive bifocals** have an intersection in which the visual axis is bisected by the top of the lower segment crossing the lower portion of the pupil. The upper segment should contain correction for any hypermetropic refractive error. The lower segment contains the minimum amount of extra 'plus' needed to relax the drive for accommodative convergence at near fixation, allowing the child to maintain fusion at near fixation (often started at +3.00 D). Once worn, the aim is to reduce the strength of the bifocal by 0.50 D every 6 months, until binocular single vision is achieved for both near and distance vision with single focus lenses

Surgery may be chosen if it is not possible to reduce the power of the bifocal segment, in cases of very high AC/A, or because of doctor/parent preference. Surgery consists of bilateral medial rectus recessions and/or posterior fixation suture (Faden suture), depending on the size of the deviation. It is important to emphasize to the parents that surgery may not always correct the convergence excess.

Other intermittent esotropias

Near esotropia

Near esotropia is a concomitant esotropia that is manifest for near vision but straight or latent for distance vision, with a normal AC/A ratio and insignificant refractive error. Differential diagnosis is convergence excess esotropia. Treatment is surgical with bilateral medial rectus recessions.

Distance esotropia

Distance esotropia is an esotropia that is present for distance only. It may be associated with age (70 and above) or related to myopia. The presenting sign is diplopia for far distance vision, either intermittent or constant. Over time, the esotropia increases and surgical intervention may need to be considered if prisms are no longer sufficient to maintain single vision. Differential diagnoses include sixth nerve palsy, divergence paralysis and convergence and accommodative spasm.

Non-specific esotropia

Non-specific esotropia is an intermittent esotropia that is not related to accommodation or to fixation distance. Fusion is present but may be weak. It may be seen in adults as well as children, although such a finding is unusual.

Cyclic esotropia

Cyclic esotropia is an esotropia usually affecting 3–6 year olds and which is intermittent in nature. The angle is equal for both near and distance vision, and the squint is manifest for 24 hours and then disappears for 24 hours. It has also been reported after a number of ocular procedures and invariably becomes constant. Treatment is with surgery (medial rectus recession and lateral rectus resection) before the esotropia becomes constant, with the aim of preserving binocularity.

Secondary esotropia

A **secondary esotropia** may develop because of vision loss or impairment in early childhood via congenital cataracts, macular scars, trauma, or optic atrophy. If it is not possible to improve the vision, treatment for psychosocial benefit and to correct ocular alignment can be achieved with botulinum toxin injections or horizontal rectus surgery.

Consecutive esotropia

Consecutive esotropia rarely develops spontaneously from primary exotropia and is mostly likely caused by surgical overcorrection of an exotropia. A small-angled esotropia is frequently the desired outcome following squint surgery for an exotropia. If significant esotropia occurs in the post-operative period after intermittent exotropia correction and does not resolve, then any diplopia may be managed with base-out prisms or botulinum toxin injections to the medial rectus muscle. However, further surgery is required if esotropia persists for more than 6–9 months and causes functional impairment.

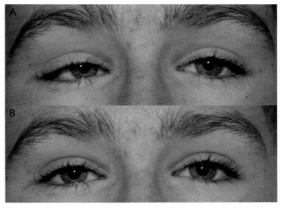

Fig 9.20 Intermittent esotropia
A Right esotropia when fixating an accommodative target
B Orthophoric when fixating on a non-accommodative target

Exotropia is a manifest divergent squint.

Pseudo-exotropia

Anatomical variations may mimic exotropias:
* Large positive-angle kappa
* Wide interpupillary distance
* Facial asymmetry
* Globe and orbit abnormalities
* Pupil abnormalities, e.g. corectopia

Classification of exotropia

* Primary exotropia: constant or intermittent; can be subdivided into:
  – Near, distance (true and stimulated), and non-specific
  – Secondary or sensory exotropia: following loss or impairment of vision
  – Consecutive exotropia: following previous esotropia, with or without prior surgery

Primary intermittent exotropia

Distance intermittent exotropia

Distance intermittent exotropia usually presents before the age of 2 years. The patient is asymptomatic but may be aware of an increase in the visual field or the sensation that the eye is diverging. Clinical features are:
* No amblyopia,
* Exotropia present for distance or far distance fixation, and binocular single vision for near
* The angle of deviation is greater for distance fixation than for near fixation by >10 D.
* Exotropia may be precipitated by daydreaming, tiredness, or bright light, and the child may close the affected eye.
* Hemiretinal suppression is present for distance to prevent diplopia.
* V patterns with underacting superior recti may be present.
  Divergence excess may be true or simulated, and the two types require different surgical approaches.
* In **true divergence excess**, the near angle is consistently less than the distance angle, and the AC/A ratio is normal. This type responds to bilateral lateral rectus recessions.
* In simulated divergence excess, the underlying angle is the same for both near and distance fixation but is partially controlled by accommodative or fusional convergence for near fixation. The near angle will measure less than the distance angle with both eyes open but, if +3.00 D lenses are placed over both eyes to interrupt accommodative convergence, or one eye is occluded to interrupt fusional convergence, the near angle increases. This type responds to unilateral medial rectus resection and lateral rectus recession in the diverging eye.

Near intermittent exotropia

Near intermittent exotropia typically presents in teenagers or young adults, with headaches, 'eye strain' symptoms, or diplopia for near vision. It may be due to a low AC/A ratio or associated with poor fusional convergence. Clinical features are:
* The near angle measures at least 10 D more than the distance angle does.
* Equal visual acuities but limited binocular function and poor convergence
* Associated with acquired myopia
* May become constant with time
  Any myopia should be corrected. Convergence exercises and base-in prisms may help control the condition. However, surgery may be required to preserve binocular function for near vision and distance vision; unilateral or bilateral medial rectus resection is the usual technique.

Non-specific intermittent exotropia

Non-specific intermittent exotropia is very similar to distance intermittent exotropia but the child intermittently manifests an exotropia of the same angle for both near and distance vision. Treatment, if needed, is usually with lateral rectus recession and medial rectus resection in the affected eye.

Primary constant exotropia

Primary constant exotropia presents early in life or may result from decompensation of an intermittent exotropia. Infantile cases presenting at <6 months are associated with a high incidence of ocular and CNS abnormalities. True primary congenital constant exotropia is quite rare. Clinical features are:
* Constant large angle for both near and distance vision
* Amblyopia may be absent if there is alternating deviation
* Binocular function generally absent depending on age of onset
* May be associated with facial and developmental abnormalities
  Treatment consists of botulinum toxin therapy or horizontal surgery.

Secondary exotropia

An exotropia may develop because of loss of vision in the diverging eye, usually in adults. If it is not possible to improve the vision, treatment for social and cosmetic benefit can be achieved with botulinum toxin injections or horizontal rectus surgery.

Consecutive exotropia

Consecutive exotropia can occur at any time after an esotropia but usually has a gradual onset, years to decades after surgery. Management is dependent on whether the initial aim for surgery is cosmetic or functional. If cosmetic, then further surgery may be required depending on the size of the deviation. If the initial aim of surgery is functional, and the deviation has not resolved, diplopia may be managed with base-in prisms, orthoptic exercises, or further surgery.

In **incomitant strabismus**, the angle of deviation differs depending on the direction of gaze or on which eye is fixing. It may be associated with restriction or paralysis of ocular movements in given directions. These conditions (congenital or acquired) have typical features depending on their underlying aetiology (see Table 9.6) and are often classified as:

* Neurogenic
* Mechanical
* Myogenic

Patients may have **ophthalmoplegia**, that is, paresis of two or more extraocular muscles.

Neurogenic disorders

Neurogenic incomitant strabismus may be caused by any pathology of the third, fourth, or sixth cranial nerves, or their nuclei (see also Chapter 10 for clinical evaluation, examination, differential diagnosis, and management). This type of strabismus may be congenital—for example, developmental hypoplasia of cranial nerve nuclei—or acquired following head trauma. Clinical features are:

* Ductions are greater than versions.
* Saccades are slow in the paretic direction.
* Full sequelae develop in agonist and antagonist muscles with time.
* The Hess chart shows proportional inner and outer fields. The smaller of the two fields indicates the affected eye, although the size difference between the fields may reduce with time as sequelae develop.
* Forced duction testing shows full passive movement, although antagonists of the affected muscle(s) may show contracture.

Mechanical disorders

Mechanic incomitant strabismus occurs when there is a mechanical limitation restricting eye movement in the affected direction(s). Clinical features are:

* Ductions and versions are of equal magnitude.
* Saccades are of normal speed but come to an abrupt stop at a point of restriction.
* Attempted eye movements may be painful.
* Intraocular pressure (IOP) increases with attempted gaze in paretic direction.
* The globe may retract on looking in the paretic direction (Duane retraction syndrome).
* The inner and outer fields of the Hess chart are compressed in the paretic direction.
* Forced duction testing shows reduced passive movement in the direction of limitation.

Causes of mechanical incomitant strabismus include congenital disorders such as developmental abnormalities, fibrosis, or adhesions of the extraocular muscles (e.g. Brown syndrome), or acquired causes such as trauma to the orbit, or extraocular or iatrogenic adhesions after previous surgery.

Myogenic disorders

Myogenic incomitant strabismus may be due to abnormalities in the neuromuscular junction or in the extraocular muscles.

Myasthenic

Myasthenia gravis, an autoimmune disorder of the neuromuscular junction, can cause ocular dysmotility of virtually any pattern. It may mimic other ocular motility disorders, but the dysmotility is characteristically variable and fatigable (see Chapter 10). Clinical features are:

* Fatigable ptosis demonstrated by sustained up-gaze of more than 1 minute, or rapid saccades
* Hess chart may show high variability.
* May have associated ptosis
* Full passive movement on forced duction test
* Cogans twitch: after the patient looks down for 20 seconds and then returns to the primary position of gaze the upper lid may initially overshoot
* May have systemic involvement

Myopathic

Inherited myopathies such as chronic progressive external ophthalmoplegia may cause gradual, symmetrical, non-fatigable loss of ocular motility. Other disorders of extraocular muscles, such as thyroid eye disease and myositis, generally cause a mechanical pattern of incomitant strabismus.

385

Table 9.6 Differential diagnosis of unilateral mechanical and neurogenic strabismus

	Neurogenic	Restrictive
Deviation in primary position	Depending on extent of sequelae, angle may be marked	Small deviation
Ocular movements	Ductions>versions	Ductions=versions
Saccade velocity	Slow in paretic direction	Normal with sudden stop
Sequelae	Full sequelae with time	Sequelae limited to overaction of contralateral synergist
IOP change	IOP may go up or down but stays constantly up or down; no change with direction of gaze	IOP increases in direction of limitation
Pain	None	Pain on ocular movements
Globe	No change	May retract on movement in direction of limitation
Hess/Lees screen	Inner and outer fields are proportional; the smaller of the two fields is of the affected eye	Inner and outer fields are compressed in direction of limitation
Forced duction testing	Full passive movement	Reduced passive movement in direction of limitation

IOP, intraocular pressure.

Mechanical (restrictive) disorders are caused by factors that interfere with muscle contraction or relaxation, or free movement of the globe.

Thyroid eye disease

Thyroid eye disease is an acquired disorder that affects the extraocular muscles in two phases. Initially there is an **inflammatory phase** in which they become swollen and infiltrated with inflammatory cells. Eye movements may be very variable in this phase but immunosuppressive treatment may be effective. This phase is followed by a **cicatricial phase**, in which the inflammation subsides, leaving affected muscles scarred, fibrotic, and tight. This condition can lead to any pattern of ocular motility, but the medial and inferior recti are the muscles most commonly affected. Clinical features may include:

* Visual loss in extreme cases (optic nerve compression)
* Diplopia, depending on the extent of restriction
* Restriction of up-gaze (tight inferior rectus), with chin elevation for comfort
* Restriction of abduction (medial rectus involvement)
* A combination of vertical and horizontal restriction (inferior rectus and medial rectus affected)
* Restriction of depression (superior rectus restriction)
* Lid lag
* Lid retraction
* Normal binocular functions with abnormal head posture

It is essential to ensure that the disease is stable and that the patient is euthyroid for 9–12 months, before any squint surgery is considered. Until then, any diplopia can be managed conservatively with prisms or with occlusion, depending on the extent of involvement of the extraocular muscles. If orbital decompression is required, it must be done before squint surgery is performed.

The aim of squint surgery in restrictive thyroid eye disease is to improve function by maximizing the field of binocular single vision in the primary position, in down-gaze, and to each side.

Orbital blowout fractures

Fractures to the bony orbit can affect extraocular muscle actions in a number of ways by causing:

* Incarceration of muscles within a fracture (especially the inferior rectus in orbital floor fractures)
* Entrapment of orbital fibrous septae
* Haemorrhage or oedema of extraocular muscles
* Muscle ischaemia via a compartment-syndrome-type mechanism
* Damage to the nerve supply of the muscle

All patients sustaining an orbital fracture must be examined for ocular motility defects and diplopia. The most common defect is restriction of up-gaze (plus or minus limited down-gaze) via incarceration of the inferior rectus or, more commonly, the surrounding orbital fibrous septae in an orbital floor fracture.

CT scanning should be performed to identify the cause of the dysmotility. If required, fracture repair should be performed before squint surgery is undertaken. Extraocular muscle restriction after blowout factures often resolves spontaneously as soft tissue swelling reduces but, if diplopia in primary position or down-gaze persists beyond about 6 months after the injury, then surgery may be required.

Forced duction tests should be performed to identify the pattern of restriction. Strabismus surgery may be required to correct diplopia after blowout fractures.

Brown syndrome

In Brown syndrome, there is a limitation of elevation in adduction of the affected eye; this limitation is thought to be caused by a short superior oblique tendon sheath, although other aetiological factors have been reported. Brown syndrome may be congenital or acquired.

* Congenital: most cases; due to abnormal development of the superior oblique muscle/tendon or trochlea and often improves or resolves by age 12. A click or pain may be felt as the tendon moves through the trochlea.
* Acquired: due to trauma, surgery, or inflammation (e.g. rheumatoid arthritis, sinusitis)

Clinical features

* Moderate or marked limitation of elevation in adduction.
* Small limitation in direct elevation
* Muscle sequelae limited to the overaction of the contralateral synergist, the superior rectus
* V pattern
* Downshoot of the affected eye on adduction
* Small latent hypo deviation in the primary position
* Abnormal head posture: chin up, head tilt to affected side and face turned away from deviated eye
* Unilateral > bilateral
* Positive forced duction test

Differential diagnosis

* Inferior oblique underaction (full muscle sequelae)

Treatment is not usually required unless there is hypotropia in the primary position, in which case amblyopia may be present. Surgery is only performed in cases with a marked abnormal head posture, manifest deviation, or symptoms of asthenopia.

Congenital cranial dysinnervation disorders

Congenital cranial dysinnervation disorders comprise a group of congenital non-progressive disorders resulting from developmental errors in one or more cranial nerves or nuclei. Commonly recognized disorders include:

* Duane retraction syndrome
* Congenital fibrosis of the extraocular muscles (CFEOM)
* Moebius syndrome

Duane retraction syndrome

Duane retraction syndrome is a congenital 'miswiring' syndrome in which the lateral rectus is aberrantly innervated by the third cranial nerve, leading to co-contraction of the lateral and the medial recti and retraction of the globe on attempted adduction (see Figure 9.21). The sixth cranial nerve nucleus may be hypoplastic. This syndrome occurs more commonly in girls than in boys (60% and 40%, respectively) and in the left eye than in right (60% and 40%, respectively), although 20% of cases are bilateral. It accounts for about 1% of strabismus cases. There are two systems of classification for Duane retraction syndrome:

1. Brown classification (based on clinical findings):
   - Type A: convergent deviation with limited abduction > limited adduction
   - Type B: convergent deviation with limited abduction and normal adduction
   - Type C: divergent deviation with limited adduction > limited abduction
2. Huber classification (based on EMG recordings):
   - Type 1: limited abduction > limited adduction; the lateral rectus has little or no innervation on abduction but has some innervation on adduction
   - Type 2: limited adduction; the lateral rectus has innervation on both abduction and adduction, so it can abduct; on adduction, it counteracts the medial rectus, thus producing limited adduction and globe retraction
   - Type 3: limited abduction and adduction; the lateral rectus has little or no innervation on abduction but is innervated on adduction

Clinical features

- Amblyopia in about 20% of cases if strabismus is present.
- Limitation of adduction, abduction, or both
- Esotropia is most commonly seen in primary position but the patient may be exotropic or orthotropic
- Abnormal head posture: face turned towards direction of most limited movement
- Globe retraction on attempted adduction
- Narrowing of palpebral fissure on adduction, and widening on abduction
- Up- or downshoots on attempted adduction
- Usually suppress in lateral gaze, so binocular single vision is preserved in the primary position, and diplopia is rare

Differential diagnosis

- Sixth nerve palsy
- Localized inflammation
- Medial wall fracture
- Moebius syndrome

Systemic abnormalities

- Deafness: perceptive with associated speech disorders.
- Goldenhar syndrome: abnormalities of external ear, hemifacial microsomia, dermoids, and scoliosis; may have learning disability
- Klippel–Feil syndrome: short, webbed neck, decreased range of movement of cervical spine, low hairline
  The combination of Duane retraction syndrome, Klippel–Feil syndrome, and deafness is termed **Kirkhams triad**; Duane retraction syndrome plus Goldenhar syndrome and deafness is **Wilderwank syndrome**.

  Treatment of Duane retraction syndrome is not usually necessary unless amblyopia is present. Surgery is not usually undertaken but may be desirable for abnormal head posture, disfiguring up-/downshoots, severe globe retraction, loss of binocular single vision in the primary position, or manifest deviation in the primary position. Surgery is with a combination of horizontal muscle recessions; resections should be avoided as they may exacerbate the retraction. Parents must be warned that restoration of normal eye movements following surgery will not occur.

Moebius syndrome

Moebius syndrome is a very rare congenital syndrome of varying degrees of loss of motor function in the sixth through the twelfth cranial nerves. Ocular features are:

- Bilateral sixth nerve palsies: 50% of cases are esotropic in the primary position; cross-fixation may develop since convergence is intact.
- About 50% of cases have a horizontal gaze palsy.

Other features are:

- Lack of facial expression due to bilateral upper motor neuron seventh cranial nerve palsies
- Paresis of the ninth and eleventh nerves can cause feeding and swallowing difficulties; some affected children die in infancy.
- IQ usually low
- Abnormal digits

CFEOM

CFEOMs are non-progressive, rare, congenital eye movement disorders caused by dysfunction of the third cranial nerve.

- CFEOM 1 (autosomal dominant) causes bilateral restrictive ophthalmoplegia and ptosis, with impaired elevation
- CFEOM 2 (autosomal recessive) restricts horizontal motility and causes a large exotropia plus ptosis
- CFEOM 3 causes a variety of motility anomalies

Strabismus following retinal detachment surgery

Retinal detachment surgery may restrict ocular movements via direct damage to extraocular muscles or pressure on a muscle from an explant. This restriction often improves spontaneously,

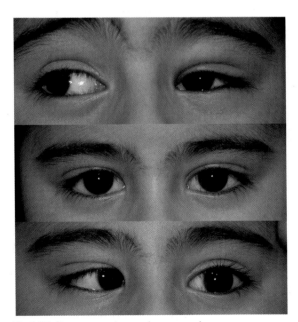

Fig 9.21 Duane retraction syndrome type A
Top photo: right gaze, showing left eye globe retraction, narrowing palpebral fissures, and slight limitation in adduction. Middle photo: shows primary position small esotropia. Bottom photo: limitation of left eye on abduction with widening palpebral fissures

but treatment with prisms, botulinum toxin injections, or surgery may be required.

Myopic restrictive strabismus

In large, highly myopic eyes, a progressive eso-hypotropia may develop where abduction and elevation become increasingly restricted. It has been proposed that, because the elongated globe is too long to fit into the muscle cone, it causes a downwards dislocation of the lateral rectus. The Yokoyama surgical procedure aims to restore the integrity of the muscle cone by joining together the muscle bellies of the superior rectus and the lateral rectus, with an optional medical rectus recession.

Strabismus fixus

Strabismus fixus is a very rare congenital condition in which the eyes are fixed tightly in convergence or divergence by fibrosis in and around the horizontal rectus muscles.

Surgical principles in management of restrictive strabismus

A number of principles should be borne in mind when considering surgery for restrictive strabismus.

- Differentiate restricted muscles from weak muscles by using the forced duction test.
- Always recess restricted muscles, as resection can reduce their action.
- Recession of overacting ipsilateral antagonists may also be required.
- Use adjustable sutures, as results may be unpredictable.
- Consider leaving restriction of up-gaze untreated if there is no deviation in the primary position.
- Problems on down-gaze lead to disabling diplopia, e.g. when reading or walking downstairs, and need particularly careful evaluation and management.

9.19 Principles of strabismus surgery I

Indications for strabismus surgery

All patients presenting with strabismus require a full examination, refraction, and fundal check as part of their assessment. In some cases, further investigations may be needed to rule out an underlying neurological cause. Non-surgical treatments such as refractive error correction, prisms, and botulinum toxin injections should be considered prior to proceeding with surgery, which may be avoided in many patients. In children, amblyopia should also be addressed prior to considering surgery.

Surgery is performed for functional reasons and/or to restore normal ocular alignment. There are considerable psychosocial effects of having strabismus, and these can have a marked impact on the patient.

Surgical indications

* To promote or restore development of binocular single vision in children
* To eliminate diplopia or visual confusion
* To restore and maximize binocular single vision in patients in whom it was previously present
* Intolerance of glasses or prism
* Restoration of visual field
* Elimination or improvement of abnormal head posture
* Psychosocial function/vocational status

Preoperative considerations

Once non-surgical treatment has been maximized, full visual potential reached following treatment of amblyopia, and the deviation is stable over time, then strabismus can be surgically treated.

Squint surgery is usually carried out under general anaesthetic, since it is more comfortable for the patient and allows the anaesthetist to monitor and treat any episodes of bradycardia induced by the oculo-cardiac reflex (which occur quite commonly when extraocular muscles are pulled or handled).

Although each patient will have a specific surgical plan, certain techniques are common to many strabismus procedures:

1. Traction tests
2. Conjunctival incisions
3. Identification, hooking, and exposure of the muscle
4. Muscle suturing
5. Recess/resect techniques

Techniques common to most strabismus surgery

Traction tests

Passive forced duction test

A passive forced duction test is often performed prior to commencement of surgery but may also be done under local anaesthetic in adults. It is used to assess the passive range of movement of the globe when active movement is limited and to confirm the presence or absence of restriction.

* The eye is grasped with two pairs of toothed forceps at the limbal conjunctiva.
* The eye is moved as far as possible in the direction of interest.
* If passive movement is full, there is weakness of the muscle(s) moving the eye in that direction.
* Resistance and limitation of passive movement indicates restrictive pathology.

Forced generation test

A forced generation test is used to differentiate muscle paresis (partial weakness) from palsy by evaluating the amount of contraction force generated by the weak muscle. The test is done under local anaesthetic, as patient cooperation is required.

* The patient is asked to move the eye as far as they can in the direction of limited movement.
* The anaesthetized conjunctiva is gripped with toothed forceps, and the examiner attempts to move the eye in the opposite direction.
* If the eye can be moved but resistance is felt, there is muscle paresis.
* If the eye can be moved without resistance, this result suggests that there is a palsy of the muscle.

Conjunctival limbal incisions

The conjunctiva and Tenons capsule fuse together 1.0–2.0 mm from the limbus. Tenons capsule is thick in children and becomes progressively thinner during adulthood such that it is barely identifiable in the elderly

* Identify the site of incision, which will usually be 10 or 2 o'clock for horizontal recti.
* Use a pair of non-toothed forceps (Moorfields) to grip the conjunctiva.
* Make a small radial incision with a pair of spring scissors through the conjunctiva and Tenons capsule down to the sclera.
* Use blunt dissection to open the sub-Tenons space and extend the incision round the limbus.
* Enlarge the superior radial incision and make a further radial incision inferiorly.
* Open the sub-Tenons space above and below the muscle.

Identification, hooking, and exposure of the muscle

* Under direct vision, identify the borders of the rectus muscle insertion.
* Pass a round-bodied squint hook into the opening created in the sub-Tenons space and slide underneath the muscle, just posterior to the insertion. Aim for the tip of the squint hook to emerge just posterior to the opposite border of the muscle into the other opening you have created.
* Clean off any Tenons capsule that has got hooked from the tip of the hook until the edge of the muscle is visible.
* Replace the squint hook with a Chavasse hook to spread the muscle.
* Lift the conjunctiva from the muscle with a pair of non-toothed forceps.
* Remove any adhesions of Tenons capsule from the muscle by using blunt or sharp dissection until the muscle is clean.

Muscle suturing

A number of different suturing techniques can be used and are preferred by different surgeons. These sutures can be either continuous or interrupted and are commonly used for straightforward rectus muscle recess/resect procedures.

Continuous suturing

- Use a double-ended 6-0 Vicryl suture, with quarter-circle needles.
- Place the suture through the middle third of the muscle with two passes, locking the second pass.
- Pass the needle from the middle to the outer third, partial thickness through the muscle.
- Make another two similar passes, full thickness, locking the suture each time.
- This process then needs to be repeated on the other side of the muscle.
- The muscle is now ready to disinsert.

Interrupted suturing

- Use a double-ended 6-0 Vicryl suture, with quarter-circle needles, cut in half.
- Pass the needle from the middle to the outer third, partial thickness through the muscle.
- Make another two similar passes, full thickness, locking the suture each time.
- Tie a knot to secure the suture.
- This procedure then needs to be repeated on the other side of the muscle.
- The muscle is now ready to disinsert.

Recess/resect techniques

Recess/resect techniques are most commonly used to weaken the medial rectus and strengthen the lateral rectus in esotropias or to weaken the lateral rectus and strengthen the medial rectus in exotropias.

Recession

For recession, the muscle is detached at its insertion and moved posteriorly towards its origin. The amount of recession is dependent on the preoperative size of the deviation.

- Once the muscle has been secured by the suture, it can be detached from its insertion using spring scissors.
- The desired amount of recession is measured with calipers and marked on the sclera.
- The muscle is resutured onto the sclera at the marked distance posterior to the original insertion, with interrupted sutures or, alternatively, secured with hang-back sutures to its initial insertion, where an adjustable technique can be utilized (see Figure 9.22).
- The conjunctiva is closed with 8-0 Vicryl.

This technique can be adapted to both the inferior and the superior rectus to treat hypo/hypertropia.

Resection

Resection involves the excision of a length of a rectus muscle, hence shortening it and strengthening its action. It should be avoided in strabismus with restrictive aetiology such as occurs in thyroid eye disease and Duane retraction syndrome.

- The muscle is identified and cleaned as previously described.
- A second Chavasse hook is placed under the muscle and moved away from the insertion.
- The desired amount of resection is measured with calipers and marked on the muscle.
- The muscle is sutured at this site with interrupted sutures unless an adjustable technique is used.
- The muscle is then diathermied or clamped near the suture and cut.

- The remaining muscle stump is removed from the insertion, and the resected muscle is sutured directly to the original insertion (see Figure 9.23).
- The conjunctiva is closed with 8-0 Vicryl.

Advancement

Advancement is used to strengthen a muscle that has previously been recessed if the patient subsequently develops a consecutive deviation; for example, medial rectus advancement for consecutive exotropia following medial rectus recession for childhood esotropia.

The muscle is identified in its recessed position, and the insertion moved anteriorly. It should be noted when calculating the amount of surgery to be performed that advancement has a slightly greater effect and may also need to be combined with resection of the muscle if a pseudotendon is present. Thus, a repeat calculation may be required perioperatively, depending on findings. This procedure is often paired with a recession of antagonist muscle on an adjustable suture, which allows postoperative modification if necessary.

Transposition procedures

A number of procedures have been devised that transpose rectus muscles away from their usual positions and utilize them to do some of the work of another weak or paretic muscle. Transposition techniques are for weak muscles and do not overcome limitations of movement that are restrictive in aetiology. Transposition procedures can be combined with recessions and it should be noted that if three muscles are operated on, there is a significant risk of anterior segment ischaemia.

Vertical muscle transposition to improve abduction

Vertical muscle transposition to improve abduction may be used to treat conditions such as sixth nerve palsy. Transposition procedures are only indicated if there is no abduction past the midline, or worse.

- The superior and inferior recti are identified and secured with sutures.
- Both muscles are disinserted and transposed to the upper and lower border of the lateral rectus.

Modifications

- Toxin transposition: the vertical recti are transposed and the medial rectus is weakened with botulinum toxin
- Hummelsheim procedure: the muscles are split and only the lateral halves of the superior and the inferior recti are disinserted and reattached to the superior and inferior margins of the paretic lateral rectus muscle. The medial rectus may also be recessed.
- Jensen procedure: the superior and inferior recti are split along their lengths and attached to the belly of the lateral rectus, which is also split lengthways. The medial rectus must also be recessed.

Vertical transpositions can also be used to try and reduce an abnormal head posture associated with Duane syndrome. Surgery in this condition is, however, extremely unpredictable.

Horizontal muscle transposition

To improve elevation

Horizontal muscle transposition may be used to treat such conditions as double elevator palsy.

- Knapp procedure: the horizontal recti are disinserted and transposed upwards to the superior rectus insertion.

To improve depression

- Inverse Knapp procedure: the horizontal recti are disinserted and transposed downwards to the inferior rectus insertion.

Weakening procedures not affecting primary position

In certain incomitant situations, it may be desirable to weaken or limit a muscle in its direction of action, without affecting primary position. A Faden procedure (posterior fixation suture) and a Scott procedure can be used for this purpose

Faden procedure, or posterior fixation suture

In a Faden procedure, a non-absorbable suture is passed through the belly of the muscle and tethers it to the sclera in a post-equatorial position. This suture should have no effect in the primary position, but the muscle action becomes progressively weaker as it moves into its direction of action. The suture should be passed 15.0–18.0 mm posterior to the limbus for the medial and inferior recti, and 18.0–24.0 mm for the lateral and superior recti.

Indications

- The medial recti in convergence excess esotropia.
- The contralateral inferior rectus after blowout fracture if there is persistent diplopia in down-gaze despite good depression in the affected eye
- The contralateral medial rectus in recovered sixth nerve palsy if diplopia persists in abduction
- The contralateral medial rectus for diplopia on contralateral gaze following surgery for exotropia

Scott procedure

The Scott procedure achieves a result similar to that obtained via the Faden procedure by combining recession and resection of the same muscle; a portion of the muscle is resected but, rather than suturing it back to its insertion, it is recessed. This technique has the advantage that it can be done with adjustable sutures and modified post-operatively to avoid precipitating any deviation in the primary position.

Inferior oblique surgery

Myectomy and disinsertion

Both myectomy and disinsertion reduce the action of the inferior oblique muscle, in cases of inferior oblique overaction, without requiring reinsertion.

The inferior oblique is identified and hooked. In a disinsertion, the muscle is clamped and simply disinserted from its attachment to the sclera. In a myectomy, a portion of the muscle is also removed.

Inferior oblique recession

The inferior oblique is identified and hooked, and sutures are placed into the muscle. It is then disinserted and sutured at 'Parks point', which is 4.0 mm lateral and 4.0 mm inferior to the border of the inferior rectus. All three weakening techniques have similar efficacy.

DVD

DVD is often associated with infantile or childhood esotropia. It is commonly bilateral, and the most common surgical treatment for it is inferior oblique anterior positioning. The muscle is isolated and sutures placed; the muscle is then disinserted from its insertion and resutured at the lateral border of the inferior rectus, just adjacent to the insertion.

Superior oblique surgery

Harada–Ito procedure (Fells modification)

Superior oblique paresis with excyclotorsion commonly occurs with an acquired fourth nerve palsy, often following head trauma, and is frequently bilateral. To treat the torsion, the superior oblique tendon is split and the anterior half, sutured with 6-0 Vicryl, is advanced temporally and sutured to the sclera as close as possible to the upper aspect of the lateral rectus. Leaving the posterior fibres in place prevents an iatrogenic Brown syndrome from occurring.

Tenotomy

Tenotomy is the division of the tendon of a muscle to weaken the tendon's action. Posterior tenotomy of the superior oblique involves the disinsertion of the posterior 80% of the tendon fibres. It is used in A-pattern exotropia with superior oblique overaction, to weaken the depressor action of the muscle whilst preserving intorsion (which occurs in the anterior fibres). Free tenotomy of the whole superior oblique tendon is sometimes performed to treat Brown syndrome.

Tucking

Tucking is specific to the superior oblique and involves tightening a lax superior oblique tendon to improve its function. It is most useful for congenital superior oblique palsy. The tendon is identified and folded over; then, a non-absorbable suture is placed around the tuck to hold it in place. Care must be taken not to induce an iatrogenic Brown syndrome, but this can be checked for during the procedure using adjustable sutures.

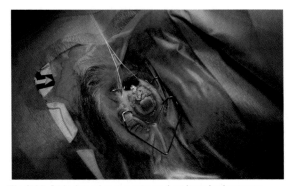

Fig 9.22 Right lateral rectus recessed on hang-back sutures

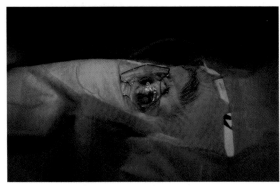

Fig 9.23 Right medial rectus resection

Serious complications are fortunately rare in strabismus surgery. Problems that may occur can be divided into preoperative, early post-operative, and late post-operative complications. The national British Ophthalmological Surveillance Unit audit suggests that serious sight-threatening complications occur in approximately 1 in 2000 strabismus procedures.

Surgery to wrong muscle

A clearly written preoperative plan that is agreed prior to surgery and reconfirmed in theatre during the WHO timeout check should avoid surgery to the wrong muscle. It may happen if a muscle is incorrectly identified during surgery. The potential risk is greatest when operating on the inferior oblique, as the inferior and lateral recti are in close proximity. This complication can be avoided by good exposure during surgery and by methodically identifying the adjacent muscles. As soon as such a mistake is identified, the operation should be reversed or other corrective procedure performed as required. This complication should be fully discussed with the patient post-operatively.

Globe perforation

Globe perforation is rare but may occur during muscle detachment or more commonly when resuturing muscles to the sclera. It can be avoided by careful technique and by the use of hang-back sutures during recessions if access for suturing posteriorly is difficult or the sclera is especially thin. If perforation occurs, dilated fundoscopy should be performed after the surgery to look for retinal breaks, and treatment should be administered as appropriate.

Haemorrhage

Some bleeding is common during squint surgery but it should be carefully controlled and rarely causes an adverse outcome. It can be minimized by preoperative administration of vasoconstrictor drops (adrenaline or phenylephrine), judicious use of diathermy, and careful avoidance of vortex veins. Inferior oblique surgery is particularly prone to haemorrhage.

Lost muscle

A muscle may be lost and retract back down its sleeve if it has no controlled attachments anteriorly; for example, if it slips off its sutures or if the body of a flimsy muscle tears. This complication usually occurs at the time of surgery, when it can be rectified, but may also occur in the early post-operative period. It is more common in redo squint surgery and with tight muscles such as in thyroid eye disease. A lost muscle can be extremely difficult to correct and requires urgent surgical attention.

Early post-operative complications

Immediate undercorrection

A small undercorrection is often the desired result with esotropia surgery and reduces the risk of consecutive exotropia. Unplanned undercorrections may occur for a number of reasons:

* The surgery performed was insufficient for the angle of the squint.

* Restriction due to scarred muscles, if this was not the first surgery to the eye
* A slipped muscle
* Ongoing excessive drive to squint, e.g. a high AC/A ratio.

Immediate overcorrection

A small overcorrection is often the desired result immediately post-operatively for correction of exotropia, to reduce the chance of redivergence over time. However, unplanned amounts of overcorrection may occur because of:

* Excessive surgery for the angle of deviation
* Resection or advancement of a scarred, tight muscle
* A slipped muscle
* Ongoing controlling drive despite correction of an intermittent strabismus, e.g. decompensated exophoria

The use of adjustable sutures in adult squint surgery greatly reduces the risk of unwanted surgical outcomes, as they allow modification on the day of surgery, following orthoptic measurement of the post-operative angle.

Diplopia

Despite thorough preoperative assessment of the risk of post-operative diplopia, some patients experience unpredicted diplopia after surgery. In the majority of cases, this condition settles over 48 hours. Diplopia may be due to an inability to suppress with the eye in different alignment or to unmasking of an unsuppressed area of retina. If it does not resolve, further treatment with prisms, botulinum toxin, or surgery may be indicated.

Infection

Inflammatory conjunctivitis is quite common after surgery but post-operative topical antibiotics usually prevent infectious conjunctivitis. Orbital cellulitis and endophthalmitis have been reported after squint surgery but are rare.

Anterior segment ischaemia

Anterior segment ischaemia occurs if the blood supply to the anterior segment is compromised when surgery is performed to three or more rectus muscles (with their associated anterior ciliary arteries). It presents with pain, visual blurring, corneal oedema and thickening, and anterior chamber flare. It is managed with topical steroids and analgesics but rarely persists, as the blood supply is restored within a few months by hypertrophy of the remaining long posterior ciliary arteries.

Later complications

Suture granuloma

Suture granuloma is a raised red area in the region of a suture. It is less common with modern absorbable sutures than in the past when catgut sutures were used. It may resolve with topical steroids but often requires surgical excision.

Residual, recurrent, or consecutive deviation

Patients or their parents should be warned when consented that consecutive deviations are common and may occur many years after the primary surgery. Reoperation may be needed if there is persistent over- or undercorrection.

9.21 **Other procedures in strabismus**

Adjustable suture techniques

Surgery with adjustable sutures is increasingly popular for operations to the rectus muscles in adults and cooperative teenagers. The amount of surgery performed is the same as for non-adjustable techniques, but the sutures are tied in such a way that the muscle can be manipulated under local anaesthetic post-operatively to adjust for any unexpected under- or over-correction. Once the eyes are in correct ocular alignment, the suture is tied off and cut, as would be the case at the end of surgery. Adjustable techniques are particularly useful in situations where the outcome may be unpredictable, for example:

* Nerve palsies
* Restrictive strabismus
* Reoperations
* Risk of post-operative diplopia
* Complex strabismus

Botulinum toxin in strabismus management

Injection of botulinum toxin into extraocular muscles is a useful and reversible tool in diagnosis and treatment of strabismus. It should be noted that, whilst widely accepted, these techniques are an off-licence use of the drug and should be given on a 'named patient' basis.

Indications

Diagnostic
Examples include the following:

* To assess the likelihood of post-operative diplopia following a positive post-operative diplopia test; an injection is used to mimic the effects of surgery temporarily to see whether symptomatic diplopia is induced
* To align the eyes to look for useful binocular function.
* To assess residual function in a paretic muscle

Therapeutic
Examples include the following:

* To improve the ocular deviation in a squint where no further surgery is possible or general anaesthetic contraindication

on medical grounds; injections need to be repeated every 4–6 months
* As a functional cure of strabismus in patients who have binocular function but have a motor cause for the strabismus, e.g. decompensating phorias, sudden-onset childhood esotropia
* To manage strabismus which is not stable in the long term, e.g. in early thyroid eye disease
* To treat small post-operative over- or undercorrections, with and without diplopia
* To treat deviations secondary to poor vision, either because the eye is likely to rediverge following surgery or in hypotonous eyes where surgery is contraindicated

Injection technique

* A number of topical anaesthetic drops are instilled.
* Electrodes are connected to the forehead to monitor an EMG signal.
* The patient looks in the opposite direction to that of the action of the muscle to be injected.
* The needle, connected to another EMG electrode, is passed towards the muscle via a transconjunctival approach (or transcutaneous for the inferior rectus).
* The patient is then asked to look in the direction of action of the muscle, and an EMG signal should be detected if the needle is correctly positioned in the muscle.
* The toxin is injected (2.5 units of Dysport® in 0.1 ml) and left in situ for 30 seconds to reduce the spread of the toxin.

Complications of toxin injection

* Ptosis
* Diplopia
* Spread to other recti, causing vertical deviations
* Infection
* Globe perforation (rare)

Development is a continual process that begins in utero and is related to the maturation of the central nervous system. Development is generally divided into the following areas:

- Gross motor: locomotion
- Fine motor : manipulation
- Vision
- Hearing and speech/language: cognitive
- Behaviour, personality, and play: social and personal

An infant will demonstrate primitive reflexes (see Table 9.7). As a child grows, these primitive reflexes give way to reactions and then definite actions and responses.

Development is a continuous sequence that is the same in all children, although the rate of development varies between children. Development occurs in a cranial to caudal direction and a proximal to distal direction, for example, head control, then sitting, and then standing. As an ophthalmologist, you will not be expected to have detailed knowledge of child development nor how to assess and examine development; however, it is useful to have some idea of some developmental milestones, as impaired vision can impact on all areas of development. Tables 9.8–9.11 contain the significant developmental milestones that can be seen or easily assessed in an ophthalmology clinic. Table 9.12 details the warning signs that should prompt a referral of the child for a full developmental assessment regardless of their ophthalmological problem.

Within the United Kingdom, all children will have several assessments in early childhood that screen for actual or potential developmental problems.

- Newborn examination: paediatrician, midwife, or GP
- Six-to-eight week check: GP or paediatrician
- Two to two and a half years: health visitor
- Five-year (school entry) height, weight, hearing, and vision: school nurse

Outside of these checks, children may also have contact with other health professionals, thus having additional opportunities for developmental assessment:

- Midwife: pregnancy to 2 weeks old
- Health visitor: 2 weeks to 5 years or reception class entry

Table 9.8 Normal developmental milestones: Vision

1–4 weeks	• Looks at faces, starts to recognize parents
6 weeks	• Follows object through 90°
3 months	• Follows object through 180° • Converges on near objects
6 months	• Visually attentive for far and near objects • Full conjugate eye movements • Watches small rolling ball 2.0 m away
12 months	• Sustained visual interest for near and far objects
2 years	• Letter-matching test, from 2 years and 6 months
4 years	• Letter-matching with each eye

Table 9.9 Normal developmental milestones: Motor

	Gross motor	Fine motor
3 months	• Lifts head and chest when placed prone	• Brings hands together in midline
4–5 months		• Reaches for objects
6 months	• Sits with support with a straight back • Will stand with legs straight and weight bearing if held up supported	• Mouthing (toys taken to mouth) • Passes toy from hand to hand
12 months	• Walks with hands held or by holding furniture (cruising)	• Casting (deliberate throwing) of objects/toys • Uses a pincher grasp
18 months	• Walks well; stoops down without over-balancing	• Looks at pages in book and turns pages
2 years	• Runs; climb stairs by using two feet per step	• Circular scribble
3.5 years	• Hops on one foot	• Copies drawing of a cross
4 years	• Climbs stairs by using one foot per step. • Stands on one foot for 5 seconds	• Holds pen with a tripod grip, i.e. mature pen hold
5 years	• Skips	• Copies a square

Table 9.7 Primitive reflexes

Grasp	• Tightly grasps finger or object placed onto palm
Moro	• Extends and then flexes arms and legs on being startled
Walking/ stepping	• Seems to 'walk' when soles of feet touch a flat surface
Root	• When lightly touched on the cheek, the baby turns his/her head in the direction of the cheek that was touched
Suck	• The baby sucks when an object is placed in his/her mouth
Atonic neck	• Fencers posture when the head turned to one side

Table 9.10 Normal developmental milestones: Behaviour and play

6 weeks	• Social smile
6 months	• Plays 'peek-a-boo'
12 months	• Drinks from cup with help and holds spoon
18 months	• Drinks from cup and uses spoon
3.5 years	• Dresses with help
4 years	• Dresses on own; can do up buttons

Table 9.11	Normal developmental milestones: Hearing, speech, and language
1–4 weeks	• Startled by sudden loud noises
6 months	• Turns to parent's voice across a room
	• Tuneful babble; single and double syllables
12 months	• Babble sound, conversational
	• Knows and responds to own name
	• Waves bye-bye, can follow simple commands
18 months	• Has 6–20 recognizable words and understands many more
2 years	• Simple sentences formed of two or more words
3.5 years	• Uses personal pronouns
	• Knows some colours
	• Begins to understand concepts of size and number
4 years	• Uses full name
5 years	• Asks 'why', 'when', and 'how'

Table 9.12	Warning signs that should prompt referral for a full developmental assessment
At any age	• Excessive floppiness (hypotonia) or stiffness (hypertonia)
	• Marked asymmetry of posture, tone, or movements
	• Abnormal movements
	• Tendency to push head back and arch trunk
	• Parental concern about hearing
	• Regression or loss of any milestones
4 weeks	• Not fixing on mother's face
3 months	• Not fixing and following
	• Not smiling
	• Not holding a toy placed in hand
4 months	• Persistence of primitive reflexes
	• Poor head control
	• Not bringing hands to midline
6 months	• Persistent hand regard
	• Not interested in surroundings
	• Doesn't turn head to sounds
7 months	• Not reaching for toys
	• Not transferring toys from hand to hand
	• Not mouthing toys
9 months	• Not sitting unsupported
10 months	• No tuneful babble
12 months	• Not rolling or crawling
	• No pincher grasp
	• Hand preference seen before 12 months
	• Babbling not started or has stopped
18 months	• Has not stopped mouthing or casting
	• Not demonstrating wants/needs
2 years	• Walking unsteadily, not running
	• Poor social interaction, no imaginative play
2.5 years	• Not using two-word phrases
	• Does not understand simple commands
3 years	• Not using four-word phrases
	• Throws or kicks a ball but falls
4.5 years	• Cannot follow stories
	• Cannot follow several step commands
	• Unable to balance on one leg for 3–5 seconds

- School nurse
- GP
- Community/developmental paediatrician
- Hospital-based paediatrician: generalists and specialists
- Child and Adolescent Mental Health Services

Visual impairment and development

Visual impairment can impact on all areas of development, generally because learning is more challenging with visual impairment than without. However, it often causes a delay rather than a deficit or difficulty, as the child often catches up by school age. The caveat is, of course, whether the visual impairment is due to a condition that itself causes developmental delay. Generally, the more severe the visual impairment is, the greater the delay.

Visual impairment can also impact on the development of vision and result in a failure to achieve full visual potential. The aim of any input is to stimulate cognitive interest and to move the child from light perception to visual awareness.

For children with visual impairment, it is important to refer them to the local visual impairment team (VI service), to ensure early and appropriate input to promote development. Such a referral may be done even without a confirmed diagnosis or cause for the visual impairment. There should be an agreed policy within your local unit for referrals, but remember that the VI service is based within the education system and so you will need to obtain consent from the parents or carers to send the referral.

Concerns about development

If there is concern that a child may have developmental delay, the local community/developmental paediatrician or general paediatrician will be happy to accept a referral for a developmental assessment. Please do not forget to include details about the child's visual acuity and ophthalmological condition. Community paediatricians tend to be based at a central child developmental centre, although they may see the child at a health centre or clinic closer to the child's home. In some regions, the community paediatricians have merged with the acute general paediatrics service.

The Red Book

Each parent/carer is given a handheld record called 'The Red Book' (although the colour of the cover varies depending on the region) for their child by the midwife or health visitor within the first few weeks of the child's life. This A5-sized book contains useful information about the child, including vaccinations, height, weight, growth charts, and routine assessments. Many also contain tables that the family can complete about the child's developmental milestones. Parents and carers should be encouraged to bring this record book to all consultations, and health professionals should be encouraged to use information from within it and to add to it (a short (legible) note in the 'contact with health professional' section) for each consultation.

Special educational needs

Under the 1996 Education Act, a child has special educational needs if he/she has a learning difficulty which calls for special educational provision to be made for him/her. It does not matter what the cause of the learning difficulty is but causes can include visual problems, chronic medical conditions, and physical disabilities. A small minority of children with learning difficulties will require a medical assessment that will then form part of a **'Statement of Special Educational Needs'**. The medical assessment is usually carried out by a community paediatrician, but he/she may ask for reports from other health professionals involved in the care of the child. The Statement of Educational Needs is to ensure the local education authority provides the support the child needs in a suitable school. It is reviewed annually, so it is important to send copies of any clinic correspondence to the paediatrician if you see a child with a Statement of Special Educational Needs, including any child attending a 'special school'.

Vaccination schedule

For up-to-date information, please use:

1. 'The Green Book': http://immunisation.dh.gov.uk/category/the-green-book
2. The Health Protection Agency website: http://www.gov.uk/government/publications/routine-childhood-immunisation-schedule

9.23 Retinopathy of prematurity

Retinopathy of prematurity can lead to severe childhood visual loss, which is largely preventable. A number of severely premature babies will develop some degree of retinopathy of prematurity, but the majority resolve spontaneously without treatment and do not progress to severe disease. Screening and treatment of sight-threatening retinopathy of prematurity with peripheral retinal ablation is successful in preventing sight loss in the majority of babies.

Embryology

Retinal vascularization begins in the sixteenth week of gestation. Retinal vessels grow out of the optic disc as a wave of mesenchymal cells. Endothelial and capillary proliferation follows. Capillaries eventually form mature retinal blood vessels. The nasal ora serrata is vascularized by 32 weeks but the temporally portion is usually not vascularized until term and rarely before 37 weeks.

Pathogenesis

The pathogenesis of retinopathy of prematurity is not fully understood. One theory suggests that an initial hyperoxic stimulus after birth leads to vasoconstriction and irreversible cell death. The resultant ischaemia triggers the release of angiogenic factors, such as vascular endothelial growth factor (VEGF), which causes new, immature vascular channels to develop that do not respond to proper regulation. Although there are many causative factors, genetics play an important role, as babies of African origin are less likely to develop retinopathy of prematurity than white babies, whilst babies of Indian/Asian origin are more likely.

Epidemiology

Some retinopathy of prematurity is present in 66%–88% of extreme preterm babies, but most of these cases are mild (Stage 1–2). Severe disease (Stage 3 onwards) occurs in around 18% of extreme preterm babies, but only 6% reach threshold and require treatment. From 1985 to 1990, 5%–8% of childhood visual impairment was as a result of retinopathy of prematurity. In 2000, it had fallen to 3%.

Clinical evaluation of retinopathy of prematurity

The Royal College of Ophthalmologists have produced evidence-based guidelines for the screening and treatment of retinopathy of prematurity:

Screening criteria

- All babies less than 32 weeks gestational age or less than 1501 g (guidelines for best practice)
- Strongest evidence for babies less than 31 weeks gestational age or less than 1251 g

Screening protocol

- If <27 weeks: screen at 30–31 weeks
- If 27–32 weeks: screen at 4–5 weeks postnatally.
- If >32 weeks, <1501 g: screen at 4–5 weeks
- Weekly screening if:
  - Vessels end in Zone 1/posterior Zone 2
  - Any plus or pre-plus
  - Any Stage 3 disease
- Screening every two weeks in all other cases until criteria for terminating screening reached

Screening examination

- Dilate pupils with cyclopentolate 0.5% and 2.5% phenylephrine (allow 30–60 minutes)
  - Binocular indirect ophthalmoscope with 28 D lens, sterile lid speculum, and neonatal scleral depressor
  - RetCam digital imaging
  - Nursery staff present to assist and monitoring of vital signs
  - Determine presence of plus disease, zone, extent, and stage of retinopathy of prematurity

Retinopathy of prematurity grading

Retinopathy of prematurity is described:

- By severity: 5 stages
  - Stages 1 and 2 are considered mild.
  - Stages 3–5 are considered severe.
  - Stage 3 is the first stage that presents a significant risk of poor visual outcome.
- By location: Zones 1–3
- By extent: clock hours or sector quadrant
- By the presence or absence of plus or pre-plus disease

Retinal zones

- Zone 1: the area within a circle for which the radius is twice the distance from the disc to the macular
- Zone 2: the area extending concentrically from the edge of Zone 1 to the nasal ora serrata and to an area near the temporal equator
- Zone 3: the residual area temporal to Zone 2
  See Figure 9.24 for a diagram showing the zones.

Stages of retinopathy of prematurity

- Stage 1: fine thin demarcation line between vascular and avascular retina
- Stage 2: broad thick ridge; clear separation between vascular and avascular retina; ominous if Zone 1; consider as threshold if vessel engorgement present
- Stage 3: extraretinal fibrovascular proliferation; may be present on the ridge, on the posterior surface of the ridge, or anterior to the vitreous cavity (see Figure 9.25)
- Stage 4: subtotal retinal detachment beginning at the ridge; the retina is pulled anteriorly into the vitreous by the fibrovascular ridge
  - 4A: fovea involved (see Figure 9.26)
  - 4B: extra foveal (see Figure 9.27)
- Stage 5: total funnel retinal detachment

Plus disease

- Arteriolar tortuosity and venous engorgement of the posterior pole (see Figure 9.25)
- Iris vascular engorgement
- Pupillary rigidity and poor dilatation
- Vitreous haze (always an ominous sign)

Pre-plus disease
- Vascular abnormalities of posterior pole insufficient for a diagnosis of plus
- More tortuosity and dilatation than normal
- If seen early, is more likely to require laser treatment

Treatment criteria

Treatment for retinopathy of prematurity should be undertaken if any of the following indications are reached:
- Zone 1, any retinopathy of prematurity with plus disease.
- Zone 1, Stage 3 without plus disease
- Zone 2, Stage 3 with plus disease

Treatment for retinopathy of prematurity should be seriously considered if the following indication is reached:
- Zone 2, Stage 2 with plus disease

Treatment
- Usually transpupillary diode laser
- Near confluent burn width to entire avascular retina.
- Often up to 3000 laser burns per eye
- Treatment time 1–2 hours

Post-treatment review
- Five to seven days following treatment
- If failure of regression, re-treat within 10–14 days.
- Weekly review until signs of decreasing activity or regression

Termination of retinopathy of prematurity screening

If no retinopathy of prematurity is seen, screening can be stopped when vessels reach Zone 3 (not before 36 weeks). If retinopathy of prematurity is seen, termination of screening can occur if the following are seen on two successive examinations:
- Lack of increase in severity
- Partial/complete resolution
- Change in colour of the ridge from pink to white
- Transgression of vessels through the demarcation line
- Replacement of active retinopathy of prematurity lesions by scar tissue

No fundal view possible

It is extremely rare in the United Kingdom to find no fundal view visible on retinopathy of prematurity examination; however, if this is the case, an ultrasound B-scan should be performed and the following differential considered:
- Retinoblastoma (retinal mass on ultrasound)
- Familial exudative vitreoretinopathy (dominant family history)
- Incontinentia pigmenti (female, X-linked dominant)
- Norries disease (male, X-linked recessive)
- Congenital cataract (examination)
- Persistent fetal vasculature (unilateral, microphthalmia)
- Strabismus (up to 30%): observe during first year

Complications
- Retinopathy of prematurity examination in infants may cause apnoea, and retinal or vitreous haemorrhage. Topical anaesthetics may cause epithelial toxicity. General anaesthesia may have mortality because of systemic comorbidities.
- Cryotherapy may lead to anterior segment ischaemia, delayed rhegmatogenous retinal detachment, and cataract.
- Laser photocoagulation may cause anterior segment ischaemia or cataract. Five per cent progress to Stage 4 disease despite treatment at threshold level.
- Preterm babies are at a higher risk of strabismus and refractive errors (usually myopia).

Prognosis
- Functional visual acuity (4/60 or better) in approximately 85% at 9 years, and favourable anatomical outcome in approximately 90% at 2 years, with laser treatment at prethreshold levels.
- Untreated threshold disease is associated with unfavourable anatomical outcomes in 48% at 10 years.
- Vitrectomy in Stage 4A may prevent progression to Stages 4B or 5.

Further reading

1. Good WV, Early Treatment for Retinopathy of Prematurity Cooperative Group: Final results of the Early Treatment for Retinopathy of Prematurity (ETROP) randomized trial. *Trans Am Ophthalmol Soc* 2004 Dec; **102**: 233–48
2. Royal College of Paediatrics and Child Health, Royal College of Ophthalmologists, British Association of Perinatal Medicine, BLISS: UK Retinopathy of Prematurity Guidelines May 2008. London: Royal College of Paediatrics and Child Health, 2008.

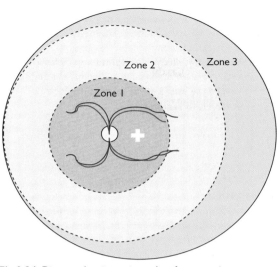

Fig 9.24 Diagram showing retinopathy of prematurity zones

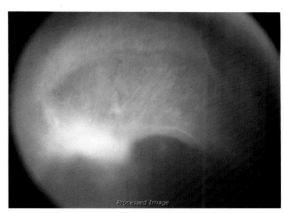

Fig 9.27 Stage 4 disease showing extraretinal neovascularization

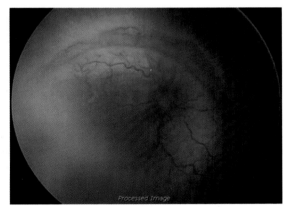

Fig 9.25 Stage 3 retinopathy of prematurity with plus disease, manifesting as posterior pole vascular dilatation and tortuosity

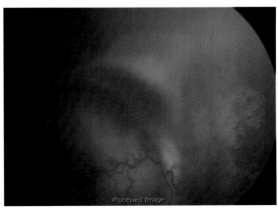

Fig 9.26 Stage 4 disease with laser scars in the avascular zone

Retinoblastoma is the most common primary intraocular malignancy in childhood.
* Age: birth to 5 years
* Sex: M = F
* Ethnic group: any
* Incidence: 1 : 15 000 live births

Care of a child with retinoblastoma and his/her family involves an intensive multidisciplinary approach involving ophthalmologists, paediatricians, oncologists, geneticists, specialist nurses and orthoptists, and counsellors. In the United Kingdom, retinoblastoma care is undertaken in two treatment centres: the Royal London Hospital and Birmingham Children's Hospital.

Aetiology

A mutation in both alleles of the *RB1* tumour suppressor gene (Chromosome 13q14) is required for the development of retinoblastoma (Knudsons two-hit hypothesis). In hereditary (germline) retinoblastoma, one mutant allele is inherited, and one normal allele subsequently undergoes mutation following conception. In nonhereditary retinoblastoma, both alleles are normal after fertilization, but spontaneous mutations subsequently inactivate both alleles.

The majority of the mutations in the *RB1* tumour suppressor gene lead to a truncated, unstable protein product and a consequent 50% reduction in the amount of retinoblastoma protein. Germline mutations in retinoblastoma protein and possibly other tumour suppressor proteins may result in retinoblastoma development in early life (with 80%–90% penetrance), osteogenic and soft tissue sarcoma in the teenage years (20%–30% risk), cutaneous melanoma and brain tumours in the fourth decade, and lung and bladder carcinoma in later life (60%–70% risk). The risk of a child developing retinoblastoma if the parent has a heritable retinoblastoma (germline mutation) is 40%–45%.

Pathology

Retinoblastoma cells are derived from neuroepithelial cells that have the potential to differentiate into rod and cone photoreceptors or Müller cells. A tumour arises from the retina and may invade the vitreous (endophytic growth), the subretinal space (exophytic growth), or the optic nerve. Tumour calcification and necrosis are common. The retinoblastoma cells are highly mitotic, forming retinal structures of increasing maturity (Homer–Wright rosettes, from neuroblasts; Flexner–Winsteiner rosettes, which are early retinal cells; and fleurettes, which are immature photoreceptor cells; see Figure 9.28).

Clinical evaluation

* Can the condition be something other than retinoblastoma (e.g. PHPV, cataract, retinal detachment)?
* Is there a germline mutation (implying that there may be a second malignancy, that siblings are possibly at risk, and that genetic counselling for heritability may be required)?
* Staging (to guide further investigation and treatment)

History

* Leucocoria (the presenting feature in 60% of cases)
* Strabismus (exotropia or esotropia)
* Painful red eye and/or swollen red eyelids with proptosis
* Hyphaema, hypopyon, heterochromia

* Family history of retinoblastoma present in 6% of all new cases. Family history of sarcoma, melanoma, and carcinoma also confer an increased risk of germline mutations.

Examination and staging

See Table 9.13.
* White intraretinal mass, multifocal or bilateral in 30% of cases
* Rubeosis, raised IOP, hyphaema, vitreous seeding
* Preseptal or orbital cellulitis, proptosis

Investigations

* Examination of both parents for retinoma/retinocytoma: a benign lesion associated with retinoblastoma and seen in disease-free relatives
* Examination under anaesthesia for detailed evaluation of both eyes
* Ocular ultrasound (see Figure 9.28)
* Perform an MRI of the head if suspicious of extraocular spread or if the intracranial pressure is raised, because of the possibility of trilateral retinoblastoma (bilateral hereditary retinoblastoma with intracranial neuroblastoma, most often pinealoma).
* CT should be avoided in patients already at increased risk of secondary malignancy because of the radiation used for it.
* Cerebrospinal fluid and bone marrow aspiration if extraocular spread suspected

Differential diagnosis

* Leucocoria: cataract, PHPV, Coats disease, toxocariasis, retinopathy of prematurity.
* Vitritis: pars planitis, endophthalmitis, leukaemia.
* Retinal mass: astrocytic hamartoma, capillary haemangioma.

Management

Screening of children of parents with heritable retinoblastoma and of siblings of patients

* Preimplantation genetic diagnosis
* Regular fundus examination (from birth to 4 years old)

Family and genetic counselling

* Identify germline mutations and educate regarding risk to siblings and potential later development of sarcoma, melanoma, or carcinoma
* Some 30%–40% of patients with retinoblastoma have a germline mutation. Those with a family history of retinoblastoma (parent or sibling) or multifocal/bilateral tumours will have a germline mutation. A family history of sarcoma, melanoma, carcinoma, or the development of a second tumour also suggests the presence of a germline mutation. 15% of sporadic unifocal unilateral tumours are due to a spontaneous germline mutation

Treatment

Treatment is dependent on the classification of the retinoblastoma at presentation.

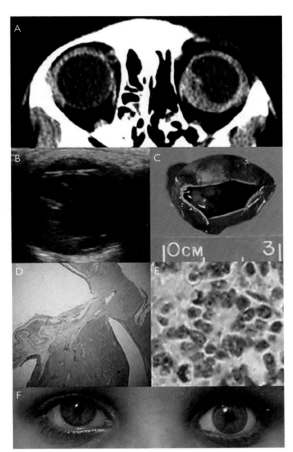

Table 9.13 The ABC classification will replace the Reese–Ellsworth classification, as the former is the based on outcome following current therapeutic approaches, and the latter on outcome from external beam radiotherapy

Group	Description
A	Small tumours away from foveola and disc
	• Tumours <3 mm in greatest dimension confined to the retina
	• Located at least 3 mm from the foveola and 1.5 mm from the optic disc
B	All remaining tumours confined to the retina
	• All other tumours confined to the retina and not in group A
	• Subretinal fluid (without subretinal seeding) <3 mm from the base of the tumour
C	Local subretinal fluid or vitreous seeding
	• Subretinal fluid alone >3 mm and <6 mm from the tumour
	• Vitreous or subretinal seeding <3 mm from the tumour
D	Diffuse subretinal fluid or seeding
	• Subretinal fluid >6 mm from the tumour
	• Vitreous or subretinal seeding >3 mm from the tumour
E	Presence of any one or more of these poor prognosis features
	• More than two-thirds of the globe filled with tumour
	• Tumour in the anterior segment or anterior to the vitreous
	• Tumour in or on the ciliary body
	• Iris neovascularization
	• Neovascular glaucoma
	• Opaque media from haemorrhage

Reprinted from *Ophthalmology Clinics of North America*, 18, Murphree AL, 'Intraocular Retinoblastoma: the Case for a New Group Classification', pp. 41-53, 2005 with permission from Elsevier.

Fig 9.28 This 4-year-old child presented with unilateral pan-uveitis and no fundus view. (a) CT and (b) ocular ultrasound revealed an intraocular mass arising from the retina, with no optic nerve infiltration. (c) Enucleation specimen showed endophytic chalky white retinal mass. (d) Microscopy showed basophilic cells infiltrating the retina but not the optic nerve head. Under high power magnification (e), retinoblastoma cells formed a Homer–Wright rosette, with the lumen filled with eosinophilic cytoplasmic processes. (f) Left prosthetic eye shell after enucleation

- Groups B/C/D: primary chemotherapy (carboplatin, etoposide, and vincristine) and focal consolidation with laser or cryotherapy. Plaque brachytherapy is also used.
- Unilateral tumours, Group C or better: primary chemotherapy with focal consolidation, focal laser, cryotherapy only, or brachytherapy
- Unilateral tumours, Group D or worse: enucleation
- Group E eyes: enucleation is used; if evidence of poor prognostic indicators (massive choroidal invasion and retrolaminar invasion), systemic chemotherapy should be used.
- If relapse continues, intra-arterial chemotherapy should be considered before using external beam radiation therapy. Intra-arterial melphalan is increasingly used with good effect; however, there can be significant local side effects (third cranial nerve palsy, vitreous haemorrhage, retinal detachment, orbital oedema, and changes in the retinal pigment epithelium) which may be temporary or permanent.
- Intra-vitreal therapy is considered a treatment that can only be given in a research setting at present.
- Orbital extension: primary chemotherapy with radiotherapy and delayed enucleation (rare in the United Kingdom).

Follow-up and monitoring
- Response to treatment may follow one of five patterns:
  - Complete disappearance
  - Complete calcification
  - Homogenous, semi-translucent 'fish-flesh' lesions
  - A combination of 'fish-flesh' and calcification
  - A flat chorioretinal scar with prominent retinal pigment epithelium hyperplasia
- The last three patterns require further focal consolidation.
- Side effects of radiotherapy:
  - Hypoplasia of midface
  - Cataract
  - Radiation retinopathy

— Retinal detachment
— Neurocognitive deficits
— Second malignancy

Complications and prognosis

* Survival rates are improving because of earlier diagnosis than before, prompt treatment, and reduced rates of treatment failure or tumour recurrence.
* Greater than 90% retinoblastoma-free survival is generally achievable.

* Group A and B eyes are salvaged in more than 90% of cases. Group C, D, and E eyes are salvaged in 70%, fewer than 50%, and 2% of cases, respectively.

Further reading

1. Muen WJ, Kingston JE, Robertson F, Brew S, Sagoo MS, Reddy MA: Efficacy and complications of super-selective intra-ophthalmic artery Melphalan for the treatment of refractory retinoblastoma. *Ophthalmology* 2012 Mar; **119**(3): 611-16
2. Shields CL, Shields JA: Basic understanding of current classification and management of retinoblastoma. *Curr Opin Ophthalmol* 2006 Jun; **17(3)**: 228–34

9.25 Congenital cataract

Bilateral congenital cataract is the most common cause of treatable childhood blindness. The management of congenital cataract is considerably different to that of acquired cataract in adults. The most critical difference is that congenital cataracts carry a risk of stimulus deprivation amblyopia and so must be treated urgently. The incidence is approximately 3 per 10,000.

Aetiology

Bilateral cataract
* Idiopathic
* Hereditary, with no associated systemic disease.
* Associated with ocular disease
  — Aniridia
  — Coloboma (lens and/or iris)
  — Peters anomaly
* Associated with systemic disease (see Table 9.14)

Unilateral cataract
The majority of cases are idiopathic, and association with systemic disease is uncommon. There may be an association with other lens abnormalities such as:
* Lenticonus
* Lentiglobus
* Persistent fetal vasculature

Clinical evaluation

History
History obtained from parents may include:
* Family history of congenital cataract
* Observation of a white pupil
* Squint
* Abnormality found at baby check (at birth and 6 weeks)

Examination
General inspection
* Presence of dysmorphic features suggesting a systemic association
* Leucocoria (white pupil; see Figure 9.29).

Visual function assessment
* Visual behaviour
* Objection to occlusion of either eye
* Formal assessment of vision (see Section 9.4)

Ocular examination
* Nystagmus
* Strabismus
* Red reflex, with a direct ophthalmoscope
* IOP, with a Tono-Pen, an iCare tonometer, or by air puff tonometry
* Corneal diameter
* Presence of congenital cataract in the fellow eye
* Coexisting ocular disease, e.g. PHPV, coloboma

Investigations
Paediatric referral to exclude underlying systemic disease is advised. Potential investigations include:
* Serology for intrauterine infections (a TORCH screen; see Table 9.14)
* Chromosomal analysis
* Blood sugar and calcium
* Urine tests; for reducing substances after milk feeding (galactosaemia) and for amino acids (Lowe syndrome)
* B-scan ultrasound for:
  — Axial length measurement (microphthalmia)
  — Biometry in children old enough to cooperate in preparation for surgery
  — Assessment of gross retrolenticular pathology if a dense cataract precludes adequate fundal view
* Doppler ultrasonography to assess for vascularized persistent fetal vasculature

Common morphological types

Nuclear cataract
* Located in the centre of the crystalline lens, in the embryonic and fetal nuclei
* Often very dense centrally
* Present at birth
* Non-progressive
* Bilateral in 80% of cases
* Autosomal dominant inheritance

Posterior cataract
* Associated with PHPV, posterior lenticonus, and posterior lentiglobus
* Abnormal retrolental vasculature results in abnormal posterior lens development
* Develops after 2–3 months of age
* Usually unilateral
* Sporadic
* Risk of posterior capsular defects and haemorrhage from abnormal vasculature during surgery

Lamellar cataract
See Figure 9.30.
* Opacity occurs in the layer between the nucleus and cortex.
* Bilateral

Table 9.14 Systemic associations of bilateral congenital cataracts	
Metabolic	Galactosaemia (oil droplet cataracts) Galactokinase deficiency Lowe syndrome Hypocalcaemia (diffuse lamellar punctate cataract) Hypoglycaemia
Chromosomal	Down syndrome (Trisomy 21; snowflake cataract) Turner syndrome Patau syndrome (Trisomy 13) Edward syndrome (Trisomy 18)
Infection	Toxoplasmosis Syphilis Rubella Cytomegalovirus Herpes simplex virus Varicella-zoster virus (known collectively as TORCH)
Medication	Steroids (e.g. long-term topical use for eczema)

- Progressive
- Autosomal dominant inheritance

Other less common types

- Sutural cataract (see Figure 9.31)
- Anterior polar cataract
- Blue dot cataract
- Coronary cataract
- Membranous cataract

Management

Management depends on cataract location, density, and laterality.

Visually insignificant cataracts

When the retinal vasculature is visible though the central portion of a cataract, it may be considered visually insignificant.

- Bilateral cases can be managed with close monitoring.
- Unilateral cases can be managed with occlusion therapy (patching).
- Electrodiagnostic tests are useful in determining the effect of a cataract on vision.

Visually significant cataracts

Early identification and surgery is essential in order to prevent stimulus deprivation amblyopia. If untreated, visually significant congenital cataracts result in dense amblyopia. Surgery for cataracts identified at birth or shortly after needs to be performed at around 6 weeks. Bilateral cataracts should be removed individually in rapid succession (within 1–2 weeks) in order to prevent the development of amblyopia in the second eye.

Surgical technique for congenital cataracts

Surgical management of paediatric cataract is more difficult than adult cases for the following reasons:

- The small dimensions of paediatric eyes.
- The lens capsule is highly elastic, making continuous curvilinear capsulorrhexis more difficult.
- Significantly higher rates of posterior capsule opacification occur in paediatric eyes; thus, most surgeons perform both anterior and posterior capsulorrhexes.
- Post-operative inflammation is more pronounced.
- It is impossible to stop children from rubbing their eyes; therefore, tight suturing of both the main incision and the paracentesis is required.

Variation in surgical technique

Taking the above factors into consideration, there are several differences in technique when operating on paediatric cataracts as opposed to adult cataracts. The precise operative plan is determined in part by the age of the patient and the preferred practice of the surgeon, but variations include:

- Use of a high-viscosity viscoelastic such as Healon GV
- Soft lens aspiration, as phacoemulsification is not required
- Primary posterior capsulorrhexis
- Anterior vitrectomy to remove the anterior hyaloid face
- Tight suturing of the surgical wound and the paracentesis

Timing and choice of intraocular lens implant

In the past, intraocular lens (IOL) implantation was only performed as a secondary procedure in children. More recently, lens implantation has become commonplace in children over the age of 2 years. Many surgeons also implant lenses into younger children, often from 6 months onwards, but there is considerable variability of practice.

IOL power

The globe continues to grow until approximately 10 years of age. For this reason, it is normal practice to aim for a hypermetropic IOL prescription, which is initially corrected with glasses. This approach allows the child to 'grow into' the refractive power of the IOL, aiming for emmetropia when ocular growth is complete. Nomograms are available to predict the IOL power required.

Contraindications to IOL implantation

Microcornea, microphthalmos, and uveitis are contraindications to IOL implantation.

Complications of congenital cataract surgery

In principle, all of the complications of adult cataract surgery apply to paediatric cataract surgery. Some complications are exaggerated in paediatric eyes.

Posterior capsular opacification

Eighty per cent of paediatric eyes with an intact posterior capsule develop posterior capsule opacification. This condition can be addressed by performing a primary posterior capsulorrhexis and an anterior vitrectomy in young children and those children who are unlikely to cooperate with Nd:YAG laser capsulotomy. Posterior capsule opacification can recur despite Nd:YAG capsulotomy, and sometimes secondary surgical intervention is required.

Post-operative uveitis

Brisk inflammation following cataract surgery is more common in children than in adults, with a significant risk of posterior synechiae. Intensive post-operative topical steroids and regular cycloplegia are used.

Glaucoma

The risk of glaucoma is greatest in eyes operated in the first 9 months of life and in those that remain aphakic. Glaucoma may not develop for many years and thus lifelong monitoring is required.

Post-operative ametropia

Ametropia must be addressed immediately after surgery, especially in aphakic eyes. Parents should be counselled from the beginning regarding the lifelong need for glasses, in particular for reading, and bifocal/varifocal lenses should be used from the outset in pseudophakic eyes.

Further reading

1. Solebo AL, Russell-Eggitt I, Nischal KK, Moore AT, Cumberland P, Rahi JS: Cataract surgery and primary intraocular lens implantation in children ≤2 years old in the UK and Ireland: finding of national surveys. *Br J Ophthalmol* 2009 Nov; **93**(11): 1495–8

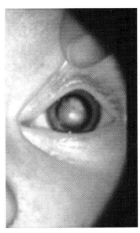

Fig 9.29 Leucocoria of the left eye
courtesy of GGW Adams

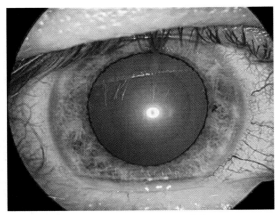

Fig 9.30 Congenital cataract: lamellar morphology
Courtesy of E Hughes

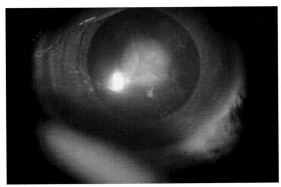

Fig 9.31 Congenital cataract: sutural morphology
Courtesy of L Amaya

9.26 Paediatric glaucoma

Paediatric glaucomas are classified as primary or secondary. Primary glaucomas are due to an isolated developmental anomaly of the angle, whereas secondary glaucomas are associated with other ocular or systemic abnormalities.

Causes of secondary paediatric glaucoma

- Aphakia
- Aniridia
- Peters anomaly
- Axenfeld–Reiger anomaly (see Figure 9.32; also see Chapter 8, Section 8.22)
- Uveitis (see Section 9.27 and Chapter 7)
- Sturge–Weber syndrome (see Section 9.28)

The diagnosis and management of paediatric glaucoma is very different from that for adults.

Clinical evaluation

History

Children may attend because of parental concerns that 'our child has a large eye', concerns about visual behaviour, tearing or 'squinting' with light, or a family history of glaucoma or an associated condition such as aniridia. The child with high IOP may be either asymptomatic or irritable and not feeding well.

Examination

- Assess visual behaviour and acuity.
- Look for strabismus or nystagmus.
- Assess external appearance: secondary glaucomas may have features such as a port-wine stain in Sturge–Weber syndrome.
- Measure the corneal diameter: a diameter >11.5 mm in a newborn is abnormal; buphthalmos, or global enlargement, occurs with increased IOP up to about 3 years of age (see Figure 9.33).
- Corneal examination: look for corneal oedema, and Haabs striae (breaks in Descemets membrane).
- IOP assessment: may need to use a device such as a rebound tonometer (iCare). In children old enough to cooperate, the slit lamp Goldmann tonometer can be used. If the child is crying or squeezing, falsely high pressures might be obtained.
- Optic disc examination
- Look for abnormalities of the iris, pupil, and lens.
- Perform gonioscopy and cycloplegic refraction.

Investigations

- Ultrasound measurement of axial length is useful for diagnosis and assessing progression.
- Pachymetry.
- Consider examination under anaesthesia. IOP measurement should be done immediately after sedation, as anaesthetics (except ketamine) lower IOP.

Primary congenital glaucoma

Primary congenital glaucoma (PCG) is the commonest glaucoma in infants. It most commonly presents at 1 month to 2 years of age.

Pathophysiology

Developmental arrest of the anterior chamber angle leads to a high anterior insertion of the iris and ciliary body, impaired aqueous outflow, and raised IOP.

Prevalence

- 1 in 10 000 births
- Sixty-five to eighty per cent of cases are bilateral.

Risk factors

- Ten per cent of cases are familial (autosomal recessive inheritance).

Clinical evaluation

- Triad of epiphora, photophobia, and blepharospasm

Examination

- High iris insertions on gonioscopy
- Sustained high IOP associated with increasing axial length and myopic change in refraction

Management

- Treat associated amblyopia and ametropia.

Medical treatment

- May be used preoperatively in PCG to help clear corneal oedema
- Children are at greater risk of systemic side effects than adults are.
- Brimonidine should not be given to children less than 6 years of age as it can cross the blood–brain barrier and cause CNS depression.

Surgical treatment

1. Goniotomy
   - Goniotomy involves incision of 90°–120° of the angle under direct vision using a gonioscopy lens.
   - This procedure spares the conjunctiva but requires the cornea to be relatively clear.
2. Trabeculotomy.
   - Conjunctival and scleral flaps are made, preferably in the inferior quadrants, and Schelmms canal is located.
   - A metal probe (trabeculotome) or suture is gently threaded into the canal and swept into the anterior chamber, rupturing the trabecular meshwork and the internal wall of Schlemms canal.
3. Trabeculectomy.
   - Trabeculectomy is used for secondary paediatric glaucomas or in PCG when angle surgery has failed.
   - There is a higher risk of high- and low- pressure failures and of intraoperative complications than in adults as children have more aggressive healing, thinner scleras and lower scleral rigidity compared to adults.
   - An anterior chamber maintainer should be used intraoperatively.
4. Tube surgery
   - Tube surgery is useful for refractory paediatric glaucoma.
   - Tube surgery is also indicated if future cataract surgery is needed and has an advantage over trabeculectomy in that it allows use of contact lenses in aphakia.

Aphakic glaucoma

Glaucoma is an important complication of congenital cataract surgery (whether the eye is aphakic or pseudophakic). The incidence ranges from 6% to 70% depending on a variety of factors including length of follow-up.

- Proposed risk factors include early age at surgery (especially during the first month of life), microphthalmos, microcornea, and surgical complications.
- Some cases are due to angle closure with pupil block, but for most there is an open angle and the cause of glaucoma is not known.
- Glaucoma may present many years after surgery, so lifelong follow-up is needed.
- If glaucoma develops, surgery is usually required.

Aniridia

Pathophysiology

Aniridia is a bilateral, congenital condition due to mutations in the *PAX6* gene on Chromosome 11. It may occur in isolation or in association with other syndromes. Glaucoma occurs because of a developmental abnormality of the drainage angle (synechial angle closure or trabecular meshwork abnormalities).

Prevalence

- Between 1 : 64 000 and 1 : 100 000 births.

Classification

- AN1: familial aniridia (autosomal dominant), no systemic associations, most common variant (two-thirds of cases).
- AN2: non-familial (sporadic), associated with Wilms tumour (nephroblastoma) in 30% of cases before the age of 5 (one-third are bilateral). Other systemic associations include mental retardation, genitourinary abnormalities, and craniofacial dysmorphism. The incidence of Wilms tumour is higher if these features are present than if they are absent.
- AN3: Gillespie syndrome; autosomal recessive, with mental retardation, ptosis, and cerebellar ataxia

Clinical features

- There is a spectrum of disease, from complete absence of the iris, partial absence, mild stromal hypoplasia (transillumination defects), to a normal-looking pupil. Even in total clinical aniridia, a peripheral frill of iris is seen with gonioscopy (see Figure 9.34).
- May present at birth with an absence of the iris (large pupil/prominent red reflex, nystagmus) or later in life with keratopathy. If glaucoma develops, it is usually in the preadolescent or early adolescent years.
- Aniridic keratopathy (20%): secondary to stem cell failure; results in progressive conjunctivalization and vascularization of the cornea, eventually leading to subepithelial fibrosis and stromal scarring, causing recurrent erosions, corneal ulcers, and pain

  Other features include:
- Symptoms due to iris deficiency:
  - Photophobia
  - Reduced vision
- Nystagmus: also due to associated foveal and optic nerve hypoplasia (10%)
- Cataracts: 50%–85% of eyes

Investigations

- Corneal impression cytology: conjunctival phenotype in epithelium with the presence of goblet cells
- Testing for mutation of the *PAX6* gene
- Pachymetry: aniridic eyes have corneas that are thicker than average.

Differential diagnosis

- Loss of iris secondary to trauma
- Stem cell failure due to chemical/thermal injury, Stevens–Johnson syndrome, ocular cicatricial pemphigoid, contact lens, surgery

Treatment

- Conservative management, e.g. goggles, a wide-brimmed hat, lubricants, a painted contact lens, tarsorrhaphy, and a bandage contact lens in the early stages
- Treat glaucoma medically (usually inadequate in most cases). Surgery may be required, often in the form of glaucoma drainage device insertion. Cycloablation may be necessary.

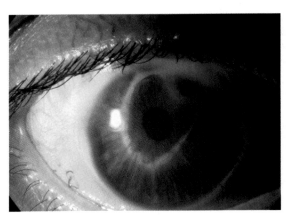

Fig 9.32 Axenfeld–Reiger syndrome
Courtesy of Prof A T Moore

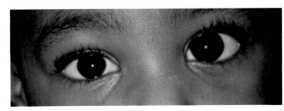

Fig 9.33 Primary congenital glaucoma with left buphthalmos
Courtesy of Prof Peng Tee Khaw

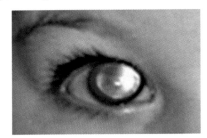

Fig 9.34 Total aniridia
Courtesy of J Brookes

- In the late stages of stem cell failure, kerato-limbal graft/ stem cell transplantation with/without a penetrating graft may be needed to restore vision.
- Cataract extraction can be combined with implantation of an iris prosthesis or a painted IOL, to reduce photophobia.

Peters anomaly

Pathophysiology

Peters anomaly is a rare disease in which patients are born with an opaque cornea.

Genetics

Most cases are sporadic (a few are autosomal recessive or autosomal dominant). Mutations described include those in *PAX6* (a gene associated with aniridia), *PITX2* and *FOXC1* (genes associated with Axenfeld–Rieger syndrome), and *CYP1B1* (a gene associated with PCG).

Clinical features

Peters anomaly is bilateral in 80% of cases.

Cornea

- Corneal impression cytology: conjunctival phenotype in epithelium, with the presence of goblet cells
- A central white opacity of variable density

- Iridocorneal adhesions at the margin of opacity, and a posterior corneal defect involving the posterior stroma/Descemets membrane and the endothelium

Lens

- Cataract, with corneal–lens touch or even with the lens in the normal position

Glaucoma

- Occurs in 50%–70% of cases
- Mostly infantile but can develop at any time of life; most cases have a normal trabecular meshwork

Other ocular abnormalities

- Microphthalmos
- Persistent hyperplastic primary vitreous
- Systemic abnormalities (developmental delay, congenital heart disease, CNS, genitourinary, etc.) have been described.

Treatment

- The main problem is amblyopia due to opaque cornea.
- Keratoplasty is required but has a poor prognosis.
- Manage glaucoma medically or with surgery; it is difficult to control.

9.27 Uveitis in children

Uveitis in children is uncommon. In 2003, the incidence in a UK district general hospital setting was 4.9 : 100 000. The most common cause of uveitis in children is juvenile idiopathic arthritis (JIA); however, infective causes such as toxoplasmosis underlie a significant proportion of cases. Management of uveitis due to infective causes is covered in Chapter 7. Masquerade syndromes should also always be considered in any uveitis in children, as it may be a feature of an underlying diagnosis such as leukaemia (see Table 9.15).

JIA

JIA is a chronic arthritis in children who are normally rheumatoid factor negative. The incidence of JIA in the United Kingdom is 1 : 10 000, and the prevalence is 1 : 1000. Disease may be oligo-/pauciarticular (four or fewer joints in first 6 months), polyarticular, or systemic (also known as Still disease). The prevalence of uveitis in JIA is 8%–30% overall but increases to 45%–57% in the oligo-/pauciarticular group. Females with pauciarticular disease and positive for anti-nuclear antibodies (ANAs) are at greatest risk of uveitis. Systemic JIA (presenting with fever, rash, and hepatosplenomegaly) is very rarely associated with uveitis.

Clinical evaluation

History

Uveitis is usually chronic, bilateral, and painless. Blurring of vision may be noticed incidentally, or the parents may notice a strabismus or altered pupil (synechiae or dense cataract). However, many cases are referred for screening by paediatricians. The lack of redness and pain and the unreliability of symptom reporting in children necessitate screening of JIA patients on the basis of risk.

Examination

* Cells and flare in anterior chamber
* Posterior synechiae
* Vitreous cells and macular oedema occasionally
  Later features:
* Band keratopathy (see Figure 9.35)
* Cataract (see Figure 9.36)
* Glaucoma or hypotony

Investigations

Refer to paediatrician if the patient has undiagnosed joint symptoms. Exclude other causes of uveitis (e.g. juvenile sarcoidosis, *Toxocara*, tuberculosis, human leukocyte antigen B27). Frequent review (at least every three months) in those with identified uveitis.

Screening

Because of the asymptomatic nature of uveitis in JIA, screening is necessary, and frequency depends on type, age of onset, and ANA positivity. Current recommendations from the UK Royal College of Ophthalmologists and the British Society of Paediatric and Adolescent Rheumatology include:

Table 9.15 Causes of uveitis in children	
Anterior	• Juvenile idiopathic arthritis
	• Human leukocyte antigen B27
	• Varicella
	• Kawasaki disease
	• Tubulointerstitial nephritis and uveitis syndrome
Intermediate	• Idiopathic
	• Toxocara
	• Lyme disease
Posterior	• Toxoplasma
	• Toxocara
	• Tuberculosis
	• Syphilis
	• Sarcoidosis
	• HIV
	• Behçets disease
Vasculitis	• Cat scratch
	• Systemic lupus erythematosus
	• Herpes simplex virus
	• Varicella-zoster virus
	• Cytomegalovirus

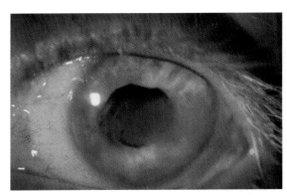

Fig 9.35 Band keratopathy from chronic uveitis in juvenile idiopathic arthritis

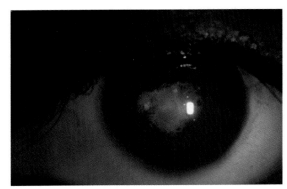

Fig 9.36 Extensive posterior synechiae and a white cataract secondary to chronic uveitis in juvenile idiopathic arthritis

Table 9.16 UK Royal College of Ophthalmologists and the British Society of Paediatric and Adolescent Rheumatology screening guidelines for juvenile idiopathic arthritis

Oligoarticular JIA, psoriatic arthritis onset, and enthesitis-related arthritic, irrespective of ANA status; age at onset <11 years

Age at onset	Length of screening
<3 years	8 years
3–4 years	6 years
5–8 years	3 years
9–10 years	1 years

Polyarticular JIA, ANA positive; age at onset <10 years

Age at onset	Length of screening
<6 years	5 years
6–9 years	2 years

Polyarticular JIA, ANA negative; age at onset <7 years

All children need 5 years of screening

Children presenting for the first time and aged >11 years

All children need 1 year of screening

ANA, anti-nuclear antibody; JIA, juvenile idiopathic arthritis juvenile idiopathic arthritis.
Data from Guidelines for Screening for Uveitis in Juvenile Idiopathic Arthritis (JIA) Produced jointly by BSPAR and the RCPOphth 2006

- Initially screening no later than 6 weeks after diagnosis of JIA.
- Subsequent screening should take place every 2 months for 6 months and then every 3–4 months, as guided by the clinical risk (see Table 9.16).
- Symptomatic patients or those suspected of having synechiae or cataract should be seen within 1 week of referral.
- Uncooperative patients should undergo an urgent examination under anaesthetic.

- Patient and parental education is essential owing to the asymptomatic nature of the disease.
- Treatment with methotrexate or other immunosuppressants may control the disease; however, cessation of treatment may precipitate a flare-up of uveitis. Screening should therefore take place every 2 months for 6 months after stopping treatment before reverting back to the screening regime based on risk.

On discharge from screening, the family should be reminded that ending screening does not mean the risk of uveitis is now 0%. Discharge from screening assumes that the patient is now capable of detecting any vision change which might signify a flare-up.

Treatment

- Topical steroids: mainstay of treatment (check IOP).
- Steroid-sparing agents:
  - Methotrexate
  - Ciclosporin
  - Mycophenolate mofetil.
- Anti-tumour necrosis factor alpha agents.
  - Etanercept
  - Infliximab
- Surgery for cataract, band keratopathy, and/or glaucoma

Further reading

1. British Society of Paediatric and Adolescent Rheumatology, The Royal College of Ophthalmologists: Guidelines for screening for uveitis in juvenile idiopathic arthritis (JIA). 2006. https://www.bspar.org.uk/DocStore/FileLibrary/PDFs/BSPAR%20Guidelines%20for%20Eye%20Screening%202006.pdf
2. Edelsten C, Reddy MA, Stanford MR, Graham EM: Visual loss with pediatric uveitis in English primary and referral centers. *Am J Ophthalmol* 2003 May; **135**(5): 676-80

Sometimes also known as the neuro-oculocutaneous syndromes, phacomatoses are a group of conditions consisting of ocular, dermatological, and neurological features. The term **phacomatosis** was first used in 1923 in a paper comparing neurofibromatosis with tuberous sclerosis and is derived from the Greek word *phaco*, originally referring to the multiple 'spotty' lesions associated with both conditions. There is no universally accepted definition of phacomatoses, nor is there a consistently accepted list of conditions; but the following syndromes are all commonly considered to fall within the category.

Neurofibromatosis type 1

Also known as **von Recklinghausen disease**, neurofibromatosis type 1 (NF1) is inherited in an autosomal dominant fashion with 100% penetration but variable expressivity. The diagnostic criteria are described in Box 9.1.

Ocular features

Lisch nodules

Lisch nodules are iris hamartomas which are seen as small, dome-shaped lesions that may occur anywhere on the anterior iris surface, including in the angle. They increase in number with age: they are seen in approximately a third of two-and-a-half-year-olds, half of five-year-olds, and almost all adults with NF1.

Glaucoma

The cause of glaucoma in NF1 is not completely understood. It occurs with increased frequency in individuals with an ipsilateral upper lid plexiform neurofibroma.

Other anterior segment features

Ectropion uveae, iris heterochromia, structural angle anomalies, and posterior embryotoxon may all occur and may also predispose to glaucoma. Plexiform neurofibromas may affect the upper lid and are classically described as feeling like a 'bag of worms'. Complete surgical excision is difficult, and the patient/parents should be warned that recurrence is common.

Retinal features

Rarely, astrocytic hamartomas or combined hamartoma of the retina and pigment epithelium can occur. Multifocal choroidal naevi, central retinal vein occlusion secondary to optic nerve glioma, and retinal haemangiomas have been reported.

Optic glioma

Optic gliomas are slow-growing tumours of astrocytic origin that can affect any part of the visual pathway. They can occur in isolation but have a strong association with NF1. The child may develop reduced acuity, optic disc swelling or pallor, and proptosis of the globe. Treatment consists of monitoring with MRI scans unless severe proptosis or pain is a feature, as surgery involves sacrificing the optic nerve. Chiasmal or midbrain involvement may be an indication for chemo- or radiotherapy.

Bony defects

Hypo- or dysplasia of the greater and/or lesser wing of sphenoid may occur, resulting in pulsating proptosis.

CNS involvement

As well as gliomas, intracranial vascular lesions are not uncommon. Sixth cranial nerve palsy, dorsal midbrain syndrome and headache may result. Neurofibromas can also affect other cranial nerves, causing isolated nerve palsies.

Neurofibromatosis type 2

Limited to the central nervous system, neurofibromatosis type 2 (NF2) was previously known as central neurofibromatosis. It is also autosomal dominant with high penetrance but is ten times rarer than NF1. The diagnostic criteria are described in Box 9.2.

Ocular features

Visual loss in NF2 has the added dimension that uni- or bilateral deafness is often a feature because of the presence of vestibular schwannomas.

Ocular features include:

* Lisch nodules: rare but have been documented in NF2
* Corneal hypoaesthesia: secondary to trigeminal schwannoma

Box 9.1 Diagnostic criteria for neurofibromatosis type 1 (National Institutes of Health)

NF1 is diagnosed if two or more of the following criteria are met:

1. 6 or more café-au-lait macules over 5 mm in greatest diameter in prepubertal individuals and over 15 mm in greatest diameter in postpubertal individuals
2. 2 or more neurofibromas of any type *or* one plexiform neurofibroma
3. Freckling in the axillary or inguinal regions
4. Optic glioma
5. 2 or more Lisch nodules (iris hamartomas)
6. A distinctive osseous lesion such as sphenoid dysplasia or thinning of long bone cortex, with or without pseudoarthrosis
7. A first-degree relative with NF1

NF1, neurofibromatosis type 1.
Reproduced from *GeneReviews*, 'Neurofibromatosis 1' (2014) with permission from University of Washington, Seattle, © 1993-2015. http://www.ncbi.nlm.nih.gov/books/NBK1109/. Accessed 12/06/2015

Box 9.2 Diagnostic criteria for neurofibromatosis type 2

Neurofibromatosis type 2 (NF2) is diagnosed if one or more of the following criteria are met:

1. Bilateral vestibular schwannomas
2. A first-degree relative with NF2 and either a unilateral vestibular schwannoma or any two of the following:

   * Neurofibroma
   * Meningioma
   * Glioma
   * Schwannoma
   * Juvenile posterior subcapsular cataract

NF2, neurofibromatosis type 2.
Reproduced from *GeneReviews*, 'Neurofibromatosis 1' (2011) with permission from University of Washington, Seattle, © 1993-2015. http://www.ncbi.nlm.nih.gov/books/NBK1201/. Accessed 12/06/2015.)

- Cataract: a feature in up to 87% of individuals with NF2; may present in childhood; most commonly posterior subcapsular or cortical in nature
- Lagophthalmos: secondary to facial nerve involvement
- Combined hamartoma of the retina and pigment epithelium
- Epiretinal membrane
- Cranial nerve palsies: most commonly third cranial nerve palsy but fourth nerve palsy and sixth nerve palsy have been reported.

Tuberous sclerosis

Tuberous sclerosis is inherited in an autosomal dominant fashion with a high spontaneous mutation rate. A high number of cases therefore do not have a family history. It has major and minor diagnostic criteria, which are described in Box 9.3. A diagnosis is confirmed if two major criteria or one major criterion and two minor criteria are seen. The presence of a single major criterion and a single minor criterion constitutes a probable but not definitive diagnosis.

Epilepsy, due to the presence of intracranial lesions, is a major feature of tuberous sclerosis. Any child with unexplained epilepsy, developmental delay, or learning difficulties should be investigated for tuberous sclerosis.

Ocular features

Retinal astrocytic hamartomas are seen in 50% of patients with tuberous sclerosis, and a third of these patients may have bilateral lesions. The lesions are most commonly flat, grey, and translucent and frequently overly retinal vessels; however, the classic, calcified, white, 'mulberry' lesion is seen in approximately 50% of patients with retinal involvement (see Figure 9.37). In 80% of cases, the lesion is located on or within two disc diameters of the optic disc.

Box 9.3 Diagnostic criteria for tuberous sclerosis
Major criteria
• Facial angiofibromas
• Ungual fibroma
• Shagreen patch
• More than three hypomelanotic macules
• Cortical tuber
• Subependymal nodule
• Subependymal giant cell astrocytoma
• Retinal hamartoma
• Cardiac rhabdomyosarcoma
• Lymphangiomyomatosis
Minor criteria
• Multiple pits in dental enamel
• Hamartomatous rectal polyps
• Bone cysts
• Cerebral white matter radial migration lines
• Gingival fibromas
• Retinal achromatic patch
• 'Confetti' skin lesions
• Multiple renal cysts

Vigabatrin therapy and monitoring

The epilepsy of tuberous sclerosis responds well to vigabatrin but this approach requires regular monitoring of the patient to identify significant visual fields changes that can occur with use of vigabatrin. The typical field change is bilateral concentric constriction beginning in the nasal field. Cooperative children should be monitored with perimetry (Humphrey 120° or Goldmann perimetry) every 6 months for 5 years and then annually. Children unable to perform accurate perimetry represent a challenge, as do uncooperative adults. Electrodiagnostic testing may be used, with cautious interpretation of the results.

Von Hippel–Lindau disease

Von Hippel–Lindau disease (vHL) is inherited in an autosomal dominant fashion with very high penetrance. It is rare, with an incidence of 1 : 35 000. The diagnostic criteria for vHL are described in Box 9.4.

Screening of patients with vHL is vital, as the lesions are progressive and may be treatable in early stages. The major cause of death in vHL is renal cell carcinoma (seen in up to 45% of patients by the age of 60 years) and CNS haemangiomas (seen in 70% of patients by the age of 60 years).

Ocular features

Retinal capillary haemangiomas are diagnosed by retinal biomicroscopy and fundus fluorescein angiography and can be classified descriptively into:

- Peripheral or juxtapapillary
- Endophytic, exophytic, or sessile
- Exudative or tractional

Treatment consists of observation only for non-exudative lesions that do not pose a threat to vision. Small (<1.5 mm) visually threatening lesions can be treated with laser photocoagulation, whereas lesions >1.5 mm may require cryotherapy. Anti-VEGF has been used with good results but does not yet form a mainstay of treatment.

Sturge–Weber syndrome

Sturge–Weber syndrome is a very rare, sporadically occurring condition affecting 1 in 40 000–50 000 live births. It is classified as:

- **Type 1:** Most common; patients have the classical facial capillary malformation ('port-wine stain') and intracranial

Box 9.4 Diagnostic criteria for von Hippel–Lindau disease
A diagnosis is made when there is a positive family history and any one of the following:
• Retinal capillary haemangioma
• CNS haemangioma
• Visceral lesion (includes phaeochromocytoma, renal cell carcinoma, renal or pancreatic cyst, islet cell tumour, or epididymal cystadenoma)
A diagnosis is made when there is a negative family history and any one of the following:
• Two or more retinal capillary haemangiomas
• Two or more CNS haemangiomas
• Single retinal or CNS haemangioma with a visceral lesion

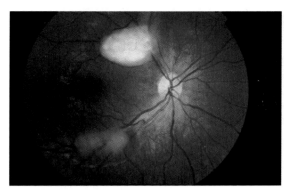

Fig 9.37 Retinal astrocytoma in tuberous sclerosis

Courtesy of Prof A T Moore

leptomeningeal vascular malformations; they may or may not develop ocular features.

- **Type 2:** Patients have a port-wine stain along with ocular features but no CNS involvement.
- **Type 3:** Patients have CNS lesions but no dermatological or ocular involvement.

The CNS lesions most commonly affect the occipital and temporal lobes and can lead to epilepsy, progressive mental retardation, contralateral hemiplegia, and/or hemianopia.

Ocular features

Glaucoma is relatively common in Sturge–Weber syndrome, occurring in up to 71% of cases. It is more likely to be seen in individuals with a port-wine stain affecting the ipsilateral upper lid. It is bimodal in presentation:

- **Early onset:** Considered to be due to trabeculodysgenesis.
- **Late onset:** Secondary to raised episcleral venous pressure.

Management of glaucoma in Sturge–Weber syndrome is challenging. Goniotomies are used in the early onset group. Standard medical and surgical management is used but requires close and careful monitoring (see Section 9.26).

Choroidal haemangiomas also feature in this condition. They may be localized to the posterior pole or diffuse; the latter type is commonly described as a 'tomato ketchup fundus' because of the diffuse, deep red discolouration seen across the entire retina. The lesions are slowly progressive in nature and may result in secondary degenerative changes in the overlying retina, and serous retinal detachment.

Wyburn–Mason syndrome

Wyburn–Mason syndrome is a sporadically occurring condition consisting of unilateral retinal arteriovenous malformations (AVMs), known also as racemose haemangiomas, with associated ipsilateral intracranial AVMs.

The lesions may be detected incidentally, as they frequently cause no change to visual acuity; however, symptomatic lesions may cause a subtle or severe loss of vision. Intracranial lesions may cause a variety of neurological features, depending on the site of the AVM.

Treatment

There is no effective treatment for the retinal lesions. Intracranial AVMs have been successfully treated by surgery, radiotherapy, or embolization.

Multiple types of metabolic diseases affect the eye. In depth discussion of the individual conditions is beyond the scope of this chapter and is more than the average ophthalmologist requires for general practice. However, as children with metabolic diseases may present for diagnosis or monitoring, a general overview of these diseases and their effects on the eye is provided.

Albinism

The term 'albinism' refers to a heterogeneous group of genetic disorders resulting in abnormality of melanin synthesis and pigment deficiency in the eye, skin, and hair. Oculocutaneous albinism (OCA) involves all three tissues, whereas ocular albinism involves the eye alone.

Ocular features

For both ocular albinism and OCA, ocular features may include:

* Reduced visual acuity (variable severity).
* Nystagmus
* Foveal hypoplasia
* Abnormal fundal pigmentation
* Delayed visual maturation
* Strabismus
* Iris translucency
* Photophobia
* Reduced proportion of uncrossed fibres at optic chiasm

Ocular albinism

Usually inherited in an X-linked recessive fashion, ocular albinism represents 10% of all albinism and is also known as Nettleship–Falls albinism. It involves the *OA1* gene (Chromosome Xp22.3–22.2) and its prevalence is 1 in 50,000.

OCA

OCA results from abnormal melanogenesis and can be divided into three main types:

* **Type 1:** Caused by an abnormality in the tyrosinase gene (Chromosome 11q14–21); usually autosomal recessive; typical characteristics of white hair, pale skin, pink/pink-blue eyes, and classic ocular features
* **Type 2:** Caused by an abnormality in Substance P (Chromosome 15q11–q13). Patients have features that are similar to those seen in type 1 but generally have more pigment and better vision.
* **Type 3:** Caused by an abnormality in tyrosine-related protein 1; rare

Systemic associations of albinism

* **Prader–Willi syndrome:** type 2 OCA with learning difficulties, obesity, and hypotonia
* **Angelman syndrome:** type 2 OCA with learning difficulties, ataxia, and abnormal facies
* **Chédiak–Higashi syndrome:** type 2 OCA with immunocompromise and recurrent bacterial infections, hepatosplenomegaly, and peripheral and cranial neuropathies
* **Hermansky–Pudlak syndrome:** type 2 OCA with platelet dysfunction and easy bruising/bleeding

Other disorders of metabolism

Features of other disorders of metabolism and their effects on the eye are summarized in Tables 9.17–9.21. Please see Chapter 6, Section 6.19 for a detailed description of gyrate atrophy.

Disorders of connective tissues

Children with connective tissue disorders are not uncommonly seen in paediatric ophthalmology clinics (see Table 9.22). Ectopia lentis and/or high myopia require regular and experienced refraction, and sports goggles are often recommended for children with angioid streaks. It is important to remember the potential systemic associations in any child presenting with features suggestive of any of these disorders, particularly Marfan syndrome, where cardiology review is essential.

Table 9.17 Disorders of carbohydrate metabolism

Syndrome	Deficiency	Ocular features	Systemic features
Galactosaemia (AR)	Galactose-1-phosphate uridyltransferase	Oil droplet cataracts	Low IQ Failure to thrive
Galactokinase deficiency (AR)	Galactokinase	Cataracts	Normal
Mannosidosis (AR)	Alpha-mannosidase	Spoke-like cataracts	Low IQ MPS-like changes but clear corneas

AR, autosomal recessive, MPS, mucopolysaccharidosis.
Adapted from Denniston and Murray, *Oxford Handbook of Ophthalmology*, 2014 with permission from Oxford University Press

Table 9.18 Disorders of amino acid metabolism

Syndrome	Deficiency	Ocular features	Systemic features
Homocystinuria 1–3 (AR)	Cystathione synthetase	Ectopia lentis Myopia Glaucoma	Low IQ Marfanoid habitus Thromboses Fine, fair hair
Cystinosis (AR)	Lysosomal transport protein	Crystalline keratopathy	Renal failure Failure to thrive
Lowe syndrome (XLR)	Unknown	Microphakia Cataracts Blue sclera Anterior segment dysgenesis Glaucoma	Low IQ Failure to thrive Rickets (Vitamin D resistant)
Zellweger syndrome (AR)	Unknown	Flat brow Optic nerve hypoplasia Pigmentary retinopathy Glaucoma	Dysgenesis of brain, liver, and kidneys Metabolic acidosis
Albinism	Melanin	Reduced visual acuity Nystagmus Foveal hypoplasia Abnormal fundal pigmentation Delayed visual maturation Strabismus Iris translucency Photophobia Reduced proportion of uncrossed fibres at optic chiasm	Pigment deficiency in the eye, skin, and hair May be associated with Prader–Willi syndrome, Angelman syndrome, Chédiak–Higashi syndrome, or Hermansky–Pudlak syndrome
Alkaptonuria (AR)	Homogentisic acid dioxygenase	Scleral darkening	Ochronosis Arthritis
Sulphite oxidase deficiency (AR)	Molybdenum cofactor	Spherophakia Ectopia lentis	Neurodegeneration LE <2 years
Tyrosinaemia type 2 (AR)	Tyrosine transaminase	Herpetiform corneal ulcers	Low IQ (in some) Hyperkeratosis of palms/soles
Gyrate atrophy	Ornithine aminotransferase	Decreased visual acuity Progressive night blindness Peripheral visual field loss Scalloped chorioretinopathy Myopia Cataract Cystoid macular oedema Epiretinal membrane	Mild muscle weakness Fine, straight hair Patches of alopecia Hearing loss Slow wave background changes on EEG Peripheral neuropathy

AR, autosomal recessive; LE, life expectancy; XLR, X-linked recessive.
Adapted from Denniston and Murray, *Oxford Handbook of Ophthalmology*, 2014 with permission from Oxford University Press

Table 9.19 Disorders of lipid metabolism

Syndrome	Deficiency	Ocular features	Systemic features
Abetalipoproteinaemia (AR)	Triglyceride transfer protein	Cataract Pigmentary retinopathy	Spinocerebellar degeneration LE <50 years
GM₁ gangliosidosis, types 1 and 2 (AR)	Beta-galactosidase	Cloudy corneas Cherry-red spot Optic atrophy	Neurodegeneration Visceromegaly LE (type 1) <4 years LE (type 2) <40 years
Tay–Sachs disease (AR)	Hexosaminidase A	Cherry-red spot Optic atrophy	Visceromegaly LE <3 years
Sandhoff disease (AR)	Hexosaminidase A and B	Cherry-red spot Optic atrophy	Visceromegaly Neurodegeneration LE <3 years
Gaucher disease (AR)	Beta-glucosidase	Supranuclear gaze palsy	Visceromegaly Neurodegeneration
Niemann–Pick disease, type A (AR)	Sphingomyelinase	Cherry-red spot Optic atrophy	Visceromegaly Neurodegeneration LE <3 years
Fabry disease (XLR)	Alpha-galactosidase	Vortex keratopathy Cataract Tortuous vessels	Angiokeratomas Painful episodes Renal failure Vascular disease LE = middle age
Metachromatic leucodystrophy (AR)	Arylsulphatase-A	Optic atrophy Nystagmus	Neurodegeneration
Krabbe disease (AR)	Galactocerebrosidase	Optic atrophy	Neurodegeneration
Farber disease (AR)	Ceramidase	Macular pigmentation	Granulomas Arthropathy
Batten disease (Neuronal ceroid lipofuscinosis) (AR)	Unknown	Macular discolouration RP-like changes Optic atrophy	Neurodegeneration Reduced LE
Refsum syndrome (AR)	Phytanic acid alpha-hydroxylase	Pigmentary retinopathy	Neuropathy Ataxia Deafness Icthyosis

AR, autosomal recessive, LE, life expectancy; RP, retinitis pigmentosa; XLR, X-linked recessive.
Adapted from Denniston and Murray, *Oxford Handbook of Ophthalmology*, 2014 with permission from Oxford University Press

Table 9.20 Disorders of mineral metabolism

Syndrome	Deficiency	Ocular features	Systemic features
Wilson disease (AR)	Cu binding protein	Kayser–Fleischer ring Cataract	Neurodegeneration Ataxia
Menke syndrome (AR)	Cu transport syndrome	Optic atrophy	Kinky hair Neurodegeneration Ataxia

AR, autosomal recessive; Cu, copper.
Adapted from Denniston and Murray, *Oxford Handbook of Ophthalmology*, 2014 with permission from Oxford University Press

Table 9.21 Disorders of glycosaminoglycan metabolism (mucopolysaccharidoses)

Syndrome	Deficiency	Ocular features	Systemic features
MPS I (Hurler/Scheie/Hurler–Scheie syndrome; AR)	Alpha-iduronidase	Cloudy corneas Pigmentary retinopathy Optic atrophy	Skeletal/facial dysmorphism Low IQ Severity: H>H/S>S
MPS II (Hunter syndrome; XLR)	Iduronate sulphatase	Pigmentary retinopathy Optic atrophy	Variably low IQ Dysmorphism
MPS III (Sanfilippo syndrome; AR)	Heparan N-sulphatase	Pigmentary retinopathy Optic atrophy	Neurodegeneration Hyperactivity Mild dysmorphism
MPS IV (Morquio syndrome; AR)	Galactose-6-sulphatase	Cloudy corneas	Skeletal dysplasia Normal IQ/facies
MPS VI (Maroteaux–Lamy syndrome; AR)	N-Acetyl-galactosamine-4-sulphatase	Cloudy corneas	Skeletal/facial dysmorphism Normal IQ
MPS VII (Sly syndrome; AR)	Beta-glucoronidase	Cloudy corneas	Skeletal/facial dysmorphism Low IQ

AR, autosomal recessive, MPS, mucopolysaccharidosis; XLR, X-linked recessive.
Adapted from Denniston and Murray, *Oxford Handbook of Ophthalmology*, 2014 with permission from Oxford University Press

Table 9.22 Disorders of connective tissues

Syndrome	Deficiency	Ocular features	Systemic features
Marfan syndrome (AD)	Fibrillin	Ectopia lentis Glaucoma Blue sclera Keratoconus	Long limbed Arachnodactyly High-arched palate Mitral/aortic regurgitation Aortic dissection
Osteogenesis imperfecta	Collagen, type 1	Blue sclera Keratoconus	Brittle bones
Stickler syndrome (AD)	Collagen, type 2	Myopia Liquefied 'empty' vitreous Retinal detachment	Arthropathy Midfacial flattening Cleft palate
Ehlers–Danlos syndrome	Collagen, types 1 and 3	Blue sclera Keratoconus Angioid streaks	Hyperflexible joints Hyperelastic skin Vascular bleeds
Pseudoxanthoma elasticum	Elastin fragility	Angioid streaks	'Chicken skin' GI bleeds
Weill–Marchesani syndrome (AR)	Fibrillin-1	Ectopia lentis Microspherophakia	Short stature Brachydactyly Low IQ

AD, autosomal dominant; AR, autosomal recessive; GI, gastrointestinal.
Adapted from Denniston and Murray, *Oxford Handbook of Ophthalmology*, 2014 with permission from Oxford University Press

Chapter 10

Neuro-ophthalmology

Lucy Barker, Gordon T. Plant, and Indran Davagnanam

419

Visual pathway anatomy

The visual pathway extends from the globe through to the visual cortex. As the anatomy of various aspects of the globe is covered elsewhere, this section focuses on the visual pathway from the optic nerve to the striate and extra-striate cortex.

Optic nerve

The optic nerve extends from the globe to the optic chiasm and can be divided into four parts: intraocular, intraorbital, intracanalicular, and intracranial. The intraocular part is 1 mm long and includes the optic disc. It contains retinal ganglion cell axons and exits posteriorly through the lamina cribrosa. The intraorbital part is 25 mm long and myelinated. It exceeds the distance from the globe to the optic foramen by approximately 8 mm, thus permitting free ocular movement except in severe proptosis. The intracanalicular segment is 5 mm long and begins at the optic foramen within the lesser wing of the sphenoid. Finally, the intracranial part is 12–16 mm long and passes upwards, backwards, and medially to reach the optic chiasm. The blood supply of the intraocular segment is from the short posterior ciliary arteries, via the anastomotic circle of Zinn. The remaining parts are supplied by the ophthalmic artery via the pial plexus. The intracranial optic nerve also receives blood supply from the superior hypophyseal artery.

Optic chiasm

The optic chiasm sits within the suprasellar cistern, approximately 10 mm above the pituitary gland, which itself sits within the sella turcica of the sphenoid bone. In 80% of cases, the chiasm is situated directly above the sella turcica and pituitary gland. Owing to variability in the length of the intracranial segment of the optic nerves, however, in 10% of cases the chiasm is pre-fixed (short optic nerves) and lies over the tuberculum sellae, and in another 10% the chiasm is post-fixed (long optic nerves) and overlies the dorsum sellae. Tumours arising in the pituitary gland therefore classically compress the chiasm; however, they may also compress the optic tract in pre-fixed cases, and optic nerves in post-fixed cases.

The supraclinoid segments of the carotid arteries lie lateral to the chiasm, and the cavernous sinus lies infero-lateral to the chiasm. Posteriorly, the chiasm forms the anterior wall of the third ventricle, and its blood supply is from a pial plexus via the circle of Willis.

Optic tracts

The optic tracts connect the optic chiasm to the lateral geniculate nuclei. Each optic tract conveys nerve fibres from the ipsilateral temporal and contralateral nasal retina. Lesions in the optic tract therefore produce incongruous homonymous hemianopia, as the optic tracts do not maintain strict retinotopic architecture. The blood supply is from pial arteries with branches from the anterior choroidal, the posterior communicating, and the middle cerebral arteries.

Lateral geniculate nuclei

The lateral geniculate nuclei are situated on the under surface of the pulvinar of the thalamus. Each nucleus is divided into six neuronal layers. The axons from the contralateral eye synapse in Layers 1, 4, and 6, and those from the ipsilateral eye synapse in Layers 2, 3, and 5. In addition, Layers 1 and 2 represent magnocellular layers (fast motion/low acuity), and Layers 3 to 6 represent parvocellular layers (slow motion/high acuity and chromatic processing) enabling further visual information processing. Blood supply is via the middle and the posterior cerebral arteries.

Optic radiations

The optic radiations convey information from the lateral geniculate nuclei to the striate cortex. Superior optic radiations (carrying projections of superior retina) pass through the parietal lobe and terminate on the superior lip of the calcarine fissure in the striate cortex. Each inferior optic radiation (carrying projections of inferior retina) sweeps around the inferior horn of the lateral ventricle within the temporal lobe (including the Meyer loop) and terminates in the inferior lip of the calcarine fissure. Anteriorly, the optic radiations are supplied by the anterior choroidal branch of the internal carotid artery, and posteriorly by the middle and the posterior cerebral arteries.

Striate and extra-striate visual cortex

The visual cortex is situated in the occipital lobe and is divided into striate and extra-striate visual areas. Each striate (primary) visual area represents the contralateral visual field. Furthermore, the superior visual field is represented below the calcarine sulcus, and the inferior visual field above it. The anterior part of the striate cortex represents the visual periphery and is supplied by the posterior cerebral artery. The macula is represented posteriorly just lateral to the tip of the calcarine fissure, and is supplied by the middle cerebral artery. The extra-striate visual areas surround the primary visual areas on the medial and lateral surfaces of each hemisphere. They assist in the interpretation and recognition of images. Visual processing can broadly be divided into the dorsal and ventral streams. The dorsal stream extends into the parietal and superior temporal cortical areas and is responsible for spatial orientation, movement, and location of objects and depth perception (the 'where' of visual information processing). The ventral stream extends to the inferior temporal cortex and is responsible for recognition of objects, colours, and text, as well as the association of meaning to objects (the 'what' of visual information processing).

Pupil reflex pathways

The pupil responses to light, near targets, and sympathetic stimulation occur via different anatomical pathways.

Parasympathetic pathway (light reflex)

See Figure 10.1.

1. Afferent impulses originate in the intrinsically photosensitive (melanopsin-containing) retinal ganglion cells of the retina and travel to the pretectal nucleus, which lies close to the superior colliculus. Nasal retinal impulses from each eye are conveyed by neurons that decussate at the chiasm, terminating in the contralateral pretectal nucleus. Temporal retinal impulses terminate in the ipsilateral pretectal nucleus.

2. Each pretectal nucleus connects with both of the Edinger–Westphal nuclei (parasympathetic nuclei) of the oculomotor nerve. This connection allows bilateral pupil constriction on uniocular light stimulation.

3. Parasympathetic preganglionic fibres travel through the inferior division of the oculomotor nerve, reaching the ciliary ganglion in the orbit.

4. Postganglionic parasympathetic fibres pass through the short ciliary nerves to innervate the constrictor pupillae muscles of the iris.

Parasympathetic pathway (near reflex)

1. Afferent impulses pass from the retina, through the visual pathway to the visual cortex. The visual cortex is connected to the frontal eye field, from where cortical fibres descend through the internal capsule to the oculomotor nuclei in the midbrain.
2. The oculomotor nerve travels to supply the medial recti, allowing convergence, with some fibres synapsing with the Edinger–Westphal nuclei to mediate pupil constriction. Accommodation is also stimulated through impulses from the short ciliary nerves to the ciliary muscles.

Sympathetic pathway

See Figure 10.2.

1. Impulses originate in the posterior hypothalamus and descend the brainstem to the ciliospinal centre of Budge, in the intermediolateral horn of the spinal cord, around T1.

2. Preganglionic neurons then carry signals to the superior cervical ganglion, in the upper part of the neck.
3. Postganglionic neurons travel along the internal carotid artery, entering the cavernous sinus to join the ophthalmic division of the trigeminal nerve. Sympathetic fibres then travel with the nasociliary nerve. These fibres continue as the long ciliary nerve to reach the ciliary body, the dilator pupillae, and the Müller muscles. Other sympathetic fibres pass through the ciliary ganglion without synapsing and continue with the short ciliary nerves to the ciliary body and iris.

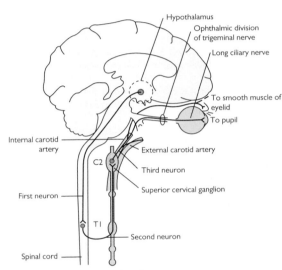

Fig 10.2 Sympathetic pupil pathway

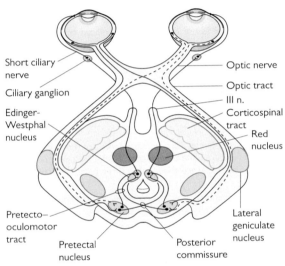

Fig 10.1 Pupil light reflex pathway

10.2 Cranial nerve anatomy

Aside from the optic nerve, the other cranial nerves that are most relevant in ophthalmology are the third (oculomotor), fourth (trochlear), fifth (trigeminal), and sixth (abducens) nerves. An understanding of the anatomy and function of these cranial nerves is helpful in recognizing clinical signs and using these to locate underlying pathology.

Third cranial nerve

The third nerve, or oculomotor nerve, supplies all the extraocular muscles except the superior oblique and lateral rectus. It also gives innervation to the levator palpebrae superioris and carries pupillary fibres.

Nuclei

The third nerve has two motor nuclei: the main motor nucleus and the accessory parasympathetic nucleus (the Edinger–Westphal nucleus).

The main motor nucleus is situated in the midbrain, at the level of the superior colliculus. It is subdivided into the following subnuclei:

* **The central caudal nucleus:** this single nucleus innervates both of the levator palpebrae superioris muscles
* **The superior rectus subnuclei:** each subnucleus innervates the contralateral superior rectus
* **The medial rectus, inferior rectus, and inferior oblique subnuclei:** these subnuclei provide innervation to their respective ipsilateral extraocular muscles

The accessory parasympathetic nucleus is situated posterior to the main motor nucleus and receives fibres from the pretectal nucleus for the light reflexes, and from the corticonuclear fibres for the accommodation reflex.

Course

The fascicle of the third nerve leaves the nucleus and passes through the midbrain, traversing the medial longitudinal fasciculus, the red nucleus, the substantia nigra, and the crus cerebri before emerging into the subarachnoid space from the anterior aspect of the midbrain, medial to the cerebral peduncle (see Figure 10.3). It then moves forwards and laterally, passing between the posterior cerebellar and superior cerebellar arteries, and runs alongside the posterior communicating artery. On the lateral side of the anterior clinoid process, the third nerve perforates the dura mater, entering the cavernous sinus, where it runs along the lateral wall, superior to the fourth nerve (see Figure 10.4). In the anterior cavernous sinus, the third nerve divides into superior and inferior divisions, both of which enter the orbit through the superior orbital fissure (within the tendinous ring). The superior division ascends lateral to the optic nerve, supplies the superior rectus, and then terminates by supplying the levator palpebrae superioris. The inferior division divides into three branches to supply the medial and inferior recti and the inferior oblique muscles. The nerve to the inferior oblique gives rise to a further branch that carries parasympathetic fibres to the ciliary ganglion.

Fourth cranial nerve

The fourth cranial nerve, or trochlear nerve, supplies the contralateral superior oblique muscle. It is the thinnest cranial nerve, with the longest intracranial course, and is the only one to exit from the dorsal brainstem.

Nuclei

The fourth cranial nerve nucleus lies inferior to the third nerve nuclei, at the level of the inferior colliculus in the midbrain. The nuclei receive input from the vestibular system and the medial longitudinal fasciculus.

Course

The fascicle of the fourth nuclei travels dorsally and exits the midbrain just caudal to the inferior colliculus. The nerve immediately decussates and passes forwards and laterally within the subarachnoid space, around the cerebral peduncle. It runs along with the third nerve, between the posterior and superior cerebellar arteries, and pierces the dura mater just below the free border of the tentorium cerebelli. It then passes forwards along the lateral wall of the cavernous sinus, lying below the third nerve and above the ophthalmic division of the fifth cranial nerve (see Figure 10.4). The nerve enters the orbit through the superior orbital fissure (outside the tendinous ring) and passes medially above the origin of levator palpebrae superioris before reaching the superior oblique muscle.

Fifth cranial nerve

The fifth cranial nerve, or trigeminal nerve, supplies the muscles of mastication and sensation to the face and anterior scalp.

Nuclei

The sensory nuclei of the trigeminal nerve are the largest of the cranial nerve nuclei and extend through the midbrain, pons, and medulla. The nuclei are divided into three parts, from rostral to caudal:

* The mesencephalic nucleus receives proprioceptive information from the jaws and teeth.
* The chief sensory nucleus receives information from the touch and position fibres.
* The spinal trigeminal nucleus receives information from pain and temperature fibres.

The motor nucleus of the trigeminal nerve lies medial to the chief sensory nucleus in the pons.

Course

A single large sensory root and smaller adjacent motor root emerge from the pons. Both pass anteriorly to enter Meckels cave, an arachnoidal pouch filled with cerebrospinal fluid and sitting posterolateral to the cavernous sinus on either side of the sphenoid bone. Here, the sensory nerves from the face synapse, forming the trigeminal ganglion. The motor nerve passes directly through the ganglion without synapsing. From the trigeminal ganglion, the nerve forms three main divisions: ophthalmic, maxillary, and mandibular. The ophthalmic division (V_1) passes anteriorly in the lateral wall of the cavernous sinus and gains access to the orbit via the superior orbital fissure. It supplies sensation to the eyeball, the lacrimal glands, the nasal mucosa, and the skin of the upper eyelid, forehead, and scalp as far posteriorly as the vertex. The maxillary division (V_2) exits the skull base via the foramen rotundum infero-lateral to the cavernous sinus. It enters the pterygopalatine fossa, where it gives off several branches. The main trunk continues anteriorly along the orbital floor as the infraorbital nerve to supply sensation to the middle third of the face, the upper jaw, and the teeth of the upper jaw. The mandibular division (V_3) runs laterally across the skull base to exit the skull via the foramen ovale into the masticator space. Here, it divides into several sensory branches which supply sensation to the lower jaw, the teeth of the lower jaw, the tongue, the floor of the mouth, and the lower third of the face. The motor division divides to supply the muscles of mastication: the masseter, the temporalis, the mylohyoid, the medial pterygoids, and the lateral pterygoids.

Sixth cranial nerve

The sixth cranial nerve, or abducens nerve, supplies the ipsilateral lateral rectus muscle. However, 40% of the cells in its nuclei are interneurons which project (via the medial longitudinal fasciculus) to the contralateral medial rectus subnucleus to mediate conjugate gaze.

Nuclei

The sixth nerve nuclei lie in the pons, just beneath the floor of the upper part of the fourth ventricle. The fascicle of the seventh cranial nerve wraps around the sixth nerve nucleus, and damage in this area can result in an associated facial palsy.

Course

The sixth nerve fascicle traverses the paramedian pontine reticular formation (involved in horizontal eye movement) and the corticospinal tract before leaving the anterior surface of the brain between the lower pons and the medulla oblongata (see Figure 10.5). The nerve then runs upwards, forwards, and laterally, piercing the dura mater just lateral to the dorsum sellae of the sphenoid bone. Here, it makes an acute bend forwards across the sharp upper border of the petrous part of the temporal bone, near its apex. It then passes forwards within the cavernous sinus, running infero-lateral to the internal carotid artery (see Figure 10.4). It enters the orbit through the superior orbital fissure, between the two divisions of the third nerve, and terminates on the medial surface of the lateral rectus.

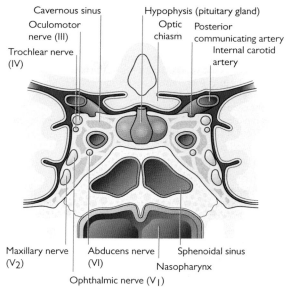

Fig 10.4 Relationship of cranial nerves within the cavernous sinus (coronal section)

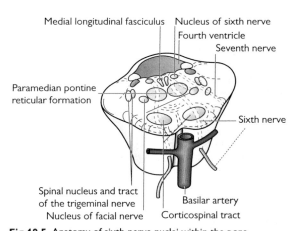

Fig 10.5 Anatomy of sixth nerve nuclei within the pons

Adapted from *Ophthalmology*, 2nd Edition, Yanoff M. and Duker J.S., copyright (2004) with kind permission of Elsevier

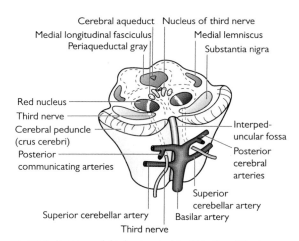

Fig 10.3 Anatomy of third nerve nuclei within the midbrain

Adapted from *Ophthalmology*, 2nd Edition, Yanoff M. and Duker J.S, copyright (2004) with kind permission of Elsevier

10.3 Central control of ocular motility

The ocular muscles, like other muscles, are under both reflex and voluntary control. The frontal eye fields in the frontal cortex are thought to regulate voluntary initiation of eye movements whilst the occipital cortex and superior colliculus serve as coordinating centres for reflex movements.

Supranuclear ocular motor control can be considered to consist of four separate subsystems:

- The saccadic (fast fixation) system
- The pursuit (tracking) system
- The vergence system
- The vestibular system

However, these systems feed into a shared final common pathway and may represent different outcomes from a cascade of related sensory–motor functions, rather than acting as truly distinct neural systems. In normal circumstances, it is the direction of the eyes in space that is important (gaze) not the position of the eyes in the orbit. Hence, most eye movements will be a combination of pursuit or saccades with vergence, vestibular movement, and/or head movement. However, in assessing disorders of eye movements clinically, it is necessary to examine separately each of the four types of eye movement.

Saccadic eye movements

Saccades are fast, fixating eye movements that rapidly place the object of interest onto the fovea or switch fixation from one object to another. They must be fast (around 600°/second), brief (30–100 milliseconds) and accurate to support clear vision. They are triggered by an object in the peripheral visual field and may be under voluntary or reflex control.

Initiation of voluntary saccades occurs in the contralateral premotor frontal cortex, from which impulses pass down to the midbrain via the anterior limb of the internal capsule to synapse in the brainstem. However, the saccades themselves are generated in the brainstem reticular formation, with the paramedian pontine reticular formation in the pons predominantly controlling horizontal saccades, and the rostral interstitial nuclei of the medial longitudinal fasciculus in the midbrain controlling vertical movements and torsional movements.

Two types of burst neurons in the brainstem control saccades. Glutaminergic **excitatory** burst neurons trigger saccades and project to the nuclei of the third, fourth, and sixth cranial nerves, as well as having projections via the medial longitudinal fasciculus to coordinate with the other eye. **Inhibitory** burst neurons are glycinergic in the horizontal system and GABAergic in the vertical system; they fire to inhibit the antagonist muscles during a saccade (hence, they tend to mediate Sherringtons law of reciprocal innervation; see Section 9.1).

Other structures that influence saccades include the basal ganglia and the superior colliculus, which consists of neurons laid out in a retinotopic map and seem to be involved in selecting a target for fixation, and the cerebellum, which plays a role in steering and stopping saccades and thus influencing their accuracy.

Pursuit eye movements

Pursuit movements are slow, smooth eye movements that maintain fixation on a target once it has been foveated by the saccadic system. Gaze velocity is matched to target velocity. Smooth pursuit is a continuous movement that slowly rotates the eyes to compensate for the motion of the viewed object, minimizing blur that might otherwise compromise visual acuity. The major stimulus for pursuit movements is movement of the image near the fovea. Pursuit movements have shorter latency than saccades do (125 milliseconds) but their velocity is much slower, at 20°–70°/second.

Pursuit movements are initiated from the occipital striate cortex, which receives input from the lateral geniculate nucleus. The cortex projects ipsilaterally via the dorsolateral pontine nuclei to the flocculus and the ventral paraflocculus of the cerebellum and then to the motor nuclei of the third, fourth, and sixth cranial nerves.

Vergence eye movements

Vergence eye movements are smooth, disconjugate movements of convergence and divergence, such that the eyes move in different directions to maintain fixation and fusion. The stimulus is target displacement or motion along the visual surge axis (towards or away from the observer).

The higher control areas for the generation of vergence eye movements are poorly understood. However, vergence movements may take the form of saccadic or pursuit movements. Therefore, the cortical areas involved in saccadic or pursuit movements may also be responsible for vergence eye movements. Vergence eye movements have a latency of about 160 milliseconds and a velocity of 20°/second.

Vestibular eye movements

Vestibular movements compensate for changes in head and body position, allowing fixation to be maintained despite head and body movement. They are conjugate or vergence, smooth movements with a latency of 10–100 milliseconds and a peak velocity of 300°/second.

Head movement stimulates the vestibulo-ocular response via inputs from:

- The semicircular canals, with output from the horizontal canals producing horizontal eye movements (in response to movement in the yaw axis), the anterior canals producing vertical movements (in response to movement in the pitch axis), and the posterior and anterior canals together producing torsional movements (in response to movement in the roll axis)
- The neck proprioceptors

Afferent fibres synapse in the vestibular nuclei and then pass to the third, fourth, and sixth nerve nuclei. Thus, the vestibulo-ocular reflex (or oculo-cephalic reflex if neck proprioceptors are involved) is mediated via only three synapses and does not involve the cerebral hemispheres in the way that other classes of ocular movement do. Hence, it is the fastest ocular motor system and also can be used to assess brain stem function. The vestibular system can respond only to relatively fast head movements. For slower movements, the optokinetic system (which relies on visual input) operates (see Section 10.16). It is the utricle that is involved in signalling translational (non-rotational) movements of the head such as the surge axis mentioned in 'Vergence eye movements' (naso-occipital movement) but also the bob (dorsal–ventral) and heave (interaural) axes.

10.4 **Neuro-ophthalmic history taking**

Introduction

The optic nerve and visual pathways are potentially subject to a variety of ocular, intracranial, and systemic pathologies. Although a high proportion of ophthalmic conditions can be diagnosed on clinical examination alone, accurate history taking is of particular importance in neuro-ophthalmic disorders, as several different conditions may present with similar clinical signs (e.g. in optic neuropathies). Good history taking is more likely to help reach the correct diagnosis with the avoidance of unnecessary investigations.

Presenting complaint

Symptoms that could indicate a neuro-ophthalmic aetiology include visual disturbance, diplopia, headache, and pain on eye movements.

Visual disturbance

Key aspects to elicit from a history of visual disturbance include the following.

Unilateral or bilateral visual disturbance

Uniocular visual loss is suggestive of ocular or optic nerve pathology whereas binocular visual disturbance occurs following lesions at or posterior to the optic chiasm.

With binocular loss, it is important to ascertain whether it is bitemporal (in chiasmal disorders) or homonymous (retrochiasmal lesions). Homonymous hemianopia may be asymptomatic. When it is abrupt in onset or transient (as in transient ischaemic attacks or migraine), patients may be aware that they can only see one-half of a fixated object such as a face. Patients with a right homonymous hemianopia may complain of difficulty reading because they are unable to follow a line of text efficiently (hemianopic alexia). Patients with a left homonymous hemianopia may complain that they cannot return to the next line of text efficiently.

Bitemporal hemianopia may be asymptomatic until visual acuity begins to deteriorate. Patients may, however, complain of post-fixational blindness or hemifield slide. Awareness of temporal field loss is unusual.

Extent of visual loss

Severe visual loss affecting the majority of the uniocular visual field can occur with optic neuropathies. Altitudinal visual field loss is common with anterior ischaemic optic neuropathy. Unilateral, segmental visual loss is more common with retinal disorders such as retinal detachment and branch retinal artery or vein occlusion.

Speed of onset

Sudden-onset visual disturbance suggests an ischaemic cause; gradual onset is more typical of compressive causes. Visual loss progressing over a few hours to days can occur in optic neuritis.

Duration of visual loss/any recovery

Visual recovery occurs within several weeks in typical cases of optic neuritis, whereas spontaneous improvement in vision is less common with ischaemic optic neuropathies.

Disturbance of colour vision

Optic nerve disorders typically result in decreased colour vision, and this decrease may be disproportionate to the level of visual acuity loss. Patients may complain of a 'greying' of their vision.

Positive or negative scotomas

Positive scotomas, where patients are aware of a particular part of the visual field being obstructed, occur in retinal lesions. Such scotomas may be coloured or be perceived as a region of flickering lights which are more visible in the dark. In contrast, with negative scotomas, patients are not specifically aware of an area of diminished vision; thus, this condition may only be identified with visual field testing, although patients may be aware of a gap when presented with repeating images such as printed text or the Amsler grid test.

Associated pain

Retrobulbar pain and pain on eye movements can occur in optic neuritis.

Transient visual loss

Transient visual loss is most commonly due to thromboembolic disease. However, important neuro-ophthalmic associations include temporal arteritis and papilloedema, both of which can cause intermittent episodes of visual disturbance prior to more permanent visual loss. An important distinction between embolic transient monocular visual loss and transient loss in papilloedema is that the former may last many minutes more than the latter, which lasts for less than 1 minute and is precipitated by a change in posture. This is also the case with giant cell arteritis (GCA) and other conditions where the problem is poor perfusion of the eye. Retinal arterial vasospasm can cause transient monocular visual loss in young people.

Visual loss in children

Children are commonly referred to ophthalmologists regarding concerns about their visual development. Assessment can be difficult, as children rarely complain of even severe unilateral visual loss, up to the age of approximately 10 years. In addition, bilateral visual loss may not be symptomatic until very advanced. A full pregnancy, birth, developmental, and family history is essential. In children old enough to give a reliable history, one should ask about specific symptoms of headache, diplopia, and pain on eye movement.

Diplopia

With diplopia, it is important to ascertain whether it is binocular or, more rarely, monocular, when it is likely to be due to a refractive cause and is 'ghosting' rather than true diplopia.

Other aspects of diplopia to enquire about include the following.

Vertical, horizontal, or torsional diplopia

Vertical diplopia is usually a result of vertical recti or oblique muscle disorders (e.g. in fourth nerve palsies, where patients can have difficulty whilst looking down when descending stairs). In the case of oblique muscle palsies (usually superior oblique), one image may be tilted (torsional diplopia). Horizontal diplopia typically arises following horizontal recti involvement (e.g. in sixth nerve palsies, where patients have horizontal diplopia that is worse when looking to the side of the affected muscle than in primary position or to the side of the unaffected muscle, and for distance as compared to near vision).

Speed of onset

Diplopia of abrupt onset is more likely to be vascular in origin, whereas progressive diplopia suggests a compressive cause.

In reality, diplopia is always of abrupt onset but may be preceded by blurred vision if progressive. It is important to enquire whether the double vision has progressed or changed in any way since the patient first became aware of it.

Variability

Variability of diplopia may occur in myasthenia gravis and is typically worse with fatigue. Breakdown of phorias can also give intermittent diplopia, as can thyroid eye disease.

Pain

Diplopia associated with pain can occur in compressive third nerve lesions, cranial nerve infarction in temporal arteritis, and inflammatory orbital conditions such as myositis and pseudotumour.

Pupil involvement

A dilated pupil in the presence of diplopia should raise suspicion of a compressive third nerve lesion. Patients may also have a new-onset ptosis, and headache.

Associated neurology

Diplopia in the context of multiple cranial nerve palsies implies either brainstem disease or peripheral lesions such as cavernous sinus or orbital apex pathology. Symptoms of weakness, dizziness, bladder dysfunction, and hearing problems should also be enquired about.

Headache

Headache (see Section 10.19) is a common presenting complaint, with a wide differential diagnosis, but features that are of particular concern include:

* Temporal pain and tenderness, with other symptoms of jaw ache, malaise, and joint pains (e.g. in temporal arteritis)
* Headache worse in morning and associated with nausea and vomiting (e.g. in raised intracranial pressure)
* Association with visual disturbance (e.g. intermittent visual loss in papilloedema)
* Headache which occurs on standing, relieved by lying flat (low intracranial pressure, e.g. post lumbar puncture or cerebrospinal leak)
* Sudden-onset and severe headache (may represent an intracranial aneurysm or other source of bleeding)
* Systemic features such as weight loss, night sweats, or fever
Other features of headache to consider include the following:
* Preceding visual aura (migraine)
* Unilateral headache associated with nausea, vomiting, phonophobia, and photophobia (migraine)
* Unilateral headache or retrobulbar pain associated with dysautonomic features such as lacrimation, nasal congestion, or Horner syndrome (cluster headache, short-lasted unilateral neuralgiform headache with conjunctival injection and tearing, paroxysmal hemicrania)
* Headaches which are unremitting over weeks or months without even momentary relief, not responding to analgesics and often associated with insomnia (chronic daily headache)

Red eye versus white eye

A wide range of ocular conditions can give rise to headache in the presence of a red eye, providing clues to the diagnosis. Non-ocular conditions such as cluster headache can similarly produce headache with a red eye. In addition, early iritis can sometimes be missed when assessing patients with headache and who have a seemingly normal ocular examination.

Facial pain

Facial pain often presents to ophthalmology. The significant differential diagnoses are:

* Trigeminal neuralgia: lancinating paroxysmal pain triggered by touch, cold, wind, etc.
* Sinusitis: associated with local tenderness, post-nasal drip, evidence of infection
* Cluster headache: paroxysmal pain centred on the eye, each attack lasting approximately 30 minutes, occurring in clusters, associated with dysautonomic features such as lacrimation
* Atypical facial pain: absolutely constant localized pain, no effect of analgesics, associated with insomnia

Past medical history

Enquire about any atherosclerotic risk factors that are common in vascular neuro-ophthalmic conditions (e.g. ischaemic optic neuropathies, visual pathway infarction). Ask about any history of cancer, which may be relevant in space-occupying intracranial lesions or compressive optic neuropathies. Previous trauma or surgery to the head and neck region should also be elicited. Any psychiatric history may be relevant in functional visual loss.

Drug history

A variety of medications can result in optic neuropathy, including ethambutol, isoniazid, amiodarone, and ciclosporin. Recreational drug use should also be asked about, especially in the context of atypical pupil abnormalities.

Family history

A family history of multiple sclerosis is found occasionally in patients with optic neuritis, and often patients are particularly anxious about this association. Congenital optic disc disorders may also have a family association, and enquiring about other family members can help reveal inheritance traits that can be helpful in future genetic counselling.

In the case of bilateral optic neuropathy, familial disorders may show inheritance which is mitochondrial (Leber hereditary optic neuropathy) or nuclear (autosomal dominant optic atrophy).

Social history

Alcohol and tobacco consumption are relevant in nutritional causes of optic neuropathy. Previous exposure to toxins such as lead and carbon monoxide can also cause optic nerve dysfunction. Occupation is important, as visual loss may severely affect eligibility to continue working in certain professions. Sexual behaviour may need to be enquired about if neuro-ophthalmic manifestations of sexually transmitted diseases (e.g. syphilis, AIDS) are present.

Systems enquiry

* Multiple sclerosis may also have symptoms of weakness, paraesthesia, and bladder dysfunction.
* Thyroid eye disease can result in optic nerve compression, and patients may have symptoms of hyperthyroidism, with heat intolerance, weight loss, irritability, and anxiety.
* Proximal weakness, dysphagia, and worsening of symptoms towards the end of the day can occur in myasthenia gravis.

- Emboli may occur in patients with atherosclerotic disease, and MRI is contraindicated in patients with pacemakers.
- Hypertensive or diabetic nephropathy may be relative contraindications to the use of contrast in CT or MRI scanning.

- Hearing loss, tinnitus, and balance problems may occur in conditions such as vestibular schwannoma (acoustic neuroma) and often have neuro-ophthalmic manifestations.
- Joint pains and skin rashes may occur in underlying rheumatological and collagen vascular diseases.

Visual field examination

A thorough visual field examination is important, as identifying any defects can help to locate important intracranial pathology. Lesions at various parts of the visual field pathway tend to produce characteristic field defects. Visual field defects detected by confrontation should be confirmed using quantitative perimetry.

Examination routine

See Figure 10.6.

1. Observe the patient generally for any signs of a stroke (e.g. hemiplegia) or pituitary lesion (e.g. features of acromegaly).
2. Sit approximately 1 m away from patient, with eyes at a similar level.
3. Ask patient to cover his/her left eye (with palm of their hand) and to look at your face. Enquire whether any face parts are missing or blurred, to detect any gross visual abnormality in the right eye.
4. It is often helpful to begin by assessing whether the patient can see a moving hand or count fingers in all four quadrants of the visual field. This procedure will detect e.g. a dense homonymous hemianopia or a severely depressed peripheral field. If the patient cannot see a moving hand, there is no point in testing with a target smaller than that in that region of the visual field, although it will still be necessary to do so in the remainder of the visual field.
5. Test the peripheral visual field of the right eye by using a white pin, as follows. Whilst the patients looks at your left eye, bring the white pin in from the periphery and ask the patient to say 'yes' when the white pin first comes into view. Repeat for each of the four quadrants. If a field defect is detected, map out the defect by moving the white pin into the defect area from an adjacent normal area, asking when the white pin disappears. Pay attention to the size of the defect and whether it crosses or respects the vertical or horizontal midline. Repeat Steps 3–5 with the patient covering his/her right eye.
6. Test the central (30°) visual field of the right eye by using a red pin. With the patient's left eye covered, ask the patient to again look at your left eye with his/her right eye. Show the patient the red pin and confirm that he/she can see it as being red. Now bring the red pin in from the periphery and ask the patient to say 'yes' when the pin if first seen as being red (not just when it is first seen). Continue moving the red pin towards the centre, checking whether the patient can still see the pin as red. Repeat for each of the four quadrants and then test the other eye.
7. Using the red pin, test the patient's blind spot by comparing it with the size of your own blind spot. Move the red pin in nasally from the periphery until the patient's blind spot is located. Then, move the red pin slowly upwards, downwards, left, and right and each time ask the patient to say 'gone' when the pin disappears and 'back' when it returns to view. Repeat for other eye.
8. If no peripheral or central field defect has been found, test for red desaturation (which is present in early chiasmal compression). Hold up two red pins on either side of the vertical midline. Ask the patient whether both pins are the same shade of red, or whether one pin is less red than the other.

Assessment of optic nerve function

Optic nerve disease can result in impairment of visual acuity, colour vision, and visual fields. An accurate assessment of the optic nerve is important in identifying and monitoring any dysfunction that may be due to serious local and systemic causes.

Examination routine

1. Measure best-corrected visual acuity for distance and near (acuity can be affected by a variable amount depending on the underlying pathology).
2. Measure colour vision (Ishihara colour plates are most commonly used for convenience; see Figure 10.7):
   — Perform the test in adequate light (daylight if possible)
   — Start with the control plate (first plate) and allow several seconds to read each of the subsequent 16 test plates. Record the number of correct plates read (out of 17).
   — Young children or illiterate patients can be asked to trace the line on the non-numerical plates (see Figure 10.7, *bottom panel*).
3. Check for a relative afferent pupillary defect (RAPD; see Figure 10.8).
4. Examine the optic disc, looking for any disc swelling, haemorrhage, atrophy, collateral vessels, and cupping.
5. Perform perimetry (confrontation, manual, automated) to detect any characteristic field defects (see Table 10.1).
6. Other tests: visual evoked potential may detect any subtle optic nerve impairment. An electroretinogram and/or optical coherence tomography may be helpful in confirming loss of retinal ganglion cells and excluding maculopathy.

Other colour vision tests

- Farnsworth–Munsell 100-hue test: the most sensitive and time-consuming colour vision test, involving 85 coloured caps which the patient arranges by hue between two reference tiles
- Farnsworth D15 test: similar to the Farnsworth–Munsell 100-hue test but only uses 15 caps
- City University test: consists of ten plates containing a central colour and four peripheral colours; subjects are asked to match which peripheral colour most closely matches the central colour

Differentiating optic nerve from macular disease

Macular disease can result in reduced visual acuity and colour vision, so it can sometimes have overlapping presentations with optic nerve disease. Features that can help differentiate between the two are detailed in Table 10.2.

Table 10.1 Visual field defects in optic nerve disorders

Visual field defect	Causes
Central scotoma	Demyelinating optic neuropathy
	Compressive optic neuropathy
	Toxic/nutritional optic neuropathy
Enlarged blind spot	Papilloedema
	Congenital disc anomalies
Respecting horizontal midline, e.g. altitudinal, arcuate, nasal step	Anterior ischaemic optic neuropathy
	Glaucoma
	Optic nerve drusen
Bitemporal (not respecting vertical midline)	Tilted optic discs
Junctional scotoma	Anterior chiasmal lesion
Peripheral field loss	Optic perineuritis
	Advanced atrophic papilloedema

Table 10.2 Features of optic nerve and macular disease

Feature	Optic nerve	Macular
Main complaint	Dark/grey cloud	Distortion
Pain	Sometimes on eye movement	Never
Scotoma	Negative	Positive
Vision	Variably decreased	Very decreased
Colour vision	Very decreased	Normal/mild decrease Severe in cone dystrophy
Relative afferent pupillary defect	Present in unilateral or asymmetrical disease	Absent
Refractive error	Unchanged except in papilloedema or retrobulbar mass lesion	Sometimes towards hyperopia
Perimetry	Variable	Central scotoma
Amsler chart	Central scotoma most common but variable	Distortion Central scotoma
Visual evoked potential latency	Large delay with preserved amplitude typical of demyelinating optic neuropathy Variable in other pathologies	Minor delay Reduced amplitude in accordance with reduced acuity
Pattern electroretinogram	N95 amplitude reduction	P50 amplitude reduction
Optical coherence tomography	Retinal nerve fibre layer loss	Involvement of outer retinal layers

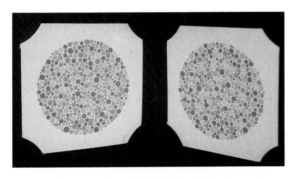

Fig 10.6 Photograph demonstrating examination of the visual field

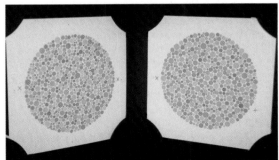

Fig 10.7 Top: standard Ishihara colour vision plates. Bottom: alternative plates for use in children or illiterate patients. Patients are asked to trace the line with their finger

Pupil examination

Pupil abnormalities can result from a variety of conditions and include anisocoria or impaired reflexes to light and accommodation. A thorough pupil examination can help to identify and locate important underlying disorders.

Examination routine

1. Ask the patient to fixate on a distant target.
2. General observation: look for any anisocoria, heterochromia, ptosis, or ocular deviation.
3. Dark response: measure pupil sizes with a ruler and then dim the room lights and repeat the measurements. If anisocoria is present, the larger of the two pupils in bright conditions is likely to be the abnormal one and vice versa in dark conditions.
4. Check the direct pupil light response: shine a torch into one eye and observe the pupil reaction in that eye. Repeat for the other eye.
5. Check the consensual pupil response: shine a torch into one eye and observe the pupil reaction in the other eye.
6. Check for an RAPD: shine the light into one eye for 2–3 seconds and then quickly swing the light into the other eye. Observe for any initial pupillary dilatation, which would indicate an afferent visual pathway defect (see Figure 10.8).
7. Check accommodation reflex: hold up an accommodative target (e.g. an optotype) in front of the patient and observe for pupil constriction as the patient looks from a distant object to the near target.
8. Other: examine the patient on the slit lamp, looking for vermiform iris movements (e.g. in Adie pupil). Perform an eye movement examination, looking for associated nerve palsies. Assess optic nerve function in the presence of an RAPD. Perform a full neurological examination, particularly checking for absent deep tendon reflexes (in Holmes–Adie syndrome).

RAPD

When light is shone into the normal eye, both pupils constrict normally. However, when the light is swung into the affected eye, both pupils will initially dilate (swinging flashlight test; see Figure 10.8). This result is because the effective luminance signalled by the abnormal optic nerve is lower.

An RAPD can still be detected if one eye is pharmacologically dilated. Observation should be on the undilated pupil to assess whether an initial dilatation occurs.

If the visual loss is severe, an afferent pupillary defect can be detected without the need for the swinging flashlight test. A blind eye will have no direct pupillary light reflex (amaurotic pupil). If there is bilateral symmetrical optic neuropathy, it is not helpful to use the swinging flashlight test as it is reliant upon there being unilateral or asymmetrical optic neuropathy.

Nystagmus examination

The examination of patients with nystagmus or other abnormalities of fixation can initially be daunting and confusing. Using a systematic approach whilst considering important questions during the examination process can help to identify the key features and aid the diagnosis of underlying pathology.

Examination routine

1. Observe the patient generally, looking for any:
   - Abnormal head posture (most commonly, but not exclusively, in congenital causes)
   - Signs of visual developmental disorders (e.g. oculocutaneous albinism, aphakic glasses in congenital cataracts)
   - Signs of vestibular disease (hearing aids, associated facial nerve palsies)
   - Cerebellar signs
2. Carefully observe the eyes in the primary position and consider whether the nystagmus is:
   - Unilateral or bilateral
   - Conjugate (both eyes move together) or disconjugate.
   - Symmetrical (both eyes involved to the same degree) or asymmetrical
   - Jerky (slow initial movement followed by fast recovery movement) or pendular (to and fro or with torsional movements of equal speed)
   - Characterized by other patterns (e.g. see-saw or periodic alternating)
   - Also evaluate the frequency and amplitude of nystagmus and, if jerk nystagmus is present, assess which direction is the fast phase movement.
3. Observe the eyes in all cardinal positions of gaze, checking whether the nystagmus:
   - Only occurs on deviation of gaze from primary position with the fast phase in the direction of gaze (gaze-evoked nystagmus)
   - Occurs with fast phase opposite to the direction of gaze (third-degree nystagmus, typical of vestibular nystagmus)
   - Occurs in all positions of gaze, or whether there is a position where the nystagmus reduces (null point)
4. Check whether nystagmus alters with near fixation.
5. If no obvious nystagmus is present, perform a cover test in each position of gaze, checking for latent nystagmus.

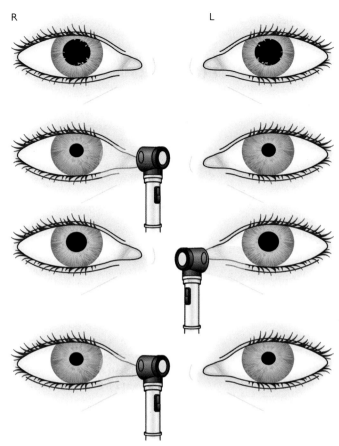

R   L

Fig 10.8 Swinging flashlight test showing a left relative afferent pupillary defect
Note that, if one pupil is paralysed (e.g. in an oculomotor nerve palsy), the test can be carried out by observing only a single functioning pupil; L, left eye; R, right eye

CT

CT works by assessing the X-ray attenuation of different tissues. It involves an X-ray tube and an array of detectors which rotate around a patient, allowing multiple contiguous images to be acquired at different levels, in the coronal or the axial plane. The images can then be reconstructed in any of the standard orthogonal or complex oblique planes. The attenuation of tissues is represented on a greyscale image, with structures of high attenuation (e.g. bone, fresh blood) appearing white, and tissues of lower attenuation (e.g. fat, soft tissue) appearing grey (see Figures 10.9a and 10.10m).

Indications for CT

* Evaluation of bony lesions (trauma, erosion)
* Orbital inflammation (thyroid eye disease) or tumour (lymphoma)
* Acute haemorrhage
* Detecting intraocular or intraorbital calcification (optic nerve sheath meningioma, retinoblastoma, optic nerve drusen)
* When MRI is contraindicated (ferromagnetic foreign bodies)

Disadvantages of CT

* Radiation exposure (as opposed to MRI)
* Bony artefacts can occur
* Possible adverse reaction to iodinated contrast

CT angiography and CT venography

The contrast-enhanced techniques CT angiography and CT venography are now commonly used for the assessment of the intracranial vasculature. They are of superior spatial resolution and of equal or greater sensitivity compared to magnetic resonance angiography and magnetic resonance venography in detecting aneurysms and dural venous sinus thrombosis, respectively (see Figure 10.10d).

MRI

MRI involves the use of magnetic fields to disrupt the alignment of hydrogen atoms within tissues. Strong magnetic fields cause hydrogen atoms to become more uniformly aligned, parallel to the magnetic field. A radio frequency pulse is then applied, causing the hydrogen atoms to change their alignment. When the radio frequency pulse is terminated, the hydrogen atoms return to their previous position and, in doing so, emit magnetic energy which is picked up by receivers surrounding the patient. Computer analysis then converts these signals into information on signal intensity and spatial location (see Figures 10.9c and 10.10a).

Signal intensity

The signal intensity of tissues refers to whether the structure appears bright (high signal) or dark (low signal). The intensity is dependent on the 'weighting of the scan' (T1 or T2), which refers to the method of measuring relaxation times of excited hydrogen atoms.

T1-weighted scans give better anatomical detail. Cerebrospinal fluid and vitreous emit a low-intensity signal and therefore appear dark (see Table 10.3).

T2-weighted scans are considered better for assessing pathological detail, as most pathology is associated with intrinsic or surrounding oedema, which appears bright, as does cerebrospinal fluid and vitreous in these scans (see Table 10.3).

Fat suppression

Fat suppression techniques (e.g. short-time inversion recovery) are particularly useful when imaging the orbits, as the high signal emitted from orbital fat can obscure adjacent structures, making interpretation difficult (see Figure 10.9c and g).

Fluid-attenuated inversion recovery sequence

The fluid-attenuated inversion recovery, or FLAIR, sequence is T2 weighted with nulling of the signal from fluids. It is useful in neuroimaging to suppress the signal from the cerebrospinal fluid so as to accentuate the signal from periventricular lesions in multiple sclerosis.

Gadolinium enhancement

Gadolinium is a paramagnetic agent that is used as contrast medium in T1-weighted scans. It is able to pass through breakdowns in the blood–brain barrier and is therefore used to help detect tumours and other vascular lesions (see Figures 10.9d and 10.10k and l). Side effects of gadolinium use include nausea, vomiting, and hypotension. Contraindications to its use include pregnancy, haemolytic or sickle cell anaemia, and renal failure.

Indications for MRI

MRI is more useful in the evaluation of soft tissue pathology:

* Optic nerve and brain tumours (e.g. glioma)
* Pituitary tumours
* Optic nerve and brain-demyelinating disease

Disadvantages of MRI

* Contraindicated in patients with metallic objects (e.g. pacemakers, aneurysm clips, foreign bodies)
* Noisy, and patients can feel claustrophobic
* Requires patient to remain motionless
* Recent haemorrhage can be missed.
* More expensive than CT

Magnetic resonance angiography

Magnetic resonance angiography is a non-invasive way of imaging the intracranial and extracranial circulations and assesses signal differences between moving blood and stationary tissue. It is useful in detecting pathology such as aneurysms, arteriovenous malformations, and carotid stenosis (see Figure 10.10 i and j). Time-of-flight magnetic resonance angiography may fail to detect aneurysms less than 5 mm in diameter, but resolution can be improved by using contrast-enhancement magnetic resonance angiography techniques.

Magnetic resonance venography

Magnetic resonance venography is similar to magnetic resonance angiography but is more effective in evaluating venous flow. It is particularly useful for identifying venous sinus thrombosis (see Figure 10.10f).

System for evaluating ophthalmic-related neuroradiology images

* Basics:
  — Check name, age, and sex of patient, and scan date.
  — Confirm whether it is a CT (bone is white) or MRI scan.
  — Check whether it is a T1 or T2 image (MRI), whether signal from fat has been suppressed (low signal), and whether contrast has been used.

- Check whether axial, coronal, or sagittal images have been used.
- Assess the following:
  - Globe: present/enucleated, phakic/aphakic, vitreous opacities, retinal calcification
  - Optic nerve: demyelination (T2 hyperintense lesion; associated with swelling if acute, and atrophy if chronic), compressive lesions, trauma
  - Extraocular muscles: enlargement, tendon involvement, entrapment
  - Orbit: masses, vascular lesions, wall fractures
  - Other bony structures: sphenoid wing
  - Pituitary region: enlargement, masses, infarction
  - Posterior visual pathway: space-occupying lesions/vascular lesions in optic radiations/occipital cortex

Table 10.3 Appearance of different tissues on T1- and T2-weighted scans

Body tissue	Appearance in T1 scan	Appearance in T2 scan
Bone	Dark	Dark
Vitreous	Dark	Bright
Cerebrospinal fluid	Dark	Bright
White matter	Bright	Dark
Grey matter	Dark	Bright

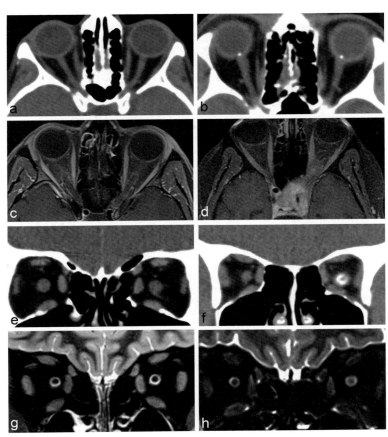

Fig 10.9 Imaging through the orbits
Axial CT demonstrating normal orbits (a) and bilateral optic nerve calcified drusen (b). Axial, post-contrast, fat-suppressed MRI of normal orbits (c) and an enhancing optic pathway glioma extending through the left intraorbital, intracanalicular, and intracranial segments of the left optic nerve (d). Coronal reformatted CT of normal orbits (e) and an enlarged left optic nerve sheath complex with the characteristic peripheral calcification of an optic nerve sheath meningioma (f). Coronal short-time inversion recovery (STIR) MRI of normal orbits (g), and a swollen and T2-weighted hyperintense intraorbital segment of the left optic nerve in an acute left optic neuritis (h)
Courtesy of Dr Indran Davagnanam

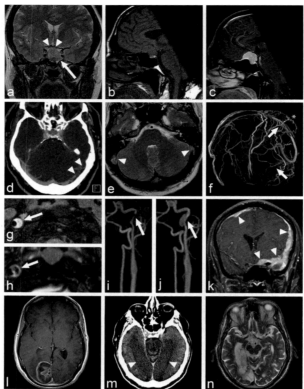

Fig 10.10 Coronal T2-weighted MRI through the sella turcica (a), demonstrating a pituitary macroadenoma extending into the left cavernous sinus (white arrow) and suprasellar cistern, extension into the latter causing displacement and compression of the optic chiasm (white arrowheads). Sagittal pre- (b) and post- (c) Gadolinium contrast T1-weighted MRI demonstrating an enhancing suprasellar meningioma extending along the planum sphenoidale. Note the difficulty in detecting the meningioma pre-contrast. Axial CT venography (d), illustrating a lack of contrast opacification of the left transverse dural venous sinus (white arrowheads), indicative of venous sinus thrombosis. The subsequent axial T2-weighted MRI (e) demonstrates lack of the normal 'flow-voids' in the sinuses bilaterally (arrowheads), with an absence of signal on the sagittal maximal intensity projection magnetic resonance venogram (f) in the superior sagittal, transverse, and sigmoid sinuses (white arrows). Note the extensive scalp venous collaterals (asterisk). Axial fat-supressed T1- (g) and T2- (h) weighted MRI of the distal cervical internal carotid artery, illustrating the 'crescent' of abnormal signal (white arrows) representing attenuated flow within the false lumen of an arterial dissection. The subsequent contrast-enhanced magnetic resonance angiography of this region initially demonstrates near occlusion of the internal carotid artery (i) and then, after several weeks, interval recanalization (j; white arrows). Coronal, post-contrast, fat-supressed T1-weighted MRI (k), demonstrating extensive dural thickening (white arrowheads) in a patient with intracranial sarcoidosis. Axial, post-contrast, T1-weighted MRI (l) of a heterogeneously enhancing right occipital lobe abscess. Axial CT of the brain in a patient with basilar artery thrombosis (m), showing hypodensity in the pons and in the medial temporal and the occipital lobes (white arrowheads), representing extensive posterior circulation infarction. Axial T2-weighted MRI (n) showing mature encephalomalacia of the right medial temporal and occipital regions from a mature right posterior cerebral artery infarct

Courtesy of Dr Indran Davagnanam

Lesions occurring in the visual pathway from the optic chiasm to the occipital cortex can result in characteristic visual field defects, providing information about the likely anatomical site of underlying pathology. An awareness of the various patterns of visual field defect and possible causative lesions is an important part in the evaluation of visual field disorders.

Optic chiasm lesions

Chiasmal lesions typically produce a bitemporal hemianopia (which respects the vertical midline) as a result of compression of decussating nasal retinal fibres. However, different clinical presentations may occur depending on the specific site and type of lesion.

Aetiology

Causes of chiasmal lesions include:

* Tumours:
  - Pituitary adenomas
  - Craniopharyngiomas
  - Meningiomas
  - Gliomas
  - Lymphoma
  - Metastases
* Vascular:
  - Aneurysms (internal carotid artery)
  - Cavernous haemangiomas
* Trauma
* Post-radiation
* Inflammation (e.g. sarcoidosis, multiple sclerosis, neuro-myelitis optica (NMO; also Devic syndrome), pituitary hypophysitis)
* Others: Rathke pouch cysts, sphenoid sinus mucoceles, arachnoid cysts

Clinical evaluation

Patients are often asymptomatic (especially in early stages of disease); however, they may have the following:

History

* Symptoms of raised intracranial pressure (headache, nausea, vomiting, pulsatile tinnitus)
* Symptoms of pituitary dysfunction
* Post-fixation blindness (disappearance of objects during close work, as object is then projected into an area of blindness beyond fixation)
* Diplopia or vertical splitting of visual scene (may arise in patients with pre-existing phoria, as separation of hemifields can occur, known as hemifield slide)

Examination

* Bitemporal field defects (the nature and extent will depend on the precise location of lesion
* Central visual loss if macular fibres affected
* Involvement of other cranial nerves (e.g. third, fourth, and/or sixth in cavernous sinus lesions)
* Colour desaturation in temporal hemifields
* Optic atrophy, which may have a 'bow-tie' configuration
* See-saw nystagmus

Localization of visual field defect patterns

Table 10.4 shows the different types of visual field defects arising from chiasmal lesions, with the corresponding anatomical lesional site and possible causative conditions.

Pituitary adenomas

Pituitary adenomas account for 15% of intracranial tumours and can be functioning or non-functioning. Functioning adenomas often produce systemic symptoms and signs (depending on the resulting hormonal secretion; see Table 10.5) prior to the onset of visual field defects. Non-functioning pituitary adenomas are usually larger than 10 mm and have extended beyond the suprasellar cistern before they result in visual field defects. Both CT and MRI will identify a pituitary adenoma. For such a lesion to be responsible for visual loss, it must be in contact with and elevating the chiasm (see Figure 10.10a).

Pituitary apoplexy

Pituitary apoplexy occurs when infarction or haemorrhage causes sudden enlargement of a pituitary adenoma. It can present with features of subarachnoid haemorrhage, such as acute headache and vomiting, along with reduced vision, superior bitemporal field loss, and ophthalmoplegia. This life-threatening

Table 10.4 Visual field defects resulting from chiasmal lesions	
Visual field defect	**Lesion site**
Superior bitemporal	Inferior chiasmal, e.g. pituitary adenoma (initially compresses infero-nasal fibres)
Inferior bitemporal	Superior chiasmal, e.g. craniopharyngioma (initially compresses supero-nasal fibres)
Junctional syndrome (central scotoma with either contralateral supero-temporal loss or ipsilateral temporal hemianopic scotoma)	Anterior chiasmal lesion ipsilateral to side of central scotoma, e.g. sphenoid meningioma
Bitemporal central hemianopic scotomas	Posterior chiasmal, e.g. hydrocephalus due to dilated third ventricle

Table 10.5 Clinical features of the various types of functioning pituitary adenomas	
Pituitary adenoma type	**Clinical features**
Prolactinoma (↑ prolactin)	Women: ↓ libido, weight gain, amenorrhoea, galactorrhoea Men: impotence, galactorrhoea, ↓ facial hair
Somatotrophic adenoma (↑ growth hormone)	Acromegaly: deep voice, large hands and tongue, prognathism, teeth spacing
Corticotrophic adenoma (↑ adrenocorticotrophin)	Cushing features: ↑ weight, moon face, central obesity, purple striae
Thyrotrophic adenoma (↑ thyroid-stimulating hormone)	Sweating, anxiety, ↑ appetite, ↓ weight, heat intolerance
Gonadatroph adenoma (↑ luteinizing/follicle-stimulating hormone)	Infertility, obesity, hirsutism

↓, decreased; ↑, increased.

condition requires treatment with high-dose corticosteroids and hormone replacement therapy. Transsphenoidal tumour decompression may be required if no improvement occurs within 48 hours but, in many cases, surgery is not required.

Craniopharyngiomas

Craniopharyngiomas arise from vestigial epithelial remnants of the Rathke pouch (an embryonal precursor to the adenohypophysis). They are slow-growing tumours occurring mostly in children but with a second peak in older adults. Treatment is with surgical resection (with or without radiotherapy); however, recurrences are frequent. CT may reveal calcification, which can be helpful in differential diagnosis, but MRI better demonstrates the relationship of the tumour to the anterior visual pathways.

Meningiomas

Sphenoid meningiomas causing optic chiasm compression can arise specifically from the tuberculum sellae, resulting in compression of the junction of the anterior chiasm and optic nerve, with a subsequent junctional syndrome. Meningiomas can also arise superiorly from the olfactory groove, laterally from the medial sphenoidal ridge, and posteriorly from the diaphragma sellae. Both CT and MRI will identify a meningioma; CT may show calcification of the tumour itself or associated hyperostosis, which may be helpful in differential diagnosis. MRI better shows the relationship between the tumour and the anterior visual pathway (see Figure 10.10b and c).

Investigations

* Formal visual field testing to assess field loss at presentation, with repeat testing required to monitor progress
* Endocrinology assessment and appropriate pituitary function tests are required if a pituitary adenoma is suspected or pituitary failure due to metastasis, craniopharyngioma, or extrinsic inflammatory lesions (sarcoidosis or hypophysitis).
* Urgent MRI scanning (discuss with radiologist) is required in suspected chiasmal involvement, although CT may show bony involvement such as erosion due to slow-growing tumours, hyperostosis due to meningioma, or calcification in the tumour itself (meningioma or craniopharyngioma).

Management

Management will depend on the underlying cause, with options including:

* Medical treatment of pituitary tumours (e.g. bromocriptine use in prolactin-secreting tumours)
* Hormone replacement
* High-dose steroids (in pituitary apoplexy and inflammatory lesions)
* Surgical resection
* Transsphenoidal decompression
* Radiotherapy
* Gamma knife radiosurgery

10.9 Retrochiasmal visual pathway disorders

Retrochiasmal lesions of the visual pathway result in homonymous hemianopic field defects, as each side carries ipsilateral temporal and contralateral nasal retinal nerve fibres. Homonymous hemianopic defects may be complete or incomplete, depending on the extent of the underlying lesion. They may also be described as congruous (similar) or incongruous, with increasingly posterior lesions resulting in increased congruity as retinotopic arrangements become more manifest towards the posterior visual pathway.

Retrochiasmal visual field defects are most commonly due to vascular events (e.g. strokes) and tumours, with other causes including trauma, demyelination, abscesses, and migraine (see Figure 10.10l and n). Retrochiasmal lesions can be separated into the specific part of the visual pathway affected (optic tract, lateral geniculate nucleus, optic radiation, and visual cortex) and may result in other neurological features, as nearby structures can also be affected.

Optic tract lesions

Features of a right optic tract lesion can include:
* Left incongruous homonymous hemianopia (see Figure 10.11)
* Left RAPD (in complete lesions)
* Optic atrophy (band atrophy in the left eye)
* Wernicke pupil (abnormal pupil light reflex when light is shone into the affected hemiretina)

Lateral geniculate nucleus lesions

Features of a left lateral geniculate nucleus lesion include:
* A right, congruous, 'wedge-shaped' horizontal sectoranopia
* No RAPD or optic atrophy (although nerve fibre layer thinning can be detected on OCT)
* Contralateral mild hemiparesis

Optic radiation lesions

The optic radiations carry neurons from the lateral geniculate nuclei to the visual cortex. Inferior retinal fibres travel via the temporal lobe radiations, and superior retinal fibres travel via the parietal lobe radiations to the visual cortex.

Features of a right temporal radiation lesion include:
* Left superior incongruous homonymous quadrantanopia ('pie in the sky' defect; see Figure 10.11)
* Associated neurological features:
  - Partial seizures (auditory, olfactory, gustatory, déjà vu, and formed visual)
  - Memory loss (if bilateral)

Features of a left parietal radiation lesion include:
* Right inferior incongruous homonymous quadrantanopia ('pie on the floor' defect)
* Associated neurological features:

- contralateral hemiparesis and hemianaesthesia (posterior limb of internal capsule damage)
- Visual inattention in surviving contralateral hemifield
- Impaired pursuit movement to the left, giving rise to optokinetic nystagmus (OKN) asymmetry when an OKN drum is rotated to the left

Striate cortex lesions

Striate cortex lesions result in a congruous homonymous hemianopia, which may be macular sparing or macular involving. The anterior visual cortex represents the peripheral visual fields and is supplied by the posterior cerebral artery, with impairment of its blood supply resulting in a macular-sparing homonymous hemianopia (see Figure 10.11). The lateral side of the posterior tip of the striate cortex represents central macular function and is supplied variably by the middle cerebral artery, with interruption of this blood supply causing a macular-involving homonymous hemianopia. A contralateral temporal field defect (temporal crescent) may occur following a lesion to the most anterior part of the visual cortex, as this region normally represents the extreme temporal field in the contralateral eye. This representation is monocular.

Associated features of striate cortex lesions include:
* Riddoch phenomenon (can see moving but not stationary targets)
* Cortical blindness (if bilateral) which may be associated with Anton syndrome (denial of blindness, a form of anosagnosia)

Extra-striate cortex lesions

Damage to extra-striate cortex, particularly if bilateral, may result in an impairment of processing of specific submodalities of vision; such impairments include:
* Alexia (inability to recognize word shapes)
* Prosopagnosia (inability to recognize faces)
* Achromatopsia (inability to recognize colours)
* Balint syndrome (inability to localize objects visually)
* Ocular apraxia (inability to move eyes to command); occurs with bilateral parietal or frontal lobe damage

Management

* Full neuro-ophthalmic history and examination
* Investigate for any vascular risk factors
* Urgent neuroimaging
* Referral to stroke, neurosurgical, or oncology teams, depending on cause
* Driving advice
* Referral for visual rehabilitation
* Certificate of visual impairment

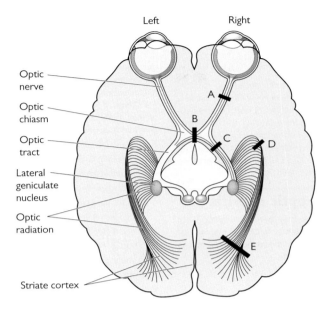

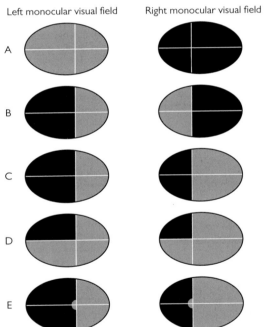

Fig 10.11 Visual field defects caused by lesions at various locations in the visual pathway

Optic neuritis

Optic neuritis is inflammation of the optic nerve and is more specifically termed papillitis when the nerve head is swollen, retrobulbar neuritis if the nerve head appears normal, and neuroretinitis when there is retinal oedema leading to the formation of a macular star. The most common form of optic neuritis in the United Kingdom is acute demyelinating optic neuritis, but infective and other inflammatory causes occur and compressive lesions can occasionally mimic optic neuritis.

Acute demyelinating optic neuritis

Acute demyelinating optic neuritis may occur in isolation but more commonly occurs in the context of multiple sclerosis. Incidence is 5 : 100,000 in the UK general population but occurs in 70% of patients with multiple sclerosis.

Risk factors

* Female sex (3 : 1, female : male)
* Age 20–50 years
* Caucasian
* Incidence increases with distance from the equator

Clinical evaluation

History

* Retrobulbar pain (may be worse on eye movement)*
* Usually unilateral, subacute worsening of vision*
* Recovery may start within 2 weeks*
* Worsening of symptoms following exercise (Uhthoff phenomenon)
* May have weakness, numbness, tingling, and other symptoms of multiple sclerosis, either currently or in the past

Examination

* Vision usually decreased but can vary between 6/6 and no perception of light
* RAPD* (may be symmetrical in bilateral cases)
* Reduced colour vision and contrast sensitivity*
* Visual field defect: central, caecocentral, arcuate, or altitudinal
* Normal optic disc appearance in two-thirds of cases (as retrobulbar)
* Papillitis in one-third of cases

Differential diagnosis

Other causes of optic neuropathy:

* Anterior ischaemic optic neuropathy
* Compressive lesion (e.g. meningioma)
* Leber hereditary optic neuropathy
* Infections (e.g. syphilis, Lyme disease)
* Sarcoidosis
* Toxic/nutritional (e.g. vitamin B_{12}, folate deficiency; always bilateral)
* Post viral
* NMO

Investigations

If the episode is typical, then diagnosis can be made on clinical grounds. However, MRI is useful in confirming optic neuritis and also in determining whether patients are at high risk of developing

*Represents the typical features.

multiple sclerosis, with two or more white matter lesions present on scanning being highly predictive of developing clinically definite multiple sclerosis in the future (see Figures 10.9h and 10.12).

If atypical features are present (e.g. not improving after 2 weeks) then the following tests may be required to exclude other serious underlying pathology:

* Bloods: full blood count (FBC), erythrocyte sedimentation rate (ESR), C-reactive protein (CRP), urea and electrolytes, glucose, vitamin B_{12}/folate, angiotensin-converting enzyme, anti-nuclear antibodies, anti-neutrophil cytoplasmic antibodies, the Venereal Disease Research Laboratory test, anti-aquaporin 4 antibodies (for NMO), and mitochondrial DNA analysis (for Leber hereditary optic neuropathy)
* Chest X-ray
* Lumbar puncture

Management

In most cases, spontaneous visual improvement occurs, with the majority of patients obtaining at least 6/9 vision, although persistent visual disturbances (such as reduced colour vision) may occur.

Numerous trials, including the Optic Neuritis Treatment Trial (ONTT), have shown that visual recovery may be hastened by giving intravenous methylprednisolone (1 g/day for 3 days) followed by oral prednisolone (1 mg/kg for 11 days, then a 4-day taper). This regime has no effect on final visual outcome and is therefore usually only recommended in cases when there is pre-existing poor vision in the other eye or bilateral disease. This regime should not be used if conditions other than optic neuritis associated with multiple sclerosis are suspected.

The ONTT also showed that intravenous methylprednisolone can reduce the rate of development of clinically definite multiple sclerosis in patients with two or more white matter MRI lesions, but only during the first 2 years of follow-up. At 4 years, there was no significant difference between the group treated with intravenous methylprednisolone and the control group.

The Controlled High-Risk Avonex Multiple Sclerosis Prevention Study (CHAMPS) showed that interferon beta 1a use following an acute episode (or other initial demyelinating event) significantly reduced the 3-year rate of clinically definite multiple sclerosis development in patients with two or more white matter lesions.

Similarly, the Early Treatment of Multiple Sclerosis Study (ETOMS) showed a reduced development rate of clinically definite multiple sclerosis (in the first 2 years) in patients who received interferon beta 1a within 3 months of an initial demyelinating event.

The management of optic neuritis not related to multiple sclerosis is very different. Treatment with corticosteroids is mandatory in cases of optic neuritis due to sarcoidosis or NMO, to prevent permanent visual loss. Some conditions, such as chronic relapsing inflammatory optic neuropathy, may require long-term immunosuppression.

Prognosis

* Patients with a normal MRI at presentation have a 16% chance of developing clinically definite multiple sclerosis at 5 years.
* Patients with two or more white matter lesions on initial MRI scanning have a 51% chance of developing clinically definite multiple sclerosis at 5 years.

Compressive optic neuropathies

The most common intrinsic tumours of the optic nerve are gliomas, particularly pilocytic astrocytomas, which may be associated with neurofibromatosis type 1. Rarely, the optic nerve may be infiltrated by lymphoma or leukaemia. Extrinsic tumours within the orbit are most commonly optic nerve sheath meningiomas. Other meningiomas arising from the sphenoid wing or anterior clinoid process may compress the intracanalicular/intracranial segments of the nerve. Extrinsic compression may be due to metastases, lymphoma, or other orbital lesions, including thyroid eye disease (see Chapter 11).

Patients typically present with a progressive visual loss and may notice reduced colour vision. An RAPD is usually present, and the optic disc may appear normal, atrophic, or swollen with retinochoroidal collateral vessels visible. Central scotomas are common.

MRI scanning is needed to evaluate the extent of the lesion and, in particular, whether intracranial extension has occurred (see Figure 10.9d and f).

With optic nerve gliomas and optic nerve sheath meningiomas, if the vision is good and only intraorbital involvement is present, observation with regular visual field testing and MRI scanning is appropriate. Other, more aggressive tumours may require urgent radiotherapy or neurosurgical intervention.

Nutritional/toxic optic neuropathies

Nutritional/toxic optic neuropathies typically present with a bilateral, painless, and gradual loss of vision. Optic discs can be normal at presentation or show temporal pallor. Reduced colour vision and bilateral central/centrocaecal visual field defects are characteristic.

Nutritional causes are commonly due to chronic alcohol and/or tobacco abuse, both of which may lead to vitamin B and folate deficiencies; however, in many cases, specific micronutrient deficiencies cannot be identified. Treatment involves thiamine, folate, vitamin B_{12}, and multivitamin supplements, in addition to reducing alcohol intake and eating a healthier diet.

Causes of toxic optic neuropathy include drugs such as ethambutol, isoniazid, and amiodarone (see Table 10.6). Visual recovery following cessation of the offending agent can be variable and may be dependent on dose and duration of taking the drug.

Traumatic optic neuropathies

Head and facial trauma may result in optic nerve damage through primary and secondary mechanisms. Primary causes include direct transection of the optic nerve by orbital bony fragments, or optic nerve ischaemia following avulsion of its nutrient vessels. Secondary mechanisms include optic nerve compression from oedema and haemorrhage surrounding the nerve. Indirect injury to the optic nerve refers to the occurrence of optic neuropathy

Table 10.6 Causes of nutritional/toxic optic neuropathy	
Nutritional	B_1 (thiamine) deficiency
	B_2 (riboflavin) deficiency
	B_6 deficiency
	B_{12} deficiency
	Folate deficiency
Toxic	Amiodarone
	Ethambutol
	Isoniazid
	Chloramphenicol
	Cimetidine
	Vincristine
	Digitalis
	Chloroquine
	Quinine
	Methotrexate
	Ciclosporin
	Methanol
	Ethylene glycol (antifreeze)
	Carbon monoxide
	Lead
	Cyanide

following a blow to the brow; loss of vision is instantaneous, the blow may not be severe, and the exact mechanism is uncertain.

Full ocular examination is warranted to exclude a penetrating eye injury or globe rupture, and a new RAPD (not accounted for by any other ocular pathology) is essential for diagnosis.

High-resolution CT scanning is helpful in determining the precise nature of the injury.

There is no treatment for primary or indirect optic nerve damage. Surgical decompression is rarely indicated. Orbital or optic nerve sheath haematoma with secondary optic nerve involvement represents a situation where surgical decompression is indicated but attempts to decompress a nerve apparently compressed by a bony fragment are not effective. High-dose corticosteroid treatment has also been shown to be of benefit.

Leber hereditary optic neuropathy

Leber hereditary optic neuropathy is a rare disorder resulting from mutations in maternal mitochondrial DNA and typically affects males aged 15–30, although it can occur at any age and also affect women. Transmission is by women to all offspring, with up to 70% of sons and 15% of daughters manifesting the disease.

Presentation is usually with an acute, unilateral, and painless visual loss, with the other eye becoming affected within days or weeks.

Vision is typically 6/60 to hand movements, with central scotomas. The optic disc may be normal or show mild disc swelling with telangiectatic vessels and progressing to optic atrophy over weeks.

Blood tests for mitochondrial DNA analysis should be performed, with G11778A being the commonest mutation.

No effective treatment is available although treatment with idebenone is currently under investigation. Visual recovery is usually poor. Genetic counselling should be offered.

Further reading

1. Comi G, Fillippi M, Barkhof F, et al.: Effect of early interferon treatment on conversion to definite multiple sclerosis: a randomised study. *Lancet* 2001 May; **357**(9268): 1576–82
2. Jacobs LD, Beck RW, Simon JH, et al.: Intramuscular interferon beta-1a therapy initiated during a first demyelinating event in multiple sclerosis. *N Engl J Med* 2000 Sept; **343**(13): 898–904
3. Kidd D, Burton B, Plant GT, Graham EM: Chronic relapsing inflammatory optic neuropathy (CRION). *Brain* 2003 Feb; **126**(2): 276–84
4. Levin LA, Beck RW, Joseph MP, Seiff S, Kraker R, International Optic Nerve Trauma Study Group: The treatment of traumatic optic neuropathy: the International Optic Nerve Trauma Study. *Ophthalmology* 1999 Jul; **106**(7): 1268–77
5. Optic Neuritis Study Group: Visual function five years after optic neuritis: experience of the Optic Neuritis Treatment Trial. *Arch Ophthalmol* 1997 Dec; **115**(12): 1545–52
6. Shams P, Plant GT: Optic neuritis: a review. *Int MS J* 2009 Sept; **16**(3): 82–9

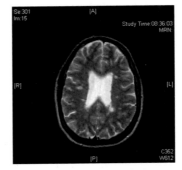

Fig 10.12 T2-weighted MRI showing multiple periventricular white matter lesions

A, anterior; L, left; P, posterior; R, right

Arteritic anterior ischaemic optic neuropathy

Arteritic anterior ischaemic optic neuropathy (AION), which is a potentially sight-threatening condition, is caused by GCA and typically affects people over 50 years of age, with incidence (1 : 100,000) peaking in the eighth decade.

Pathophysiology

GCA is a systemic granulomatous inflammatory disorder affecting large and medium-sized arteries, causing destruction of the internal elastic lamina and vessel occlusion. The superficial temporal arteries, the ophthalmic arteries, and the posterior ciliary arteries are particularly at risk; GCA in these arteries results in arteritic AION.

Clinical evaluation

History

* Sudden, severe, unilateral visual loss (which may be preceded by transient visual disturbances)
* Associated symptoms of GCA: scalp tenderness, temporal headache, jaw claudication, malaise, joint pains, weight loss, and fever

Examination

* Reduced visual acuity
* RAPD
* Pale, swollen disc with flame haemorrhages (see Figure 10.13)
* Temporal tenderness with thickened and often non-pulsatile superficial temporal artery
* Optic atrophy in chronic cases
* May have associated central retinal artery occlusion (CRAO), cotton wool spots, and/or oculomotor deficits

Differential diagnosis

* Non-arteritic AION
* Other causes of acute optic neuropathy (see Section 10.10)
* Other causes of acute visual loss (central retinal vein occlusion (CRVO), CRAO)

Investigations

* Increased ESR (>47 mm/hour) and increased CRP (>2.45 mg/dl) have a 97% specificity for GCA.
* Platelet count may also be raised.
* Temporal artery biopsy is the gold standard test for GCA, with focal areas of granulomatous arteritis seen. A negative biopsy does not exclude GCA, as skip lesions along the temporal artery may be present. Ideally, a temporal artery biopsy should be performed within 3 days of presentation (although biopsy may remain positive for several weeks after), and treatment should not be withheld pending a biopsy.

Management

High-dose systemic corticosteroids are required to prevent visual loss in the unaffected eye and to prevent systemic disease progression. The following steroid regime is recommended:

* Intravenous methylprednisolone 1 g/day for 3 days, followed by 1–2 mg/kg oral prednisolone daily, reduced by 5 mg weekly depending on reduction in ESR, CRP, and symptoms.

* Low-dose steroid maintenance for several years is often required, so osteoporosis prophylaxis is important.

Prognosis

* Visual recovery in the affected eye is generally poor.
* Untreated, the fellow eye can be affected in up to 95% of cases, with this frequency reducing to 13% on steroid treatment.
* It should be noted that GCA can also cause a posterior ischaemic optic neuropathy (no disc swelling) or visual loss due to choroidal ischaemia, or CRAO.

Non-arteritic AION

Non-arteritic AION is the most common acute optic neuropathy (incidence 10 : 100,000, peaking in the seventh decade) and results from occlusion of the short posterior ciliary arteries.

Pathophysiology

It is proposed that atherosclerotic changes in the short posterior ciliary arteries, particularly in the context of a crowded optic nerve head, result in an infarction of the anterior optic nerve. Many cases, however, have no evidence of atherosclerosis, and disc morphology may be the primary cause.

Risk factors

* Hypertension
* Diabetes
* Crowded disc with small cup
* Anaemia
* Smoking
* Hyperlipidaemia
* Hypotensive events
* Collagen vascular disorders
* Obstructive sleep apnoea
* Surgical procedures (especially long, prone procedures such as spinal surgery); posterior ischaemic optic neuropathy may also occur in this situation

Clinical evaluation

History and examination

* Sudden, painless loss of vision (may occur overnight and can be progressive)
* RAPD
* Diffuse/sectorial disc swelling or pallor (splinter haemorrhages may be present)
* Visual field defect: typically altitudinal

Investigations

* ESR/CRP to investigate for GCA
* Check for atherosclerotic risk factors: blood pressure, FBC, glucose, and cholesterol.
* Collagen vascular screen in younger patients

Management

* No proven effective treatment, although corticosteroid treatment whilst the disc is swollen has been proposed
* Whether low-dose aspirin is beneficial in reducing the risk of other vascular events is unknown; evidence suggests that aspirin does not reduce the risk of second eye involvement.
* Treat any underlying abnormalities.

Prognosis
- In 40% of patients, vision improves by two or more Snellen lines.
- There is a 20% chance of the other eye being affected within 5 years.

Temporal artery biopsy

The frontal branch of the superficial temporal artery is commonly chosen for biopsy because of its accessibility and high degree of involvement in GCA. The artery lies in the superficial temporal fascia, just deep to the subcutaneous fat.

Complications of this procedure include bleeding (intra- and post-operatively), stroke, facial nerve damage, and scar formation.

Procedure
- Identify site for biopsy: use signs of temporal artery tenderness, skin erythema, absent pulsations, and arterial nodularity as a guide.
- Mark the biopsy site (see Figure 10.14): mark the course of the vessel on the skin with a pen. Hair may need to be shaved off and occasionally Doppler ultrasound may be required to aid identification.
- Anaesthetize the skin by using 1% lignocaine with adrenaline (see Figure 10.14).
- Make a skin incision: use a Number 15 blade to incise just into the subcutaneous fatty layer.
- Exposing the artery (see Figure 10.15): lift up the wound edges and use blunt dissection to expose at least 3 mm of the artery from surrounding connective tissue.
- Removing the artery: tie a single throw of a knot of 4–0 Vicryl to the proximal end of the artery and check that the patient can still speak and move fingers and toes (i.e. cerebral ischaemia has not been precipitated). Tie the knot fully and place a further knot on the distal end (see Figure 10.16). Tie off any additional branches. Then cut the artery and remove it, being careful to avoid creating crushing artefacts; send it for histology.
- Closure (see Figure 10.17): use 5–0 Vicryl for deep layers, and 6–0 Vicryl for skin closure. Apply pressure dressing for 24 hours.

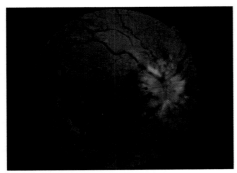

Fig 10.13 Disc swelling and haemorrhage in arteritic anterior ischaemic optic neuropathy

Courtesy of Masoud Teimory

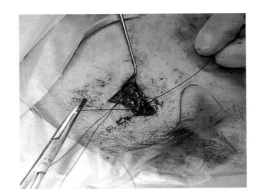

Fig 10.16 Artery exposed and ligated

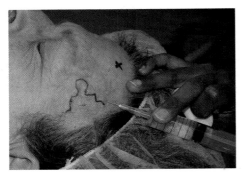

Fig 10.14 Marked left temporal artery and local anaesthetic injection

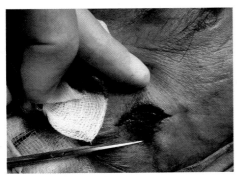

Fig 10.15 Exposed temporal artery

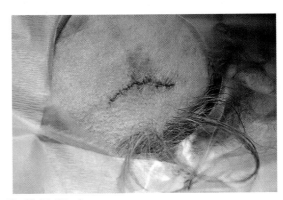

Fig 10.17 Skin closure

10.12 Papilloedema and idiopathic intracranial hypertension

Papilloedema

Papilloedema is optic disc swelling secondary to raised intracranial pressure and is usually bilateral. Its presence should raise the suspicion of serious intracranial pathology.

Pathophysiology

The optic nerve sheath is continuous with the subarachnoid space. As intracranial pressure rises, pressure is exerted onto the optic nerve, causing impairment of axoplasmic flow. This impairment leads to a build-up of axoplasmic material at the level of the lamina cribrosa, and subsequent optic disc swelling. An alternative or additional mechanism is increased pressure in the central retinal vein (which has a short course in the subarachnoid space), leading to congestion/ischaemia at the optic nerve head.

Aetiology

Causes of raised intracranial pressure are listed in Table 10.7.

Clinical evaluation

History

Symptoms are usually those of raised intracranial pressure and include:

* Headache: typically worse in the mornings, and increased by coughing/Valsalva manoeuvres
* Nausea and vomiting
* Pulsatile tinnitus

Visual symptoms may also occur and include:

* Transient visual obscurations (e.g. momentary loss/greying of vision; may be precipitated by change of posture)
* Diplopia (if sixth nerve involved)
* Blurring of vision/reduced colour vision (late atrophic papilloedema)

Optic disc signs of the different stages of papilloedema

* Early: hyperaemia and elevation of the disc, thickened peripapillary nerve fibre layer obscuring vessels
* Fully developed acute (see Figure 10.18): greater elevation of the nerve head than for early papilloedema; engorged veins; peripapillary nerve fibre layer haemorrhages and cotton wool spots; Paton lines (peripapillary circumferential retinal folds)

* Chronic (see Figure 10.19): reduced hyperaemia, reduced haemorrhages and cotton wool spots, drusen-like bodies within the optic nerve head, retinochoroidal collateral venules, retinochoroidal folds due to flattening of the posterior globe by the distended optic nerve sheath
* Atrophic (see Figure 10.20): the disc is pale and no longer swollen, arterioles are attenuated, extensive retinal nerve fibre layer thinning; indicates severe and irreversible visual loss.

Differential diagnosis

* Optic neuropathies with papillitis
* Pseudopapilloedema (e.g. drusen, hypermetropic discs, tilted discs)
* Malignant hypertension
* Uveitis causing optic disc vasculitis
* Graves compressive ophthalmopathy

Investigations

* Urgent neuroimaging with magnetic resonance venography to exclude venous thrombosis (see Figure 10.10d–f)
* Lumbar puncture if cause unclear (exclude space-occupying lesions first)
* B-scan to exclude drusen
* Visual field testing (enlarged blind spots, infero-nasal loss, generalized constriction)
* Fundus fluorescein angiography (FFA): late leakage of dye seen in early papilloedema

Management

Management depends on the underlying cause, and referral to neurosurgery/neurology is usually required.

Idiopathic intracranial hypertension

Idiopathic intracranial hypertension (previously known as benign intracranial hypertension or pseudotumour cerebri) is a common cause of papilloedema but remains a diagnosis of exclusion. The pathophysiology of idiopathic intracranial hypertension is unclear; both resistance to cerebrospinal fluid absorption across arachnoid villi, and intracranial venous hypertension, have been suggested to occur.

Aetiology

Idiopathic intracranial hypertension typically affects young (in their third decade), obese women. Associated risk factors include:

* Recent, substantial weight gain
* Drugs: tetracyclines, steroid withdrawal
* Obstructive sleep apnoea
* Intracranial venous thrombosis
* Intracranial venous sinus stenosis

Clinical evaluation

Clinical features are similar to those for other causes of raised intracranial pressure.

Investigations

Criteria for diagnosing idiopathic intracranial hypertension include:

* Symptoms and signs of raised intracranial pressure

Table 10.7 Causes of raised intracranial pressure	
Mechanism	**Underlying cause**
Space-occupying lesions (mass effect)	Tumours
	Haemorrhage
	Haematoma
Increased cerebrospinal fluid production	Choroid plexus tumour (very rare)
Reduced cerebrospinal fluid resorption due to intracranial venous hypertension	Venous sinus thrombosis
	Arachnoid villi damage (meningitis, subarachnoid haemorrhage)
	Idiopathic intracranial hypertension
Obstructive hydrocephalus	Mass lesions
	Aqueduct stenosis
Communicating hydrocephalus	

- Normal neuroimaging, other than changes due to raised intracranial pressure and venous sinus stenosis
- Raised cerebrospinal fluid pressure with normal composition

Management

The aims of treatment are to relieve headaches and prevent irreversible optic nerve impairment. Options include:

- Reducing weight if obese
- Medically reducing intracranial pressure: acetazolamide, other diuretics
- Optic nerve sheath fenestration if vision is threatened, particularly if headaches are not a feature
- Lumboperitoneal or ventriculoperitoneal shunts in severe, resistant headache
- Venous sinus stenting in suitable cases

Prognosis

- Idiopathic intracranial hypertension is a usually a self-limiting condition, but can last up to several years with recurrences.
- Visual prognosis is good in appropriately managed patients and therefore regular optic nerve assessment is important.

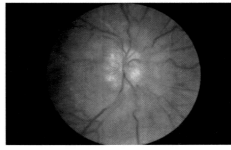

Fig 10.19 Chronic papilloedema

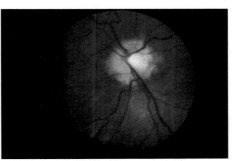

Fig 10.20 Optic atrophy secondary to papilloedema

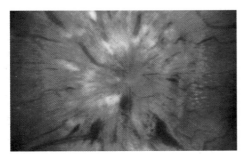

Fig 10.18 Fully developed acute papilloedema

Congenital optic nerve disorders include a range of conditions that can affect visual function to varying degrees and may be associated with systemic abnormalities.

Optic disc pit

An optic disc pit appears as a small depression in the optic disc and is usually located temporally (see Figure 10.21). Histologically, there is herniation of retina and surrounding fibrous tissue into a depression within the optic nerve.

Patients may be asymptomatic, although 45% of cases develop macular retinoschisis and subsequent serous retinal detachments, with the subretinal fluid thought to arise from the vitreous or subarachnoid space surrounding the nerve.

Vitrectomy with gas tamponade may be required when spontaneous resolution of the maculopathy does not occur. Visual field defects may also be present and may not necessarily correlate with the location of the pit.

Congenital tilted disc syndrome

Congenital tilted disc syndrome, which is normally bilateral, is due to an oblique entry of the optic nerve through the scleral canal and local fundus ectasia (see Figure 10.22). The inferonasal disc is displaced posteriorly, and thinning of the adjacent retinal pigment epithelium may also be present.

Visual field defects are common, affecting the superotemporal quadrants in nasal fundus ectasia. These defects tend not to progress or respect the vertical midline and may often be eliminated after correcting for any myopic refractive error which is associated with this condition. It must be understood that if, say, the nasal fundus is ectatic, then a higher myopic correction will be required for this region of the visual field than for the fovea.

Optic nerve hypoplasia

Optic nerve hypoplasia, which can be unilateral or bilateral, may have systemic associations and is characterized by a reduced number of optic nerve axons. Risk factors for developing optic nerve hypoplasia include young maternal age, maternal smoking, alcohol use during gestation, and preterm birth.

Vision can be normal; however, optic nerve hypoplasia is a common cause of blindness in children. On examination, a small, grey disc, often surrounded by a yellow peripapillary halo, is seen, flanked on either side by a ring of pigment (double-ring sign; see Figure 10.23).

Systemic associations include de Morsier syndrome (septo-optic dysplasia), which comprises optic nerve hypoplasia, absence of the septum pellucidum, and partial or complete agenesis of the corpus callosum. Other associations include pituitary dysfunction and cerebral hemispheric abnormalities.

Sectorial hypoplasia is also seen, possibly due to infarction in utero. There will be a visual field defect corresponding to the hypoplastic sector. There is an increased incidence of maternal diabetes in such cases.

Optic disc coloboma

In optic disc coloboma, which can be unilateral or bilateral, the optic disc appears as a clearly demarcated bowl-shaped excavation that is usually decentred and thinner in the inferior region of the disc than in the superior region (see Figure 9.5). It arises from abnormal fusion of the two sides of the proximal end of the optic cup. It may occur sporadically or be inherited in an autosomal dominant pattern, and it can be associated with multiple congenital abnormalities.

Visual acuity is reduced depending on the degree of foveal involvement by the coloboma. Defects may be present in the superior visual field, and other ocular features can include colobomas of the iris, ciliary body, and fundus.

Systemic associations include CHARGE syndrome, Aicardi syndrome, Goldenhar syndrome, Goltz syndrome, and Meckel–Gruber syndrome.

Morning glory anomaly

Morning glory anomaly, which is a rare, sporadic condition, is usually unilateral and is characterized by a funnel-shaped excavation of the optic disc, with central glial tissue and chorioretinal pigmentary disturbance surrounding the disc (see Figure 10.24). Retinal blood vessels are increased in number, arise from the disc periphery, and run an abnormally straight course over the peripapillary region.

The pathogenesis of this condition is unknown, although one theory is that it arises from a failure of closure of the fetal fissure and is possibly a variant of coloboma. Visual acuity is usually poor, and serous retinal detachments occur in one-third of patients.

This condition can be associated with transsphenoidal enchephalocele and hypopituitarism, with patients displaying hypertelorism, a wide head, and a flattened nasal bridge. Also, hypoplasia of ipsilateral intracranial vasculature may be present.

Optic disc drusen

Optic disc drusen are refractile, often calcified bodies within the substance of the optic nerve head, possibly arising from abnormalities in axoplasmic flow. They may mimic papilloedema, as the drusen may lie beneath the disc surface. The disc can therefore appear elevated, with a 'scalloped' margin and a minimal cup (see Figure 10.25). Anomalous retinal vessels with increased branching and tortuosity may accompany the disc changes. Disc drusen usually become more obvious in the early teen years, when they appear as waxy, yellow irregularities on the disc surface.

Visual field defects may accompany disc drusen as a result of nerve fibre bundle defects. Rarely, visual acuity can be affected by juxtapapillary choroidal neovascular membrane formation.

B-scan ultrasound is particularly useful in detecting the calcific elements of disc drusen. FFA can show autofluorescence (prior to dye injection) and late disc staining, although these features may be less apparent in buried drusen. Calcification at the optic nerve head may also be visible on high-resolution orbital CT (see Figure 10.9b). Using currently available protocols, optic disc drusen are not well seen on optical coherence tomograph; however, this technique may confirm that the disc is elevated but the nerve fibre layer is thinned; in contrast, in papilloedema and other causes of optic disc swelling, the nerve fibre layer will be thickened. Retinitis pigmentosa and angioid streaks are associated with optic disc drusen.

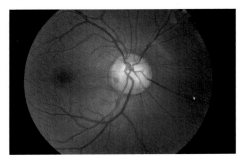

Fig 10.21 Optic disc pit
Courtesy of Prof A T Moore

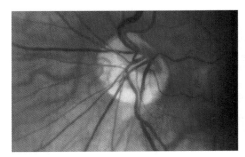

Fig 10.22 Tilted disc in the left eye
Note the thinning of the retina infero-nasal to the optic disc (lower left in the image)

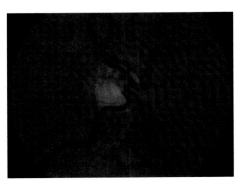

Fig 10.23 Optic nerve hypoplasia
The size of the optic nerve head can be judged to be small in comparison with the width of the vessels emerging from it. There is also a gap between the edge of the disc and the margin of the retina (double-ring sign)

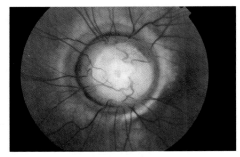

Fig 10.24 Morning glory anomaly
Courtesy of Prof A T Moore

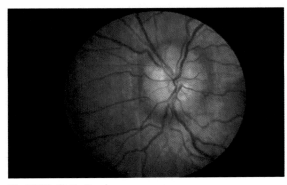

Fig 10.25 Optic disc drusen
The disc is elevated but there is no swelling of the retinal nerve fibre layer; therefore, the vessels are not obscured

Eye movement disorders and other ocular abnormalities can arise from lesions to the third, fourth, and/or sixth cranial nerves. Lesions can occur anywhere, from the nucleus, to the fascicle (as the nerve passes through the brainstem), to the peripheral nerve. As cranial nerves lie in close proximity to one other, other neurological manifestations can arise, resulting in particular presentations that can help locate the underlying lesion. A full cranial nerve and neurological examination is therefore mandatory in patients presenting with ophthalmic cranial nerve problems.

Third nerve palsies

Aetiology

Causes include:

* Microvascular disease (diabetes, hypertension)
* Trauma (e.g. extradural/subdural haematomas)
* Aneurysm (e.g. posterior communicating aneurysm at the junction with the internal carotid artery)
* Tumour
* Demyelination
* Vasculitis (e.g. GCA)
* Congenital
* Ophthalmolplegic 'migraine'
* Inflammatory (e.g. granuloma)
* Idiopathic

Clinical evaluation

As the third nerve supplies the levator muscle and all the extraocular muscles (except the lateral rectus and superior oblique), the following features can be present to varying degrees, depending on whether the nerve damage is partial or complete:

* Diplopia: usually the primary symptom
* Ptosis
* Onset painful in aneurysm and granuloma
* Affected eye abducted and usually depressed (owing to unopposed lateral rectus and superior oblique action; see Figure 10.26)
* Reduced action in all other gaze movements
* Pupil dilatation (in compressive lesions)
* Reduced accommodation
* Aberrant regeneration (with recovery following trauma or compressive lesions):
  - Lid-gaze synkinesis: lid elevation on attempted adduction or depression
  - Pupil-gaze synkinesis: pupil constriction on attempted adduction or depression

Pupil involvement versus pupil-sparing lesions

As a general rule, 'surgical' causes of third nerve lesions (e.g. aneurysms, trauma, tumours) result in pupil dilatation, as the parasympathetic pupillomotor fibres are not spared.

'Medical' causes of third nerve lesions (e.g. diabetes, hypertension) typically spare pupil involvement, as the resulting ischaemia only affects the central vascular supply of the nerve, thus sparing superficial pupillary fibres, which are supplied by pial vessels.

However, absence of pupil involvement on presentation does not exclude a compressive cause, as the lesion may be evolving and yet to manifest pupillary signs.

Localizing lesions

In addition to ipsilateral third nerve involvement, the following features can give information on the likely anatomical site of the nerve lesion.

Nuclear lesions

* Bilateral ptosis (levator subnucleus)
* Contralateral superior rectus weakness (superior rectus subnucleus)

Fascicle lesions

See Table 10.8.

* Contralateral tremor and ataxia (red nucleus lesion in Benedikt syndrome)
* Contralateral hemiparesis (cerebral peduncle lesion in Weber syndrome)

Subarachnoid lesions

* Headache, pain, neck stiffness (and other signs of meningism) following aneurysm rupture

Intracavernous lesions

* Fourth, fifth, and/or sixth nerve involvement may occur, because of the close proximity of these nerves in the cavernous sinus.

Superior orbital fissure and intraorbital lesions

* Isolated elevation defect and ptosis (superior division lesion)
* Adduction and depression deficits with mydriasis (inferior division lesion)

Investigations

* Urgent CT angiogram and neurosurgical review if an aneurysm or other compressive lesion is suspected
* Blood pressure, and bloods for vascular risk factors (FBC, glucose, lipids, ESR, CRP)

Management

Management depends on the underlying cause. Options include:

* Posterior communicating aneurysms require endovascular coiling.
* Diplopia may be controlled by using patching, inducing ptosis (if not already present), or using Fresnel prisms.
* Strabismus and/or lid surgery may be required if spontaneous improvement has not occurred (after 12 months).

Prognosis

* Spontaneous recovery rate is high in microvascular ischaemic causes (approaches 100%).
* Recovery (or partial recovery) is also common in compressive cases but is variable depending on the underlying cause and may take longer than in microvascular cases. Any manifestations of aberrant regeneration are permanent.

Fourth nerve palsies

Each fourth cranial nerve supplies the contralateral superior oblique muscle, which intorts, depresses, and abducts the eye. Nerve palsies usually present with binocular vertical diplopia, with torsion. These conditions may arise from congenital or acquired causes and be unilateral or bilateral; the unilateral and bilateral forms have differing clinical features.

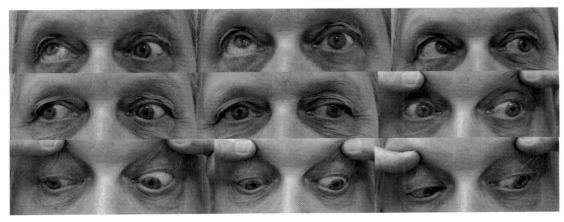

Fig 10.26 Left, pupil-sparing third nerve palsy in the major positions of gaze
Note the partial ptosis with limitation of elevation, depression, and adduction, and sparing of abduction of the left eye

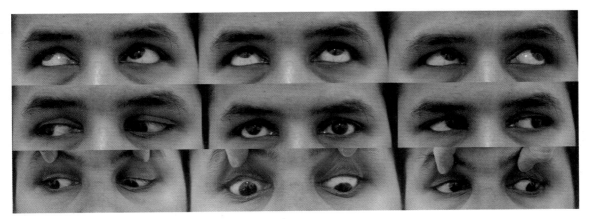

Fig 10.27 Right superior oblique palsy in the major positions of gaze
Note the right hypertropia in primary position and that it is worse on left gaze. Note also the limitation of laevodepression of the right eye

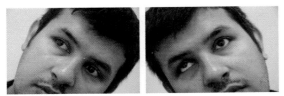

Fig 10.28 Right superior oblique palsy with increased right hypertropia on head tilt to right

Aetiology

- Congenital
- Acquired:
  - Trauma (often causes bilateral features)
  - Microvascular disease
  - Demyelination
  - Idiopathic
  - Vasculitis (e.g. GCA)
  - Tumour
  - Inflammatory (e.g. granuloma)

General clinical features

- Diplopia (vertical, torsional, or oblique), which is usually worse on down-gaze
- Affected eye is hypertropic; hypertropia increases with:
  - Adduction (see Figure 10.27)
  - Head tilt towards the ipsilateral shoulder (see Figure 10.28)
- Affected eye is excyclotropic
- Limited depression in adduction
- Compensatory head tilt (to relieve diplopia) may be present with:
  - Head tilt towards contralateral shoulder
  - Face turn towards unaffected side
  - Chin depression

Congenital features

Congenital fourth nerve palsies may present in children or only become apparent in adulthood following decompensation. Patients typically develop large vertical fusion ranges and can develop concomitance, with muscle sequelae. Torsional diplopia is rare, and abnormal head postures may have developed, of which patients are sometimes unaware.

Acquired features

Usually, there is a sudden and recent onset of symptoms, which also tend to be severe and include torsion. A history of trauma is common, with the fourth nerve being particularly vulnerable as it passes close to the rigid tentorial edge. Onset may be painful with an underlying granuloma. Variability is seen in myasthenia gravis.

Bilateral features

Bilateral fourth nerve palsies are usually caused by trauma. Other features include:

- Chin-down head posture
- Small vertical deviation in primary position

- V pattern
- Alternating adduction hypertropia
- Large excyclotorsion (>10°)

Parks–Bielschowsky three-step test

The Parks–Bielschowsky three-step test is useful for identifying the underacting muscle in vertical deviations and is therefore helpful in the diagnosis in superior oblique palsies. It involves performing cover tests in the following positions (in the example of a right superior oblique palsy).

Assess which eye is hypertropic in the primary position

Right hypertropia implies that the following four muscles could be impaired:

- The right superior oblique or the right inferior rectus
- The left superior rectus or the left inferior oblique

Assess in which lateral gaze direction the hypertropia is worse

The finding that right hypertropia is worse on left gaze implies that the following two muscles could be impaired:

- The right superior oblique
- The left superior rectus

Assess in which head tilt position the hypertropia is worse

The finding that right hypertropia is worse on right head tilt implies that the right superior oblique is affected.

Investigations

- Look at old photographs to check for congenital causes.
- Blood pressure and blood tests to exclude vascular causes
- Consider neuroimaging in cases with no vascular risk factors, trauma, or congenital causes.

Management

Aside from treating any underlying causes, options include:

- Occlusion or prisms to control diplopia
- Strabismus surgery in non-resolving palsies (after 12 months); options include:
  - Inferior oblique weakening
  - Superior oblique tuck
  - Contralateral inferior rectus recession

Prognosis

- Spontaneous recovery is high in microvascular cases, with complete resolution occurring within 2–3 months.
- Full recovery is less common in traumatic cases than in non-traumatic cases, although over 50% of patients in traumatic cases show some improvement.

10.15 Cranial nerve palsies II

Sixth nerve palsies

The sixth cranial nerve supplies the ipsilateral lateral rectus muscle, resulting in abduction defects when innervation is impaired. Lesions to the sixth nerve can occur at various sites along its course, producing localizing signs. Various other conditions can also result in abduction defects and therefore imitate a sixth nerve palsy.

Aetiology

* Microvascular disease
* Raised intracranial pressure (usually bilateral)
* Tumour (acoustic neuroma, nasopharyngeal tumours, cavernous sinus masses, pontine gliomas in children)
* Trauma (basal skull fractures)
* Idiopathic
* Demyelination
* Vasculitis (e.g. GCA)
* Inflammatory (e.g. granuloma)
* Congenital (rare)

Clinical evaluation

* Typical presentation is with binocular, horizontal diplopia that is worse for looking into the distance and in the direction of affected muscle.
* Esotropia of affected eye in primary position (see Figure 10.29)
* Limitation of abduction (see Figure 10.29)
* Compensatory face turn to the ipsilateral side to relieve diplopia may be present.
* The minimal sign of a mild lateral rectus underaction is a distance esophoria.

Differential diagnosis

The following conditions can also cause reduced abduction:

* Thyroid eye disease (look for other signs): here, the defect is restrictive because of the involvement of the medial rectus; there is no lateral rectus underaction.
* Myasthenia gravis (variability of symptoms, especially towards the end of the day): it would be unusual for the signs to remain limited to one muscle only.
* Medial wall blowout fracture: will show the signs of a restrictive rather than paretic limitation
* Duane syndrome (narrowing of palpebral fissure and globe retraction on adduction): no diplopia
* Orbital inflammatory disease (proptosis, chemosis, pain)
* Accommodative spasm: a distance esotropia seen in hypermetropia: this condition is adaptive, to improve visual acuity
* Convergence spasm: inappropriate vergence action usually only seen during examination of eye movements; confirm by observing miosis and full ductions

Localizing lesions

In addition to an ipsilateral abduction defect, the following features can give information on the likely site of underlying pathology.

Nuclear lesions

The sixth nerve nucleus lies in the pons, in close association to the seventh nerve fascicle, the paramedian pontine reticular formation (horizontal gaze centre), and first-order sympathetic fibres which travel in the pons. In addition, the sixth nerve nucleus provides innervation to the contralateral medial rectus via the medial longitudinal fasciculus. Pontine lesions can therefore cause:

* Ipsilateral gaze palsies
* One-and-a-half syndrome (ipsilateral gaze palsy plus ipsilateral internuclear ophthalmoplegia)
* Ipsilateral facial weakness or myokymia, in demyelination
* Foville syndrome (dorsal pontine infarct involving first-order sympathetic fibres and the fifth nerve nucleus):
  - Ipsilateral gaze palsy
  - Ipsilateral facial weakness
  - Ipsilateral facial analgesia (fifth nerve damage)
  - Horner syndrome
  - Deafness (eighth nerve damage)

Fascicle lesions

See Table 10.8.

Table 10.8 Eponymous brain stem syndromes

	Features	Location of lesion
Weber syndrome	Third nerve palsy with contralateral hemiparesis	Cerebral peduncle Third nerve fascicle
Benedikt syndrome	Third nerve palsy with contralateral tremor	Red nucleus Third nerve fascicle
Claude syndrome	Third nerve palsy with ipsilateral ataxia and tremor	Superior cerebellar peduncle
Foville syndrome	Contralateral hemiplegia with facial sparing Ipsilateral facial nerve palsy Horizontal gaze palsy ± ipsilateral sixth nerve palsy	Dorso-caudal pons Sixth nerve nucleus or fascicle Seventh nerve nucleus
Millard–Gubler syndrome	Contralateral hemiplegia with facial sparing Ipsilateral sixth and seventh nerve palsies	Ventro-caudal pons Sixth nerve fascicle Seventh nerve fascicle
Raymond syndrome	Contralateral hemiplegia with facial sparing Ipsilateral sixth nerve palsy	Ventral medial pons Sixth nerve fascicle
Wallenberg syndrome	Ipsilateral facial and corneal anaesthesia Ipsilateral ataxia Nystagmus Vertigo Nausea and vomiting Dysphagia Ipsilateral palate, pharyngeal, and vocal cord paralysis ± ipsilateral central Horner syndrome (75%) ± ipsilateral sixth nerve palsy ± ipsilateral seventh nerve palsy	Lateral medulla Fifth nerve spinal nucleus Eighth nerve vestibular nuclei Tenth nerve nucleus First-order oculosympathetic neurone

Fascicle lesions involve damage to the sixth nerve as it passes through the pyramidal tract and can be associated with Millard–Gubler syndrome, which has the following symptoms:
* Ipsilateral sixth nerve palsy
* Ipsilateral facial weakness
* Contralateral hemiplegia

False localizing signs
Raised intracranial pressure (e.g. from posterior fossa tumours) may result in downward displacement of the brainstem, causing pressure on the sixth nerve as it passes over the petrous bone and thus leading to unilateral or bilateral sixth nerve palsies.

Investigations
* Blood pressure and blood tests, to exclude vascular causes
* ESR and CRP in older patients, to exclude GCA
* Consider MRI if:
  – Other cranial nerve/brainstem abnormalities are present
  – Palsy is not resolving after 3 months
  – Patients are under 40 years old
* Consider lumbar puncture and cerebrospinal fluid examination if no cause found.

Management
Aside from treating any underlying causes, options include:
* Occlusion or prisms, to control diplopia
* Botulinum toxin to the ipsilateral medial rectus
* Strabismus surgery in non-resolving palsies (after 12 months):
  – Resect/recession surgery may be sufficient in partial sixth nerve palsies.
  – Vertical muscle transposition surgery is often needed in complete sixth nerve palsies.

Prognosis
The prognosis for sixth nerve palsy depends on the underlying cause, with full recovery being high in microvascular causes.

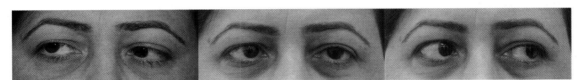

Fig 10.29 Right sixth nerve palsy
Note the right esotropia in primary position, and the limitation of abduction of the right eye

10.16 Nystagmus

Nystagmus is an involuntary, rhythmic oscillation of the eyes, arising from congenital or acquired causes. It can be further classified according to whether the movements have a fast (saccadic) component and a slow phase (jerk nystagmus), whether the speed of movement is slow and equal in both directions (pendular nystagmus), or saccadic in all directions (flutter and opsoclonus).

Pathophysiology

Highest visual acuity requires images to be held steady over the fovea and is dependent on four mechanisms: fixation, the vestibulo-ocular reflex, the optokinetic reflex, and the neural integrator. Fixation refers to (a) the visual system's ability to detect drift of the desired retinal image from the fovea and instigation of corrective eye movements (saccades) and (b) suppression of unwanted movements that would take the eyes off the target. The fixation mechanism is physiologically identical to the pursuit mechanism (See Sections 10.3 and 10.17). The vestibulo-ocular system helps generate compensatory eye movements in response to high-velocity changes in head position. This task is performed by the optokinetic reflex at slow velocities. The neural integrator (comprising the cerebellum, the ascending vestibular pathways, and the ocular motor nuclei) maintains eccentric eye positions despite the actions of the globe's muscles and suspensory ligaments (these actions are known as orbital elastic forces), as they return the eye to the primary position. Lesions affecting any of these mechanisms or their control can result in the various types of nystagmus. The optokinetic reflex generates physiological jerk nystagmus (also known as railway nystagmus). The vestibular system can also generate physiological nystagmus, such as that seen after rotation.

Downbeat nystagmus

Downbeat nystagmus is usually caused by posterior fossa lesions at the level of the craniocervical junction (e.g. Chiari malformations and space-occupying lesions). Ischaemic and inflammatory lesions are rare causes; however, downbeat nystagmus infrequently occurs in association with cerebellar degeneration. Features include:

* Nystagmus in primary position, with the fast phase beating downwards
* Maximum nystagmus amplitude on lateral down-gaze

Upbeat nystagmus

Upbeat nystagmus can be caused by cerebellar, medulla, and/or thalamic lesions and produces a nystagmus in the primary position, with the fast phase beating upwards.

See-saw nystagmus

See-saw nystagmus usually results from large parasellar tumours but can also arise from infarction and trauma to the subthalamic region. It can also occur in bitemporal hemianopia. Features include a pendular nystagmus with, in the first half of the cycle, one eye elevating and intorting whilst the other eye depresses and extorts, and a reversal in direction in the second half of the cycle.

Periodic alternating nystagmus

Periodic alternating nystagmus is a consequence of cerebellar dysfunction and its features include:

* Horizontal jerk nystagmus with fast phase beating in one direction for about 90 seconds (amplitude gradually increases and decreases during this period), an intervening neutral period of about 10–20 seconds, and then recommencement of nystagmus, with the fast beat in the other direction
* Repetition of this alternating cycle
* May be congenital, in which case the cycle may be much shorter

Gaze-evoked nystagmus

Gaze-evoked nystagmus may be physiological or due to cerebellar dysfunction (including that induced by drugs such as anticonvulsants and alcohol). Features include a horizontal jerk nystagmus on eccentric gaze, with the fast phase being in the direction of gaze. Physiological end-point nystagmus usually only becomes apparent at gaze of 45°–50°, so gaze-evoked nystagmus occurring at an angle less than that is likely to be pathological. A similar nystagmus results from extraocular muscle paresis.

Pathological gaze-evoked nystagmus usually diminishes in amplitude with sustained eccentric gaze because of adaptation. This adaptation results in rebound nystagmus on return to primary position.

Vestibular nystagmus

Eye movements are intricately linked to the vestibular system, and both central and peripheral vestibular lesions can produce nystagmus with differing features.

Central vestibular nystagmus

Central vestibular nystagmus arises from lesions in the vestibular nuclei, in the cerebellum, or in the interconnections between the vestibular nuclei and the cerebellum. Features include:

* Pure horizontal, vertical, or torsional nystagmus
* Bidirectional fast phase in the direction of gaze
* Nystagmus not attenuated by fixation

Peripheral vestibular nystagmus

Features include:

* Horizontal jerk nystagmus, increasing in amplitude with gaze in direction of the fast phase (Alexander law)
* Fast phase in the direction of gaze but often also the same direction in primary position (second degree) or even in contralateral gaze (third degree); this condition cannot occur in gaze-evoked nystagmus, which cannot be present in primary position.
* May have a torsional component (usually second- or third-degree nystagmus)
* The fast phase beats away from the side of the lesion in destructive disorders (e.g. labyrinthitis).
* The fast phase beats towards the side of the lesion in irritative disorders (e.g. Ménière disease).
* Is suppressed by fixation

Congenital nystagmus

Congenital nystagmus usually presents in the first few months of life and can be idiopathic (autosomal dominant, autosomal recessive, or X-linked inheritance) or secondary to disorders that impair visual development (e.g. albinism, congenital

cataracts, congenital glaucoma, foveal/optic nerve hypoplasia), with both types of the condition resulting in similar features:
- Horizontal and usually jerk nystagmus (although may be pendular)
- Increases in amplitude with fixation
- Amplitude may be dampened by convergence.
- A null point (where nystagmus movement is least) may be present in a particular position of gaze.
- An altered head position may be adopted to facilitate the null point.
- OKN may be reversed.

Latent nystagmus

Latent nystagmus is associated with strabismus (usually infantile esotropia), with the nystagmus only becoming apparent when one (either) eye is occluded. Occlusion of a single eye produces a horizontal jerk nystagmus, with the fast phase in the direction of the uncovered eye.

Spasmus nutans

Spasmus nutans, which is a rare condition, comprises the following triad of symptoms:
- Nystagmus
- Head nodding
- Torticollis

It usually presents within the first year of life and resolves spontaneously by 2–3 years. The nystagmus is typically horizontal, with high frequency and low amplitude. The cause is normally idiopathic, although chiasmal and third ventricular gliomas can produce similar features.

Acquired pendular nystagmus

Pendular nystagmus may be acquired in cases of severe visual loss. Rarely, monocular blindness may result in monocular pendular blindness.

A particular type of pendular nystagmus occurs in multiple sclerosis; this type is often asymmetric and severely degrades vision.

Convergence–retraction nystagmus

Convergence–retraction nystagmus is not, strictly speaking, a nystagmus. In Parinaud syndrome (see Section 10.17), there is a loss of upwards saccades. On attempted up-gaze, there is a rhythmic saccadic impulse to all four horizontal recti, causing rhythmic retraction of the globes.

Management of nystagmus

- A thorough neuro-ophthalmic history and examination is essential in eliciting any possible causes or associations.
- Consider neuroimaging when other neurological deficits are present or when no cause is found.
  Treatment can include:
- Refractive correction and amblyopia treatment (if needed) in children
- Prisms may help to induce convergence and move the null point into the primary position in congenital cases.
- Baclofen may help reduce periodic alternating nystagmus.
- Gabapentin is often helpful in pendular nystagmus due to multiple sclerosis.
- Retrobulbar or intramuscular botulinum injections are recommended very rarely in severe cases.
- Surgery is generally reserved for congenital cases where extraocular muscle adjustments to shift the null position into the primary position can help reduce the nystagmus. However, the null position may again become eccentric.

Coordination of eye movements originates at a supranuclear level (i.e. central to the ocular motor nuclei) and involves gaze centres for the control of horizontal and vertical movements. In addition, saccadic movements (which bring an object of interest on to the fovea) and pursuit movements (that maintain fixation on a target) are initiated supranuclearly. This section briefly describes the pathways of these eye movements and the disorders associated with them.

Horizontal gaze palsies

For horizontal gaze, impulses originate in the pontine paramedian reticular formation, adjacent to the sixth nerve nucleus. The pontine paramedian reticular formation activates the ipsilateral sixth nerve nucleus and thereby innervates the lateral rectus. The sixth nerve nucleus also communicates with the contralateral medial rectus subnucleus, via the medial longitudinal fasciculus (see Figure 10.30). Horizontal gaze disorders include the following:

Horizontal gaze palsy

Pontine paramedian reticular formation lesions produce a gaze palsy to the affected side. This type of gaze palsy can be differentiated from that produced by lesions in the sixth nerve nucleus by oculocephalic and caloric testing, which produce vestibular input at the nuclear level and are therefore normal in pontine paramedian reticular formation lesions (i.e. a supranuclear horizontal gaze palsy).

Internuclear ophthalmoplegia

Internuclear ophthalmoplegia results from medial longitudinal fasciculus lesions (e.g. demyelination, vascular disease, trauma, and brainstem tumours); features of a right internuclear ophthalmoplegia include:

* An adduction deficit of the right eye on attempted left gaze
* Horizontal jerk nystagmus of the abducting left eye
* Normal right gaze
* Upbeat and torsional nystagmus may be present
* Convergence is preserved
* Skew deviation

Bilateral internuclear ophthalmoplegia (see Figure 10.31) is usually due to demyelination, with upbeat nystagmus on up-gaze and downbeat nystagmus on down-gaze as constant features. A variant is the WEBINO syndrome (**w**all-**e**yed **bi**lateral **i**nternuclear **o**phthalmoplegia), so called because of the large exotropias that can feature.

One-and-a-half syndrome

One-and-a-half syndrome is caused by pontine paramedian reticular formation lesions (or sixth nerve nucleus lesions) extending to ipsilateral medial longitudinal fasciculus lesions. Features of a right-sided one-and-a-half syndrome include:

* Gaze palsy on attempted right gaze
* Adduction deficit on attempted left gaze
* Abduction of the left eye is the only normal horizontal movement

Vertical gaze palsies

Vertical eye movements are generated in the rostral interstitial nucleus of the medial longitudinal fasciculus, which consists of paired nuclei, with the lateral portion of each initiating up-gaze, and the medial portion initiating down-gaze. Vertical gaze disorders include the following.

Parinaud syndrome

Parinaud syndrome occurs in dorsal midbrain lesions that involve the posterior commissure. Causes include demyelination, vascular disease, aqueduct stenosis, arteriovenous malformations, and tumours. Clinical features include:

* Up-gaze disturbance
* Convergence–retraction nystagmus
* Light-near dissociation of the pupils
* Lid retraction (Collier sign)
* Convergence paralysis

Progressive supranuclear palsy

Progressive supranuclear palsy is a progressive neurodegenerative condition affecting the elderly and initially impairs down-gaze. Subsequently, up-gaze also becomes affected, followed by the loss of horizontal and then saccadic and pursuit eye movements. Patients may also develop pseudobulbar palsy, Parkinsonism, and dementia. The palsy is supranuclear, resulting in normal vertical movements on oculocephalic testing.

Skew deviations

Skew deviations are vertical tropias that are usually small and can occur following brainstem or cerebellar lesions. The vertical deviation is usually concomitant, and the hypertropic eye ipsilateral to the side of the lesion. They are usually associated with other features that allow localization, for example, unilateral internuclear ophthalmoplegia in pontine lesions, or Horner syndrome plus lateropulsion in medullary lesions.

Saccadic disorders

Saccades are fast eye movements (up to 800° per second) that can occur in any direction and may be voluntary or involuntary. They require an initial strong **pulse** signal to overcome orbital viscous forces, followed by a **step** signal to maintain the eye in its new position. The pathway for horizontal saccades originates in the frontal eye fields and superior colliculus, and from here signals pass to the contralateral pontine paramedian reticular formation. Vertical saccades originate in either the frontal eye fields or the superior colliculus, and impulses then pass to the contralateral rostral interstitial nucleus of the medial longitudinal fasciculus. Saccadic disorders can arise from:

* Frontal lobe lesions: can cause difficulty in generating horizontal saccades and result in a preferential gaze to the ipsilateral side (however, as there are other pathways to generate saccades, such lesions do not cause permanent saccadic palsies)
* Cerebellar disease: can cause hypometric saccades where the eye fails to reach its new target, or hypermetric saccades when overshoot of initial target occurs
* Degenerative conditions such as Huntington disease, olivopontocerebellar degeneration, and Wilson disease
* Ocular myopathies: cause slow saccades

Square-wave jerks

Square-wave jerks are sporadic saccades away from the fixation point, followed by a corrective saccade between 100 and 200 milliseconds later. They are named after their appearance on eye movement recordings and are usually pathological if the

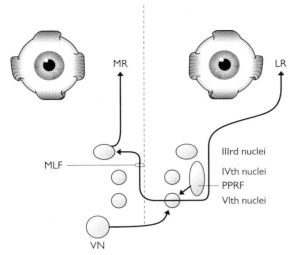

Fig 10.30 Control of horizontal eye movements
LR, lateral rectus; MLF, medial longitudinal fasciculus; MR, medial rectus; PPRF, paramedian pontine reticular formation; VN, vestibular nucleus

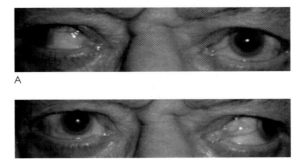

Fig 10.31 Bilateral internuclear ophthalmoplegia: (a) right gaze and (b) left gaze

jerks are greater than 1°. They are suggestive of cerebellar disease but also occur in healthy individuals.

Ocular flutter and opsoclonus

Ocular flutter consists of intermittent, rapid horizontal oscillations around a fixation point and can also occur in cerebellar disease. However, they differ from square-wave jerks as no intersaccadic interval between saccades occurs. Opsoclonus is similar to ocular flutter, although the saccades are multidirectional. Opsoclonus is due to antibodies possibly against prenuclear saccadic pause cells, although this hypothesis has never been proven. The disorder is either post-infectious (often in childhood) or paraneoplastic (mostly in adults). Ataxia and myoclonus are often associated. The pathogenesis of ocular flutter is more varied than that of opsoclonus, with some cases being due to discrete brain stem lesions. 'Voluntary nystagmus' is indistinguishable from ocular flutter but can be generated at will by some healthy individuals.

Pursuit movement disorders

Pursuit movements allow tracking of visual targets and are integrated with the vestibular system. They consist of smooth conjugate movements from 20° to 70° per second. The pathway is complex but thought to originate in the parieto-occipito-temporal junction and then projects to the ipsilateral pontine paramedian reticular formation. Lesions to the pursuit pathway can be demonstrated by failure to follow an OKN drum when rotated with the stripes moving towards the side of the lesion. In posterior cerebral hemisphere lesions, this phenomenon underpins the Cogan rule, which states that, in a patient with a hemianopia, if his/her OKN is normal, the lesion will be an infarct (posterior cerebral artery occlusion; parietal lobe spared); if the patient's OKN is absent when the stripes are rotated towards the side of the lesion, the lesion is likely to be a tumour (i.e. likely to involve the parietal lobe).

Isolated disorders of the pursuit system are less common than gaze palsies are in the case of brain stem lesions. The most commonly encountered abnormality of smooth pursuit is 'saccadic' or 'broken' pursuit, in which there is failure of the eye to keep up with a moving target, and saccades are generated to catch up. Saccadic pursuit is a common feature of cerebellar dysfunction.

10.18 Pupil abnormalities

Pupillary disorders can be divided into two main groups: afferent and efferent defects. Afferent pupillary defects are due to an interruption of light stimulus in the anterior visual pathway (retina to pretectal area), resulting in a reduction in amplitude of the pupil light reflex bilaterally when light is shone into the affected eye. Efferent pupillary defects affect constriction or dilatation of the pupil because of damage to the midbrain or to the nerves supplying the iris muscles (or to the iris muscles themselves) and often result in anisocoria.

Afferent pupillary defects

RAPD

RAPD results from unilateral or asymmetric lesions in the anterior visual pathway. Causes include:

- Gross retinal pathology (e.g. CRVO, retinal detachment)
- Optic neuropathy (e.g. optic neuritis, compressive lesions)
- Homonymous hemianopia due to optic tract lesions (infarcts, demyelination); in this situation, the RAPD is seen in the eye with the temporal hemifield loss.

Absolute afferent pupillary defect (amaurotic pupil)

Absolute afferent pupillary defect occurs following a complete optic nerve or retinal lesion. Both pupils will constrict normally when light is shone into the healthy eye, but neither pupil will constrict when light is shone into the affected eye.

Efferent pupillary defects

Horner syndrome

Horner syndrome results from an interruption (at any level) of the sympathetic nerve supply to the eye (see *Chapter 1, Figure 1.15*).

Aetiology

1. First-order neuron (central) lesions:
   - Basal skull tumours
   - Syringomyelia
   - Brainstem disease (vascular, demyelination)
2. Second-order neuron (preganglionic) lesions:
   - Apical lung tumours (Pancoast tumour)
   - Neck disorders (trauma, surgery, tumour)
   - Carotid and aortic aneurysms/dissection
   - Cervical rib
3. Third-order neuron (postganglionic) lesions:
   - Internal carotid artery dissection, usually acute onset and painful, a medical emergency in view of stroke risk (see Figure 10.10g),
   - Middle ear disease (otitis media, herpes zoster)
   - Cavernous sinus disease (thrombosis, mass)
   - Headaches (cluster, migraine)

Clinical features

- Miosis with anisocoria, which is more apparent in dark conditions than in bright light
- Normal pupil reactivity to light and near
- Mild upper lid ptosis (reduced innervation of the Müller muscle)
- Apparent enophthalmos, due to a slight elevation of the inferior eyelid (inferior tarsal muscle weakness)

- Ipsilateral facial anhydrosis in first- and second-order lesions
- Iris hypochromia in congenital lesions

Investigations

Pharmacological pupil tests can help to confirm a diagnosis of Horner syndrome and identify the location of the underlying lesion. Classic teaching dictates that cocaine 4% drops are used but apraclonidine 0.5% (Iopidine) is more readily available and now widely used.

Apraclonidine 0.5% confirms the diagnosis:

- **Method:** measure the pupil sizes in ambient light and dimmed light. Instil one drop in each eye and measure pupil sizes after 20 minutes.
- **Findings:** reversal of the anisocoria; the apraclonidine dilates the affected pupil and may lift the ptosis but has minimal effect on the normal eye.
- **Reason:** loss of sympathetic innervation in Horner syndrome results in denervation hypersensitivity on the affected side. The weak alpha 1 adrenergic properties of apraclonidine have little effect on the normal pupil but cause a supernormal response in the denervated muscle.

Hydroxyamphetamine 1% identifies the level of the underlying lesion:

- **Method:** instil two drops in each eye (at least 48 hours after the cocaine/apraclonidine test) and measure pupil sizes after 60 minutes.
- **Findings:** in first- and second-order neuron lesions, the Horner pupil will dilate similarly to the normal pupil. In third-order neuron defects, the abnormal pupil will dilate poorly.
- **Reason:** hydroxyamphetamine potentiates the release of noradrenaline from postganglionic nerve endings; as these endings are damaged in third-order neuron lesions, poor dilatation results.

Further investigations including chest X-ray, carotid Dopplers, CT, and MRI may be warranted to diagnose the underlying cause, and subsequent treatment will be dependent on this.

Adie (tonic) pupil

Adie pupil results from denervation of the parasympathetic supply from the ciliary ganglion to the iris and ciliary muscle. Young women are mostly affected, and onset may follow a viral illness. However, the condition is often subclinical in onset and unnoticed by the patient until some time later.

Clinical features

- Large pupil, with poor reactivity to light
- Exaggerated response to near stimuli, with miosis persisting for longer and with slower re-dilation (tonic pupil) than in the normal pupil
- Vermiform iris movements seen at the slit lamp (hippus in a pupil with sectorial denervation)
- The affected pupil can become the smaller of the two in chronic cases.
- Diminished deep tendon reflexes in Holmes–Adie syndrome

Investigations

Dilute (0.125%) pilocarpine can be used to confirm the diagnosis.

- Instil one drop into each eye and measure pupil sizes after 30 minutes.

- The abnormal pupil will constrict because of denervation hypersensitivity.

Argyll Robertson pupil

Argyll Robertson pupils are small and irregular pupils that react poorly to light but accommodate. The condition occurs secondary to neurosyphilis (which causes damage to the midbrain tectum region) but diabetes and alcohol abuse can produce similar pupils. Appropriate management should be undertaken to assess whether active syphilitic disease is present.

Anisocoria

Physiological anisocoria occurs in approximately 20% of the population. Here, the anisocoria is usually less than 1 mm and remains constant in light and dark conditions, with pupil reactivity also being normal. Non-physiological causes of anisocoria include the following.

Abnormal pupil is constricted

- Horner syndrome
- Chronic Adie pupil
- Unilateral miotic use
- Iritis
- Argyll Robertson pupil

Abnormal pupil is dilated

- Adie pupil
- Iris trauma
- Mydriatic agent
- Pupil-involving third nerve palsy

Light-near dissociation

Light-near dissociation is a condition in which the pupil reaction to near objects is greater than that caused by light stimulus. Causes include:

- Afferent conduction defect (e.g. optic neuropathy)
- Adie pupil
- Aberrant regeneration of the third nerve
- Argyll Robertson pupil
- Parinaud syndrome
- Chronic alcohol use

Further reading

1. Davagnanam I, Fraser CL, Miszkiel K, Daniel CS, Plant GT: Adult Horner's syndrome: A combined clinical, pharmacological, and imaging algorithm. *Eye* 2013 Feb; **27**(3): 291–8

Headache

Headache is one of the most common clinical complaints, and patients are often referred for an ophthalmological opinion. The ophthalmologist's role in such cases is first to diagnose any ocular cause of the headache and second to help distinguish between benign causes of headache and those due to serious intracranial/systemic conditions.

Aetiology

Causes of headache include:

* Raised intracranial pressure*
* GCA*
* Malignant hypertension*
* Subarachnoid haemorrhage*
* Migraine
* Tension headache
* Cluster headache

General considerations

Although the majority of headaches are caused by benign conditions that can be elicited with a thorough history taking, clinical features that suggest serious intracranial/systemic pathology include:

* Headache characteristics:
  — New onset in a previously asymptomatic patient
  — New pattern/type of headache
  — Severe ('worst headache I've ever had')
* Focal neurological signs
* Change in personality/mental status
* Recent head trauma
* Signs of meningism
* Temporal tenderness

Migraine

Migraine is a common, recurrent condition affecting up to 20% of males and 40% of females, with the initial episode occurring before 10 years of age in 25% of patients (see Table 10.9). Current theories of the pathogenesis of migraine are centred on the concept that a particular type of abnormal electrical activity known as spreading depression is the primary underlying abnormality. There is good evidence that spreading depression is responsible for the aura and for cluster headache. Vascular changes and the release of neuropeptides and vasoactive substances may be responsible for the headache.

Migraine incorporates a variety of symptoms and has been classified by the International Headache Society into (1) migraine without aura and (2) migraine with aura.

* These are serious/life-threatening causes.

Migraine without aura

Migraine without aura usually begins with a prodrome phase of symptoms such as mood alterations, food cravings, and drowsiness, lasting for hours to days. A unilateral, throbbing headache then normally follows, building in intensity over 1–2 hours and which can last for several days. Photophobia, phonophobia, nausea, and vomiting are common with the headache. Termination of the headache is followed by a postdrome phase, characterized by fatigue.

Migraine with aura

In migraine with aura, a headache (which is similar to that in migraine without aura) usually follows an aura that can last from several minutes up to 1 hour. Most auras are visual, occurring in 99% of cases of migraine with aura, but other types include somatosensory (tingling, numbness), motor (hemiparesis), and speech (dysphasia) auras.

Visual auras are limited to one hemifield in 70% of cases and may consist of positive and negative visual phenomena. Symptoms can include foggy vision, tunnel vision, hemianopia, and even complete blindness. However, the most commonly described form of visual aura is the 'fortification scotoma', features of which include:

* Central visual disturbance evolving into a scotoma in several minutes
* Multiple silver, coloured, or zigzag lines surrounding the scotoma
* Enlargement and migration of the visual aura across the visual field
* Aura seen with eyes either open or closed

Although migraine is normally a benign condition, it has been associated with ophthalmic complications such as retinal artery occlusion, ischaemic optic neuropathy, and normal tension glaucoma. A causative association with these conditions has not been established.

Investigations

Migraine can, in the majority of case, be diagnosed with history taking, in the presence of a normal neurological examination. Cases with atypical clinical features require referral to a neurologist, with further workup possibly including a vasculitic screen, carotid Dopplers, and neuroimaging.

Management

* Avoid triggering factors (e.g. certain food types, flickering lights).
* Acute attacks: rest in dark/quiet room; 5-hydroxytryptamine agonists (e.g. sumatriptan) in severe episodes
* Recurrent episodes: prophylaxis with beta blockers, calcium channel blockers, or anticonvulsants

Table 10.9 Classifications of migraine by the International Headache Society	
Migraine type	**Features**
Migraine with prolonged aura	Aura lasting >60 minutes, with full recovery
Migraine aura without headache	Aura with no headache: diagnosis of exclusion
Ophthalmic migraine	Two to three days of headache followed by a unilateral third, fourth, or sixth nerve palsy, which usually recovers fully in 6–8 weeks. Attacks may be recurrent. The condition may not be related to migraine at all.
Retinal migraine	Cases of non-embolic transient monocular visual loss are sometimes referred to as 'retinal migraine' but may be due to vasospasm involving the central retinal artery. Whether this is related to migraine is uncertain.
Basilar migraine	Headache follows bilateral visual disturbance, dizziness, and weakness.
Complications of migraine	Permanent visual loss may occur with migraine but the cause is uncertain. In some cases, it may be that an occipital lobe infarction has occurred for another reason and provoked migraine aura.
Atypical migraine	Migraine not filling other criteria

10.20 Non-organic visual loss

Non-organic visual loss refers to visual loss that is not attributable to any organic cause and is therefore a diagnosis of exclusion. It is divided into two types: conversion reaction (previously known as hysterical blindness), and malingering. In conversion reaction disorders, patients truly believe they have lost vision and this is usually associated with environmental stresses (e.g. impending exams) and is considered to be a method of coping with such pressures. Malingering patients, however, consciously mimic visual loss to obtain an external secondary benefit such as financial or legal gain. Malingerers can be uncooperative during the examination process and may even try to actively deceive the examiner.

Although the ophthalmologist's role in patients with non-organic visual loss is to exclude any attributable, organic cause for their visual symptoms, it is important to remember that non-organic visual loss can coexist with genuine pathology, and to have caution in making a diagnosis of non-organic visual loss in children (see section 9.5).

Differential diagnosis

Ocular pathologies that may have subtle clinical signs and should therefore be considered in the differential diagnosis of unexplained visual loss include:

* Amblyopia
* Keratoconus
* Retrobulbar neuritis
* Cone–rod dystrophy
* Cortical blindness
* Early chiasmal tumours

Clinical evaluation

Non-organic visual loss may affect one or both eyes and be of total or near total blindness. Suspicion should be raised in patients who claim total visual loss and cannot perform tests of proprioception (e.g. touching index fingers together or signing one's name), yet can navigate smoothly around the hospital.

Further ways of assessing the validity of claimed total visual loss include:

* Response to a visual threat indicates some degree of vision.
* The mirror test: rotating a mirror before a patient and observing for pursuit movements
* OKN elicited with a rotating OKN drum indicates a visual acuity of 6/60 or better.

Investigations

The following tests can also be useful in the assessment of non-organic visual loss.

* Fogging test: plus lenses of progressively increasing power are placed in front of the 'good' eye, and visual acuity is measured; this process is repeated until a plus lens will sufficiently blur the vision in the 'good' eye so that the patient must have been reading from their 'bad' eye.
* Prism shift test: a 4 D base-out prism is placed in front of the 'bad' eye whilst the patient fixates on a Snellen chart; any movement detected or acknowledged diplopia equates approximately to the acuity of the Snellen letter read.
* Stereoscopic tests: patients with 40" of arc stereopsis must at least have a visual acuity of 6/6.
* Preferential looking: the patient's fixation is observed whilst various grating acuity cards are shown to them.
* Tangent visual field testing: visual field defects in non-organic visual loss typically remain the same size irrespective of the test distance (tunnelling visual field loss); may also be seen on confrontational visual field testing
* Humphrey automated perimetry may show a 'cloverleaf' pattern as performance deteriorates during the test. The first four points tested then stand out on the greyscale plots.
* Goldmann visual field testing may show 'spiralling' of the isoptre as performance deteriorates during the test.
* Electrophysiological testing: electroretinography and visually-evoked potential tests should be performed if the diagnosis remains in doubt.
* Neuroimaging may be required to further investigate reproducible visual field defects or suspected cortical blindness.

Management

* Reassurance that no abnormality with the eyes or brain is present and that a full visual recovery is expected is important.
* Psychiatric assessment may be indicated in some cases, although non-organic visual loss alone is not sufficient for referral.

Prognosis

Good prognostic factors include:

* Young age
* Absence of any psychiatric disease

10.21 Neuromuscular junction disorders

Myasthenia gravis

Myasthenia gravis is an autoimmune disorder of neuromuscular transmission, characterized by fatigability and weakness of muscles and which can include ocular and systemic features. Myasthenia gravis can occur at any age, although incidence peaks in the third decade for females, and in the sixth and seventh decades for males.

Pathophysiology

In most cases, antibodies are directed against the postsynaptic acetylcholine receptors (anti-AChR antibodies), resulting in a decreased number and altered structure of these receptors. A small number of cases have been shown to have an antibody against a protein in the postsynaptic membrane known as muscle-specific kinase (anti-MuSK antibodies). The amount of acetylcholine released from the presynaptic terminal normally decreases with successive nerve impulses (presynaptic rundown) and this, combined with the reduced function of the postsynaptic membrane, results in muscle fatigability. Myasthenia gravis is associated with thymoma (in 10%–15% of cases), thymic hyperplasia (85% of cases), and other autoimmune disorders such as hyperthyroidism and pernicious anaemia.

Clinical evaluation

History and examination

Weakness in myasthenia gravis typically increases during the day and improves with rest. Systemic features include dysphagia, dysarthria, and facial and limb weakness. Myasthenic crisis with severe respiratory difficulty is rare but can result in death.

Ocular features are present initially in 70% of patients with myasthenia gravis and later develop in up to 90% of cases. These include:

* Diplopia: variable and can result from weakness of one or more extraocular muscles
* Ptosis:
  - Unilateral or bilateral; rarely symmetrical
  - Most prominent or may increase on sustained up-gaze due to fatigability
  - In unilateral ptosis, lifting the ptotic lid may relieve retraction of the contralateral lid (because of Herings law of equal innervation).
  - Cogan lid twitch sign is pathognomonic of myasthenia. If the levator muscle is weak, with reduced excursion, an attempted upwards saccade will generate a low-amplitude but high-velocity saccade. 'Overshoot' may also be seen, but this feature is not specific to myasthenia.

Investigations

* Ice pack test: ice placed over a ptotic lid for 2 minutes, with a 2 mm or more reduction in ptosis considered significant
* Edrophonium test: used to assess whether any improvement in ptosis or diplopia occurs following intravenous edrophonium injection. Asystole can occur rarely during this test, so cardiac monitoring and immediately available intravenous atropine (0.5–1 mg) are essential. Intravenous edrophonium (2 mg) is initially given and, if no improvement (or adverse effect) occurs after 1 minute, up to 8 mg of edrophonium can be further given. The atropine can be given routinely before the edrophonium.

* Anti-AChR antibody assays are positive in 50% of patients with ocular myasthenia gravis and in 80% of patients with generalized myasthenia gravis.
* Anti-MuSK antibodies are found in 40%–50% of seronegative (negative for anti-AChR antibodies) patients.
* Anti-striated muscle antibodies are present in 84% of patients with thymoma and who are less than 40 years old.
* Chest CT to investigate thymic involvement
* Repetitive supramaximal nerve stimulation produces a progressive decremental response in the action potential.
* Single-fibre electromyography produces a characteristic 'jitter' because of variable synaptic transmission.

Management

Treatment depends on the severity of symptoms. If the ocular symptoms are disturbing to the patient, options include:

* Pyridostigmine (an anticholinesterase inhibitor): 30–60 mg every 4 hours initially, increasing up to 120 mg three times a day
* Immunosuppression with agents including corticosteroids, azathioprine, and ciclosporin may be needed in patients not managed with anticholinesterase inhibitors.
* Intravenous immunoglobulin infusions may also be used.
* Thymectomy: indicated in all patients with a thymoma, but improvement in myasthenia occurs in patients with thymic hyperplasia rather than thymoma
* Plasma exchange is effective in myasthenic crisis and prior to thymectomy.

Prognosis

* In patients with ocular myasthenia gravis, 10%–20% undergo spontaneous remission, whereas 50%–80% go on to develop generalized myasthenia gravis, usually within 2 years.
* Risk factors for poor prognosis include age >50 years, thymoma, and a short history of progressive disease.

Lambert–Eaton myasthenic syndrome

Lambert–Eaton myasthenic syndrome occurs as a result of impaired acetylcholine release at the neuromuscular junction, following an autoimmune attack on presynaptic calcium channels. Nearly 50% of cases are associated with small-cell carcinoma of the lung.

Patients can develop proximal muscle weakness and autonomic dysfunction including dry mouth, constipation, and postural hypotension. Ocular features may include dry eye resulting from reduced lacrimation, and intermittent ptosis and diplopia.

Investigations should include imaging of the chest to exclude any lung carcinoma, and calcium channel antibodies are present in over 50% of cases. In contrast to myasthenia gravis, repetitive nerve stimulation produces increased muscle contractions.

Aside from removal of any underlying carcinoma, treatment options include 3,4-aminopyridine (acetylcholinesterase inhibitors are less effective than in myasthenia gravis) and immunosuppressive agents to help increase muscle strength.

Ocular myopathies can cause disorders of ocular motility, ophthalmoplegia and ptosis, and arise from pathology affecting the extraocular muscles. Acquired causes such as thyroid eye disease and other orbital inflammatory conditions are covered elsewhere, with this section focusing on inherited causes.

Chronic progressive external ophthalmoplegia

Chronic progressive external ophthalmoplegia (CPEO) is a rare condition, characterized by a slowly progressive paresis of the extraocular muscles and ptosis. It occurs as a result of impaired protein synthesis within mitochondria. Most cases are due to mutations in mitochondrial DNA (sporadic or maternally inherited) but some cases result from nuclear DNA mutations (autosomal inheritance). CPEO can occur in isolation but can also occur with systemic features, as in Kearns–Sayre syndrome.

Clinical evaluation

Ptosis is usually the first clinical sign and is typically bilateral and symmetrical. A reduction in ocular motility then follows, although patients are often not aware of any diplopia, as the impairment is often symmetrical. Saccadic slowing is typical (in contrast to myasthenia and dysthyroid ophthalmopathy). Down-gaze is usually the last to be affected.

Kearns–Sayre syndrome includes the triad of CPEO, pigmentary retinopathy (typically salt-and-pepper retinal pigment epithelium changes occurring at the macular), and heart block. Patients may also have proximal muscle weakness, endocrine dysfunction, cerebellar signs, and deafness. CPEO may also be a feature of a variety of other mitochondrial syndromes such as stroke-like episodes, epilepsy, and myoclonus.

Investigations

* The demonstration of a pathogenic mutation in mitochondrial or nuclear DNA is the definitive test.
* Muscle biopsy is often helpful showing 'ragged red fibres' with a modified Gomori trichome stain. However, not all cases will show this.
* ECG to exclude any conduction defects
* PCR may reveal mitochondrial DNA mutations.
* Blood lactate and pyruvate levels are usually raised in Kearns–Sayre syndrome.

Management

* Ptosis may be helped with lid crutches or surgery.
* Diplopia may be resolved with strabismus surgery.
* Cardiac pacemaker insertion may be required in conduction defects.
* Coenzyme Q$_{10}$ has been of some benefit with the systemic features in Kearns–Sayre syndrome, although the effects are often transient.

Prognosis

* Poor in Kearns–Sayre syndrome, with death commonly occurring in the third to fourth decades
* In pure CPEO, life expectancy is normal, with many patients presenting late in life.
* Most cases of CPEO and Kearns–Sayre syndrome are due to sporadic mitochondrial DNA deletions and are not inherited.

Point mutations in mitochondrial DNA are much less likely and will show maternal inheritance.

Myotonic dystrophy

Myotonic dystrophy is an uncommon autosomal dominant condition characterized by a delay in muscle relaxation following contraction. It arises following a genetic defect consisting of a trinucleotide CTG repeat sequence in Chromosome 19. As the repeat sequence can be repeated further in offspring, the condition shows 'anticipation', that is, worsening in successive generations.

Clinical evaluation

Ocular features include:
* Bilateral ptosis
* Polychromatic 'Christmas tree' or posterior subcapsular cataracts (see Figure 10.32)
* External ophthalmoplegia (not commonly severe)
* Pigmentary retinopathy (rarely)

Systemic features include:
* Mournful facial expression due to bilateral weakness of facial muscles (facial myopathy)
* Wasting of temporalis and masseter muscles (characteristic and distinguishes from other causes of facial myopathy)
* Muscle weakness, difficulty in releasing grip following handshake, percussion myotonia
* Slurred speech from weakness of tongue and pharyngeal muscles (bulbar myopathy)
* Premature frontal baldness and testicular atrophy in males.
* Cardiomyopathy that can lead to cardiac failure

Investigations
* DNA analysis
* Electromyography shows spontaneous, high-frequency discharges.
* Muscle biopsy (rarely required) reveals characteristic changes including rows of nuclei down the centre of muscle fibres.
* Serum creatine kinase is mildly elevated.

Management

The treatment of muscle weakness is mainly supportive, with a multidisciplinary approach including neurologists, cardiologists, physiotherapists, and speech therapists often required to manage the systemic features. Genetic counselling should be offered, as should cataract surgery, if required.

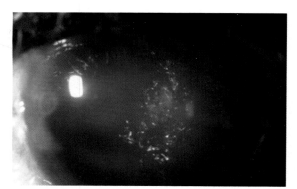

Fig 10.32 Christmas tree cataract

Chapter 11

Orbit

Tarang Gupta and Daniel Ezra

Bony and soft tissue anatomy

The orbit cavity contains the globe and all surrounding soft tissues. It is pyramidal in shape, with the apex at the postero-medial aspect, conducting the optic nerve to the cranial cavity. The walls of the orbit (see Figure 11.1) consist of the following components:

- Floor: orbital plates of maxilla, zygomatic, and palatine bones
- Roof: orbital plate of frontal bone and lesser wing of sphenoid
- Lateral wall: zygomatic bone and greater wing of sphenoid
- Medial wall: frontal process of maxilla, lacrimal, ethmoid, and sphenoid bones

The ethmoidal bone along the medial wall is paper-thin and is perforated by several foramina transmitting blood vessels and nerves. It is a common entry site for infection from the ethmoid sinus; such infection causes orbital cellulitis. The orbital rim is made of thick bone, but the walls are thinner and more likely to fracture with a direct blow to the orbit than the rim is.

The optic canal is contained within the lesser wing of sphenoid and connects the middle cranial fossa with the orbit. It transmits the optic nerve, the ophthalmic artery, and the sympathetic plexus within the surrounding dural–arachnoid sheath.

The superior orbital fissure is a slit-like division between the greater and lesser wings of sphenoid (see Figure 11.2). The superior orbital fissure is divided by the fibrous ring of the origins of the recti muscles. The superior part of the fissure lies outside the ring and transmits the lacrimal nerve, the frontal nerve, the trochlear nerve, and the superior ophthalmic vein. The inferior part of the fissure lies inside the ring and transmits the oculomotor nerve, the abducens nerve, and the nasociliary nerve, along with the sympathetic fibres. Any disease at the apex or involving the superior orbital fissure can therefore result in ophthalmoplegia, proptosis, and/or chemosis because of venous congestion.

The inferior orbital fissure divides the greater wing of sphenoid and maxilla. It connects the orbit to the pterygopalatine and infero-temporal fossae. It transmits branches of the pterygopalatine ganglion and the inferior ophthalmic vein. Orbital lymphoma and fungal infections may infiltrate this area. The infraorbital artery, vein, and nerve pass through the infraorbital foramen onto the zygoma.

The orbit is bound anteriorly by the orbital septum, which is attached to the orbital rim periosteum peripherally to the tarsi of the upper and lower lids. The orbital septum also invests the lacrimal sac to form the lacrimal fascia. The orbital septum is an important structure, as it limits the spread of infection from the eyelids into the orbit. Its relative inextensibility can result in increased intraorbital pressure in the event of haemorrhage within the orbit, and this pressure can compromise optic nerve function.

The lacrimal gland is situated in the supero-temporal anterior orbit (in the lacrimal fossa) and is divided by the lateral horn of the levator aponeurosis into the orbital and palpebral lobes.

Orbital blood supply

The ophthalmic artery is a branch from the internal carotid and enters the orbit through the optic canal; it usually lies infero-lateral to the optic nerve (see Figure 11.3). It is the main arterial supply to the orbit and globe. It is encased within the dural sheath of the optic nerve. As the optic nerve emerges from the optic canal, the ophthalmic artery pierces the optic nerve sheath and travels anteriorly along the medial wall of the orbit. There is significant variability in the terminal branching of the ophthalmic artery, and many anastomoses between the internal and external carotid systems are made at the orbito-facial interface.

- Globe branches: central retinal and ciliary arteries
- Orbital branches: lacrimal and muscular arteries
- Superficial branches: supraorbital, supratrochlear, medial palpebral, dorsal nasal, ethmoidal arteries

The anterior and posterior ethmoid arteries pass through their respective foramina in the medial orbital wall and are important surgical landmarks, as they correspond with the level of the cribriform plate.

The venous drainage of the orbit is through the superior and inferior ophthalmic veins. The majority of orbital and ocular veins (including the inferior ophthalmic vein) drain into the superior ophthalmic vein, which subsequently drains into the cavernous sinus. The veins of the eyelids drain into the ophthalmic and angular veins medially and the superficial temporal vein laterally. Numerous anastomoses are present which connect the orbital venous system flow to the facial vein and pterygoid venous plexus.

Orbital nerve supply

The efferent motor supply to the extraocular muscles is from the oculomotor nerve, the trochlear nerve, and the abducens nerve. The oculomotor nerve and the abducens nerve enter the orbit via the apex within the tendinous ring of the recti muscles. The oculomotor nerve supplies all the extraocular muscles apart from the superior oblique and the lateral rectus. The abducens nerve supplies the lateral rectus muscle. The trochlear nerve enters the orbit via the superior orbital fissure above the tendinous ring before travelling anteriorly to the superior oblique muscle.

The general sensory innervation of the orbit is supplied by the first and second branches of the trigeminal nerve (the ophthalmic nerve and the maxillary nerve, respectively). The ophthalmic nerve enters via the superior orbital fissure as it branches into the lacrimal nerve, the frontal nerve, and the nasociliary nerve (see Figure 11.2). Postganglionic parasympathetic fibres join the lacrimal nerve en route to the lacrimal gland. The frontal nerve divides into the supraorbital nerve and the supratrochlear nerve. The supraorbital nerve exits the orbit at the supraorbital notch, which is palpable on the superior orbital rim medially, and supplies the skin of the forehead to the middle of the scalp. It is important to identify these nerves during brow surgery to avoid injury. The supratrochlear nerve passes medial to the supraorbital nerve, above the trochlea of the superior oblique muscle. Both supraorbital nerve blocks and supratrochlear nerve blocks are useful for the repair of scalp lacerations and for frontal cranial surgery. The nasociliary nerve gives rise to both the short and the long ciliary nerves to the globe.

The infraorbital and zygomatic branches arise from the maxillary branch of the trigeminal nerve. The infraorbital nerve, which supplies cutaneous sensory innervation to the cheek, is commonly injured in an orbital blowout fracture.

Optic canal Supraorbital notch
Lesser wing of sphenoid Orbital plate of frontal
Superior orbital fissure Anterior ethmoidal foramen
Greater wing of sphenoid Superciliary ridge
Zygomatic

Trochlear fossa

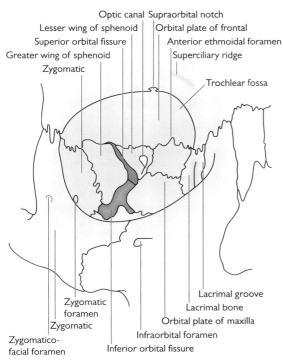

Zygomatic
foramen Lacrimal groove
Zygomatic Lacrimal bone
Orbital plate of maxilla
Zygomatico- Infraorbital foramen
facial foramen Inferior orbital fissure

Fig 11.1 Bony anatomy of the orbit

Dorsal nasal artery
Medial palpebral artery
Supraorbital artery
Lateral palpebral
artery
Supratrochlear
artery
Lacrimal
gland
Anterior
ethmoidal
artery
Short
posterior
ciliary artery
Posterior
ethmoidal
artery
Lateral rectus
muscle
Lacrimal artery
Long posterior
ciliary artery
Central
artery of
retina
Ophthalmic
artery
Optic nerve
Internal carotid
artery

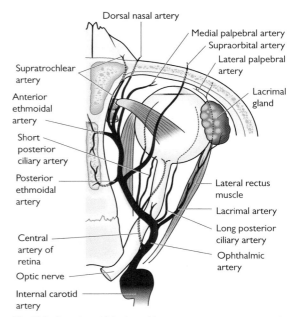

Fig 11.3 Arteries within the orbit

Superior branch of oculomotor nerve III
Trochlear nerve IV Superior rectus
Frontal nerve V₁ Lavator palpebrae superioris
Lacrimal nerve V₁ Superior oblique

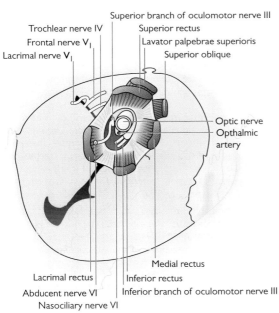

Optic nerve
Opthalmic
artery

Medial rectus
Lacrimal rectus Inferior rectus
Abducent nerve VI Inferior branch of oculomotor nerve III
Nasociliary nerve VI

Fig 11.2 Superior orbital fissure

History taking

Presenting complaint

When taking a history for orbital disease it is vital to ascertain any change in optic nerve function (decreased visual acuity, colour vision, visual field loss), speed of symptom onset, pain, and the presence of diplopia. Pain may support a diagnosis of inflammatory disease and is often a feature of destructive lacrimal gland carcinoma. Paraesthesia and pain may indicate nerve involvement secondary to carcinoma or a neuroma. Examination of old photographs is often useful in differentiating new changes in physiological appearance.

The presentation of orbital tumours varies with the location of the mass, as anterior masses cause a visible and palpable localized eyelid swelling whereas tumours in the posterior half of the orbit cause progressive proptosis and are often associated with ill-defined periocular swelling.

Past ophthalmic history

Enquire about previous surgery or trauma that may result in facial asymmetry, enophthalmos, or globe displacement.

Past medical history

Include direct questions about any history of thyroid dysfunction (even if this has not been clinically diagnosed): ask about weight loss or gain, flushing, tremor, palpitations, sweating, heat intolerance, or hair loss. A patient with thyroid eye disease may be euthyroid, hyperthyroid, or hypothyroid. Smoking history is relevant as it is known to exacerbate thyroid eye disease. Orbital inflammatory disease may be associated with systemic diseases such as sarcoidosis and Wegeners granulomatosis.

Primary tumours may invade from adjacent structures; for example, nasopharyngeal carcinoma with associated sinus symptoms. Metastatic orbital disease often has a history of carcinoma (e.g. breast, lung, bowel), chemo- or radiotherapy, or recurrence of the tumour elsewhere.

Drug history

Long-term immunosuppression with steroids or other agents may mask inflammatory diseases. Anticoagulants may cause bleeding from vascular lesions within the orbit. If the patient is dysthyroid, it is important to know their thyroid status as it may influence the activity of thyroid eye disease.

Family history

It is important to determine familial idiopathic proptosis, strabismus, telecanthus, and so on.

Examination of orbit

First assess vision and optic nerve function (indicated by * in the list below). The following must always be included in an orbital examination:

- Best-corrected visual acuity*
- Presence of an afferent pupillary defect*
- Colour vision*
- Visual fields to confrontation*
- Facial appearance: obvious orbital dystopia, scars, hemifacial asymmetry
- Orbital dystopia (axial and non-axial proptosis, hyper- or hypoglobus)
- Palpable masses (supero-temporal region for lacrimal gland and medial canthal for lacrimal sac mucocele)

- Localized swelling (colour, e.g. haemangioma may be bluish), fixation to tissue (bony or skin), variability with Valsalva manoeuvre
- Tenderness and ease of globe retropulsion
- Bony rim in trauma
- Upper lid position and function (see Section 1.5); note any lagophthalmos, eyelid hang-up, or corneal exposure
- Lower lid malpositions, especially inferior scleral show (the most reliable sign for relative proptosis)
- Ocular motility (may require a Hess chart to differentiate between mechanical restriction and underacting muscles)
- Note injected episcleral vessels that indicate abnormal orbital blood flow
- Intraocular pressure (IOP) in primary position and on upgaze (IOP increases in conditions where ocular motility is restricted, e.g. thyroid eye disease)
- Dilated fundoscopy for disc swelling/pallor/venous congestion* and chorioretinal folds
- Lymphadenopathy
- Sensation; e.g. infraorbital nerve with blowout fractures, supraorbital nerve in infiltrative disease

Assessing globe dystopia

The direction of globe displacement can give vital information regarding the location of an orbital lesion. Axial proptosis (in which the globe is displaced along the visual axis) indicates a lesion within the muscle cone (intraconal) or of the muscles themselves. Its causes include orbital inflammatory disease (most commonly thyroid eye disease), cavernous haemangioma, gliomas, metastases, and meningiomas. Enophthalmos (posterior displacement of the globe) is most commonly caused by orbital fractures and rarely by scirrhous inflammation or by carcinoma.

Lesions outside the muscle cone (extraconal) can lead to displacement of the globe away from the lesion. Dermoid cysts and lacrimal gland tumours (such as pleomorphic adenomas) cause infero-medial globe displacement. Sinus disease may cause displacement of the globe superiorly if it originates in the maxillary sinus, laterally if the ethmoid sinus is involved, or inferiorly if the frontal sinus is involved. Bilateral disease suggests thyroid eye disease, lymphoma, vasculitis, or idiopathic orbital inflammation.

Measuring axial proptosis

Axial proptosis is measured with an exophthalmometer, of which there are many types. Bilateral proptosis is suspected if the reading is over 22 mm in Caucasians, and 24 mm in Afro-Caribbean populations. The difference between the two eyes is normally equal to or less than 2 mm. The basic process is as follows:

1. Sit opposite the patient at a similar eye level.
2. Rest the exophthalmometer on the patient's lateral orbital rim and note the horizontal width (see Figure 11.4A). This value will vary with different types of exophthalmometer; therefore, document the distance (in millimetres) and the make of instrument (e.g. Keeler, Oculus). The same horizontal width should be used for subsequent measurements to allow for accurate comparisons.

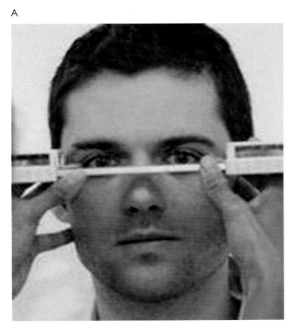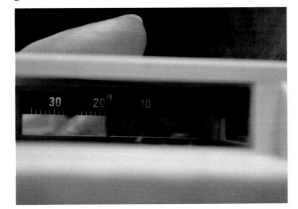

A

B

Fig 11.4
A Positioning the exophthalmometer against the lateral orbital rims
B The reading is 19 mm when the parallax marker is aligned

3. Ensure you are level with the patient's face. To measure the patient's right globe position: close your right eye and ask the patient to look at your open (left) eye.
4. Align the parallax marker on the exophthalmometer and measure where the patient's corneal apex appears on the scale (see Figure 11.4B).
5. Repeat for the left eye.

Pseudoproptosis

Causes include:

• Contralateral enophthalmos
• Contralateral ptosis
• Ipsilateral upper or lower lid retraction
• Axial myopia
• Facial asymmetry

Measuring non-axial globe displacement

To measure horizontal globe displacement, a ruler is placed horizontally over the bridge of the nose at the lateral canthi level. The distance between the corneal light reflection and the middle of the nasal bridge is measured on both sides. A cover test must first be performed to ensure there is no heterotropia. If a manifest deviation is present, the patient's right globe should be measured with the left eye occluded and then vice versa.

Vertical displacement is measured using two rulers. The first is placed horizontally at the level of the lateral canthi. The distance from the horizontal ruler to the corneal reflection is measured by using a second ruler held vertically.

11.3 Orbital infections

Preseptal cellulitis

The orbital septum is a tough, fibrous structure which forms a barrier that can limit the spread of infection from the skin and subcutaneous tissues and keep it from entering the orbit proper. Preseptal cellulitis is an infection that is confined to tissues anterior to the orbital septum. In children, however, the septum is thin, and infection can spread posteriorly much more readily. Orbital cellulitis is much more serious and may require aggressive treatment.

Aetiology

The most common cause of preseptal cellulitis is *Staphylococcus aureus* or *Streptococcus pyogenes*. Infection may spread from upper respiratory tract infections, sinusitis, hordeola, trauma, post eyelid or oral surgery, and dacryocystitis.

Clinical evaluation

History

- Acute over a matter of days
- Pain, swelling, tenderness, and redness over the upper/
- lower lid
- Importantly, there is **no** deterioration in vision, diplopia, or pain on eye movement.
- There may be a conjunctivitis; however, chemosis should not be marked.

Examination

- Overlying skin is red, tender, hot, and oedematous (see Figure 11.5).
- Eyelids should be opened and ocular motility assessed; there should be no restriction of movement or diplopia.
- Optic nerve function should be normal.
- No proptosis or resistance to globe retropulsion
- Any of these features should warrant imaging studies such as CT.

Treatment

- Oral antibiotics are required for 10 days, e.g. co-amoxiclav (Augmentin) 375 mg three times a day in adults and in children over 6, or 125 mg in suspension three times a day in children under 6. Other broad spectrum antibiotics with staphylococcus and streptococcus cover are suitable.
- Regular specialist review is required in children, as the infection can spread retroseptally very quickly. Consider admission if the patient is febrile and treat with intravenous antibiotics and regular review. Consider CT scanning if there is no improvement.

Orbital (postseptal) cellulitis

Orbital cellulitis is an ophthalmic emergency and can be life-threatening as a result of cavernous sinus thrombosis and meningeal spread. Ocular complications include raised IOP, central retinal artery or vein occlusion, keratopathy due to corneal exposure, and endophthalmitis. If orbital cellulitis is suspected, a full ophthalmic and systemic assessment is essential.

Aetiology

- Infection most commonly spreads from adjacent paranasal sinuses (most commonly ethmoid). The frontal sinus usually develops after the age of 8, whilst the ethmoid sinus, the maxillary sinus, and the sphenoid sinus are usually present at birth. Organisms spread to the orbit via neurovascular foramina, bony dehiscences, valveless venous channels, and the thin orbital walls (particularly the medial wall).
- Infection may also be caused by an extension of preseptal cellulitis, dacryoadenitis, dacryocystitis (see Figure 11.6), or dental infections (anaerobic organisms). It may also occur secondary to endophthalmitis.
- Organisms may gain direct access to the orbit following surgery or trauma, e.g. via an orbital fracture that allows the spread of organisms in the sinuses.
- The most common organisms are *Staph. aureus, Strep. pyogenes, Strep. pneumonia,* and *Haemophilus influenzae* (the latter is less common with the availability of the Hib vaccination).

Chandler classification of orbital cellulitis

1. Preseptal cellulitis
2. Orbital cellulitis: infection of the orbital soft tissues without abscess formation; characterized by the obliteration of fat shadows on CT
3. Subperiosteal abscess (see Figure 11.7): a collection of purulent material between the bony wall and the periosteum (most commonly medial); generally a complication of sinusitis. Patients often have restricted ocular motility and globe displacement. Displacement of the globe should raise suspicion of a collection. CT imaging shows a homogenous mass with smooth margins and a convexity towards the orbit.
4. Orbital abscess: caused by coalescence and liquefactive necrosis within the periorbita; is secondary to orbital cellulitis rather than intraorbital extension from a subperiosteal abscess; often associated with severe proptosis, ophthalmoplegia, chemosis, and venous engorgement (and concurrent disc swelling)
5. Cavernous sinus thrombosis: the superior orbital fissure in the posterior part of the orbit forms a direct extension to the cavernous sinus. The facial veins drain into both the superior and the inferior ophthalmic veins, which in turn drain into the cavernous sinus. Infectious thrombosis is a rare complication of orbital cellulitis but carries a high mortality rate. CT and MRI are useful in confirming the diagnosis. Patients present with ptosis and facial paraesthesia. Thrombosis may occur directly from orbital cellulitis without the prior development of an abscess.

Visual loss occurs in the presence of an orbital abscess because of elevated IOP and resultant optic nerve ischaemia.

Clinical evaluation

History

- Onset is acute over hours or days, with systemic upset, nausea, vomiting, and general malaise.
- May have preceding coryzal symptoms
- Fever, pain, visual deterioration, diplopia, and pain on eye movement are typical.

Examination

Signs of preseptal cellulitis, along with:

* Pyrexia
* Conjunctival chemosis
* Ophthalmoplegia
* Proptosis may or may not be present; however, this condition is often difficult to judge because of eyelid swelling.
* Resistance to globe retropulsion, and raised IOP
* Potential optic nerve compromise (this condition may be difficult to assess in young children, especially those with marked lid swelling)
* Fundoscopy may reveal optic disc swelling and retinal venous congestion.

Investigations

* Swab purulent discharge.
* Bloods: full blood count (FBC), erythrocyte sedimentation rate (ESR), C-reactive protein (CRP), and blood cultures
* Urgent CT scan of the orbits, sinuses, and brain, with contrast (see Figure 11.7); imaging should include views of the frontal lobe to rule out brain abscesses

Treatment

* Admission with a multidisciplinary team (including paediatricians, ENT specialists, and microbiologists) and immediate intravenous antibiotics are essential. Usually intravenous ceftriaxone (1–2 g in one to two divided doses), flucloxacillin (1–2 g four times a day) and metronidazole (500 mg three times a day) are the antibiotics of choice (vancomycin if penicillin allergy).
* Regular 4-hourly recording of visual acuity, colour vision, and papillary defect is essential to look for progression, until the infection subsides.
* Surgical drainage by ENT specialists may be necessary if there is no response to antibiotic therapy or if there is a rapid deterioration of symptoms.
* The presence of an abscess is not an absolute indication for surgical drainage. In certain circumstances, resolution can occur with medical therapy alone. Young children (<9 years old) typically have single-organism infections and therefore may respond to antibiotics alone. A worsening clinical picture after 24–48 hours of adequate antibiotic therapy warrants surgical intervention. Children older than 9 years typically have polymicrobial infections with mixed aerobic and anaerobic organisms and often need surgical intervention.
* Canthotomy and cantholysis may be required as emergency procedures in cases where raised IOP compromises optic nerve function.

Mucormycosis

Mucormycosis is a rare, opportunistic, life-threatening fungal infection which may affect immunocompromised or diabetic patients. It often presents with discharge around the periorbital tissues, with black eschars along with orbital cellulitis signs. Progression is very rapid, and treatment involves urgent surgical debridement, intravenous amphotericin, hyperbaric oxygen, and daily wound cleaning.

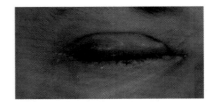

Fig 11.5 Right preseptal cellulitis

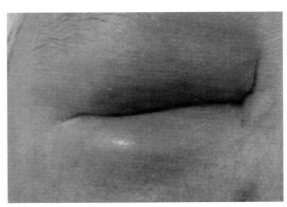

Fig 11.6 Right orbital cellulitis

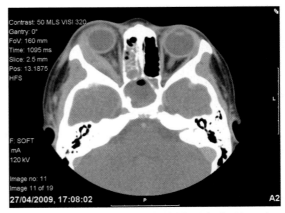

Fig 11.7 Axial CT image showing a right lateral subperiosteal abscess

Note the ethmoidal sinus opacification

Inflammation affecting the orbit may be diffuse or be localized to a specific tissue (e.g. myositis or dacryoadenitis). Causes include idiopathic orbital inflammatory disease as well as diseases associated with systemic inflammation such as Wegeners granulomatosis, sarcoidosis, polyarteritis nodosa, IgG4-related disease, xanthogranuloma, autoimmune thyroid eye disease, and systemic lupus erythematosus. Orbital infections, vascular abnormalities (such as cavernous sinus thrombosis and arteriovenous fistula), and congenital malformations (such as dermoid cysts) should also be considered in the differential diagnosis. In adults, bilateral orbital inflammation is highly suggestive of systemic inflammatory disease or lymphoproliferative disease. Bilateral idiopathic inflammation can occur in children.

It is essential for the clinician to understand that inflammation simply describes a tissue response rather than indicating any specific diagnosis. Many neoplasms such as lymphoma, haematological malignancies, orbital metastases, and lacrimal gland tumours present with signs consistent with orbital inflammation and also respond well initially to steroids. The unwary clinician starting steroid therapy for these patients without a clear diagnosis can significantly delay the diagnosis of potentially life-threatening disease, as the diagnostic yield of orbital biopsy is often significantly reduced with steroid use.

Idiopathic orbital inflammatory disease

Idiopathic orbital inflammatory disease is a diagnosis of exclusion and is made after investigations fail to identify an underlying cause. Histology is usually non-specific, with a cellular infiltrate including lymphocytes, plasma cells, and eosinophils and which sometimes leads to a reactive fibrosis.

Presentation varies according to the anatomical site of inflammation within the orbit. Posterior scleritis, myositis, and dacryoadenitis may occur in isolation, or diffuse inflammation of the orbital soft tissues may occur.

Clinical evaluation

History

* Symptoms depend on the site of inflammation and tissues affected within the orbit.
* Patients usually present with acute/subacute onset orbital pain, diplopia, and proptosis.
* Chronic, fibrosing disease may be less painful than the acute form.
* Recurrent episodes are common.
* Vision may be affected.

Examination

* Eyelids and conjunctiva are variably red and swollen.
* A careful assessment of optic nerve function should be conducted to exclude visual compromise.
* Ocular motility abnormalities may be reduced and are suggestive of associated myositis.
* An intraocular examination is essential identify any ocular inflammatory disease, chorioretinal folds, and/or retinal effusions.

Investigations

* CT scan may show diffuse or local involvement. Orbital fat may be streakier than normal. The lacrimal gland or the extraocular muscles may be enlarged, and the sclera may be thickened. Bone destruction is rare.
* B-scan may show scleritis, with scleral thickening and an acoustic hollow due to oedema in Tenons capsule ('T-sign').
* Raised ESR and white cell count are common.
* FBC with differential CRP, tests for anti-nuclear antibodies (ANAs), serum angiotensin-converting enzyme (ACE), anti-neutrophil cytoplasmic antibodies (ANCAs), and serum calcium, a Quantiferon test (for tuberculosis), and a chest X-ray (CXR) should be done to exclude systemic disease.
* Biopsy is often necessary if the clinical and imaging findings are atypical. Biopsy is essential to exclude other pathology such as malignancy, which can often mimic orbital inflammatory conditions. If biopsy is indicated, it should be undertaken before corticosteroid treatment is initiated.

Management

* NSAIDs can be highly effective (e.g. flurbiprofen 100 mg 2 to 3 times a day for a week, then tapering the dose according to clinical response).
* High-dose systemic steroids give a prompt response in cases that do not respond to NSAIDs. Orbital apex syndromes or generalized idiopathic inflammatory disease require high-dose oral or pulsed intravenous steroids.
* Radiotherapy may be used in patients who relapse frequently.

Orbital myositis

In orbital myositis, which is a variant of idiopathic orbital inflammatory disease, the extraocular muscles are affected in isolation. It may be unilateral or bilateral, and acute or chronic, and it may affect more than one muscle at a time. The main differential is thyroid eye disease, although lymphoma can also affect the extraocular muscles.

Clinical evaluation

* More common in young adults (slight female preponderance)
* Acute-onset pain, exacerbated by eye movement of the affected muscle(s)
* Periocular swelling and conjunctival chemosis
* Diplopia
* Ptosis
* Proptosis if severe

Investigations

Ultrasound and CT show fusiform enlargement of the affected extraocular muscles, usually with involvement of the muscle tendons.

Management

* Biopsy is rarely indicated; however, atypical muscle involvement warrants exclusion of infiltrative lesions.
* NSAIDs can be used for mild disease.
* Oral steroids are indicated for moderate-to-severe disease. The disease may recur once steroids are tapered, and second-line immunosuppression should be considered.
* Radiotherapy for chronic severe disease may be beneficial.

Tolosa-Hunt syndrome

Tolosa-Hunt syndrome is an idiopathic inflammation at the orbital apex, the superior orbital fissure, or the anterior cavernous sinus, causing painful ophthalmoplegia. There is variable cranial nerve involvement including motor pathways, sensory pathways, and autonomic pathways. The condition is usually unilateral. The condition is sensitive to high-dose oral or intravenous steroids.

Dacryoadenitis

Dacryoadenitis is an acute or chronic inflammation of the lacrimal gland.

Aetiology

- Inflammatory: mostly idiopathic and acute
- Viruses: herpes zoster, influenza, mumps, infectious mononucleosis
- Bacteria: *Staph. aureus, Neisseria gonorrhoeae*, streptococci, syphilis, tuberculosis
- Lymphoproliferative disorders
- Sjögren syndrome
- Sarcoidosis: a multisystem, granulomatous disease that affects the respiratory system, renal tract, skin and eyes
  - It is characterized by non-caseating granuloma formation.
  - Fifty per cent of patients will have ocular involvement.
  - A large proportion of patients have hilar lymphadenopathy and raised serum ACE levels (although these levels fall quickly with corticosteroid treatment).

Clinical evaluation

- Presents as redness, pain, and S-shaped ptosis of the lateral upper eyelid (see Figure 11.8A)
- Typically occurs in children and young adults
- Twenty-five per cent of patients who present with idiopathic orbital inflammation have dacryoadenitis.

Differential diagnosis

Differential diagnoses include ruptured dermoid cyst, adenoid cystic carcinoma, malignant pleomorphic adenocarcinoma, and plasmocytoma.

Investigations

- Conjunctival swabs
- FBC, ESR, and CRP
- ANA test, Venereal Disease Research Laboratory test (VDRL), fluorescent treponemal antibody absorption test, Quantiferon test, Epstein–Barr virus serology
- CXR

- CT: longitudinal enlargement with adjacent soft tissue inflammation is seen in idiopathic dacryoadenitis (see Figure 11.8B)
- Biopsy is not recommended if pleomorphic adenoma or dermoid cysts are suspected. The lesion should be removed en bloc, or fine-needle aspiration should be performed instead.

Treatment

- Inflammatory cases are treated with NSAIDs or steroids (see Figure 11.8C).
- Acute infective dacryoadenitis should be treated with oral Augmentin 250 mg three times a day (20–40 mg/kg/day in three divided doses in children).
- Severe infections require intravenous cefuroxime 750 mg four times a day (60 mg/kg/day in three divided doses in children).

Vasculitis

The main classification of vasculitis is based on the absence or presence of ANCAs, which are antibodies against antigens in the cytoplasm of neutrophil granulocytes. The following are found in patients with systemic vasculitides: c-ANCA, which stains the cytoplasm, and p-ANCA, which shows perinuclear staining. The primary antigen for c-ANCA is proteinase 3. The primary antigen for p-ANCA is myeloperoxidase. Patients with vasculitis usually have a raised white cell count, a raised CRP, and a raised ESR.

The most common ANCA-associated vasculitis affecting the orbit is granulomatosis with polyangiitis (also known as Wegeners granulomatosis). Granulomatosis with polyangiitis is a systemic, small-vessel vasculitis characterized by necrotizing, granulomatous inflammation in the respiratory tract and necrotizing glomerulonephritis, although any organ may be affected. The disease can present at any age but is most common in the fifth decade. The orbit can be involved in several ways. The respiratory epithelium of the nasal mucosa is a common site for severe inflammation, and associated fibrinoid necrosis with bone erosion can lead to fistulas from the nasal space to the conjunctival sac. Generalized orbital inflammation is also a feature, with areas of fibrosis and necrosis within the orbit causing proptosis, swelling, and other signs related to the tissues affected. Peripheral retinal arteritis and/or nasolacrimal duct obstruction may also be present. Up to 25% of patients have an associated scleritis. c-ANCA is present in up to 80% of patients with systemic disease, although it is less common than that in patients with solely orbital involvement. Biopsy is essential for the diagnosis, and treatment is with either steroids or cyclophosphamide

Other forms of ANCA-associated vasculitis such as microscopic polyangiitis and eosinophilic granulomatosis with polyangiitis (also known as Churg–Strauss syndrome) also affect the orbit.

A

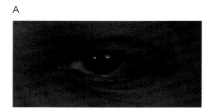

B

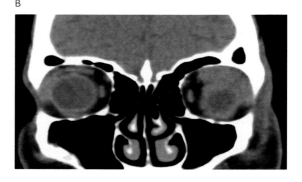

C

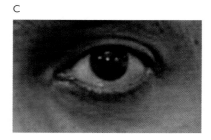

Fig 11.8 Dacryoadenitis
A An S-shaped ptosis due to lateral eyelid swelling. Note the lateral episcleral injection
B Coronal CT image showing diffuse lacrimal gland enlargement. The superior and lateral recti muscles are indistinct
C Resolution of signs following treatment with oral non-steroidal anti-inflammatory medication

11.5 Orbital vascular malformations

Cavernous haemangioma

Aetiology

* The most common benign vascular neoplasm in the adult orbit
* More common in middle-aged women than in other groups
* Can occur anywhere but most commonly in the intraconal space
* Histologically consists of blood-filled spaces separated by thin fibrous septa and lined by endothelium

Clinical evaluation

* Seventy per cent of cases develop slowly progressive, painless proptosis; however, proptosis may be accelerated during pregnancy (see Figure 11.9A).
* Although benign, haemangiomas can cause considerable mass effect resulting in choroidal folds, hyperopia, raised IOP, ophthalmoplegia, optic nerve compromise, and corneal exposure (see Figure 11.9B).

Investigations

* Ultrasound with Doppler
* CT shows a round, well-defined, homogenous mass (see Figure 11.9C).

Treatment

* Surgical excision is advocated in cases of optic nerve compromise or corneal exposure.
* Lesions are often intraconal, and the lesion is usually removed through a lateral orbitotomy approach.

Arteriovenous malformations

Carotid–cavernous fistula

A carotid–cavernous fistula (CCF) is an abnormal connection between the internal or the external carotid arteries and the cavernous sinus.

Aetiology

* High-flow (direct) CCFs:
  - Direct communication between the intracavernous internal carotid artery and the cavernous sinus; comprise the majority of fistulae
  - Usually arise from direct trauma such as a basal skull fracture that results in a trauma to the arterial wall
* Low-flow (indirect) CCFs:
  - Communication between the meningeal branches of the internal or the external carotid arteries and the cavernous sinus
  - Usually arise from spontaneous fistula formation following degeneration of the arterial wall in patients with systemic hypertension, arteriosclerosis, and/or collagen vascular disease

Clinical evaluation

* High-flow CCFs:
  - Sudden-onset pulsatile proptosis with bruit and reduced visual acuity
  - Engorged, tortuous epibulbar vessels (arterialized conjunctival vessels; see Figure 11.10A), chemosis, raised IOP, central retinal vein occlusion
  - Ocular ischaemia
  - Facial pain in the distribution of the ophthalmic branch of the trigeminal nerve
  - Ophthalmoplegia due to cranial nerve involvement at the cavernous sinus
* Low-flow CCFs:
  - Insidious onset with orbital congestion, proptosis, and mild pain
  - Patients often present with a chronic red eye and unilateral raised IOP.
  - Visual loss occurs in a third of patients, through ischaemic optic neuropathy, glaucoma, and/or central retinal vein occlusion.

Investigations

* CT shows enlarged extraocular muscles and engorgement of the superior ophthalmic vein and cavernous sinus (see Figure 11.10B and C).
* Ultrasound confirms an enlarged superior ophthalmic vein. Doppler imaging will confirm arterial waveform flow and possible flow reversal.
* MRI/magnetic resonance angiography(MRA), and angiography

Treatment

* High-flow CCFs require radiological interventional closure with coils or embolization (see Figure 11.10D).
* Low-flow CCFs often close spontaneously, but closure may be necessary if complications arise.

Primary varices

Primary varices are dilatations of **pre-existing** channels within the orbital venous system. They enlarge with increased venous pressure and can therefore present with proptosis or visible varices, both of which are often exacerbated by the Valsalva manoeuvre or a head-down posture. Complications include haemorrhage and thrombosis, both of which can lead to sudden changes in lesion size.

Contrast-enhanced CT is helpful in delineating the varices, and phleboliths (calcium deposition) may be present.

Treatment is usually conservative, with surgery reserved for patients with optic nerve compromise or severe proptosis. Surgical excision is difficult, and direct communication with the cavernous sinus makes haemorrhage difficult to control.

Lymphangioma

A lymphangioma is a hamartomatous, congenital malformation of the lymphatic system and involves skin and subcutaneous tissue. Histologically, it is composed of a large, serum-filled space lined with flattened, delicate endothelial cells.

Clinical evaluation

* Uncommon; usually present in childhood
* Superficial lesions present as cystic spaces with clear fluid (or partially filled with blood) on the lid or conjunctiva. The

lesion may enlarge on Valsalva manoeuvre or head-down posture, or during upper respiratory tract infections.

- Deep lesions may cause gradual proptosis or spontaneous haemorrhage (with loculated, blood-forming 'chocolate cysts') may occur, resulting in sudden enlargement, orbital pain, and visual loss.

Investigations

- Ultrasound, CT, or MRI

Treatment

- Spontaneous regression often occurs.
- Intralesional haemorrhage may need emergency surgical drainage but there is a high incidence of recurrence of spontaneous haemorrhage.
- If there is diffuse infiltration of the orbit, causing reduced function of orbital tissues, then debulking may be necessary but difficult.

A

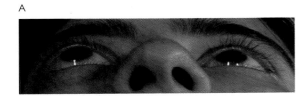

B

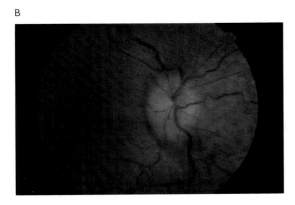

C

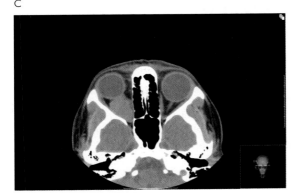

Fig 11.9 Right cavernous haemangioma
A Right sided proptosis
B The right optic nerve is swollen
C Axial CT showing an intraconal, retrobulbar mass which is enhancing heterogeneously. The optic nerve is displaced

A

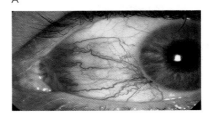

B

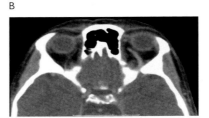

C

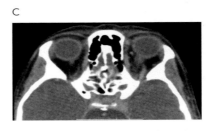

D

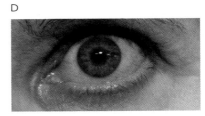

Fig 11.10 High-flow carotico-cavernous fistula
A Dilated episcleral veins
B Axial CT showing a dilated superior ophthalmic vein
C Axial CT showing an enlarged left cavernous sinus
D Resolution of episcleral vessel dilation following embolization of the fistula

Glioma

Optic nerve gliomas are slow-growing pilocytic astrocytomas and represent 4% of orbital tumours. They are commonly associated with neurofibromatosis type 1.

Clinical evaluation

* Usually presents at the end of the first decade and is more common in females than in males
* Causes slowly progressive visual loss and ultimately axial proptosis
* Optic disc pallor and optociliary shunt vessels are late signs (see Figure 11.11A).
* Possible intracranial spread to the chiasm and beyond

Investigations

* CT and MRI show fusiform enlargement of optic nerve (see Figure 11.11B).

Treatment

* Observation if slow growth and preserved visual function
* Surgery is reserved for severe proptosis, visual loss, or when posterior extension is threatened.
* Radiotherapy with adjunctive chemotherapy for intracranial extension

Prognosis

* Visual prognosis is poor, with higher mortality when there is associated posterior extension than when there is not.
* Malignant transformation into glioblastoma is very rare, occurring mostly in middle-aged males. Patients may present with symptoms of optic neuritis; if so, they will require aggressive management.

Meningioma

Meningioma is the most common adult optic nerve tumour. It appears as a diffuse tubular swelling of the optic nerve sheath. Optic nerve meningioma can occur either within the orbit or intracranially. Histologically, the two most common types are meningothelial meningiomas and psammomatous meningiomas (containing pink-staining 'psammoma' bodies). Incidence increases with age. Optic nerve meningiomas can cause gradual vision loss through optic nerve compression. Meningiomas also arise from the posterior end of the sphenoparietal fissure and from the lateral wing of the sphenoid; these kinds of meningiomas typically create hyperostosis with an orbital mass effect, and the resultant proptosis can often be the presenting feature. Cranial nerve function can also be affected by the mass effect.

Clinical evaluation

* Symptoms vary depending on the position of the tumour.
* Primary orbital meningiomas from the arachnoid of the optic nerve sheath will affect vision early. Neurofibromatosis type 2 affects around 10% of patients with optic nerve sheath meningiomas.
* A full cranial nerve assessment should be made for sphenoid wing meningiomas.
* Meningiomas are often progestogen driven and, if the patient is female, she should avoid progestogens as a contraceptive or as hormone replacement therapy.

Investigations

* CT: the tumour has a radiolucent centre (compared to optic nerve gliomas, which have a dense centre). There may be hyperostosis (thickening of bone and abnormal calcification within the tumour; see Figure 11.12). Occasionally bone absorption and destruction may occur.
* MRI can be helpful in delineating the extent of the tumour.

Treatment

* Observation, if vision is preserved
* If vision deteriorates, radiotherapy can stabilize or improve vision in a large proportion of patients.
* Surgery for optic nerve meningioma carries a high risk of blindness and is therefore deferred until intracranial structures are threatened or severe proptosis occurs.
* Lateral wall decompression can be highly effective at relieving proptosis caused by sphenoid wing meningioma.

Neurofibroma

Plexiform (diffuse) neurofibroma

Plexiform (diffuse) neurofibroma appears almost exclusively with neurofibromatosis type 1 in early childhood, with periorbital swelling of the periocular tissues. Neurofibromas can cause a mechanical ptosis and S-shaped deformity of the upper eyelid, appearing like a 'bag of worms'. Surgical excision is difficult, and repeated debulking may be necessary.

Isolated neurofibroma

Isolated neurofibromas are associated with neurofibromatosis type 1 in 10% of cases. They present in adulthood with mildly painful, gradual proptosis. Surgical excision is usually effective as a definitive treatment.

Rhabdomyosarcoma

Rhabdomyosarcoma is one of the most common primary orbital malignancies of childhood. It usually presents late in the first decade, but can occur at any age. Boys are more commonly affected than girls (5 : 3). Despite the misleading name of this condition, it usually does not affect the orbital musculature. Histologically, it can be divided into three main categories:

* **Embryonal**: most common type; usually supero-nasal, with a tumour consisting of abnormally shaped rhabdomyoblasts with little evidence of cross striations
* **Alveolar**: most malignant form; usually in the inferior orbit; malignant cells are confined by circular fibrous septa resembling lung alveoli
* **Pleomorphic**: rarest but best prognosis; is the most differentiated, with rhabdomyoblasts closely resembling striated muscle fibres; usually affects older children

Clinical evaluation

* Acute/subacute proptosis, lid oedema, and ptosis
* May present as orbital cellulitis or mimic other orbital inflammatory conditions
* Twenty-five per cent of rhabdomyosarcomas are in the superior orbit, and a palpable upper lid mass may be present.

Investigations

- Ultrasound shows a well-circumscribed mass.
- CT/MRI may show bony destruction.
- Urgent biopsy is necessary to confirm the diagnosis.
- A full workup for metastases is performed in conjunction with a paediatric oncologist.

Treatment

- Surgical excision, if well circumscribed
- Radiotherapy and chemotherapy are often required.

Prognosis

- Ninety-five per cent of patients achieve 5-year survival if the tumour is confined to the orbit.

Lymphoproliferative tumours

Lymphoproliferative disorders represent a continuous spectrum of benign to malignant disease and mainly affect the elderly. It is the most common malignant orbital tumour in adults. Orbital imaging typically shows a well-defined, homogenous mass that classically 'moulds around the globe' because of its slow growth. These tumours can be broadly divided into three categories:

Benign reactive lymphoid hyperplasia

Benign reactive lymphoid hyperplasia is a benign proliferation of lymphoid follicles; polyclonal colonization most commonly occurs in the anterior-superior orbit, and the lacrimal gland is involved in 15% of cases. Presentation is with gradual, painless proptosis, often with a palpable, firm, rubbery mass beneath the orbital rim. A 'salmon-pink' conjunctival mass may be visible in some cases. Extraocular muscles may also be involved, and suspicious, atypical thyroid eye disease in elderly patients may warrant a biopsy of the enlarged muscle. Treatment is with systemic corticosteroids or local radiotherapy. Progression to systemic lymphoma occurs in about 15% of cases by 5 years.

Atypical lymphoid hyperplasia

Atypical lymphoid hyperplasia is an intermediate between benign reactive lymphoid hyperplasia and malignant lymphoma, with histology showing sheets of lymphocytes and an absence of plasma cells. Its presentation is similar to benign reactive lymphoid hyperplasia, although it is less responsive to corticosteroids than that form is.

Malignant orbital lymphoma

Extramarginal zone lymphoma is the most common subtype of malignant orbital lymphoma and is a low-grade proliferation of monoclonal B-cells (non-Hodgkins). Follicular lymphoma, diffuse B-cell lymphoma, mantle cell lymphoma, or peripheral T-cell lymphoma may also occur in the orbit; these lymphomas behave more aggressively than extramarginal zone lymphoma does. Presentation is usually in patients aged 50–70 years, with gradual proptosis and possibly an anterior, palpable orbital mass (see Figures 11.13 and 11.14). Twenty-five per cent of cases are bilateral, and 40% are associated with systemic lymphoma at presentation. Patients require systemic workup to determine the presence of systemic disease. Radiotherapy is the standard treatment for orbital disease, and chemotherapy is required in disseminated or poorly differentiated cases.

A

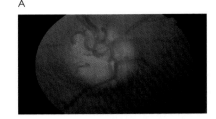

B

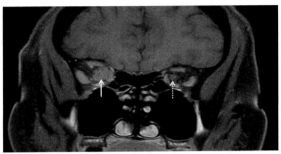

Fig 11.11
A Optociliary shunt vessels in a patient with optic nerve glioma
B Coronal MRI showing right optic nerve glioma in the same patient (solid white arrow). Compare it with the left optic nerve (dashed white arrow)

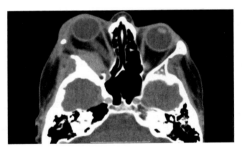

Fig 11.12 Axial CT of sphenoid wing meningioma
Note the associated hyperostosis

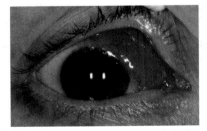

Fig 11.13 Orbital lymphoma extending into the bulbar conjunctiva

Courtesy of Mandeep Sagoo

A

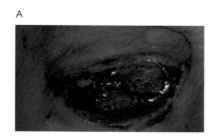

B

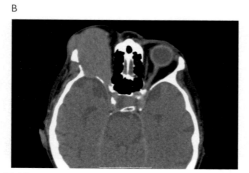

Fig 11.14
A Aggressive diffuse B-cell lymphoma
B Axial CT of the aggressive B-cell lymphoma. The lesion involves the entire orbit

Lacrimal gland lesions

Lacrimal gland swelling is most commonly due to idiopathic inflammation, which often responds to non-steroidal anti-inflammatory treatment. However, neoplastic disease can also present with primary lacrimal gland swelling. The majority of lacrimal gland neoplasms are epithelial in origin; of these, 50% are benign tumours, and 50% are malignant. CT is the investigation of choice and is particularly helpful in characterizing malignancy by identifying microinvasion of cortical bone, tumour calcification, and the macroscopic extent of the tumour.

Benign epithelial tumours

Pleomorphic adenoma (benign mixed tumour)

Pleomorphic adenoma (benign mixed tumour) is the most common epithelial lacrimal gland tumour (50%). Histologically, these tumours are comprised of epithelial and mesenchymal elements (hence the term 'mixed') and are typically circumscribed by a pseudocapsule.

They typically present in the fourth or fifth decades, with slowly progressive, painless axial proptosis and downwards medial globe displacement. Although pleomorphic adenoma more commonly affects the orbital lobe of the lacrimal gland, palpebral lobe involvement can be detected by the presence of a firm palpable 'pea-like' mass.

CT shows a slight enlargement of the lacrimal gland, with enlargement of the lacrimal gland fossa (see Figure 11.15).

Treatment is by complete, intact surgical excision. Incisional biopsy is contraindicated, as breach of the pseudocapsule leads to significant risk of seeding and recurrence, which is difficult to manage.

Malignant epithelial tumours

Malignant mixed tumour

A malignant mixed tumour is similar to a benign mixed form but contains areas of malignant transformation. It typically arises from long-standing pleomorphic adenomas and has a mortality of 50%, even with exenteration.

Adenoid cystic carcinoma

Adenoid cystic carcinoma accounts for 25% of lacrimal gland tumours (60% of malignant tumours) and is highly malignant. Several histological subtypes have been characterized, of which the cribriform variant is the most common.

Adenoid cystic carcinoma commonly presents in the fourth decade with rapid onset (less than 1 year) proptosis which may be associated with pain which is thought to be due to perineural invasion (pain is an important feature of a lacrimal gland mass as it may indicate malignancy). Ophthalmoplegia and diplopia may also be present.

CT shows a poorly demarcated lesion, often with bone destruction. Focal calcification may be present.

Treatment is controversial, although surgical excision with or without orbitectomy and adjuvant high-dose radiotherapy may be used. The prognosis depends on the histological subtype, which may predict long-term survival, with the basaloid variant having the poorest prognosis.

Metastatic tumours and sinus invasion

Adults

Orbital metastases in adults are rare, although they may be the initial manifestation of an underlying tumour. Presentation is with rapid proptosis, and ophthalmoparesis may develop. Scirrhous carcinoma of the breast or the stomach may cause enophthalmos because of orbital tissue contraction. Other primary sources include the lungs, the prostate, the gastrointestinal tract, and the kidneys. Occasionally, no source is found.

Orbital invasion by sinus tumours is rare but carries a poor prognosis unless diagnosed early. The maxillary sinus is the most common primary site and invasion there causes facial pain, congestion, epistaxis, and nasal discharge. Upwards globe displacement, diplopia, and epiphora can occur. Ethmoidal carcinoma can cause lateral dystopia, and proptosis is a late feature in nasopharyngeal carcinoma.

Children

Neuroblastoma

Neuroblastoma is the most common tumour during infancy and arises from primitive neuroblasts in the sympathetic nervous system. The tumour will have already spread in 50% of cases at the time of diagnosis. Orbital metastases present with rapid proptosis, lid swelling, and a superior orbital mass.

Granulocytic sarcoma

A granulocytic sarcoma is a localized tumour comprised of malignant cells of myeloid origin. It may occur as a manifestation of established systemic myeloid leukaemia or it may precede the disease, in which case, diagnosis can be difficult. Children and young adults are most commonly affected, and rapid proptosis, chemosis, and lid swelling are common.

Eosinophilic granuloma

Eosinophilic granuloma, one of the Langerhans cell histiocytoses, usually arises in childhood and is characterized by a proliferation of bone-marrow-derived Langerhans cells and mature eosinophils. This condition presents with intraosseous deposits in the periorbital skeleton and can cause rapid onset proptosis, and osteolytic lesions. Local involvement is treated with surgical curettage; intralesional steroids (or radiotherapy) and chemotherapy are indicated in systemic involvement. Life prognosis is good.

Cystic lesions

Dermoid cysts and epidermoid cysts

Dermoid cysts and epidermoid cysts are developmental choristomas and are both lined with keratinizing epithelium. They develop as a result of entrapped dermal or epidermal elements along the lines of embryonic ectodermal fusion. Dermoid cysts contain hair follicles, collagen, fat, and sebaceous glands. They may be superficial or deep.

- **Superficial lesions:** typically present in early infancy with a slow-growing, painless mass superiorly. They are not attached to overlying skin; this feature aids differentiation from sebaceous cysts.

- **Deep lesions:** usually present later in life, with gradual proptosis and globe restriction (see Figure 11.16A). They are associated with bony sutures and may extend into the adjacent temporal fossa, frontal sinuses, or cranium.

If the entire extent of the cyst is not palpable, CT may be useful to exclude intracranial extension, especially for medial dermoids (see Figure 11.16B).

Treatment is by complete excision. Cysts may rupture during trauma or surgery and incite a significant inflammatory response. Incomplete excision may lead to draining sinus formation or recurrence of the cyst.

Dacryops

A dacryops is a ductule cyst of the palpebral lobe of the lacrimal gland and contains clear fluid. It typically enlarges after lacrimation. The cyst is often visible through the conjunctiva, and treatment is by aspiration, de-roofing, or marsupialization.

Sinus mucoceles

Sinus mucoceles occur following obstruction to paranasal sinus drainage. Sinus mucoceles can be congenital or caused by trauma, but they are most frequently due to sinusitis. Most arise from the frontal and ethmoidal sinuses, presenting with headache, non-axial globe displacement, and occasionally a palpable lid swelling.

CT shows a soft tissue mass with thinning of the bony wall of the sinus. Surgical drainage is usually undertaken by ENT specialists, often endoscopically.

Encephaloceles

Encephaloceles are congenital defects in the skull that allow herniation of intracranial contents into the orbit. Anterior orbital encephaloceles are due to fronto-ethmoidal bony defects and may cause displacement of the globe. They are associated with other craniofacial abnormalities (e.g. hypertelorism) and ocular abnormalities (e.g. colobomas). Posterior encephaloceles cause proptosis and inferior globe displacement and are associated with neurofibromatosis type 1. Both anterior and posterior encephaloceles may exhibit pulsatile proptosis, without a bruit.

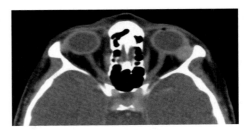

Fig 11.15 Axial CT of a pleomorphic adenoma
Note the scalloping of the bone

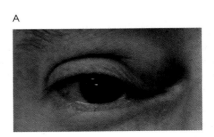

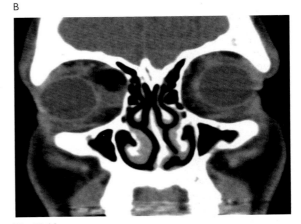

Fig 11.16
A Supero-nasal orbital dermoid causing infero-lateral globe displacement
B Coronal CT of the dermoid situated in the supero-medial extraconal space. The superior portion of the lesion shows fat density, whilst the inferior part shows soft density material

11.8 Thyroid eye disease

Thyroid eye disease, also known as Graves orbitopathy, thyroid-associated orbitopathy, or dysthyroid eye disease, affects 25%–50% of patients with Graves disease. Most patients develop orbitopathy within 18–24 months of the onset of dysthyroidism. Thyroid eye disease is also seen in patients who are euthyroid and is associated with other autoimmune conditions such as myasthenia gravis and vitiligo. Thyroid eye disease has a strong gender bias, with women much more commonly affected than men (4 : 1). The age of onset is usually in the third to the sixth decades, although rarely children and the elderly can be affected.

The symptoms and signs vary from mild disease, which can present with conjunctival injection and mild eyelid retraction, to severe disease causing marked proptosis and rarely optic nerve compression. Thyroid eye disease is often asymmetric or unilateral and is the most common cause of proptosis in adults. Smoking and poorly controlled thyroid function are significant risk factors for an increased incidence and severity of thyroid eye disease.

Pathogenesis

The pathogenesis of thyroid eye disease is poorly understood, although activated T-cells are central to the autoimmune process in the orbit. Cytokine release from activated T-cells stimulates orbital fibroblasts within orbital fat, connective tissue, and lacrimal glands to secrete hyaluronic acid, a glycosaminoglycan. Hyaluronic acid forms large, branched, gel-like macromolecular complexes with high negative charge and which are highly hydrophilic. Adipogenesis is also a prominent feature of thyroid eye disease. Together, these factors cause an increase in the volume of orbital tissues, with resulting swelling and proptosis. Histologically, the extraocular muscles show glycosaminoglycan deposition, oedema, and pleomorphic cellular infiltration. Later in the disease, fibrosis is a feature, which can affect the orbital fat compartment, levator palpebrae superioris, and extraocular muscles, leading to restriction of extraocular motility. The most important preventable causes of visual loss in this condition are corneal exposure and optic nerve compression.

Clinical evaluation

* The course of thyroid eye disease is variable but classically consists of an active phase (lasting 3–12 months) followed by a quiescent (inactive/'burn-out') phase. The length and severity of each phase varies. Occasionally, quiescent disease can reactivate, but such reactivation is uncommon.
* During the inflammatory phase, the orbits become congested, swollen, and painful.
* Patients complain of dry eye symptoms, photophobia, and retrobulbar pain. They may develop periorbital oedema, lacrimal gland swelling, and fat prolapse.
* Patients may report symptoms of dysthyroidism (tachycardia/palpitations, weight loss, tremor, heat intolerance, anxiety, and irritability).
* Other symptoms and signs include:
  - Conjunctival chemosis (see Figures 11.17 and 11.18)
  - Proptosis (see Figure 11.18)
  - Eyelid retraction (Dalrymple sign; see Figure 11.18), and lid lag on down-gaze (von Graefe sign)
  - Superior limbal keratopathy (may be a marker for severe thyroid eye disease)
  - Diplopia (most commonly hypo-or esotropia, as the inferior and medial recti are most commonly involved)
  - Corneal exposure
  - Compressive optic neuropathy (dyschromatopsia, reduced visual acuity, visual field restriction, and an afferent pupil defect)
* The disease may be asymmetrical or unilateral (see Figure 11.19).

Differential diagnosis

* Myositis
* Idiopathic inflammatory orbital disease
* Orbital mass (e.g. cavernous haemangioma)
* Low-flow carotid–cavernous fistula
* Myasthenia gravis (thyroid eye disease can coexist in myasthenia gravis in up to 5% of patients)
* Cranial nerve palsies
* Chronic progressive external ophthalmoplegia

Investigations

* Thyroid function (indicated by levels of thyroid-stimulating hormone (TSH) and free T_4) may be high, low, or normal.
* Thyroid autoantibodies (anti-TSH receptor antibody, thyroglobulin antibody, and thyroid peroxidase antibodies) are commonly elevated.
* CT is the imaging investigation of choice and can support the diagnosis by showing enlargement of extraocular muscles with sparing of the tendons (inferior > medial > superior > lateral recti; see Figure 11.20). Crowding of the orbital apex can also be observed. There may also be intraorbital fat stranding, which suggests active inflammation. CT imaging is necessary if bony decompression is planned.
* MRI can be useful in identifying active inflammation or optic nerve compression.

Classification

There are a number of published scoring systems for disease activity and severity; however, all have limitations in their use in monitoring disease activity and response to treatments.
* The NOSPECS classification is a **severity s**core:
  - (**NO**: absent signs/symptoms, **s**oft tissue involvement, **p**roptosis, **e**xtraocular muscle involvement, **c**orneal involvement, **s**ight loss)
* VISA is a **severity** score:
  - **V**ision loss (optic neuropathy), **I**nflammation/congestion and activity in thyroid eye disease, **s**trabismus/motility, and **a**ppearance/exposure
* The clinical activity score is used to measure disease **activity**:
  - One point each for pain behind the eyes (within the last month), pain on eye movement, eyelid erythema, conjunctival erythema, eyelid swelling, conjunctival chemosis, caruncular swelling, increased proptosis of >2 mm in 1–3 months, reduced ocular motility of >5° in 1–3 months, and visual loss of >1 Snellen line in 1–3 months

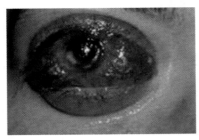

Fig 11.17 Severe active thyroid eye disease
Courtesy of Geoff Rose

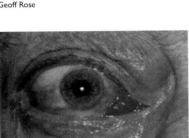

Fig 11.18 Active thyroid eye disease
Courtesy of Geoff Rose

A

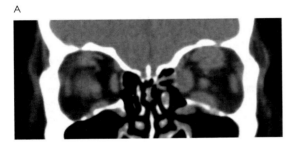

B

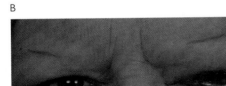

Fig 11.19 Asymmetric active thyroid eye disease
A Coronal CT showing marked enlargement of the extraocular muscles of the left eye
B Left conjunctival chemosis

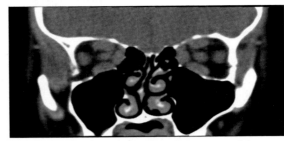

Fig 11.20 Coronal CT shows bilateral enlargement of the extraocular muscles. The inferior and medial recti muscles are preferentially involved

Treatment

Conservative

* Smoking cessation
* Lubrication with artificial tears is almost always required during the day, with ointment used at night for lagophthalmos.

Medical

* Tight control of dysthyroidism
* NSAIDs can be useful in mild disease to control symptoms of periocular discomfort.
* Oral selenium 100 µg twice a day can improve symptoms in patients with mild, active thyroid eye disease.
* High-dose corticosteroids are usually reserved for those with severe inflammation (proptosis, periorbital swelling, and chemosis) or compressive optic neuropathy. Patients should be warned of the side effects of steroids and monitored for changes in blood pressure and blood glucose levels. Bone density scans should be performed as appropriate and osteoporosis prophylaxis initiated as needed.
  - High-dose oral prednisolone (80 mg) for 3 days; then taper or pulsed intravenous methylprednisolone (500 mg weekly for 6 weeks, followed by 250 mg weekly for 6 weeks). High doses of intravenous methylprednisolone can cause hepatic failure.
  - Compressive optic neuropathy requires high doses of pulsed intravenous methylprednisolone (500 mg–1 g) given on alternate days for 3–6 days. If there is no significant response in days, then urgent surgical decompression should be considered.
* Steroid-sparing agents such as azathioprine, methotrexate, and anti-tumour necrosis factor drugs are often used in cases of extended steroid use or steroid intolerance.
* B-cell depletion is currently being evaluated and is a promising new steroid-sparing treatment.

Radiotherapy

* Orbital radiotherapy may be a beneficial adjuvant to steroids in moderate-to-severe disease.
* Irradiation affects orbital fibroblasts to reduce the inflammatory response and reduce glycosaminoglycan deposition as well as reducing cytokine release from activated lymphocytes.
* Radiotherapy takes effect in 4–6 weeks. Side effects include cataract, radiation retinopathy, and optic neuropathy.

Surgery

* Surgery is often delayed until the disease is quiescent, usually waiting for at least 6 months of stability before proceeding. However, urgent decompression may be required in cases of corneal exposure or optic nerve compression.
* Surgery for thyroid eye disease is often carried out in multiple stages with a specific sequence: decompression, followed by strabismus surgery, and lastly corrective eyelid surgery.
* Decompression is the most effective treatment for proptosis. Usually, the lateral wall is removed with or without the medial and inferior walls, as lateral wall decompression is very rarely associated with post-operative strabismus. Medial wall removal is the most effective approach for optic neuropathy and may be performed endoscopically.
* Complications include visual loss, haemorrhage, worsening diplopia, globe malposition, and periorbital paraesthesia.
* Strabismus surgery is often delayed until orthoptic measurements have been stable for at least 6 months. The main aim is to re-establish single vision in primary and reading gaze.
* Upper eyelid lowering can be achieved by either an anterior or a posterior approach.
* Lower lid retraction often requires insertion of a spacer such as hard palate or ear cartilage.
* Blepharoplasty is the final step to reduce fat prolapsed in the upper and lower eyelids.

Prognosis

* Episodes of active disease typically last for 6–18 months. If left untreated, the disease becomes progressive.
* Recurrence is uncommon and may be associated with recent loss of control of thyroid function, restarting smoking, or radioiodine treatment.

Fractures to orbital bones most commonly occur following assault, falls, road traffic accidents, and sports injuries. Depending on the point of traumatic impact, a variety of orbital fractures can occur, ranging from minimally displaced fractures that do not require intervention to major destruction of orbital architecture. Fractures can be broadly divided into three types: blowout, orbito-zygomatic, and naso-orbito-ethmoid. Sphenoidal orbital apex fractures are difficult but important to identify as there is often associated injury to the neurovascular structures within the optic canal and superior orbital fissure. Patients will present with traumatic optic neuropathy and variable cranial nerve palsies. Thirty per cent of orbital fracture cases have intraocular complications; therefore, a complete ocular examination is essential in all cases of orbital trauma. Traumatic retrobulbar haemorrhage may result in compressive optic neuropathy. CT is the investigation of choice to aid diagnosis of fractures and assist surgical planning.

Blowout fractures

Blowout fractures are fractures of the orbital walls and may or may not be associated with a fracture of the orbital rim, which is stronger than the orbital walls. Blowout fractures usually affect the orbital floor and the medial wall. High-force injuries (such as in road traffic accidents) may result in lateral wall fractures. Mechanical compression at the orbital rim transmits forces to the floor and wall, which act as 'crumple zones', causing these walls to break at their weakest points. Orbital contents such as fat, the infraorbital nerve, or extraocular muscle may prolapse through the defect to cause globe displacement, paraesthesia, or restricted ocular motility.

Clinical evaluation

* The patient is typically a young male and has been punched or hit directly in the eye.
* Patients should be assessed for airway, breathing, and circulation, as well as for cervical spine stability.
* Visual acuity **must** be recorded in all cases.
* Usually presents with pain, eyelid ecchymosis and oedema, diplopia, and occasionally surgical emphysema (due to air blowback from the sinus after nose blowing)
* Diplopia may be in any position but is most common in up- or down-gaze. Entrapment of the muscle may result in nausea or even an exaggerated oculo-cardiac reflex.
* Lower lid and/or cheek hypoaesthesia may occur in orbital floor fractures that involve infraorbital nerve injury.
* Stepping of the orbital rim may occur if the rim is fractured, as well as flattening of the malar with tripod fractures.
* Enophthalmos is often evident after oedema settles. This condition can occur after a few weeks or months. Hypoglobus may occur with significant floor fractures or with orbital roof subperiosteal haematoma.
* Ptosis may occur with injury to the levator palpebrae superioris.

Investigations

* Orthoptic assessment with Hess chart documentation at a later date (usually 2 days later) once the eye can be opened

* CT of the orbits is indicated if a fracture is associated with limitation of eye movement and suspected muscle entrapment or intraorbital foreign body (see Figure 11.21).
* Forced duction testing is performed if restriction persists beyond 1 week. Resistance felt when moving the globe away from the affected muscle suggests entrapment.

Treatment

* Oral antibiotics, e.g. cephalexin 250 mg four times a day for 1 week (risk of orbital cellulitis from sinus pathogens)
* Avoid nose blowing for 2 weeks.
* Ice packs for 48 hours
* Surgical repair is indicated if there is diplopia, enophthalmos, or globe displacement. Not all patients will require surgical intervention.
* Early repair (within 2 weeks) is considered in patients who have persistent diplopia in primary position or up-gaze, those with nausea, vomiting, or exaggerated oculo-cardiac reflex.
* Patients with large fractures or significant enophthalmos without muscle entrapment may benefit from delayed surgery once oedema has settled.

'Trapdoor' or 'white-eye' blowout fractures in children

'Trapdoor' or 'white-eye' blowout fractures usually only occur in children and young adults, because of the increased elasticity of their orbital bones. The fracture cracks open and the flexibility of the floor returns it to its normal position so that a 'trapdoor' effect occurs, trapping orbital contents in the fractured area.

A marked restriction in up-gaze as well as persistent nausea, vomiting, and excessive pain are indicative of this type of fracture. Radiology may not always confirm muscle entrapment, and restriction in up-gaze is sometimes the only sign. More urgent surgical repair (within a few days) is usually required to prevent long-term extraocular muscle damage.

Orbito-zygomatic fractures

The zygoma has a prominent position in the facial skeleton, and blows to the side of the face makes it prone to fracture. Moderate trauma usually results in minimally or non-displaced fractures, whereas severe forces result in displaced fractures which can involve the orbital rim and floor. Lateral wall fractures are generally associated with zygomatic fractures.

Clinical features include malar flattening, diplopia, trismus (pain on mastication due to masseter spasm or bony impingement of the coronoid process), pain on palpation, paraesthesia, and step deformities.

Surgical management of these fractures depends on the degree of zygomatic displacement. Non-displaced fractures can be observed, and patients should be advised to avoid nose blowing. Open reduction techniques through infraciliary or transconjunctival approaches are more favoured for displaced and/or comminuted fractures. Additional fixation may be required through a trans-oral approach, a lateral orbital wall approach, or a coronal approach to stabilize the other attachments of the zygoma. Extraocular muscle entrapment and rarely retrobulbar haemorrhage can occur following fracture repair.

Naso-orbito-ethmoid fractures

The naso-orbito-ethmoid complex describes the convergence of the frontal and the ethmoidal sinuses, the anterior cranial fossa, and the frontal and the nasal bones. Trauma in this region can result in complex fractures, making repair difficult. Fractures can be classified according to whether they are comminuted and whether medial canthal tendon disruption has occurred.

Clinical features include nasal/forehead swelling, pain, forehead paraesthesia, diplopia, telecanthus (due to lateral displacement of the medial canthal tendon), and cerebrospinal spinal fluid (CSF) rhinorrhoea.

Prompt maxillofacial surgical repair is required for optimal outcome.

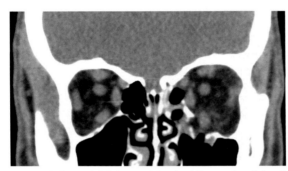

Fig 11.21 Coronal CT showing left orbital floor and medial wall fracture

Although there is prolapse of orbital fat, the inferior rectus does not appear to be entrapped on imaging; however, this observation must be correlated with clinical findings

11.10 Orbital surgery

Surgical approaches to the orbit

Orbital surgery is performed for the diagnosis and treatment of orbital disease, restoration of anatomy following trauma, and cosmetic improvement of congenital or acquired deformities.

Prior to any surgery, a full preoperative assessment should include thorough history taking and orbital, facial, and systemic examination. Photographic assessment and documentation is useful. Imaging with CT (including three-dimensional reconstruction) or MRI can give important information regarding the specific location of lesions and their relationship to adjacent structures.

The surgical approach to the orbit depends on the presumed diagnosis, location of pathology, involvement of adjacent structures, and need for adequate exposure. Orbital surgery requires the following access approaches.

Anterior orbitotomy

Superior approach

A superior approach is most commonly used for lacrimal gland biopsy and other lesions located in the supero-anterior orbit. An upper lid skin crease incision is made, and the septum identified and incised, with careful avoidance of the levator and superior oblique muscles. This approach can also be used for exposure of the orbital rim laterally, with subperiosteal dissection allowing access to the extraconal and intraconal spaces, as well as the extraocular muscles.

Inferior approach

An inferior approach provides good access to the orbital floor and extraconal and intraconal spaces. Usually a transconjunctival route is used with a lateral canthotomy (swinging lid approach). The inferior orbital rim may be exposed to dissect under the periosteum for repair of orbital floor fractures. Transcutaneous approaches via a subciliary or lid-crease incision are also used.

Medial approach

A medial approach provides excellent access to the medial wall (useful for orbital decompression in thyroid eye disease) and to the medial apex. Transconjunctival, transcaruncular, or transcutaneous (classic Lynch incision or modified dacryocystorhinostomy incision) routes can be used. This approach requires careful dissection to avoid the medial canthal tendon, the lacrimal apparatus, the superior oblique tendon, and the medial rectus.

Lateral orbitotomy

Lateral orbitotomy is used for deep orbital lesions (i.e. behind the globe equator) or lesions within the muscle cone that cannot be approached by anterior or medial routes. It is also indicated in lacrimal gland fossa lesions, when lesions need to be removed intact (e.g. pleomorphic adenoma).

The lateral orbital rim is exposed via a lateral canthotomy, and the periosteum is retracted back. The lateral wall is removed where necessary to improve access.

Orbital decompression

Orbital decompression is mainly performed in cases of thyroid eye disease when optic nerve compression or severe proptosis has developed. The aim is the removal of a combination of the lateral wall, the medial wall, and the orbital floor, allowing extra space within the orbit.

Technique

The approach can be via a swinging lid incision (i.e. canthotomy and cantholysis), an upper lid skin crease incision, or a transconjunctival inferior forniceal incision. Removal of the lateral wall allows prolapse of orbital tissue into the temporal fossa; floor removal allows expansion into the maxillary sinus, and medial wall removal allows prolapse into the ethmoidal sinus. Medial wall removal can also be carried out endonasally by ENT surgeons.

Complications

* Visual loss through optic nerve injury
* Post-operative orbital haematoma (may require immediate decompression)
* CSF leak
* Diplopia
* Lid malpositions

Evisceration, enucleation, and exenteration

Evisceration, enucleation, and exenteration are procedures which involve removal of the patient's eye. Preoperative counselling is of paramount importance in these difficult situations, and meticulous preoperative checks must be performed to avoid removing the wrong eye.

Evisceration

Evisceration involves the surgical removal of the entire contents of the globe, leaving behind a sclera shell with the extraocular muscles still attached. Evisceration is contraindicated in cases of intraocular malignancy.

Indications

* Blind, painful eye
* Phthisis bulbi
* Endophthalmitis
* Cosmetic (although other options such as a cosmetic contact lens or artificial shell should be exhausted prior to proceeding with evisceration)

Technique

* Surgery can be performed under general or local anaesthesia.
* A 360° peritomy is performed with dissection of the sub-Tenons space to allow sufficient room to operate. Relieving incisions may be made in the conjunctiva to prevent intraoperative tearing of the tissues.
* A limbal incision can then be made using a keratome, and the corneal button removed with scissors.
* The intraocular contents are then removed using an evisceration spoon, ensuring all uveal tissue is stripped. Some surgeons will use alcohol-soaked cotton-tipped applicators to remove residual pigmented tissue; however, this can be toxic to the conjunctiva.
* Anterior relieving incisions in the sclera can be made and extended posteriorly. The scleral shell is detached from the optic nerve.

- The orbital implant size is estimated using metallic sizers. The maximal ball implant size is that which can be accommodated without putting tension on the sclera or inducing excessive anterior volume changes which would make cosmetic shell fitting difficult. A typical implant size is 20 mm in diameter. The implant (either integrated, porous materials such as hydroxyapatite or non-integrated materials such as acrylic) is then inserted into the cavity using a no-touch technique (see Figure 11.22A).
- The sclera is then sutured with interrupted 5–0 Vicryl (see Figure 11.22B). Tenons capsule is closed with interrupted 6–0 Vicryl, and a running 7–0 Vicryl suture is used to close the conjunctiva.
- A clear conformer is then inserted, along with chloramphenicol ointment.
- A pressure dressing is applied for 5–7 days, and fitting of the artificial eye can begin after 4–6 weeks.

Enucleation

Enucleation involves surgical removal of the entire globe, including the sclera.

Indications

Indications for enucleation are as for evisceration but also include intraocular tumours and severe trauma with a risk of sympathetic ophthalmia. Enucleation is also important where there is any diagnostic uncertainty as to the cause of blindness.

Technique

The recti muscles are disinserted and the optic nerve transected with scissors or a Foster snare. Ball implants are inserted within the muscle cone, which is reattached to the implant anteriorly. Acrylic implants and porous polyethylene (Medpore) are commonly used. Pressure padding is applied for several days, and an artificial eye can be applied in 4–6 weeks.

Complications of enucleation and evisceration

- Implant extrusion (see Figure 11.23)
- Post-enucleation socket syndrome (volume deficiency resulting in enophthalmos, upper lid ptosis, and a deep upper lid sulcus)
- Lower lid laxity
- Evisceration may carry a high theoretical risk of sympathetic ophthalmia because of possible incomplete removal of choroidal antigens.
- Post-operative pain

Exenteration

Exenteration involves removal of all of the orbital contents. This procedure is performed either with or without removal of the eyelids. It is usually reserved for highly malignant tumours such as sebaceous cell carcinoma or malignant melanoma.

Indications

- Cutaneous tumours with orbital invasion
- Mucormycosis
- Invasive lacrimal gland malignancies
- Extensive conjunctival malignancies
- Other orbital malignancies

Technique

The technique used depends on the tumour location (i.e. anterior or posterior orbital involvement). Generally, the technique involves a skin incision at about the orbital rim to the periosteum and its reflection back from the orbital rim, continuing posteriorly within the orbit to behind the globe. The entire orbital contents, including the eyelids, globe, and muscles, are removed to the apex, including the periosteum.

Healing by granulation tissue occurs within 3–4 months but results in a shallower socket than healing with split skin grafting does. With eyelid-sparing exenteration, the eyelid skin is preserved to allow quicker healing of the socket (see Figure 11.24A).

A cosmetic prosthesis can be used once healing has occurred. This prosthesis overlies the socket and is carefully fashioned and painted to match the contralateral side. The prosthesis can be either glasses mounted (see Figure 11.24B) or held in place using osteointegrated implants with magnetic abutments.

Complications

- Severe blood loss
- CSF fluid leak through intraoperative damage to adjacent sinus walls or dura
- Sinus fistula formation
- Infection

A

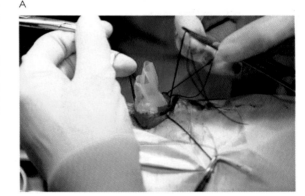

B

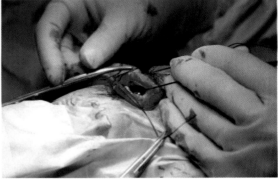

Fig 11.22 Evisceration

A The implant is inserted into the scleral shell with a no-touch technique to minimize the risk of infection

B The scleral is then closed over the implant carefully to reduce the risk of extrusion

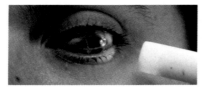

Fig 11.23 Orbital implant extrusion

A

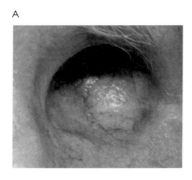

B

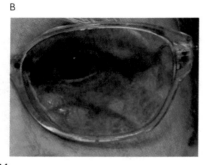

Fig 11.24
A Exenteration
B Exenteration prosthesis attached to glasses

Chapter 12

Microsurgical skills

Ronald Kam and Paul Sullivan

Surgical skills

Safe ophthalmic surgery requires the surgeon to have:
- The ability to select the best instruments for a particular task
- Knowledge of the most effective way of using each instrument
- Knowledge of the limitations and side effects of the use of each instrument

Whilst some surgical tasks may be performed with instruments that are not ideally suited to carry out the manoeuvres needed, the results obtained in a relatively unforgiving microsurgical environment may be mediocre or suboptimal. Insensitive handling of tissues may cause tissue distortion or damage or may present mechanical hindrances affecting the accurate placement of sutures or instruments. An in-depth appreciation of the reasons for the fine details of instrument design may allow a surgeon to make optimal use of specific design features to improvise in unfamiliar or difficult situations. This chapter will cover important aspects of microsurgical skills in operations both under microscopic vision and in oculoplastic practice.

Forceps, and grasping tissues

Forceps are commonly used to:
- Grasp wound edges so that they can be immobilized for sutures to be passed through them
- Hold, move, or retract tissues
- Hold strands of suture material

All the different parts of the anatomy of a pair of forceps, for example, the handles and tips, have been designed to aid the surgeon in various ways, and knowledge of these features is important to tailor the choice and use of an instrument.

Aims of proper forceps use
- To hold or immobilize tissue effectively without slipping
- The forceps design should match the tissue being grasped.
- Minimize trauma imparted to the tissue: avoid damaging tissue by crushing it or cutting through it

Grasping tissue whilst suturing
The tissue that the suture needle is going to be passed through should ideally be grasped in a direction at right angles to the wound edge, in line with the anticipated point of needle entry (see Figure 12.1). This method reduces eccentric shearing forces when the wound edge is lifted up and minimizes pivoting or rotational forces when the suture needle is passed through the wound edge.

Forceps handles

How to hold forceps
The most important piece of advice with regard to holding surgical instruments is to avoid a 'pencil grip' (see Figure 12.2). This grip may feel natural to a novice surgeon but the instrument is so effectively anchored by the middle finger and the first web space that movements in all directions and rotations about the axis of the instrument are severely restricted. Gross wrist movements are needed to achieve very small movements at the tip of the instrument. A better way of gripping the handle is shown in this section.

Round grips or flat grips
Forceps are made with either flat handle grips or round grips.

Round grips
- Allow the surgeon to roll the handle between the thumb, the index finger, and the middle finger to achieve rotational movements along the axis of the instrument

Flat grips
- Deliberately limit the amount of rotation about the instrument's axis
- Require wrist movements to produce rotational movements that cannot be achieved using the small finger joints
- Allow for rotational stability once tissue or suture material is grasped
- Usually allow forceps to be made to a lighter weight and using less metal (usually titanium for non-reusable instruments) than round grips do; large round holes are incorporated into the grips for the same reason

Length of the handles
Long handles
- Allow the instrument to be anchored at the hand in the thumb–forefinger web space if required
- Permit a greater capacity for proprioception
- Allow tissues to be held at a distance to allow close access for other instruments

Short handles
- Allow for more mobility
- Transmit force more directly and with less bending of handles than long-handled forceps do

Forceps tips

The tips of forceps can be plain, toothed, notched, grooved, or serrated (see Figure 12.3). As the fine detail of the tips can sometimes be difficult to identify with the naked eye, some instrument makers engrave a symbol on the handle (see Figure 12.4).

Plain tips
Plain tips will inevitably slip when holding tissue but are ideal for holding suture material (or eyelashes), so these tips are found in suture-tying forceps. When these forceps are squeezed with increasing pressure, at some point the flat portion of the tips come together and lie against each other completely (see Figure 12.5). This feature is useful for picking up sutures at any length of the plain tip profile. However, at high pressures, the tips may splay apart. To prevent excessive pressure from being transmitted to the tips, small struts called stops can be incorporated between the forceps handles, to limit the distance to which the handles can be compressed. Stops are usually placed underneath the point of finger contact (see Figure 12.6).

Tying blocks
It is very common for a surgeon to want to tie a knot or handle suture material without having to constantly exchange toothed or notched tissue forceps with a plain-tipped forceps. Therefore, many forceps are made with tying blocks immediately proximal to the tips. These are flat portions which, when the forceps are closed, appose immediately en bloc (see Figure 12.7) and are ideal for handling suture material.

Serrated forceps

Serrated forceps tips help to increase the friction in a direction running at right angles to the ridges. Serrations are most commonly seen on the relatively wide tips of Moorfields forceps (see Figure 12.3). The ridges work so long as the tissue being gripped is soft enough to be in contact with both the grooves and the ridges of the serrations when gripped. Moorfields forceps are specifically designed for handling conjunctiva. If the tissue grasped is too firm, only the ridges will be in contact, resulting in failure of 'biting' of the serrations, insufficient surface area of contact, decreased friction, and an increased tendency of slipping. Cornea and sclera are therefore not suited to plain or serrated forceps.

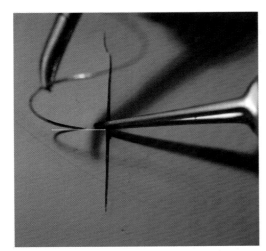

Fig 12.1 Both the gripping point and the needle entry should lie along an imaginary line at right angles to the wound edge

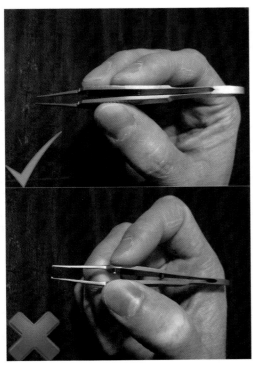

Fig 12.2 Correct and incorrect ways of holding tissue forceps

Notched forceps

Notched forceps (see Figure 12.8) are useful for grasping stepped corneal wound edges. The tips of these forceps indent the tissue and deform it so that some tissue is trapped in the notch behind the tip when the forceps are closed. A high amount of pressure can be generated at the tip, and the lack of teeth reduces the risk of tearing or cutting through thin corneal tissue. These forceps are also well suited to handling conjunctiva.

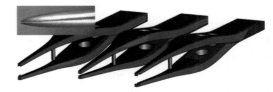

Fig 12.3 From left: serrated (inset), toothed, plain, and notched tips

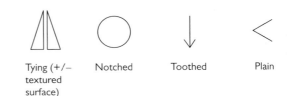

Tying (+/− textured surface)   Notched   Toothed   Plain

Fig 12.4 Symbols denoting type of forceps tip

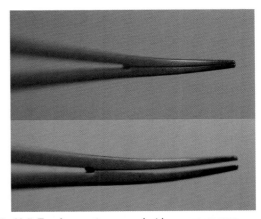

Fig 12.5 Top: forceps tips apposed with correct pressure. Bottom: forceps tips splayed apart with excessive pressure

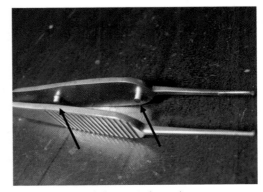

Fig 12.6 Stops beneath finger grip (arrows)

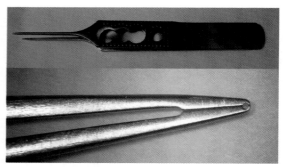

Fig 12.8 Notched forceps

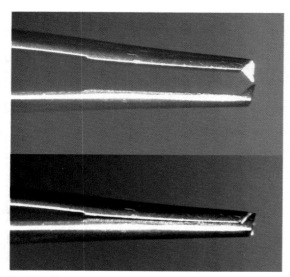

Fig 12.7 Closure of tying blocks on St Martin's forceps

Toothed forceps grasp tissue at a small area at the teeth of the forceps. The size of the teeth must be of suitable size and sharpness for the tissue being grasped. A large amount of pressure can be transmitted through the sharp tips of the teeth, which can cut through the tissue being held. As well as some deformation of the tissue whilst gripping, some penetration of the tissue is desired if toothed forceps are to hold on to relatively rigid tissues like cornea or sclera. Cornea and sclera are well suited to gripping with fine forceps possessing small, sharp teeth. Examples include the toothed Colibri forceps (see Figure 12.9) or straight corneal forceps with 0.12 mm teeth. Overly tight closure of teeth, with subsequent excessive tissue injury, can be prevented by incorporating stops. Conjunctiva is too thin and friable to handle safely with toothed forceps.

When using toothed forceps to pick up suture material, care should be taken to use the tying blocks and not the sharp teeth.

Toothed forceps in oculoplastic surgery

Tissues such as the skin, the orbicularis muscle, and the levator aponeurosis are all relatively firm and slippery tissues which require toothed tips for gripping without slipping. Efforts to hold these tissues using non-toothed forceps may result in crushing of tissue because of the excessive force required to prevent slipping. Forceps commonly used in oculoplastic surgery to grasp skin are St Martin's forceps, Jayles forceps, Lister forceps, and Adson forceps. Only the Adson forceps are made without tying blocks.

St Martin's forceps

St Martin's forceps are short-handled forceps with a wide, flat grip connected to a narrow shaft (see Figures 12.6 and 12.7). The tip is armed with 90°, sharp, angled teeth (one interdigitating with two) that are approximately 0.2–0.3 mm long. St Martin's forceps are effective for grasping skin, as the working distance is much shorter than with other forceps, offering some improvement in mobility. The wide finger grips reduce the amount of finger pressure required to transmit a certain force but conversely make it easier to transmit too much force into the tissue and macerate thin, friable tissue edges.

Jayles forceps

Jayles forceps have angled teeth and serve a similar purpose but have handles that are longer and narrower than those of other forceps and which taper gently to a narrow shaft (see Figure 12.10). The long blades of the Jayles forceps make it possible for assistants to hold or fixate tissues without their hands getting in the way of another surgeon.

Lister forceps

Lister forceps have handles that are similar to those of Jayles forceps but have slightly broader tips that usually have forwards-facing (angled) teeth (see Figure 12.11). These tips allow the forceps to exert some gripping strength on tissues ahead of the tips and allow for some fine movements such as using the teeth on an open forceps to unroll or evert a tissue edge. The teeth also may bite less deeply into the tissue substance, as the sharp points are not directed perpendicularly into the tissue.

Adson forceps

Adson forceps are larger and heavier than the other types of forceps, with flat, wide finger grips (see Figure 12.12). They are much sturdier and more resistant to bending with increased finger pressure and so are better suited to handling skin on the cheek, forehead, or scalp than other forceps are. They are commonly toothed but exist in less common variants with smooth or serrated tips. The teeth are straight and generally larger than those on St Martin's and Jayles forceps, although usually less sharp. Toothed Adsons can be used with great care to pick up vascular tissues that are not readily crushed but are easily cut into by forceps with smaller, sharper teeth. Examples of such tissue include thin, friable skin edges, the orbicularis muscle, and the levator muscle and aponeurosis.

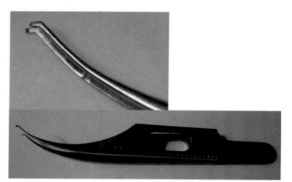

Fig 12.9 Colibri forceps, with tooth design above

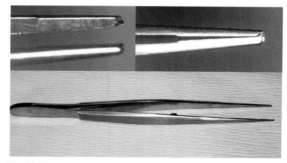

Fig 12.10 Jayles forceps

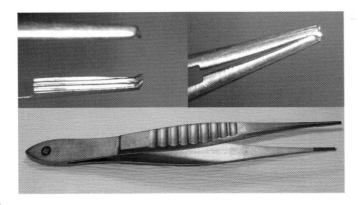

Fig 12.11 Lister forceps

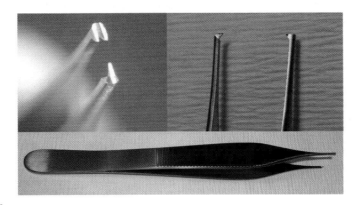

Fig 12.12 Adson forceps

12.3 Sutures

The aims of suturing tissue are to
- Appose edges or surfaces of tissue securely (but not under too much tension) until healing is complete
- Encourage healing by primary intention
- Avoid tissue deformation, even if sutures must bear some tension

The choice of suture gauge and material must suit:
- The size of the structures being united
- How much potential tension the suture will have to bear
- The intended duration of tension bearing
- The intended follow-up regimen (e.g. do you wish to avoid a second procedure to remove sutures?)

Side effects also have to be considered, including:
- The potential suture tract size left by the needle
- The amount of inflammation induced by the suture
- The amount of irritation of neighbouring structures by suture ends
- The risk of contamination of the suture thread
- The cosmetic outcome

Suture material

Absorbable versus non-absorbable; braided versus non-braided

A comparison between absorbable and non-absorbable sutures is presented in Table 12.1. For absorbable sutures, the decay time of tensile strength and time for complete absorption vary for each brand of absorbable suture and are available from the websites of manufacturers.

Sutures are made in two configurations: braided or non-braided (monofilament).

Braided sutures present more surface area for inflammation and microbial contamination but are much easier to handle and tie. There is greater friction between threads and less intrinsic memory and stiffness of the thread in braided sutures than in non-braided sutures.

Non-absorbable sutures in sizes used for ophthalmic surgery are usually **monofilaments**. If inflammation is to be minimized, for example when suturing conjunctiva during glaucoma or pterygium excision surgery or when uniting skin edges on a cosmetically sensitive part of the face or eyelids, monofilament (and non-absorbable) suture material is preferable.

Sutures are usually dyed to aid visibility. If absorbable suture is used on the face, undyed suture should be used to prevent unsightly retained pigment; alternatively, the suture should be buried.

Needle design

Needles are designed with various cross sections of tip. The three most commonly used varieties are described in this section.

Spatulated needles

Spatulated needles are designed to make it possible to first cut into tissue and then continue dissecting along a single lamellar tissue plane by using the two cutting edges on either side of the flat portion of the needle (see Figure 12.13). The flatness of this cross section minimizes the risk of the needle cutting upwards through the tissue or cutting downwards and potentially penetrating more deeply than anticipated. This feature is useful both for suturing corneal tissue, when one wants the needle to stay along a lamella of corneal stroma, and for strabismus surgery, where the depth of the needle pass must be finely controlled to achieve a sufficient bite of sclera without full-thickness penetration. The effectiveness of the spatulated needle relies on the orientation of its insertion. If the flat portion of the needle is exactly parallel to the tissue plane being dissected, it will tend to stay in this plane. However, if the needle is passed so that one of the cutting edges is tilted upwards towards the tissue surface, this cutting edge may cut obliquely through lamellae and out of the tissue.

Reverse cutting needles

Reverse cutting needles have a third cutting edge on the external radius of the needle; this edge greatly reduces the risk of the needle cutting upwards out of tissue (see Figure 12.14). The third cutting edge also confers some resistance of the needle to bending and helps the needle pass unadulterated

Table 12.1 Comparison between absorbable and non-absorbable suture materials	
Absorbable	**Non-absorbable**
No removal necessary but can nonetheless be removed post-operatively to reduce tissue reaction	Removal necessary unless permanent suture action required, in which case it is buried and/or the suture ends rotated into suture tract
'Dissolves' by hydrolysis reaction	Not permanent but may undergo very slow degradation over years
Optimal tensile strength may last less than a fortnight	Long-lasting tensile strength
Induces more inflammation around suture tract than non-absorbable material does, because of hydrolysis	Induces less inflammation around suture tract than absorbable material does
Common materials: Polyglactin 910 (Vicryl), a synthetic polyester: braided (9–0 and 10–0 available as monofilament) Poliglecaprone 25 (Monocryl): monofilament (only as 6–0 to 1) Polydioxanone (PDS II): monofilament (only as 7–0 to 2)	Common materials: Polyamide (nylon, Ethilon): monofilament Polypropylene (Prolene): monofilament Polyester (Mersilene, Dacron, Ethibond): monofilament 10–0 and 11–0, braided 6–0 to 2
Common uses: Most oculoplastic surgical procedures, particularly skin closure Closure of relatively stable, limbally placed phacoemulsification wounds	Common uses: Corneal surgery (penetrating keratoplasty) Repair of ocular trauma, e.g. corneo-scleral lacerations Deep sutures uniting deep eyelid structures Glaucoma surgery, for trabeculectomy flap closure, conjunctival closure, and securing aqueous shunt position Pterygium surgery to suture autografts Securing scleral buckles in retinal detachment surgery

through tough tissues. The path left behind within the tissue is in the shape of a triangular cross section with a broad base and an apex pointing away from the tissue surface. The cross section of this path (i.e. the size of the needle tract) is of a smaller area than that which can be achieved with a forward cutting needle edge, as there is no inadvertent upwards cutting during passage of the reverse cutting suture. When the suture is tied, it will pull up against the broad base of this triangle and thus this configuration confers a lower risk of the suture cheesewiring through the tissue than if it were lying against an apex pointing towards the tissue surface. The strength and properties of this needle make it useful in oculoplastics when suturing skin (see Section 12.7).

Round-bodied (taper) needles

Round-bodied (taper) needles have only a singular sharp taper point at the tip, with no cutting edges (see Figure 12.15). Once it has penetrated into tissue, the body of the needle simply pushes the tissue apart instead of cutting further into it. This feature reduces the risk of both the needle and suture cutting through tissue in an inadvertent direction and minimizes the size of the hole left behind by the needle after its introduction. It is particularly useful for suturing the iris and the conjunctiva, both

of which are soft tissues that can be easily perforated. It is very difficult to pass round-bodied needles through tough tissues such as the cornea or the skin.

Needle shapes

Needles also come in several shapes, which are described by the fraction of the circumference of a circle that the curvature of a needle occupies. The most commonly used is the three-eighths circle needle. Half- and quarter-circle needles also exist. Half-circle needles are useful for suturing at the bottom of tight spaces, where a small radius of bend can be very helpful, for example when suturing the tarsal strip to the lateral orbital rim periosteum in the lateral tarsal strip operation (see Section 12.7). An example of a useful quarter-circle needle is the long CIF-4 (Ethicon) needle, which can be used for suturing iris defects. The length and gentle curve of this needle enable it to reach easily from one corneal paracentesis through the iris to an opposite paracentesis, from where it can be extricated from the eye. Several irregular shapes of needle exist, such as the compound circle needle, in which the needle tip has a tighter radius of curvature than the shaft does.

All features of sutures and needles are printed on their respective packets (see Figure 12.16).

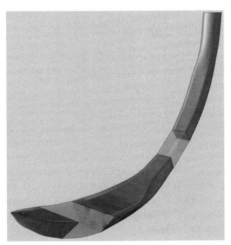

Fig 12.13 Spatulated needle

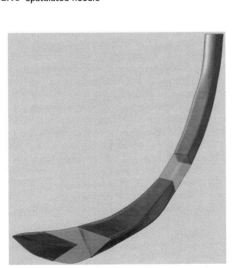

Fig 12.14 Reverse cutting needle

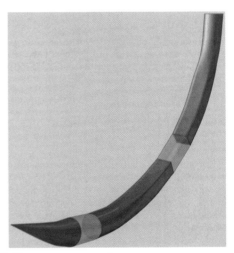

Fig 12.15 Round-bodied needle

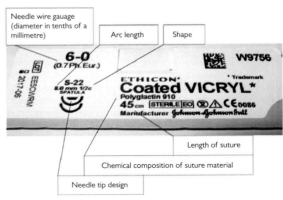

Fig 12.16 Data given on suture packet

12.4 Suturing tissues

Holding the needle in the needle holder

Ideal needle holder use achieves a secure grip on a suture needle to perform a smooth, stable pass through tissue. All types of needle ultimately possess a segment towards the swage (the attachment point between the needle and the suture material) where the needle can be grasped by a needle holder. This area is usually less circular in cross section than elsewhere on the needle, so that the needle can be held without any unwanted pivoting about its own axis during its introduction into tissue.

Holding needles properly

The best place to hold the needle is as follows: with a suitably sized needle holder, the most mechanically effective means of holding the suture needle for passage through tissue is to hold it at the junction between its distal two-thirds and the proximal third (see Figure 12.17). The needle should be mounted in a direction perpendicular to the axis of the jaws (see Figure 12.18).

Troutmans pirouette can be performed to pick up the needle so that it ends up being held in a correct position. The suture is picked up by using the tying blocks proximal to the tips of the tissue forceps, and the needle is dangled so that its convex surface rests gently on a relatively flat surface (e.g. an area of drape, or the cornea). Minor movements of the suture can bring about some spinning of the needle on the flat surface. The needle holders can then grasp the needle when it is spun to a position which closely approximates its intended position when grasped in the jaws of the needle holder.

Choosing the type of needle holder

Bear in mind the following.

The size of the needle

The jaw size should suit the size of needle and should be able to grasp it without any slipping during passage through intended tissues. Oversized needle holders can bend a needle during use or crush a curved needle flat when the jaws are closed tightly. Some needle holders possess hollowed, cylindrical jaws to avoid a flat jaw profile bending a curved needle flat (see Figure 12.19). For the very fine needle that arms a 10–0 suture, a fine-tipped needle holder is required.

The orientation of the surgeon's hands required to effectively pass the needle through the tissue

See the description in 'Needle holders with curved or straight jaws'.

Needle holders with curved or straight jaws

Needle holders used in suturing under the microscope usually have fine tips that can grasp needles mounted onto 10–0 suture thread. The jaws of these needle holders tend to be curved upwards, such as in the Barraquer curved needle holders (see Figures 12.19 and 12.20) The need for curved jaws lies in the fact that any needle should be held at right angles to the tips of the needle holders. As the needle should enter the tissue perpendicular to the surface of the tissue, a needle holder with straight jaws would therefore need to be held parallel to the plane of the tissue being sutured (see Figure 12.21). This technique may not be possible if the eye is deep set or if the patient's nose

prevents positioning of the needle holders in a parallel or tangential position. Incorporating a 30°Curve in the needle holder jaws means that only the tip of the jaws needs to be parallel to the plane of the tissue being sutured (see Figure 12.21).

Straight-tipped needle holders can be used more easily in oculoplastics than needle holders with curved jaws can, as spatial and anatomic limitations are less marked in oculoplastics than in other types of surgery. One example of a straight-tipped needle holder is the Castroviejo needle holder (see Figure 12.22). These forceps are commonly manufactured with a handle lock in the form of a catch located between the handles, under the finger grips. This locking mechanism, together with the large size of these forceps, facilitates their use with large-gauge suture needles. Many surgeons wrongly believe the catch is a toggle mechanism, that is, that it is operated by squeezing once to lock and then squeezing again to unlock. In fact, the handles lock at a certain pressure threshold and must be squeezed tighter than this pressure for the catch to be unlocked.

Suturing tissue

The aims of suturing tissue are to unite edges or surfaces of tissue securely until healing is complete.

Depth of suture

The suture must be passed deep enough within the tissue to:

* Bring together all the layers of the tissue that are intended to be united
* Reduce tissue deformation. A single interrupted suture tends to assume the shape of a circular loop when tightened. A suture within a deep, semicircular needle tract will compress a large, uniform thickness of the wound. When an interrupted suture is tightened within a very shallow needle tract, it will only compress a superficial part of the wound thickness and will be liable to cheesewiring centripetally towards the wound when tightened. Furthermore, the deep parts of the wound will not undergo any compression by the suture and may lose apposition.

Tying the knot

A knot must be tied with enough security to hold under the forces it is expected to be subjected to. Several types of knot can be employed in ophthalmic surgery. The most widely known is the surgeon's knot. This knot is an elaboration on the reef or square knot (see Figure 12.23), which is a two-loop knot formed by throwing one thread over the other, passing one of the free ends through the loop to form an overhand, initial loop (an 'approximating loop'), and then doing this a second time with an opposite overhand knot. In a surgeon's knot, two overhand throws are used in the approximating loop, to generate additional friction between the threads, before the opposing overhand loop is tied on top of it as a securing loop (see Figure 12.24). A second securing loop can be tied on top of the first securing loop. The multiple throws on the approximating loop help reduce the likelihood of the threads slipping against each other. Any properly formed square or surgeon's knot tends to have a very compact, symmetrical appearance (see Figure 12.23).

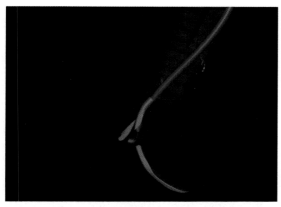

Fig 12.17 Hold the needle at the junction of the proximal third and the distal two-thirds

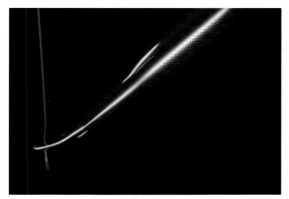

Fig 12.18 Mount the needle at right angles to jaws

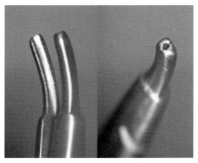

Fig 12.19 Hollowed jaws on a Barraquer needle holder

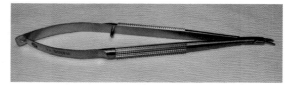

Fig 12.20 A Barraquer needle holder

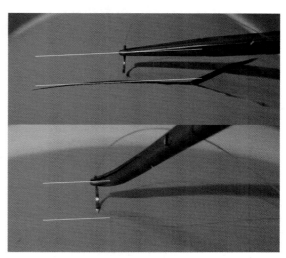

Fig 12.21 Needle holder jaw tips must be parallel to the plane of the wound

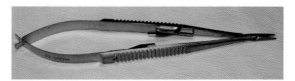

Fig 12.22 A Castroviejo needle holder

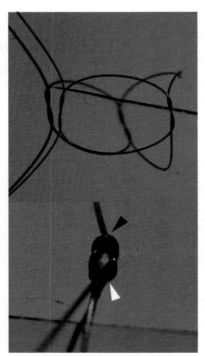

Fig 12.23 Formation of square knot (tightened form below)
Note that the suture ends of a square or surgeon's knot emerge
above the loop at one end of the knot (white arrowhead) and
below the loop at the other end (black arrowhead)

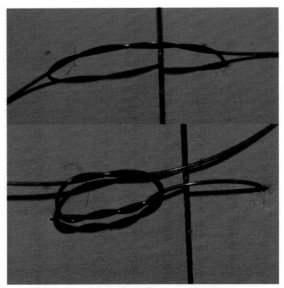

Fig 12.24 Formation of a surgeon's knot (two throws on
approximating loop, untightened)

12.5 Tying a surgeons knot with instruments

Procedure for tying a surgeon's knot with instruments

1. First, after the needle has passed through its intended tract, the suture is pulled through enough that a reasonable 'short end' is left distally.

2. Three throws are typically used in the approximating loop of the knot when suturing with a monofilament suture, and two are used with a braided suture. Imagine you have a needle holder in your dominant hand, and a suture-tying forceps or tissue forceps with tying blocks in your other hand. Grasp the long end, that is, the proximal suture length, at its end using the tying blocks of the tying forceps. Position the needle holders so that the jaws are between the two suture ends (e.g. over the wound; see Figure 12.25).

3. 'Throw' the proximal suture length over the needle holder away from you and then wrap around the closed jaws two or three times as necessary (see Figure 12.26).

4. Then, still enveloped in the suture loops, use the needle holder to pick up the distal suture length near its end and pull taut in the opposite direction (see Figure 12.27). Do not let go of the long end with your non-dominant hand.

5. The securing loops then need to be tied. In a classic surgeon's knot, the needle holder is positioned centrally between suture ends once more and the long end is looped over and around it (see Figure 12.28). The needle holder picks up the short end (see Figure 12.29), and the securing loop is tightened with the hands again going in opposing directions (see Figure 12.30). An optional second securing loop may be tied on top of this one.

Knotting difficulties

We will now offer some tips on how to overcome some common difficulties encountered when tying sutures; these tips are especially applicable to microsurgery. This advice is nonetheless also applicable to suturing other tissues and using large-gauge needles and suture material.

Sutures slipping off the needle holder

Often, when the surgeon tries to pick up the distal suture length with two or three loops of proximal suture around the needle holder to form the approximating loop, the suture slides off the needle holder jaws. Two strategies can be used to help prevent this difficulty.

The first strategy is to keep tension in the long end of the suture at all times whilst wrapping it around the needle holder. The tension can be maintained by wrapping a relatively short length of suture around the needle holder so that the instruments are relatively close together at all times. Winding a long length of suture high up the needle holder may seem intuitively to be the correct technique; however, this approach can compound the problem, as it is difficult to maintain tension in a long length of suture under an operating microscope. The suture will also risk getting trapped in the hinge of the needle holder.

Second, once the loops of the suture have been wrapped around the needle holder, keep the forceps below the needle holder and maintain tension on the proximal suture, with this taut suture pointing away from the knot (see Figure 12.31).

Keep this relative position between forceps and needle holder by moving the two instruments as a pair when you reach with the needle holder to pick up the distal suture length.

Reducing movements during microsurgical knotting

The needle holder (and thus the tying forceps with it) sometimes must move across a large angle or distance to pick up the distal thread, and it is necessary to ensure that the length of proximal suture wrapped around the needle holder does not fall off during this process. Pointing the needle holder towards the distal length of the suture before and during the throwing of the loops of proximal suture length around it will minimize the amount of swivelling movement required once the suture is precariously wrapped around the needle holder.

Suture knots slipping at the knot

Sometimes, after the approximating loop is completed, it slips and loosens before the securing loop can be tied over it. To try to prevent this problem, the approximating loop can be 'locked' by pulling the proximal suture thread upwards (whilst maintaining tension in both threads) once this loop has been tied. Both ends of the suture will end up in a distal position (see Figure 12.32). To complete the securing loops, keep the needle holder between the two ends of the suture during suture throws to construct square knots.

Incorporating a slip knot to fine-tune tension

A slip knot may be constructed by not crossing suture ends when forming the loops of what would have otherwise formed a square knot (see Figure 12.33). This type of knot is inherently insecure but can be used to lower a knot into a confined or inaccessible space. A slip knot can be converted into a square knot by reversing the direction of traction on the suture ends.

Some surgeons find it difficult to fine-tune the tension in a classic surgeon's knot, as the approximating loop may loosen whilst the securing loop is being tied and the locking procedure described in 'Suture knots slipping at the knot' may lead to an overly tight tension. This problem is more likely to occur with smooth, monofilament threads such as 10–0 nylon (polyamide). Using a slip knot for the second knot on top of the approximating loop can help the surgeon regulate the tightness of the suture before locking it.

1. Make a **one- or two**-throw approximating loop (Steps 1–4 in 'Procedure for tying a surgeon's knot with instruments'). Then use the tying forceps to hold the suture's long end, which now lies distally. To form the slip knot loop, position the needle holder underneath the distal strand of suture (see Figure 12.34) instead of centrally between the suture ends. Wrap the suture over and around the needle holder once.

2. The needle holder picks up the free end of the suture.

3. Tighten the suture by pulling the strands in the same orientation as they were facing before to form a slip knot.

If the thread of the suture is smooth enough, the knot can be progressively tightened without locking by progressively increasing tension. Pulling up at the approximating suture loop can loosen the tension. When the correct tension is reached, complete the securing loops as for Step 5 in 'Procedure for tying a surgeon's knot with instruments'.

When braided sutures are used, it is unnecessary to use slip knots for controlling suture tension. The high inter-thread friction in braided sutures should prevent the approximating loop from coming loose and thus prevent a tight slip knot from slipping.

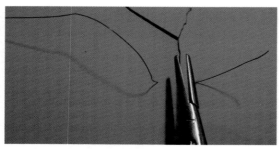

Fig 12.25 Starting position for tying a surgeon's knot with instruments

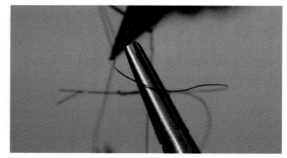

Fig 12.28 Starting the securing loop of a surgeon's knot

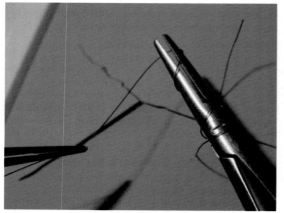

Fig 12.26 Three throws over the needle holder

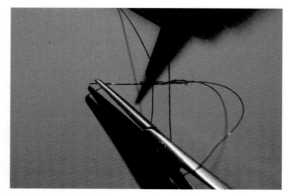

Fig 12.29 Pick up the short strand again

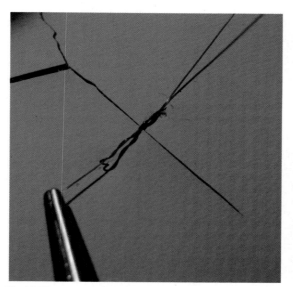

Fig 12.27 Pull taut with instruments heading in directions opposite to where they started

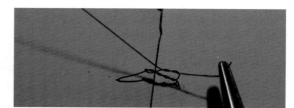

Fig 12.30 Pull taut in opposite directions

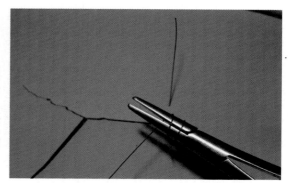

Fig 12.31 Keep the long end taut to prevent suture slipping off needle holder

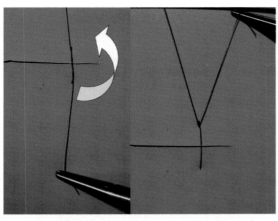

Fig 12.32 Lock the approximating loop by pulling proximal strand distally whilst keeping both ends taut

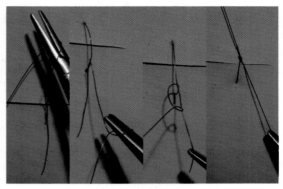

Fig 12.34 Formation of a slip knot

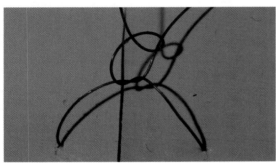

Fig 12.33 Slip knot

12.6 Scenario 1: Suturing a leaking corneal wound

The most likely situation where suturing of a corneal wound would be required is at the end of phacoemulsification surgery when a surgeon is presented with a leaking corneal section. The aims of placing this suture are:

1. To achieve watertight closure of the wound until it heals
2. To avoid distorting the wound and inducing excessive corneal astigmatism

Placing a suture to make the corneal wound watertight in this situation can be very tricky, especially if there is a wound burn or if the wound construction makes it difficult to grasp or appose the wound edges.

Grasping the cornea

It is important not to grasp the cornea at the very edge of the wound, as the tissue there is so thin that the forceps' teeth can cleave right through it or tear pieces off the wound edge. Fine-toothed or notched forceps should be used. The tips of the forceps should grasp the corneal wound edge via as close to a perpendicular approach as possible.

Suture choice

A spatulated 10–0 nylon or 10–0 absorbable (e.g. Vicryl) suture is usually chosen for suturing a corneal wound. Absorbable suture should be reserved for limbal wounds, where the effect of the suture is only needed for a week or two. Wounds significantly anterior to the limbus take longer to heal than limbal wounds do and should be closed with non-absorbable suture. If there is any doubt, non-absorbable suture should be used: it is far easier to remove a suture postoperatively than to put in a new one.

Passing the needle

A fine, curved-tipped Barraquer needle holder should be used. The site of needle entry should be somewhere along an imaginary line extending perpendicularly from the wound edge through the point where the tissue forceps have grasped the cornea (see Figure 12.1).

1. The needle should enter pointing perpendicularly down into the cornea. Once a desired depth within the cornea is reached, the tip of the needle should be directed parallel to the corneal lamellae and kept at this depth and direction across the wound gap so that it enters the proximal (i.e. more limbal) wound edge at the same tissue depth and orientation. This method helps to ensure that one wound edge does not override the other when the suture is tightened. The needle shaft should be manipulated in a plane perpendicular to the corneal surface at all times to keep the flat portion of the spatulated segment parallel to the corneal lamellae. Any oblique tilt of the needle may lead to the needle tip being guided by the tough corneal lamellae into a direction deviating towards one that is parallel to the lamellae or may lead to the needle cutting through lamellae towards the surface.
2. Entering the proximal wound edge accurately can occasionally be difficult, especially in corneal wounds constructed for the phacoemulsification probe. It is usually difficult to grasp the proximal wound edge with forceps. If the wound is a carefully constructed three-step incision, the posterior lip may be amenable to grasping. However, if the wound construction is closer to a one-step incision with an oblique pathway through the surface of the cornea, the proximal wound edge may be quite smooth and almost a flat surface. In this circumstance, the needle can usually be passed across the wound gap straight into the proximal wound to fixate it. Once the needle has penetrated some of the proximal wound in this way, it should be stable in its trajectory.
3. Just as it entered the cornea perpendicularly, the needle should exit it perpendicularly. The tissue forceps can be used to indent the limbus or sclera just ahead of the path of the needle to deform the tissue so that the needle exits in a perpendicular pathway. Care must be taken not to blunt the tip of the needle by attempting to pull out the suture by its very tip. For similar reasons, the tissue forceps must not be used to handle the needle.

Tying the suture

A surgeons knot with two to three throws in the approximating loop should be tied. Corneal suturing is unforgiving, and all the tricks outlined in this section for addressing difficulties during suturing may be employed, for example, incorporating a slip knot in the first securing loop to attain a good tension.

Trimming the ends

Once tied, the redundant ends of the suture should be cut off and the knot of the suture rotated into its suture tract in order to prevent irritation caused by the suture knot rubbing against adjacent surfaces, such as the subtarsal conjunctiva. The ends can be trimmed off using a sharp blade such as a 15° scalpel or a keratome. We recommend laying the blade flat on the knot with the sharp edge pointing away from you. Pull each suture end towards you against the sharp edge to cut, instead of moving the blade (see Figure 12.35). The position of the blade can be adjusted to alter the remaining length of suture end required. Vannas scissors may also be used to trim suture ends. However, one disadvantage of this technique is that your view of the knot will be obscured by the blades of the scissors during cutting, so it can be difficult to judge how much suture length will remain.

Rotating the knot into the tract

To rotate the knot into the suture tract, the suture is held with smooth forceps, such as tying forceps, adjacent to one suture tract and pulled along the plane of the corneal surface towards the opposite suture tract, dragging the knot forwards into this tract. Sometimes the knot seems too bulky to slip into the tract despite a swift and firm tug on the suture. Brute force should be avoided, as it will break the thread. Instead, if the eye is soft, filling the anterior chamber to firm up the eye may increase natural counter-traction when the thread is tugged, so that the knot may be advanced.

12.7 Scenario 2: Suturing skin during a lateral tarsal strip operation

A lateral tarsal strip is an oculoplastic procedure intended to shorten and return an ectropic lower lid to apposition with the globe, by performing a lateral canthotomy and releasing the lower limb of the lateral canthal tendon before fashioning a strip of tarsus and suturing it against the periosteum of the lateral orbital rim. The lateral canthus is reformed at the grey line, and the skin at the lateral canthus is then closed. To minimize scarring, it is important to achieve closure of skin using suture bites close to the wound edge, and tie sutures to produce gentle apposition of the edges without puckering.

Grasping skin

The skin should be grasped near the skin edge, close to where you are choosing to insert the suture needle.

Choice of suture material

Undyed suture should be used if absorbable suture material is chosen, as dye may get deposited in the tract as the suture hydrolyses and lead to a visible blemish or tattoo. Undyed 6–0 Vicryl would be a typical choice for this scenario. Some surgeons prefer to use non-absorbable polypropylene sutures for eyelid skin and then remove them at a suitable time, for example, after one week.

Grasping the needle

Needles used in suturing skin at the lateral canthus and in oculoplastic surgery in general are usually reverse cutting needles. As the natural tendency is for needles to be pulled upwards whilst being passed through tissue, forward cutting needles with the cutting edge pointing up at the skin will tend to create a large suture tract. Whilst skin at the lateral canthus is usually quite thin, it can be surprisingly tough and elastic. Reverse cutting needles are well suited for penetrating this kind of skin without inadvertently enlarging the suture tract. A typical choice of suture material would be 6–0 undyed Vicryl.

Passing and tying the suture

When closing the skin edges at the end of a lateral tarsal strip operation, the suture bites should be passed close to the skin edge. This technique approximates the cut skin edges more effectively, with less puckering and wound inversion when the sutures are tied than when other methods are used. Be careful to avoid unnecessary trauma to the underlying orbicularis fibres, which have a rich vascular supply and will bleed easily if provoked.

A normal surgeons knot can be used when tying the suture. No slip knots are needed, as the suture is usually braided. Often, forceps are not required in the non-dominant hand to aid tying, and the suture can be picked with by the fingers of the non-dominant hand and wrapped around the needle holder to tie the knot. Forceps can be used to tie the knot if the remaining strands of suture are too short to handle with fingers. The knot should not be tied with too much tension, as a knot that is too tight distorts the skin and may cause the tissue encircled by the knot to become devitalized. Similarly, skin edges that are too far apart to be brought together without tension should not

be forced together by sutures; otherwise, they may fail to heal correctly and may pull apart. Consider apposing the orbicularis underneath first, in order to bring the skin edges close together, before attempting to close the skin.

If sutures are to be removed, it helps to not trim the ends too short once the knot has been tied. Leaving suture ends that are long enough to be visible to the naked eye aids suture removal at a post-operative visit. For large-gauge and non-absorbable sutures, use sharp-ended straight scissors to reduce wear and tear to Westcott scissors (which can be used for small-gauge, absorbable sutures).

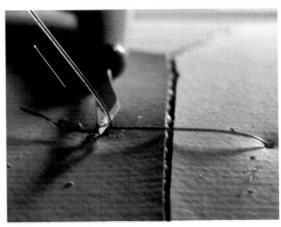

Fig 12.35 Trimming corneal sutures
Stationary blade position for trimming suture ends (note: this photo shows a large-gauge suture on a skin model only for visibility). Traction in the direction shown will cut the suture

12.8 Scenario 3: Repairing full-thickness corneal lacerations

Full-thickness lacerations of the cornea can come in a large variety of different forms. They can be simple and linear, form an angulated flap, or form a stellate wound with multiple apices, depending on the sharpness and velocity of the object or projectile which caused the injury. The aims of repair are to achieve stable closure and minimize the astigmatic side effects of both the sutures and the laceration itself.

Making a start: Preparing the wound

Placing sutures is most difficult when the eye is soft and the anterior chamber is shallowing with fluid egress from a leaking corneal wound. Iris prolapse through the laceration is common. In this circumstance, a paracentesis with a long tunnel should be made in the peripheral cornea, and viscoelastic should be injected into the anterior chamber before the iris is repositted using sweeps of the viscoelastic cannula or an iris repositor. The temptation to prod a prolapsed iris directly through the wound should be resisted, as this approach will be futile and may fray the iris tissue. It may be impossible to clear the wound entirely of prolapsed iris but aim to clear enough of the wound to place a first suture. In simple, small corneal lacerations without iris prolapse or other significant intraocular injury that requires repair, sutures may be placed whilst reforming the anterior chamber with balanced salt solution through the laceration, and a paracentesis is unnecessary.

Choosing the site of the first suture

- In simple, linear corneal lacerations not involving the limbus, suture the most perpendicular wound areas first, leaving the shelved areas until later. Perpendicular, unshelved areas of laceration are the least likely to self-seal, whereas shelved areas might inherently become watertight once sutures are placed to hold the unshelved areas.
- In lacerations with jagged edges where there are apices between linear segments, the straight segments to either side of an apex should be sutured first. The apex may then be found to be well apposed and self-sealing, in which case it should not be sutured. Very commonly, the tissue at the apex is fragile and somewhat frayed, making it difficult to suture. If there is a need to suture an apex to ensure proper closure, place a suture within a lamellar plane to balance tension across all components of the apex without distorting the anatomy away from its natural contour (see 'Grasping tissue and passing the suture').
- If the laceration runs into sclera, a peritomy must be performed to explore the full extent of injury. The first suture (an 8–0 non-absorbable suture) should be placed to realign the limbus.

Grasping tissue and passing the suture

The following instruments and materials should be used:
- Tissue forceps: fine, toothed corneal forceps or Colibri forceps should be used to grasp cornea
- Suture: 10–0 monofilament nylon
- Needle holder: fine-tipped Barraquer needle holder

Try to follow the following principles:
- Distal wound edges should be properly everted to accurately judge the depth of suture passes. The suture should be passed to 90% of the corneal stromal depth: shallow passes may result in posterior wound gape, and full-thickness sutures may allow microorganisms to track into the anterior chamber and increase the risk of endophthalmitis.
- The more perpendicular areas should be easier to appose first; use needle bites equidistant from the wound to align the anterior and posterior surfaces.
- Once this step is done, the shelved areas should lie in a natural position and should be easily closed. The needle bites in shelved areas should be equidistant from the posterior wound edge to minimize the slipping of one wound edge over the other when the suture is tightened.
- Suture bites close to the visual axis should be small but still at 90% depth. The scarring that occurs adjacent to the suture tracks therefore covers a small area.
- To achieve a more natural corneal shape (flattening towards the periphery), sutures that are more central should be tied with as little tension as necessary to achieve apposition. Peripheral sutures should be placed at higher tension to flatten the peripheral cornea.
- To suture an apex of a jagged wound, a suture should be passed deep within the corneal stroma in a near-circular path encircling the apex, with the suture pass starting and ending within a corneal groove as deep as the lamellar plane of the suture. The knot, when tied, will lie buried in the groove, and all tension will be in the plane of the lamella. This step is technically challenging. The wound edges should be everted to allow the needle to be extricated from the wound between each bite of cornea.
- To suture a stellate wound with three or more apices, small 300 μm grooves should be cut with a guarded diamond at right angles to the direction pointed to by each apex. A suture just like the one used to suture the apex of a jagged wound can then be passed within a deep stromal plane encircling all the apices. However, instead of extricating the needle within each wound edge, the needle should be passed straight across each wound edge, exiting and re-entering the cornea within each pre-cut groove.
- It is fairly common to have to replace sutures at the end, as the tension within different areas of the wound will change as it is repaired.

Tying the sutures and finishing off

Slip knots are very useful when tying sutures apposing corneal lacerations, as the tension within them can be easily regulated. Once tied, all sutures which are not buried in pre-cut corneal grooves should have their ends trimmed and knots rotated into the suture tract; ensure that the knots do not cause wound gape. Knots should be left on the side of the wound away from the visual axis. All viscoelastic should be removed from the anterior chamber before it is filled with balanced saline. The cornea should then be dried with a sponge before 2% fluorescein is used to check for any leaks.

12.9 Scenario 4: Repairing scleral lacerations

The following principles should be followed when repairing scleral lacerations:

- Explore: always explore fully any wound in the sclera or involving the limbus. This step will involve performing a localized peritomy for apparently small wounds, and a full 360° peritomy for large wounds, posterior wounds, or cases where a foreign body may have caused both an entry and an exit site. Have a low threshold for disinserting the rectus muscle nearest the wound.
- Expose gently: be careful not to extrude ocular material through the wound by placing undue pressure on the eye. It is worth taking the time to experiment gently to ascertain whether a limbal traction suture (e.g. 6–0 or 7–0 silk) might help and to establish early on whether it is easier to operate without an operating microscope than with one. Repair the immediately visible regions of the scleral laceration before proceeding posteriorly.
- Treat muscles with respect: if muscles must be moved, slinging with a 4–0 silk suture will allow gentle retraction. To disinsert a rectus muscle at its insertion, secure it with a double-armed 6–0 Vicryl suture.
- When suturing sclera, do not rotate posteriorly placed nylon sutures, as there is a risk of suture ends eroding through retina. Anteriorly, scleral sutures are difficult to bury, and consideration should be given to using Vicryl sutures or else starting the suture within the wound so as to create a buried knot.
- Clear the wound of vitreous: a scissors-swab manoeuvre may be carried out, sweeping the wound gently with the tip of a dry Weck-Cel sponge and cutting any vitreous strands stuck to it as close to the wound as possible. Do not pull on the vitreous with the sponge. If visibility is good, an automated cutter can be used.
- Use a cyclodialysis spatula wisely: the flat portion of this spatula can be used by an assistant to reposition prolapsed uvea and hold it away from the wound edge whilst sutures are placed or tightened on top to close the sclera.
- Do not penetrate full thickness through the sclera with the suture needle.
- To prevent placing undue pressure on the eye, grasp the sclera and hold it still whilst passing the suture needle through as close to the grasping site as possible. Take the needle out through the wound before passing it through the other scleral edge.
- Slide the scleral edges over any prolapsed uveal tissue; if there is uveal prolapse, try to reposition the uvea through the wound instead of excising it (excision risks inducing a haemorrhage).

For radial wounds

- Start at the limbus (or nearest to it); place an 8–0 or 9–0 non-absorbable (e.g. nylon) suture to reunite the limbus if the laceration crosses it. Rotate the knot into the suture tract.
- Then suture progressively away from the limbus: start off by using a few interrupted 8–0 Vicryl sutures to close the scleral wound aspect closest to the limbus. Absorbable sutures are used anteriorly, as knots cannot be rotated to hide the suture ends, which in monofilament non-absorbable suture materials are sharp and protrude through conjunctiva. As closure is continued heading progressively posteriorly, 8–0 nylon sutures can be used for more posterior aspects of the wound.
- As you close the sclera in a stepwise manner heading away from the limbus and taking small steps between each interrupted suture, it should be possible to slide the scleral edges shut over the prolapsed uvea in a stepwise manner. Ensure that the needle is taken out through the wound after passing through the first scleral edge, before passing it though the remaining edge so that the uvea is not entered.

For circumferential wounds

- If the laceration is circumferential with respect to the limbus, halve the wound progressively using interrupted sutures (instead of the stepwise closure described in 'For radial wounds').
- A cyclodialysis spatula may be helpful in temporarily depressing intraocular tissues out of the way whilst the sclera is sutured.

Remember to check for watertightness with a drop of 2% fluorescein at the end. Watertightness is the main objective of primary repair.

12.10 Conclusion

This chapter has illustrated, using a few common scenarios, the key surgical skills required both for extraocular surgery and for surgery under the microscope. We have seen the importance of suitable instrument selection to perform specific tasks with maximal efficacy and minimal tissue damage. Furthermore, techniques required to close wounds to achieve an optimal anatomic result have been described. These microsurgical skills and the analytical approach to evaluating the effects of actions of instruments are applicable to a wide spectrum of surgical settings in ophthalmology and should both demystify the contents of operating instrument sets and enable the reader to operate with increased understanding and an increased ability to adapt to different situations by falling back to basic surgical principles.

Chapter 13

Professional skills and behaviour

Lucy Barker, Ameenat Lola Solebo, Melanie Hingorani, and John Bladen

Professional skills

Practical skills

13.1 Good medical practice

Good Medical Practice: Working with Doctors, Working for Patients, published by the General Medical Council (GMC), outlines the standards that all doctors should strive to uphold in their clinical practice. It has been updated in 2013 and is divided into four key domains.[1]

Knowledge, skills, and performance

- Make the care of your patients your first concern.
- Maintain your professional performance.
- Maintain familiarity with relevant guidelines and developments.
- Keep knowledge and skills up to date (through personal development, attending courses or conferences, or keeping up to date with the relevant literature).
- Take part in audit, appraisal, and revalidation.
- Apply knowledge and experience to practice.
- Recognize and work within the limits of your competence.
- Ensure all documentation is clear, contemporaneous, accurate, and legible.
- Medical records must be kept securely and in accordance with any data protection requirements.

Safety and quality

- Contribute to and comply with systems to protect patients.
  - Take part in systems of quality assurance and improvement.
  - Make sure all staff for whom you are responsible are properly supervised.
  - Make sure that you or another named person retains responsibility for the continuity of care for each of your patients.
  - Provide information to enable the health and social care of your patients to be provided safely when their care is transferred.
  - Report suspected adverse drug reactions.
  - Provide information for confidential inquiries and significant event recognition.
  - Protect the interests of patients and volunteers who participate in research.
- Respond to risks to safety.
  - Take prompt action if you think that patient safety is or may be seriously compromised.
  - Protect patients from risk of harm posed by another colleague's conduct, performance, or health. Discuss your concerns with another colleague, your medical defence body, or the GMC.
  - Offer assistance in emergency situations, taking into account your own safety and competence and the availability of other options for care.
  - Consider the needs and welfare of vulnerable adults, children, and young people and offer assistance if you think that their rights have been abused or denied.

- Protect patients and colleagues from any risk posed by your health.
  - If you know or suspect that you have a serious condition that you could pass onto patients or if your judgement or performance could be affected, you must consult a suitably qualified colleague. You must not rely on your own assessment of the risk to patients.
  - You should be immunized against common serious communicable diseases.
  - You should be registered with a GP outside your family.

Communication, partnership, and teamwork

- Communicate effectively (see Section 13.6).
- Be readily accessible to patients and colleagues when on duty.
- Work constructively with colleagues and delegate effectively.
- Establish and maintain partnerships with patients.
  - Treat patients fairly and with respect, whatever their life choices or beliefs.
  - Explain to patients if you have a conscientious objection to a particular procedure. Explain their right to see another doctor and ensure they have enough information to exercise that right.

Maintaining trust

- Show respect for patients.
  - Be open and honest with patients if things go wrong. Put matters right if possible, offer an apology, and explain fully the likely short- and long-term effects.
- Treat patients and colleagues fairly and without discrimination.
  - Give priority to the investigation and treatment of patients based on clinical need.
  - Do not refuse or delay treatment because you believe that a patient's actions or lifestyle has contributed to his/her condition.
  - Respond fully and promptly to complaints and offer an apology when appropriate.
  - Do not allow a patient's complaint to adversely affect the care or treatment you provide or arrange for them.
  - Do not end a relationship with a patient solely because of a complaint they have made.
- Act with honesty and integrity.
  - You must maintain probity (defined as 'complete and confirmed integrity') in your professional practice.
  - You must make sure that your conduct at all times justifies your patients' trust in you and the public's trust in the profession.
  - When communicating publicly, including advertising your services and speaking or writing in the media, you must ensure all information is factual and you must maintain patient confidentiality.

---

[1] Adapted from *Good Medical Practice: Working with Doctors, Working for Patients*, copyright © 2013 General Medical Council

- When writing reports, completing forms or appraisals, or giving evidence in court, you must make sure any information you provide is factual and verifiable.
- You must inform the GMC without delay if you have accepted a caution or been found guilty of a criminal offence anywhere in the world.
- You must maintain honesty and openness in financial dealings.

Your personal health

Often overlooked, doctors have a duty of care to their patients that not only covers their clinical practice but their own health and well-being. You should be aware of the multiple avenues of support for healthcare workers:
  Occupational health services
- Counselling services provided by your trust.
- Your GP

- Multiple online resources:
  - The Doctors Support Network: http://www.dsn.org.uk
  - BMA Counselling and Doctor Advisor Service: http://www.bma.org.uk/doctorsfordoctors
  - Sick Doctors Trust: provides support for doctors or medical students dealing with drug or alcohol dependence; http://www.sick-doctors-trust.co.uk
  - Support4Doctors: provides support regarding dealing with stress, health and financial issues and work/life balance; http://www.support4doctors.org
  - HOPE for Disabled Doctors: help in obtaining professional equality for those with disability or chronic illness; http://www.hope4medics.co.uk

Further reading

1. General Medical Council: *Good Medical Practice*. 2013. http://www.gmc-uk.org/guidance/index.asp

13.2 Information governance

The term 'information governance' refers to the policies and practices in place to ensure the confidentiality and security of patient records and patient-identifiable information. It is a Department of Health requirement that 95% of the workforce of each healthcare trust has completed dedicated information governance training.

Data Protection Act 1998

The Data Protection Act 1998 lays out a framework for processing identifiable information. It covers all forms of media and requires all organizations involved in the processing of personal information to notify the Information Commissioner. The Act consists of eight basic principles:[2]

1. Personal information must be fairly and lawfully processed.
2. Personal information must be processed for limited purposes.
3. Personal information must be adequate, relevant, and not excessive.
4. Personal information must be accurate and up to date.
5. Personal information must not be kept for longer than is necessary.
6. Personal information must be processed in line with the data subjects' rights.
7. Personal information must be secure.
8. Personal information must not be transferred to other countries without adequate protection.

Information Commissioner's Office

The Information Commissioner's Office (http://ico.org.uk/) is the United Kingdom's independent authority responsible for upholding data information rights in the public interest. As defined by the Data Protection Act 1998, the role of the Information Commissioner includes:

* Promoting good practice in handling data and providing advice and guidance on data protection
* Keeping a register of organizations that are required to notify the Information Commissioner's Office about their information-processing activities
* Helping to resolve disputes regarding the processing of personal information
* Taking action to enforce the Data Protection Act 1998 where appropriate
* Bringing prosecutions for offences committed under the Act (except in Scotland, where the Procurator Fiscal fills this role). This function can and has resulted in some NHS trusts being fined up to £500,000 for breaching the terms of the Act.

Caldicott Guardian

The Caldicott Report was commissioned by the Chief Medical Officer of the NHS in 1997 to address concerns regarding the confidentiality of patient information. The report made a number of recommendations that concur with the subsequent Data Protection Act 1998 and established the Caldicott Principles.

Among the recommendations was the appointment of a Caldicott Guardian (senior clinician, advisory role) for each NHS organization. The Caldicott Guardian, together with the Senior Information Risk Owner, is responsible for safeguarding the confidentiality of personal information. The Caldicott 2 Report in 2013 added an additional Caldicott Principle of encouraging information sharing with relevant professionals.

Using or disclosing confidential information

When do I have to ask for consent for use or disclosure?

Use of confidential information in patient care, clinical audit, or quality improvement carries implied consent. Any other use, including teaching, requires explicit consent.

When is disclosure allowed without consent?

Statute law requires or permits the disclosure of confidential information if it is 'in the public interest' or to protect the public.

This law most frequently applies in the case of violent crime or to prevent abuse or serious harm. The advice of the trust Caldicott Guardian should be sought in such circumstances.

Freedom of Information Act 2000

The Freedom of Information Act 2000 enables public access to information held by public authorities. Members of the public are entitled to request specific information, which must be supplied within 20 days, from public authorities such as healthcare trusts. It does not cover an individual's personal information, which can only be accessed using a subject access request under the Data Protection Act 1998.

Electronic health records

First launched in 2002, the NHS National Programme for Information Technology is part of the NHS Connecting for Health programme. The aim was to create a single, centrally mandated electronic care record for each patient and which would be accessible by all NHS and social care professionals and institutions. By 2011, it was clear that the original plan had failed and major elements of it were scrapped in favour of encouraging local systems and procurement. Elements of the programme deemed successful and therefore retained include:

* The picture archiving and communication system
* Electronic prescribing
* Choose and book

Specific to ophthalmology, the Medisoft electronic patient record system is now widely used nationwide, and other similar programmes are in development (e.g. OpenEyes).

An electronic health record creates new confidentiality and information security issues, which are addressed in the NHS Care Record Guarantee 2011. Mechanisms by which confidentiality is maintained include:

* Smartcards with access controls for healthcare workers
* Recording permission to access
* Audit trails
* Patient-elected privacy controls or 'sealing information'
* Consent to create a 'Summary Care Record' for use in an emergency care situation

[2] Adapted from the Data Protection Act 1998. This information is licenced under the terms of the Open Government Licence v3.0 (https://www.nationalarchives.gov.uk/doc/open-government-licence/version/3/).

National ophthalmic audit programme

The Royal College of Ophthalmologists has been awarded a contract by the Healthcare Quality Improvement Partnership to establish a National Ophthalmology Database Audit (RCOphth NOD Audit) as part of the National Clinical Audit and Patient Outcomes Programme. The audit uses a standardized set of data items (data set) to be collected by each healthcare provider involved in the cataract pathway, with feasibility studies ongoing for macular degeneration, glaucoma, and retinal detachment surgery. Electronic patient records (EPRs) facilitate this data collection already in a number of NHS trusts around the country and local or web-based data collection tools will support non-EPR by using trusts and community optometrists to submit data. This data will provide a basis for benchmarking, research, and revalidation and generates reputable sources of risk-adjusted information for healthcare professionals and patients, as well as providing national standards for care.

The data will be available on a named consultant and named unit basis but will not identify individual trainee surgeon names.

Further reading

1. Department of Health: Confidentiality: NHS Code of Practice. 2003. http://www.gov.uk/government/uploads/system/uploads/attachment_data/file/200146/Confidentiality_-_NHS_Code_of_Practice.pdf
2. General Medical Council: Confidentiality. 2015. http://www.gmc-uk.org/guidance/ethical_guidance/confidentiality.asp
3. Information Commissioner's Office: Home. http://www.ico.gov.uk; accessed 23 Sept 2015
4. Health and Social Care Information Centre: Home. http://www.hscic.gov.uk/; accessed 24 Oct 2015
5. Care Quality Commission: Care Quality Commission. http://www.cqc.org.uk/; accessed 24 Oct 2015

13.3 Clinical governance and audit

The Department of Health White Paper *A First Class Service* introduced clinical governance to the NHS in 1997. Its importance in maintaining high-quality health care was highlighted in high-profile investigations of system failure, such as the Bristol Inquiry.

Clinical governance can be defined as:

a framework through which NHS organizations are accountable for continually improving the quality of their services and safeguarding high standards of care by creating an environment in which excellence in clinical care will flourish.[3]

The major elements of clinical governance (sometimes called 'pillars' or more recently 'domains') include:

- Clinical effectiveness, and evidence-based medicine
- Clinical audit and performance monitoring
- Risk management
- Education and training, continuous professional development
- Patient and public involvement
- Staff management
- Information governance

Clinical effectiveness, and evidence-based medicine

The use of evidence-based medicine is essential in maintaining a high standard of care. Keeping up to date with recent clinical guidelines is a requirement of the GMC 'Duties of a Doctor', and guidelines provide a gold standard against which current clinical practice may be audited.

Clinical guidelines are systematically developed recommended care pathways designed to help practitioners and patients make appropriate decisions for specific clinical conditions and circumstances (see Table 13.1). They differ from protocols, which define a rigid sequence of activities to be adhered to in managing a specific condition. The National Institute of Health and Clinical Excellence (NICE) produces clinical guidelines following referral of a topic by the Department of Health. NICE issues guidance in five categories:

- Clinical
- Diagnostic technologies

- Interventional procedures.
- Medical technologies.
- Public health.

National Clinical Guideline Centre

The National Clinical Guideline Centre (http://www.ncgc.ac.uk/) produces and publishes guidelines on behalf of NICE for use in England and Wales.

Scottish Intercollegiate Guidelines Network

The Scottish Intercollegiate Guidelines Network (http://www.sign.ac.uk) develops and publishes clinical guidelines for use in Scotland.

National Guideline Clearinghouse

The National Guideline Clearinghouse (http://www.guideline.gov) is the largest database of appraised guidelines in the world. It is biased towards US guidance but includes guidelines from other countries.

Clinical audit

Clinical audit was included as part of clinical governance in *A First Class Service* (published by the Department of Health in 1997). It was singled out as a mandatory requirement of all doctors in *The NHS Plan* (published by the Department of Health in 2000) and is now included in the *GMC Duties of a Doctor*. It is defined as:

a quality improvement process that seeks to improve patient care and outcomes through systematic review of care against explicit criteria and the implementation of change.[4]

Table 13.2 details the differences between audit and research.

The audit cycle

The audit cycle is a continuous process of review and implementation of change. The steps include:

1. Identify the aspect of care to be investigated and the question to be answered.
2. Select criteria: audit criteria are simply the explicit standards against which care will be measured.
3. Measure performance.
4. Compare performance with standards: the data are compared with the predefined criteria and performance outcomes.
5. Discuss results with all involved staff and agree on an action plan.
6. Make improvements.
7. Demonstrate improvement by re-audit.

Table 13.1 Properties of ideal clinical guidelines	
Valid	They lead to the results expected of them.
Reproducible	If using the same evidence, other guideline groups would come to the same result.
Cost-effective	They reduce the inappropriate use of resources.
Representative/ multidisciplinary	Development and application involves key groups and their interests.
Clinically applicable	Patient populations affected should be unambiguously defined.
Flexible	They should identify and include expectations, exceptions, and patient preferences.
Clear	They use unambiguous language, readily understood by clinicians and patients.
Amenable to clinical audit	They should be capable of translation into explicit audit criteria.
Reviewable	The date of review should be stated.

Table 13.2 Features of research versus clinical audit	
Research	**Clinical Audit**
Defines best practice where uncertain or unknown	Measures if known best practice is happening in clinical care
Advances knowledge	Improves quality of care given
May lead to change	Usually leads to change
Not necessarily repeated	Always repeated

[3] Scally G, Donaldson LJ: Clinical governance and the drive for quality improvement in the new NHS in England. *BMJ* 1998 Jul; **317**(7150): 61–5

[4] NICE: Principles for Best Practice in Clinical Audit. 2002. Oxford, Radcliffe Medical Press

Outcomes

Audits can examine structure (the presence of the correct set-up to deliver best practice), process (whether correct protocols or guidelines are correctly followed), and/or outcomes (results for patients in terms of better health, less complications, etc.). The new Health Act and the NHS operating framework require all NHS trusts to produce core outcome audits to demonstrate good outcomes in key areas.

Risk management

It is the responsibility of all NHS organizations to provide mechanisms for recognizing and preventing potential or actual risks to patients, staff, or the general public. Participation in risk management is a duty of **all** NHS employees, including healthcare workers, managers, and other non-clinical staff.

Definitions

* **Risk:** the likelihood/probability of harm, an adverse event, or a reduction in performance occurring
* **Harm:** injury, damage, or loss that may arise from a hazard
* **Incident:** an event or circumstance that could have resulted or did result in unnecessary damage, loss, or harm
* **Never events:** very serious, largely preventable patient safety incidents defined by the Department of Health on an annual basis and which should not occur if the relevant preventative measures have been put in place (see Table 13.3)
* **Serious incident:** significant adverse event causing, or with the potential to cause, serious harm, and/or likely to attract public or media interest

Table 13.3 Never events *

Wrong site surgery
Wrong implant/prosthesis
Retained foreign object post-operation
Wrongly prepared high-risk injectable medication
Maladministration of potassium-containing solutions
Wrong route of administration of chemotherapy
Wrong route of administration of oral/enteral treatment
Intravenous administration of epidural medication
Maladministration of insulin
Overdose of midazolam during conscious sedation
Opioid overdose of an opioid-naive patient
Inappropriate administration of daily oral methotrexate
Suicide using non-collapsible rails
Escape of a transferred prisoner
Falls from unrestricted windows
Entrapment in bedrails
Transfusion of ABO incompatible organs as a result of error
Misplaced naso-or oro-gastric tubes
Wrong gas administered
Failure to monitor and respond to oxygen saturation
Air embolism
Misidentification of patients
Severe scalding of patients
Maternal death due to post-partum haemorrhage after electing C-section

*Those most relevant to ophthalmology are in bold.

Adapted from 'The "never events" list 2012/13', Patient Safety Policy Team, Department of Health, 2011 © Crown copyright

Risk assessment

Once identified, both incidents and potential risks are classified by type (e.g. patient safety, corporate, adverse publicity, breach of confidentiality) and are then graded both by level of consequence (**what harm did it or could it have resulted in?**) and by likelihood (**how likely is it that the same event could occur again?**). Each of these is allocated a score out of 5 (0 = no harm/will never recur, 5 = catastrophic harm/almost certain to happen again) and the risk rating is calculated as:

$$Risk\ rating = Consequence \times Likelihood$$

This equation gives a score between 1 and 25; the consequent action is:

* Score = 1–6: managed within the department
* Score = 8–10: managed internally; root cause analysis to be completed within 6 weeks
* Score = 12–25, or incident is a never event: classifies as a serious incident, to be registered on the Department of Health Strategic Executive Information System, and commissioners notified. Root cause analysis to be completed by 45–60 days. External investigation (if required) to be completed within 6 months.

Duty of Candour

A statutory Duty of Candour was introduced in 2014 as a response to the Francis Report. After any patient safety event causing significant harm (includes both serious harm and moderate harm such as an unplanned return to surgery or a prolonged episode of care) a Being Open conversation, complete with explanation and apology, must occur as soon as possible (even if no fault of care identified or the risk of the complication was included in the consenting process) and must be followed by a written letter and an offer of support.

National Patient Safety Agency and NHS England safety work

The aim of the National Patient Safety Agency was to identify and analyse problems relating to patient safety and to implement appropriate solutions at a national level. It ran the National Reporting and Learning System and also mounted campaigns to improve safety, such as the *Clean Your Hands* campaign. Under the new Health Act, its powers have transferred to NHS England.

National Reporting and Learning System

The National Reporting and Learning System collects confidential reports of patient safety incidents across England and Wales to identify common risks, national trends, and opportunities to improve patient safety. It produces guidance for risk management, including the **Seven Steps to Patient Safety** (published in 2004):

1. Build a safety culture.
2. Lead and support your staff.
3. Integrate your risk management activity.
4. Promote reporting.
5. Involve and communicate with patients and the public.
6. Learn and share safety lessons.
7. Implement solutions to prevent harm.

Central alerting system

Established in 2008, the central alerting system is a web-based cascading system for issuing safety alerts (e.g. on identified problems with medical devices and drugs) to the NHS and independent providers of health and social care.

National Confidential Enquiry into Patient Outcome and Death

Following a pilot study investigating perioperative deaths in 1982, the National Confidential Enquiry into Patient Outcome and Death was established in 1988 and has been expanded to include both deaths and near misses in all specialities. It undertakes confidential enquiries and surveys and publishes the results and resultant guidance, thus enabling quality control and highlighting any areas of concern.

Education and training

In order to maintain high-quality healthcare, all healthcare professionals must have access to appropriate training and be encouraged to participate in continuing education and professional development (see Section 13.5).

Staff management

Other than appropriate and adequate education and training, staff involvement includes up-to-date registration and appraisal. The introduction of revalidation in December 2012 is aimed at ensuring that poor performance or inadequate/dangerous practices are identified (Section 13.5). Furthermore, healthcare workers are now encouraged to speak out by a process of confidential whistle-blowing if they perceive that their colleagues are performing poorly or that patients' safety is jeopardized.

National Clinical Assessment Service

The National Clinical Assessment Service acts as an independent advisory body to clarify concerns and provide recommendations and support in cases where there is suspicion or established concern regarding an individual's working practice.

Patient and public involvement

The Health and Social Care Act enshrines in law the concept of a patient-centred NHS. Feedback and input from patients and the general public (from analysis of complaints to patient suggestions, focus groups, and the involvement of the lay public in new developments in healthcare) is becoming increasingly important in shaping the health service. Patient feedback now forms part of the 360° appraisal necessary for revalidation. The concept of openness when dealing with complaints or perceived errors is also encouraged, to enable patients and relatives access to the full story and prevent the feeling that mistakes are being covered up. The Patient Advice and Liaison Service is an integral part of this interface, and patients should be encouraged to contact the Patient Advice and Liaison Service office if they have any feedback, positive or negative, that they feel would be of use in service improvement.

Further reading

1. Clinical Audit Support Centre Limited: Welcome to the Clinical Audit Support Centre. 2015. http://www.clinicalauditsupport.com
2. Department of Health: A First Class Service: Quality in the New NHS. London: Department of Health, 1997
3. Department of Health: Safety First. A Report for Patients, Clinicians and Healthcare Managers. London: Department of Health, 2006
4. Department of Health: Trust, Assurance and Safety: The Regulation of Health Professionals in the 21st Century. London; Department of Health, 2007
5. General Medical Council: Joint Statement from the Chief Executives of statutory regulators of healthcare professionals. http://www.gmc-uk.org/Joint_statement_on_the_professional_duty_of_candour_FINAL.pdf_58140142.pdf; accessed 24 Oct 2015
6. GOV.UK: Medicines and Healthcare Products Regulatory Agency. http://www.mhra.gov.uk; accessed 23 Sept 2015
7. National Patient Safety Agency: NPSA: National Patient Safety Agency. 2012. http://www.npsa.nhs.uk
8. NHS England: Patient safety. http://www.england.nhs.uk/patient-safety/; accessed 24 Oct 2015
9. NICE: Principles for Best Practice in Clinical Audit. London: NICE, 2002

Clinical leadership

There has been recognition that clinical leaders are crucial to the NHS's ability to successfully navigate the increasing challenges it faces. A leader is best defined as someone who has followers. In order to develop and deliver clinical services, the following leadership skills are needed:

- Demonstrating personal qualities (e.g. leading by example, honesty, work ethic)
- Working with others
- Managing services (such as resources or people)
- Improving services (e.g. critical evaluation and change)
- Setting direction (e.g. applying knowledge and evidence)
- Creating the vision (through developing, influencing, communicating, and embodying the vision for the organization)
- Delivering the strategy

These skills form the foundation of the Medical Leadership Competency Framework, a tool to aid the development of clinical leadership skills. As a doctor in training, you should take every opportunity to learn and apply clinical management and leadership skills to improve patient care, and map your skills and achievements to the framework.

NHS structure

In 2012, the Health and Social Care Act (HSCA) was passed, heralding a radical reform of the NHS (see Table 13.4).

- Key reported aims of the Health and Social Care Bill 2011/12:
  - To create an independent NHS board, to promote patient choice, and to reduce NHS administration costs

- Key reported principles:
  - Putting patient choice and patient reported outcomes at the centre of the NHS, empowering GPs, and changing the emphasis of measurement of 'excellent healthcare' to clinical outcome

Some care, such as screening programmes and highly specialized care, will be commissioned centrally from NHS England; other care will be commissioned locally by clinical commissioning groups. As well as the Department of Health, there will be four key national bodies within the new, post-HSCA NHS (see Table 13.5).

Other external health/care agencies:

- **National Patient Safety Agency:**
  - Role: identify problems relating to patient safety and to implement appropriate solutions. Has now been abolished and role transferred to NHS England.
- **Medicines and Healthcare Products Regulatory Agency:**
  - Role: ensuring that medicines/devices are safe and effective
- **Healthcare Quality Improvement Partnership:**
  - Role: to support and promote audit
- **NHS Litigation Authority:**
  - A not-for-profit organization within which will sit the **National Clinical Assessment Service**, which aims to support resolution concerns on professional practice

Other important programmes include:

- **The Private Finance Initiative:** scheme where private companies are involved in the development of major healthcare projects; can overcome difficulties in raising capital to fund major projects, but the long-term repayments can be crippling, leading to financial failure for some NHS trusts

Table 13.4 Old versus new: Changes to the NHS structure

Pre-HSCA implementation	Post-HSCA implementation
Secretary of State and Department of Health: overall responsibility for the health of the nation, providing strategic direction and funding	The secretary and the Department of Health oversees a national board, which will provide strategic direction and funding
One hundred and fifty-one primary care trusts commission the delivery of secondary care and are supported by ten strategic health authorities, which monitor and improve performance	Two hundred and forty clinical commissioning groups, which are led by healthcare professionals (primarily GPs), will be overseers of NHS funds, commissioning care for patients from both NHS and private providers
NHS hospitals, GPs, mental health units, dentists, and community services deliver care, funded by primary care trusts	NHS hospitals, mental health units, and community services deliver care, all of which are funded by clinical commissioning groups. All NHS trusts to be foundation trusts with greater managerial and financial freedom than before, and to be accountable to local people, who can become trust members or governors. GPs, dentists, and certain specialist services to be funded by a central National Board

HSCA, Health and Social Care Act.
Health and Social Care Act 2012

Table 13.5 National bodies in the new NHS

Name	Role
National Institute for Health and Care Excellence	Replaces the National Institute for Health and Clinical Excellence (established in 1999 to reduce variation in NHS care and social care through guidelines, technology appraisals, and cost-effectiveness judgements). New role: advisory body to the Clinical Commissioning Groups
Care Quality Commission	Independent regulator of all health and adult social care (in England), replacing the Healthcare Commission, the Social Care Inspection Commission, and the Mental Health Act Commission. Carries out regular, unannounced inspections
NHS Commissioning Board	Overseer of new clinical (disease-specific or geographic area-specific) networks, and clinical 'senates', which will work across the networks
Monitor	Economic regulator overseeing access and competition within the new NHS

- **Commissioning for Quality and Innovation:** local agreements for a percentage of income from commissioners to be dependent on fulfilling agreed quality performance standards
- **Cost Improvement Programme:** projects aiming to increase efficiency and reduce spending for trusts
- **Quality, Innovation, Productivity and Prevention:** efficiency improvement programme lead by the Department of Health

NHS economics

The overall cost of running the NHS has increased significantly over recent years, thanks to new therapies and technology, rising public expectations, and an ageing population. The NHS budget for 2015/2016 is approximately £115 billion. Over three-quarters of NHS funding comes from general taxation, approximately 10% from National Insurance contributions, and the remainder from patient charges. In 2011, the Chief Executive of the NHS called for £20 billion of efficiency savings, known as the 'Nicholson challenge'. More recently, the government has promised £8 billion more investment but will require a £22 billion efficiency savings by 2020. Recent major reviews such as the 'Dalton Review' and the 'Five Year Forward Plan' examine how the NHS needs to change in terms of prevention, efficiencies, and new integrated care networks which break down traditional boundaries of provision (e.g. health vs social care, hospital vs community care, mental vs physical care) and are supported by vanguard programmes ('New Models of Care') which are resourcing large pilots of such new integrated care pathways.

Payment by results

Payment by results has been introduced to improve efficiency within the NHS. Healthcare providers are paid a standard fixed rate (national tariff) for a particular procedure (e.g. cataract surgery) and will therefore increase profits if they are able to carry out procedures at a reduced cost. In some areas (e.g. cataract surgery), there is a move towards a 'best practice tariff', whereby the tariff covers the whole pathway, from pre-op clinics through surgery to post-op clinics.

Public Service Agreements/NHS Operating Framework

There are a number of key performance targets in the Public Service Agreements/NHS Operating Framework, for example:

- **An 18-week patient pathway:** to deliver a maximum wait of 18 weeks from GP referral to hospital treatment
- **Choose and book:** patients are given a choice of at least four healthcare providers, and an appointment at a time and date that suits them.

These targets are expected to continue within the reformed NHS but in a less centralized manner.

NHS management for trainees

Trainee ophthalmologists should aim to understand the principles of service management and should be familiar with the key local and national systems which govern the delivery of patient care. Formal NHS management courses are available, and your educational supervisor can advise you on opportunities for exposure to management experience in your unit, whether that be:

- Building a business case
- Carrying out risk assessments
- Managing services
- Service improvement work
- Shadowing a management team within the hospital

Further reading

1. BMA: The New NHS Structure. http://bma.org.uk/working-for-change/doctors-in-the-nhs/nhs-structure-new; accessed 24 Oct 2015
2. Department of Health: Liberating the NHS White Paper. 2010. http://www.dh.gov.uk/en/Publicationsandstatistics/Publications/PublicationsPolicyAndGuidance/DH_117353
3. GOV.UK: Dalton Review: Options for Providers of NHS Care. 2015. https://www.gov.uk/government/publications/dalton-review-options-for-providers-of-nhs-care
4. GOV.UK: Department of Health. https://www.gov.uk/government/organisations/department-of-health; accessed 24 Oct 2015
5. NHS England: The NHS Five Year Forward View. http://www.england.nhs.uk/ourwork/futurenhs/; accessed 24 Oct 2015

The system for medical postgraduate training has undergone enormous change following the introduction of Modernising Medical Careers, the Tooke report, and the European Working Time Directive. Following the merger of the Postgraduate Medical Education and Training Board with the GMC in 2010, the GMC is now responsible for regulating all stages of medical education in the United Kingdom. This role includes approving the Ophthalmic Specialist Training Curriculum, ensuring that the quality of the training programmes is maintained within each school of ophthalmology, and specialist registration through the Certificate of Completion of Training, a mandatory requirement to practice as a substantive or honorary NHS consultant (see Figure 13.1).

Training

Ophthalmic Specialist Training Curriculum

The Ophthalmic Specialist Training Curriculum, accessible via a web-based training system, details the knowledge and skills required of each trainee at each stage of training. Achievement is determined by specific assessments, which are monitored at the Annual Review of Competence Progression. An e-portfolio allows trainees to document and track training achievements and learning. All portfolios should contain:

- A logbook of experiences/procedures/clinics (an online e-logbook for procedures is available)
- Personal audit, personal development plans, and a continued personal development diary
- Any critical incidents
- 360° Feedback, patient feedback/complaints
- Trainer reports and outcomes of specific assessments
- Other evidence related to the key curriculum topics, e.g. publications and presentations

Schools of ophthalmology

Within each NHS deanery sits a school of ophthalmology. Each consists of the head of the school, a training programme director (responsible for managing the speciality training programme), educational supervisors, clinical supervisors, college tutors, and the school's trainees. The main aims of the schools are to deliver training and to assess and support trainees.

Continued professional development

One of the defining aspects of a profession is the acquisition and maintenance of a body of knowledge. Continuing professional development formalizes this concept and sets the standards for doctors to continue their learning and adapt to change following their formal period of postgraduate education. Continuing professional development should correlate with the areas delineated in *Good Medical Practice* and contributes to the process of revalidation.

Reflective practice is 'the capacity to reflect on action so as to engage in a process of continuous learning'. It is an integral part of your personal development: you are responsible for your personal learning, which includes identifying and addressing your continuing professional development needs.

Assessment and appraisal

Assessment is a process of evaluation ensuring that sufficient knowledge, skills, and experience have been acquired to allow progression to the next phase of training. The standardized methods of assessment used in specialty training are direct observation of procedural skills (DOPS), case-based discussions (CbD), clinical evaluation exercises (mini-CEX), and multisource feedback (MSF). These assessments should be completed in a timely manner over the training year and documented in the e-portfolio.

Appraisal aims to provide feedback on doctors' performance, record their continuing professional development, and identify future educational and developmental goals. As appraisal focuses on a trainee's developmental needs, it differs from assessment, which measures progress based on set criteria (e.g. exams). Formal individualized appraisal is a confidential process, and trainees are encouraged to discuss their developmental concerns and future plans.

An effective appraisal meeting generally incorporates the following:

1. Setting the agenda
2. Review of past performance
3. Identify current learning needs
4. Set future learning objectives and expected time to achievement
5. Agree a date for the next appraisal

Training other trainees

As an ophthalmic trainee, you are part of your school of ophthalmology, and as such you have a role as a teacher of other trainees (see Box 13.1).

Managing a trainee in difficulty

As a trainee, you will not be expected to manage a trainee in difficulty in isolation, but you may be involved in the management process and you may be the first to identify that the trainee is struggling. Consider the difficulties you faced at any stage during your training, and which interventions proved effective. Good practice includes honest but diplomatic discussion with the individual, and involvement of their senior colleague (e.g. training director or clinical lead).

Revalidation

Revalidation is a process to 'quality assure' the medical profession. Revalidation occurs every 5 years and is now mandatory for all fully trained doctors. It examines their fitness to practice with reference to the GMC's *Good Medical Practice* and allows doctors to retain their licence to practice. A robust annual appraisal including evidence of continuing professional development is the basis for revalidation. Ophthalmic specialist trainees are the responsibility of their NHS deanery or school of ophthalmology. Each trust has a responsible officer (often the medical director) to lead the process; this officer carries the

---

Box 13.1 Becoming an effective educator: Tips

Observe and discuss teaching methods with senior colleagues who have taught you well.

Understand that different trainees learn in different ways.

Experience the strengths and drawbacks of the different teaching situations: group teaching, one-on-one teaching, didactic sessions, and practical sessions.

Seek feedback from those you teach.

Know your limits.

Attend a 'training the trainers' course.

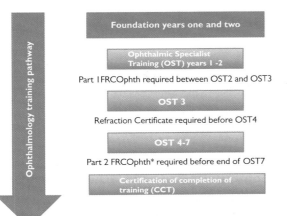

Foundation years one and two

Ophthalmic Specialist
Training (OST) years 1-2

Part 1FRCOphth required between OST2 and OST3

OST 3

Refraction Certificate required before OST4

OST 4-7

Part 2 FRCOphth* required before end of OST7

Certification of completion of
training (CCT)

Fig 13.1 Pathway of ophthalmic specialist training

responsibility for signing off all non-trainee doctors in their trust as suitable for GMC revalidation.

Non-trainee ophthalmologists are required to submit data on quality and safety for all major areas of practice over the preceding 5 years. This data should include audits of outcomes following cataract surgery, corneal graft and refractive surgery, surgery for retinal detachment, glaucoma, and strabismus, and age-related macular degeneration treatment procedures.

Further reading

1. The Royal College of Ophthalmologists: Curriculum for Ophthalmic Specialist Training. 2015. http://curriculum.rcophth.ac.uk
2. The Royal College of Ophthalmologists: RCOphth Portfolio System. https://portfolio.rcophth.ac.uk, accessed 24 Sept 2015

The move of the doctor–patient relationship from a paternalistic to a partnership footing means effective communication must be at the heart of good medical practice. The evolution of multi-disciplinary care, networks of primary and secondary care, integrated pathways, and the shift-work pattern necessitated by the European Working Time Directive has also focused attention on communication among healthcare practitioners. In order to communicate effectively, doctors must listen, respond, and inform.

Communicating with patients

Communication that is 'careless', 'insincere', or 'unclear', as perceived by patients, lies at the root of the majority of the complaints brought against the NHS. The GMC's *Good Medical Practice* guidance on patient communication and the doctor–patient partnership tallies closely with patients' expectations of a 'good' doctor as identified through commissioned polling of patients (see Boxes 13.2 and 13.3).

Individual language or communication needs should not be permitted to become obstacles to effective communication. It is the clinician's responsibility to ensure that, where practical, the necessary arrangements are made to make effective communication possible, whether that be providing translators, identifying a potential cultural barrier, or changing your language for children and young people. Ophthalmologists must also balance the need to keep relatives, carers, and partners informed and supported, whilst respecting the patient's right to confidentiality.

* Be aware of non-verbal communication: is your body language open and non-threatening?
* Be aware of alternate methods of communication, particularly when making a new diagnosis or suggesting a new

intervention: are patient information leaflets or patient support groups available? The Care Quality Commission recommends that **all** patients are directly offered patient information leaflets on their conditions.
* Be aware of your own preconceptions regarding patients' level of knowledge: e.g. not everyone knows how to instil eye drops.

Communicating with other healthcare professionals

Clinicians must also ensure that they communicate effectively with other healthcare professionals. In general, when discussing patients' care with other caregivers, it is important to follow the principals of safety critical communication:

* Address the appropriate person, at the appropriate time, using appropriate language and the appropriate medium.
* Highlight the key message, and use two types of communication media if necessary (e.g. written and verbal).
* Summarize the message to ensure comprehension.

To understand the importance of primary care and multidisciplinary care:

* Maintain communication with other professionals involved in the patient's care, particularly the patient's GP.
* Accept, process, and make clinical referrals in a timely and appropriate manner and respond to referrers with feedback or copies of letters.

When working in a team:

* Handover patients effectively.
* Inform the team of expected and unexpected leave/absence of yourself and others.
* Seek help and advice where necessary.

Documentation and record-keeping

Accurate documentation and record-keeping is important clinically, but is also a medico-legal requirement. If it isn't documented . . . it didn't happen.

* Write and sign clearly, legibly, and with a black ink pen (which allows good-quality photocopying).
* Date and time every entry, and write during or as soon as possible after the event.
* Patient records should be factual and accurate; avoid personal slurs or value judgements.

When dealing with critical documentation, such as listing forms for future surgery, or visual impairment registration forms, ensure that the paperwork is prioritized and directed towards the appropriate team.

When providing written reports, or other documentation, ensure that you are not giving false or misleading evidence:

* Within reason, verify all information.
* Do not deliberately leave out relevant information.

Dealing with complaints

A formal complaint can be oral or in writing and is an expression of dissatisfaction from a patient or third party, requiring a formal response.

Box 13.2 **What patients want from a doctor**
Patients want doctors who:
Focus their attention on you, make you feel at ease and well cared for
Introduce themselves and their colleagues
Explain things, including the reason for the consultation, and what will happen next, without using jargon
Ask what you were expecting, let you talk, seek your feedback, and understand your concerns
Treat you as an individual and involve you in decisions

Adapted from Good Medical Practice: Working with Doctors, Working for Patients, copyright © 2013 General Medical Council

Box 13.3 **General Medical Council guidance on a doctor's role in the doctor–patient partnership**
Be polite, considerate, and honest.
Treat patients with dignity and respect their individuality, privacy, and right to confidentiality.
Encourage patients to have knowledge about their condition and to use this knowledge when making decision about their care.
Support patients in caring for themselves.
Give your registered name and General Medical Council number when asked.

Adapted from Good Medical Practice: Working with Doctors, Working for Patients, copyright © 2013 General Medical Council

Managing mistakes

You must be open and honest if things go wrong; prompt and appropriate management of a medical error can prevent patient dissatisfaction and avert a complaint.

* Explain fully what has happened.
* Offer an apology.
* Put matters right if possible, and explain possible short- and long-term effects.
* Involve a senior colleague ASAP.
* Act for future patients: record, analyse, and formulate an action plan to learn from the mistake.

Managing patient dissatisfaction

Again, not all episodes of patient dissatisfaction result in a formal complaint. Most trusts offer conflict resolution courses in order to prepare you for these often challenging situations. Techniques to help prevent escalation to a formal complaint are:

* Keep calm and avoid making comments that escalate the situation.
* Acknowledge any feelings of frustration and anger with empathic statements.
* Repeat a summary of what comments have been made to show that you are listening.
* Apologize for anything that has not gone to plan: saying 'sorry' is not an admission of liability.
* Involve the Patient Advocacy and Liaison Service, which can help to resolve problems as quickly as possible.

Formal complaints procedure

Once a complaint has been made, a formal complaints procedure involves the following.

Stage 1: Local resolution

The trust will acknowledge a complaint within three working days of receipt. An investigation into the circumstances giving rise to the complaint is carried out. A reply will be sent to the complainant within 25 days.

Stage 2: Independent review by the Care Quality Commission

Complainants may ask the Care Quality Commission to review a complaint that has not been satisfactorily resolved.

Stage 3: Parliamentary and Health Service Ombudsman

Complainants who remain unhappy with the Healthcare Commission's review have the right to approach the ombudsman.

Breaking bad news

See Box 13.4.

Consent

Valid consent should always be obtained before treatment or examination of a patient by a clinician who is suitably trained and qualified and who has sufficient knowledge of the proposed procedure. It is good practice for this person to be the clinician undertaking the procedure. Patients can give consent orally or in writing, but written consent is mandatory for interventional procedures.

Valid consent

Ask the following questions when deciding whether consent is valid.

Does the patient have capacity?

You should presume that ALL adults have capacity unless demonstrated otherwise. For a patient to have sufficient capacity, they must be able to comprehend and retain information

---

Box 13.4 Breaking bad news

Breaking bad news is difficult for everyone concerned. Loss of vision is a deep-rooted human fear, second only to death or developing cancer. Mismanagement of communication of poor visual prognosis or other medical event makes a bad situation worse. Some factors to consider when breaking bad news are:

Prepare yourself: familiarize yourself with the patient's history, test results, and possible management choices. Involve nursing staff or Eye Clinic Liaison Officers if available, and if possible, consider asking the patient whether they would like a family member with them.

Prepare the environment: a quiet, private area with no interruptions. Choose an area that is free for the patient to stay in for longer if needed.

Prepare the patient: establish the patient's current understanding of the situation and their desire for further information.

Share the bad news and start to inform the patient of the consequences from their starting point.

Take time, speak clearly, and avoid jargon; repetition of key facts may be necessary, and written information is of benefit.

Recognize the patient's feelings and respond to any questions or concerns.

Plan the future care and follow-up, and share information with the multi-disciplinary team, including the patient's GP.

Document the conversation in detail.

Provide a contact number in case of questions later.

---

relevant to making the decision, and to communicate their wishes. All appropriate support must be provided to maximize their ability to do so.

If capacity is in doubt, you should seek advice from the patient's primary health carer, or a specialist (e.g. psychiatrist/speech and language therapist).

Is the consent given voluntarily?

The decision to consent has to be made voluntarily and freely by the patient. Relatives, friends, and healthcare professionals must not unduly influence or coerce the patient into making a decision.

Is the patient sufficiently informed?

Patients need to be informed of the nature and purpose of the procedure or examination. Side effects, complications, and other risks should be communicated clearly and without bias. Other options, even if less satisfactory, should be mentioned, including the option of doing nothing. Surgeons are advised to include any 'significant risk which would affect the judgement of a reasonable patient', even if the likelihood is very small, the so-called material risks. Failure to do so is negligent. For frequently undertaken procedures such as phacoemulsification cataract surgery, guidance on patient information is available from the Royal College.

Does the decision need to be reviewed?

Ideally, consent should be obtained before the day of operation or, at the very least, the patient should have begun consenting discussions and be familiar with the consent form. On the day, the healthcare team must ensure that there has been no change to the patient's state since formal consent was obtained.

Consent in different patient groups

Competent adults (over 18 years old)

* Competent adults may refuse treatment. The only exception is when the patient is detained under the Mental Health Act 1983 (see Box 13.5).

Box 13.5 The Mental Health Act 1983

There are some circumstances in which patients held under the Mental Health Act can have their mental disorder treated without their consent. It does not apply to any physical disorders they may have, for which the usual rules of consent apply.

Incompetent adults

- Incompetent patients, that is, those without mental capacity to make a valid consent decision, must be treated in their best interests, which does not necessarily equate to their best medical interests. Nobody can give or withhold consent on the behalf of such patients unless evidence of a lasting power of attorney can be shown. The medical team sign the consent form.
- Patients with fluctuating competence should have their views assessed when competent. Non-urgent treatments should be delayed until capacity is regained.
- Advanced care directives and living wills are legally binding and should be followed.
- Mental capacity assessments should be undertaken and recorded and a best interest meeting held with all key stakeholders, including relatives, mental capacity advocates, and other professionals, to make decisions on interventions with serious risk.

Children and young people (under 18 years old)

- For children under 16 years old, usually a parent or guardian signs the consent form but the child should be involved in the decision where possible.
- Children over 16 years can give consent but any decision to refuse treatment can be overruled. Under Scottish law, young people aged 16 or over have the same right to consent or refuse as adults.
- Children under 16 years can give consent if judged to have capacity (Gillick competence).
- Refusal of treatment by the parents of a child but which is deemed in the child's best interest may need a second opinion and referral to the courts.

Further reading

1. General Medical Council: Consent: Patients and Doctors Making Decisions Together. 2015. http://www.gmc-uk.org/guidance/ethical_guidance/consent_guidance_index.asp
2. General Medical Council: Good Medical Practice (2013). 2015. http://www.gmc-uk.org/guidance/good_medical_practice.asp

13.7 Research

Medical research makes significant contributions to improvement in human health. All doctors have a duty of care not only to their current patients but also to all their future patients. In other words, research is not only good for your CV, your career, and your personal development, but is also a necessary part of your role as an ophthalmologist.

The new academic career structure formalizes the integration of academic and clinical training, but 'normal' clinical trainees are also expected to be familiar with the principles of good-quality research. At an absolute minimum, doctors must be able to critically evaluate and interpret published research in order to practice evidence-based medicine.

The research process

Develop a research question

The research question is the most important step in designing a study, as it dictates the other steps. A poorly framed research question is analogous to a poorly constructed phaco wound: it sets you up to fail.

Original thought is not the first quality patients think of when asked to describe their ideal doctor, and there are no lectures on 'inspiration' at medical school. However, most doctors are excellent problem-solvers and are aware that the first step to solving a problem is identifying and defining it—and the same is true when developing a research question. Once you have framed your question, apply the 'so what' principle to the possible answer: how will this knowledge be of use?

Review the literature

A literature review allows you to create a background against which to frame your question but also stops you from wasting your time by repeating someone else's research.

- Internet search engines are useful but blunt tools when searching for medical literature.
- Take advantage of the free training on using medical databases offered by NHS hospital libraries, or the free PubMed database online tutorial.
- The Cochrane Collaboration, a useful source of high-level evidence, publishes systematic reviews of primary research in health care. A systematic review has a well-defined methodology for search, selection, and data collection and thus allows the investigators to undertake a truly comprehensive consideration of the available evidence.

When reading a paper, remember that the authors are usually inferring some general medical or surgical truth using an investigation of a specific study population. The three obstacles to this inference are:

- Chance: could the findings in fact be explained by random variation?
- Bias: has there been a systematic error in methodology, e.g. in the way the population has been selected, the disease has been classified, or measurements have been undertaken?
- Confounding: is there an alternate explanation or truth because of another association at play (e.g. is carrying matches really associated with age-related macular degeneration, or are both associated with the confounding factor of smoking history)?

Adequate sample size and statistical analysis helps reduce the first two obstacles, but good study design is the only protection against bias. Hierarchy-of-evidence scales (there are different

---

> **Box 13.6 The hierarchy of evidence**
>
> Level A: consistent randomized controlled trials or inception cohort studies
>
> Level B: consistent retrospective cohort studies, case-control studies, or individual Level A studies
>
> Level C: cross-sectional studies, a case series study, or extrapolations from level B studies
>
> Level D: Expert opinion without explicit critical appraisal or which is based on physiology

---

scales for different forms of research) rank study types according to their freedom from bias (see Box 13.6).

Develop the study methodology

When designing your study, aim to use the highest-level study methodology appropriate for your research question.

- **Case report or case series:** appropriate when reporting rare conditions or uncommon events, in order to inform a specific audience; open to bias and therefore it is difficult to generalize any study findings to a larger population
- **Cross-sectional study:** take place at a specific point in time and take a snapshot of either a whole population of patients or a representative sample; also open to bias, but useful for estimating prevalence
- **Case-control study:** two groups with different outcomes ('cases' with the target disorder, and 'controls' without) are compared on the basis of putative risk factors; can be a powerful way to demonstrate an association, but cohort studies have more power to demonstrate causation
- **Cohort study:** participants who share a common characteristic or experience are sampled and followed up to record outcome in order to determine incidence of and risk factors for the outcome. Cohort studies can be prospective (recruited before the outcome/disorder of interest) or retrospective (after the outcome/disorder). An inception cohort is made up of participants recruited near the onset of the target disorder. These studies are more time intensive than case-control studies, particularly for rare diseases, as investigators are waiting for a disease to happen rather than investigating cases which have already occurred. However, cohort studies are less time intensive than randomized trials are.
- **Randomized controlled trials:** the gold standard methodology for assessing interventions (treatments or services); randomization limits bias and ensures that confounders are randomly distributed between treatment groups

When planning methodology, consider not only logistics (what will patients and clinical staff have to do as part of the research, when, and why?) but also ethics (see Box 13.7).

Ideally, involve a statistician at the study design stage as well as at the analysis stage so that your data are collected in an appropriate manner to answer your research question, and to ensure that your study sample is large enough to allow meaningful analysis.

Write the research proposal

The research proposal should summarize the background evidence, state the research question and study aim(s), and detail the study methodology. You will also need to develop other study documentation, such as consent forms and patient information leaflets. Your local research and development department should be able to provide support at this stage.

Apply for funding

There are many sources of funding and support in the United Kingdom. Organizations directly involved in fostering UK biomedical research include the UK Clinical Research Collaboration and the Academy of Medical Sciences (for URLs, see 'Further reading', this section). Research funding comes from many different sources including the Medical Research Council, biomedical charitable organizations (e.g. The Wellcome Trust), and industry—but be aware of the conflicting interests which come along with drug company ('pharma') funding. The Royal College and smaller charities with a particular interest in the target disorder or with a broader interest in visual impairment (e.g. Fight for Sight) may also be a source of funds. The application forms and the application processes are often lengthy, so start the process as early as possible.

Obtain ethical and local research governance approval

Ethics approval is mandatory for all NHS research, which is defined by the Department of Health as activity which falls within any of these spheres:

* Intent: the aim to generate novel knowledge
* Intervention: involvement of a treatment or service which is new or which lacks firm support within the clinical community
* Allocation: the allocation of an intervention using a protocol
* Randomization

The National Research Ethics Service maintains the framework for research ethical review in the United Kingdom and supports the Integrated Research Application System, an online system for ethics and governance approval. The lengthy form for the Integrated Research Application System requires the involvement of a permanent member of hospital staff (e.g. your consultant) and a sponsor for your research (e.g. your hospital R & D department).

Collect data

Your study must meet the requirement not only of the Data Protection Act 1998 but also the principles outlined in the Caldicott Report (see Section 13.2). Collect the minimal amount of personal identifiable data, minimize the number of people who can access the data, and store it securely.

Pilot your data collection process (paper questionnaire, computer programme, diagnostic test, experiment) several times in order to refine it before using it in the field. It is important that you 'alpha test', piloting the process yourself and within the research group as well as 'beta test', piloting within a wider selected group, in order to highlight weaknesses.

Analyse the data: Statistics

Statistics allows us to see past the noise which overlies messy clinical data, enabling us to identify a possible truth and to quantify the likelihood that this truth exists. The subject is covered in Section 13.8.

Determine the impact of the data

The outcomes of the analysis may tell you how statistically significant your findings are, but they cannot tell you how clinically significant your findings are, how they may impact on patient care, or how they sit within established medical knowledge. Interpreting your results is often the most challenging, most frustrating, but also the most interesting part of research.

Report and disseminate your findings

Your work will be unable to make an impact on the field (or on your CV) unless it is disseminated. Academic writing is a skill similar to surgical dexterity: whilst a small number may be blessed with natural ability, for the vast majority of us, practice is imperative. There are some important general rules to academic writing:

* Identify target journals early on: it will help you to determine tone, style, and content.
* Ensure that the topic is relevant to the target journal: have they published on the subject before?
* Ensure that your paper offers something new, and ensure that you highlight that novelty.
* Connect the objective and conclusions.
* Editing is not the same as spellchecking; it is an important part of writing. Often, it takes a second eye to identify incoherency.

Aim also to identify scientific meetings which would provide useful platforms for disseminating your work.

Formal research training

Academic career pathway

Modernising Medical Careers formalized the integration of academic and clinical training, providing a clear, coherent, and integrated training and career path. The National Institute for Health Research Integrated Academic Training pathway has been developed to take ophthalmic trainees from the first year of specialty training to a senior lectureship or professorship (permanent posts at academic institutions, often linked with consultant posts within an associated clinical unit). This pathway proceeds via academic fellowships, with 75% clinical training and 25% academic training during the first three years of speciality training and usually leading to a PhD, and then academic clinical lectureships, in which time is equally split between academic and clinical training. These posts are advertised by the individual schools of ophthalmology.

Outside of this pathway, if you are able to identify a research topic, institution, and supervisor (which are all impressive feats), there is also the option of applying to your school to organize an out-of-training research break in order to undertake a research project which leads to an MD or a PhD. You may also need to apply for funding in order to cover your research training. The MRC, the Wellcome Trust, and the National Institute for Health Research all offer competitively awarded personal research training fellowships.

Further reading

1. Centre for Evidence-Based Medicine: Home: CEBM. 2014. http://www.cebm.net
2. Integrated Application System (IRAS): Integrated Application System. 2015. http://www.myresearchproject.org.uk
3. Medical Research Council: Home: Medical Research Council. 2015. http://www.mrc.ac.uk
4. National Institute for Health Research: Training Programmes Managed by Trainees Coordinating Centre. http://www.nihr.ac.uk/funding/training-programmes.htm; accessed 24 Oct 2015
5. National Institutes of Health, U.S. National Library of Medicine: PubMed Tutorial. 2015. http://www.nlm.nih.gov/bsd/disted/pubmedtutorial/cover.html
6. The Academy of Medical Sciences: Improving Health through Research. 2013. http://www.acmedsci.ac.uk
7. The Cochrane Collaboration: Welcome: Cochrane Eyes and Vision. http://eyes.cochrane.org, accessed 24 Sept 2015
8. United Kingdom Clinical Research Collaboration: UK Clinical Research Collaboration. 2005. http://www.ukcrc.org
9. Wellcome Trust, Wellcome Trust. http://www.wellcome.ac.uk, accessed 24 Sept 2015

13.8 Statistics

Statistics

There are three types of lies: lies, damned lies, and statistics

Mark Twain

It is easy to lie with statistics: it is easier to lie without them

Frederick Mosteller

Descriptive statistics such as median, proportion, range, and interquartile range are useful to summarize the characteristics of your data. Confidence intervals around point estimates (such as median, mean, and proportions) should be used to describe the 'precision' of your study findings. Confidence intervals, as demonstrated in Box 13.8, are partly dependent on sample size.

Statistical analysis is undertaken in order to estimate the strength of any association found between variables, or between variables and outcomes, within the study population. Analysis can also determine the likelihood that the association is not due to random variation. In statistical terms, we are testing the null hypothesis that the finding is due to random variation. This testing is at risk of two main types of errors:

* Type 1 error: a false-positive rejection of the null hypothesis, where the finding is falsely assumed to be non-random
* Type 2 error: a false negative, where the finding is falsely assumed to be due to random variation

Statistical tests can be divided into parametric (where the data are 'normally' distributed) and non-parametric tests. Normally distributed data, such as axial length in a representative sample of UK residents, are symmetrically distributed around a mean or average value. Non-parametric tests are usually the most appropriate for most ophthalmic data (such as vision in patients with age-related macular degeneration), as the data tend to be skewed at one end rather than being distributed symmetrically around a mean value. Data type also determines the test used:

* Continuous data: data which can take any value, including decimals, e.g. axial length
* Discrete: all other data, which can be:
  — Binary/binomial: only two possible values, e.g. yes/no
  — Ordinal: fitting to an arbitrary scale, e.g. the diabetic retinopathy scale

> ### Box 13.8 The importance of confidence intervals
>
> Experiment A: Toss a coin five times; it lands heads up four times. The proportion of tosses landing heads up is 80%, and the 95% confidence interval is 37%–96%: we are 95% sure that any repeated experiments will result in between 37% and 96% of tosses landing heads up. As this interval includes 50%, we have no evidence that our coin is anything other than normal.
>
> Experiment B: Toss a coin 50 times; it lands heads up 40 times. The proportion of tosses landing heads up is still 80%, but now the 95% confidence interval is 67%–89%: we are 95% sure that this coin is more likely to land heads up than tails up. These results indicate that the coin has been loaded.

— Counts: non-negative values, e.g. the number of glaucoma medications
— Categorical: non-ordinal labels, e.g. the hospital where the participant is being treated

The final determinant of which statistical test to use is whether your data are paired. Paired data consist of repeated measurements on one subject, measurements on matched subjects, or repeated experiments. Table 13.6 summarizes the general rules regarding which statistical test to use for different types of data.

Another more complex method for assessing the relationship between variables and outcomes is regression analysis. This topic is beyond the scope of this chapter (but see 'Further reading').

One peculiarity of ophthalmic data is that we tend to deal with clustered data, that is, data from two eyes which are 'clustered' within one individual. Any associations found within the data may be overstated if there is a failure to account for this clustering. In order to overcome this issue, either sacrifice some data by analysing only one eye of each participant or seek the advice of a statistician.

Further reading

1. American Journal of Ophthalmology: 2009/2010 Series on Statistics. 2015. http://www.ajo.com/content/statistics

Table 13.6 **When to use which statistical test: General rules**			
	Parametric data	**Non-parametric continuous data, non-binomial discrete data**	**Binomial data**
Comparing the results from one group to a hypothetical value	One-sample *t*-test	Wilcoxon test	Binomial test or chi-square test
Comparing results from two unpaired groups	Two-sample *t*-test	Mann–Whitney test	Chi-square test or Fishers test
Comparing results from two paired groups	Paired *t*-test	Wilcoxon test	—
There are also tests available for comparing more than two groups, e.g. ANOVA			
Quantifying associations between two variables	Pearson correlation	Spearman correlation	—
Predicting a value using the relationship with another variable	Regression analysis	Regression analysis	—

13.9 Ophthalmic Trainees' Group

Responsibility

Elected trainees from 14 regions of the United Kingdom make up the Ophthalmic Trainees' Group (OTG). The role of the OTG is to represent trainees in all aspects of decision-making within the Royal College of Ophthalmologists. This role ensures trainees are influencing not only areas pertinent to training, such as the curriculum, exams, and education, but also issues they will face in the future as providers of ophthalmic care, including professional standards. OTG members can sit on all of the Royal College committees, providing trainee persuasion and reporting back to the training community to keep it up to date.

Members of the OTG are regionally elected for a three-year term of office; their main role is to provide a two-way discussion with the Royal College to address key issues facing trainees and establishing a conduit for achieving positive outcomes. A good example was the introduction of the Advanced Subspecialty Training Opportunity programme.

The OTG want trainees to be actively engaged by regularly contacting their regional representative to express their views or concerns. In turn, the OTG members meet four times a year to discuss the issues raised by trainees as well as then information gathered from all of the Royal College committee meetings. These are then condensed into 'keypoints' and emailed to College members after each meeting. In the modern era, email will be the mainstay of communication, but there are some important annual events whereby trainees can meet their peers from across the United Kingdom, including the OTG regional representatives.

OTG Forum, Royal College of Ophthalmologists Annual Congress

The Royal College of Ophthalmologists Annual Congress is a scientific meeting attracting the best speakers in specific ophthalmic fields. The meeting is more than just lectures and offers symposia, courses, posters, DVDs, forums, and a commercial exhibition. In addition, there are associated subspecialty days with presentations solely in one field, for example, about the retina or glaucoma.

Part of the meeting encompasses the OTG Forum, where the views of trainees, gathered in the run up to the congress, are directly put to the Royal College of Ophthalmologist council officers in front of the assembly of trainees. Although it can get heated at times, it provides a satisfying method of venting issues—much more gratifying than the email route!

Ophthalmic Trainees' Annual Symposium

The Ophthalmic Trainees' Annual Symposium is an informal, relaxed day-long meeting held at different locations across the United Kingdom. In contrast to the annual congress, the symposium deliberately steers away from core academia. Instead, it covers aspects of ophthalmology that help your everyday practice, such as routes to different career paths, out-of-programme experiences, clinical management, and fellowships. Importantly, the symposium is open to anyone who is interested in ophthalmic training.

Further reading

1. The Royal College of Ophthalmologists: OTG Response to the Shape of Training Review. 2014. http://www.rcophth.ac.uk/2014/04/otg-response-to-the-shape-of-training-review/

13.10 Safeguarding

The Care Quality Commission describes safeguarding as:

Protecting people's health, well-being and human rights, and enabling them to live free from harm, abuse and neglect.[5]

Safeguarding covers children, young people, and vulnerable adults. A vulnerable adult is defined as:

Someone over the age of eighteen, who is vulnerable by reason of old age, infirmity or disability (including mental disability within the meaning of the Mental Health Act 1983) so that s/he is unable to take care of her/himself or to protect her/himself from others.[6]

A person's ability to keep themselves safe from harm is partly dependent on circumstances and may vary at different points in their life. In adults, it is therefore important to assess the present-day situation in any case of suspected abuse.

Types of abuse

There can be overlap, with an individual being subjected to more than one type of abuse:

- **Physical** abuse includes hitting, shaking, throwing, and poisoning, causing either physical harm or illness.
- **Sexual** abuse includes inappropriate physical contact, involvement in viewing adult material, or encouraging sexually inappropriate behaviour.
- **Neglect** is a failure of the child/vulnerable adult's carer to meet the physical and/or psychological needs of the child/vulnerable adult, resulting in poor health and/or development. Neglect may include inadequate shelter, food, clothing, and access to medical care.
- **Emotional** abuse involves the persistent denigration of an individual's emotional state through psychological ill treatment. It is always present to a certain degree in the other forms of abuse.
- **Financial** abuse includes theft, fraud, and exploitation, misappropriation of property, possessions, and/or benefits.
- **Discriminatory** abuse includes racism, sexism, or any other forms of harassment based on an individual's beliefs or background.

Risk factors

In children, preterm babies and infants less than 1 year old are at greatest risk. Disabled children are recognized as being at greater risk than able-bodied children are. Teenage mothers, single-parent families, mental health problems, drug and alcohol misuse, and domestic violence are all factors that increase the risk of an individual abusing a child or vulnerable adult. Old age, mental illness, and physical, sensory, and learning disability are all factors that increase the risk of vulnerability in an adult.

Domestic violence

When a case of domestic violence is suspected, **always** consider and ask whether there are children in the family and therefore at risk. Witnessing domestic violence is considered a form of emotional abuse.

- If the domestic violence involves a pregnant woman, a referral to local child-safeguarding services should be made.

- If there is a child less than 1 year old in the family, a referral to local child-safeguarding services should be made.
- If a child of any age witnessed an episode of domestic violence, a referral to local child-safeguarding services should be made.
- If a child older than 1 year did not witness the episode of domestic violence but may be at risk of violence themselves, a referral to local child-safeguarding services should be considered.

Assessing a patient where there is suspicion of abuse

General

Identify the adult accompanying the patient and their relationship to the patient:

- Identify who has parental responsibility or power of attorney and who is the day-to-day carer.
- Check the details of the GP, school and health visitor, or social worker.
- Check the child protection register or social services records to identify known issues or at risk families.

History

Try to take the history directly from the patient without influence from the carers, as well as a history from the carer. Individuals may disclose information suggesting they have been subject to abuse. Warning signs include:

- Delayed presentation or failure to seek healthcare following injury; multiple presentations with different injuries
- Poor explanation for an injury
- History not consistent with the injuries sustained
- Inconsistency of history over time or from different family members

Examination

Features of concern include:

- Poor personal hygiene and dress
- Physical signs of abuse, including slap marks and unusual bruising
- Injury patterns inconsistent with the history
- Unusual behaviour or interaction with carers and other adults
- As well as fundal examination, ensure visual acuity or responses, facial, adnexal/lid, brief anterior segment, pupil responses, and clarity of media examinations are recorded to ensure other traumatic sequelae or ocular disorders which mimic non-accidental injury are not missed.

Retinal examination

When non-accidental injury is suspected in an infant, it is common for the paediatricians to request a retinal examination to exclude retinal haemorrhage, which is a feature of **shaken baby syndrome**. In this situation, the first examination should take place as soon as possible, preferably within 24 hours, and should consist of a dilated retinal examination using an indirect ophthalmoscope with a wide view (e.g. 28 D or 30 D) lens.

[5] Safeguarding people, Care Quality Commission, 10 May 2015, © Care Quality Commission 2015. This information is licenced under the terms of the Open Government Licence (http://www.nationalarchives.gov.uk/doc/open-government-licence/version/3)

[6] 'Who Decides?' Lord Chancellor's Department, 1997 © Crown Copyright

A   B

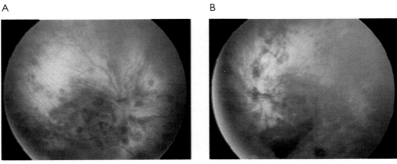

Fig 13.2 Examples of types of retinal haemorrhages seen in non-accidental injury

Courtesy of GGW Adams

Important points to document include:
- Date and time of examination
- Laterality of haemorrhages
- Location of haemorrhages (use of retinopathy of prematurity zones is helpful)
- Number of haemorrhages
- Extent/severity
- Retinal layer(s) involved (may be multiple)
- Name, signature, and designation of examiner

If no haemorrhages are found, no further action is required other than to report back to the referring paediatrician. If, however, haemorrhages are seen, then a consultant paediatric ophthalmologist should also examine the child as soon as possible, preferably within 24 hours. Ideally, retinal photographs should be taken.

It is important to remember that no ocular signs are pathognomonic for abuse. Severe, multilayered retinal haemorrhages, such as those seen in Figure 13.2A and B, can very rarely occur for reasons other than shaken baby syndrome (see Table 13.7). **All** newly found retinal haemorrhages warrant consideration of non-accidental injury, and further investigation.

Investigations

Because there is a long list of differential diagnoses for disorders which mimic non-accidental injury and because of the medico-legal implications, a large series of investigations are usually undertaken to exclude other causes; these investigations are usually coordinated by the paediatric medical team and include:
- Urinalysis
- Infection (cultures, serology) screen
- Full blood count, urea and electrolytes, clotting
- Metabolic studies
- Plain radiographs to exclude fractures and/or for skeletal survey
- CT /MRI brain

Management

Doctors caring for children have a duty to act 'single-mindedly in the interests of the child' and not the parents. The same approach should be applied to the care of vulnerable adults. Generally, concerns should be discussed with the responsible adult or carer unless this will put the patient at an increased risk of significant harm.

It is essential to keep accurate, clear, and contemporaneous notes of the initial assessment and all subsequent communications with the patient, carers, family members, and all healthcare professionals involved in the case. If possible, photography should be used to record physical signs.

Any suspicion of abuse should be discussed with the senior clinician and the paediatric medical team and brought to the attention of the local named healthcare professionals for child protection or safeguarding vulnerable adults. Appointment of both posts is a mandatory requirement of every NHS trust. The named individuals will be able to offer advice with regards to further management and escalation, where appropriate, to the police (in circumstances where a patient is in immediate danger or where there is danger to other family members at home) or to the local social services department for safeguarding.

Further reading

1. Department of Health: No Secrets: Guidance on Developing and Implementing Multi-Agency Policies and Procedures to Protect Vulnerable Adults from Abuse. 2000. London: Department of Health
2. Department of Health: What to Do if You're Worried a Child Is Being Abused. 2003. London: Department of Health
3. General Medical Council: Protecting Children and Young People: The Responsibilities of All Doctors. 2011. London: General Medical Council

Table 13.7	Some causes of retinal haemorrhages in children
Birth	Up to a third of neonates
Haematological disorders	Leukaemia, anaemia, haemorrhagic disease of the newborn, antiphospholipid syndrome
Metabolic disorders	Glutaric aciduria, cobalamin c deficiency
Vascular disorders	Arteriovenous malformations, fibromuscular dysplasia
Infection	Meningitis, malaria, Lyme disease, rubella, toxoplasmosis
Retinal disorders	Inherited telangiectasia, Bests disease, Coats disease, herpes simplex virus, cytomegalovirus
??CPR	Controversial
Tersons syndrome	Vitreous haemorrhage in association with subarachnoid haemorrhage
Osteogenesis imperfecta	Brittle bone disease
Carbon monoxide poisoning	From car fumes or faulty gas appliances
Accidental injury	Rare, usually severe other injuries

Index